Clinical De

Fenn, Liddelow and Gimson's

Clinical Dental Prosthetics

3rd edition

A. Roy MacGregor PhD, FDS, DRDRCS(Edin)

Professor of Prosthodontics, University of Glasgow; Consultant in Prosthodontics, Greater Glasgow Health Board. Formerly External Examiner, Universities of Wales, Edinburgh, London, Belfast, Lagos and Malaya. Member of Council and Examiner, Royal College of Surgeons of Edinburgh.
Formerly Visiting Professor, University of Michigan in Ann Arbor, University of Alexandria, University of Sydney and University of Witwatersrand.

WRIGHT
London Boston Sydney Singapore Toronto Wellington

Wright
is an imprint of Butterworth Scientific

PART OF REED INTERNATIONAL P.L.C.

First published 1953 by Staples
Reprinted 1955 and 1959
Second edition, 1961
Reprinted 1965, 1967, 1970 and 1974
Third edition published 1989 by Butterworths

British Library Cataloguing in Publication Data

Fenn, H. R. B. (Harold Robert Blackwell)
Fenn, Liddelow and Gimson's clinical dental prosthetics.—3rd ed.
1. Prosthetic chemistry
I. Title II. Liddelow, K. P. III. Gimson, A. P.
IV. MacGregor, A. Roy (Alastair Roy)
V. Fenn, H. R. B. (Harold Robert Blackwell).
Clinical dental prosthetics
617.6′9

ISBN 0-7236-0911-X

Library of Congress Cataloging in Publication Data

Fenn, H. R. B. (Harold Robert Blackwell)
Fenn, Liddelow, and Gimson's clinical dental prosthetics.

Updated version of: Clinical dental prosthetics/
H. R. B. Fenn, K. P. Liddelow, A. P. Gimson.
2nd rev. ed. 1961.
Bibliography: p.
Includes index.
1. Prosthodontics.
I. MacGregor, A. Roy (Alastair Roy)
II. Fenn, H. R. B. (Harold Robert Blackwell).
Clinical dental prosthetics. III. Title. IV. Title.
Clinical dental prosthetics.
[DNLM: 1. Dental Prosthesis WU 500 F334c]
RK651.F46 1989 617.6′9 88-33838

ISBN 0-7236-0911-X

Typeset by Butterworths Litho Preparation Department
Printed and bound in Great Britain by Butler and Tanner, Frome, Somerset

Foreword to the third edition

After the Second World War when the British Dental Schools began to expand and enrol increasing numbers of students, we who were teaching dental prosthetics found ourselves constrained by the lack of an up-to-date text explaining in simple straightforward terms the basic principles and techniques of the purely clinical aspects of prosthetic dentistry. Thus in 1949 the three original authors co-operated to produce the first edition of this book, covering both full and partial dentures, in one volume (published 1953).

We were gratified by its reception and by many requests that it could, with value, be expanded to cover the wider fields of prosthetic dentistry. Therefore in 1961 we produced a second edition which did this.

In the late 1970s this edition went out of print. Sadly, Professor Hal Fenn had died and we two remaining authors had retired and felt that we were too far removed from active clinical practice to produce a third up-to-date edition. We were delighted, therefore, when Wright suggested that so eminent and practical a clinician as Professor Roy MacGregor had agreed to revitalise and modernise the book into a Third edition.

Updating one's own publication is a daunting enough task; to do the same for someone else's text requires very special ability and dedication. We are truly delighted and impressed with the result which Professor MacGregor has achieved and trust that he may enjoy the gratitude of both dental students and qualified practitioners who will benefit from his work.

Kenneth Liddelow
Arthur Gimson

Preface

This book was originally published in 1953, reprinted twice, and published again in a second edition in 1961. It had wide acclaim as an undergraduate text and was extensively used in Great Britain and overseas. Its popularity lay in its practical commonsense approach to the subject together with the reputation of three well-respected teachers and clinicians of considerable experience. It is no surprise to find copies of the first and second editions of the book still on the shelves of libraries throughout the world.

As with all clinical textbooks, editions become out of date, not because of their format and principles, but rather because of changes in materials, equipment, techniques and use of terminology. For this reason I was asked by the publisher to update the last edition. This I have attempted to do without altering the basic structure or chapter arrangement. In the same theme the medical artist has freely copied the original line drawings with only minor modifications where these were considered desirable. None of the original photographs was available and so new illustrations have been used throughout.

In a book comprising 30 chapters the first 17 are devoted almost exclusively to the edentulous patient and to the design and construction of complete dentures. Some may think that this theme is rather out of date because of the increase in dental health and the decrease in edentulousness. The active clinician, however, will see things differently: an ageing population, the increase in life expectancy, ethnic attitudes to dentistry and financial constraints are all factors perpetuating the need to treat edentulous patients for many years to come. Indeed, much of this treatment will become more and more difficult because of the increasing age of patients throughout the world.

The next eight chapters are devoted, as in the earlier editions, to partial dentures. It was not thought necessary to increase the proportion of chapters on this subject because there has been in recent years a plethora of texts on partial dentures and to add excessively to these publications seemed unwise. These textbooks, together with those on complete dentures, have been listed in a Bibliography at the end of the book.

The remaining five chapters comprise other aspects which fall into the general subject matter of dental prosthetics: overdentures, complex prostheses, prefabricated attachments, cleft palate, implants, and so on. While much of this type of treatment has great appeal to the aspiring clinician and technician, it remains a fact that the basic principles of complete and partial denture prosthetics, as discussed in the first 25 chapters, serve as the foundation for good clinical practice. Without such a foundation, successful treatment and continuing care of a prosthetic patient, of whatever complexity, is liable to fail.

A. Roy MacGregor

Acknowledgements

My thanks are due to Catherine Wilson and Fiona Hunter who arranged, typed and edited the script.

I am indebted to John Davies, Kay Shepherd, Linda Scott and David Woodward for the majority of the photographs and illustrations.

Most of the artwork and line drawings were done by Anne Hughes who based her work on the original editions of this book in order to maintain continuity. She laboured long and hard in her efforts and I am deeply grateful for her help in this essential aspect of a textbook of this type.

Henry Noble and Michael MacMahon read parts of the script; Hannes Slabbert and Phillip Wragg loaned photographs in their possession; Kevin Jennings and Margaret Robinson assisted in clinical matters; Michael Broad, John Brown, Donald Cameron, John Graham, Patrick Lilly, Grant Miller and William Renwick provided technical assistance: to all these colleagues, and others who have helped in many different ways, I am sincerely grateful.

Contents

Chapter 1

Introduction to prosthetics

Definition of prosthetics

A prosthesis may be defined as an appliance which replaces lost or congenitally missing tissue. Some prostheses restore both the function and the appearance of the tissue they replace, others merely restore one of these factors.

Prosthetics is the art and science of designing and fitting artificial substitutes to replace lost or missing tissue. Dental prosthetics is a subdivision which deals with its application to the mouth.

By definition dental prosthetics (also known as prosthodontics or prosthetic dentistry) includes the replacement of any lost tissue and therefore embraces the filling of teeth and the fitting of artificial crowns. In actual practice, however, the term has come to mean the fitting of appliances such as artificial dentures, bridges, obturators and surgical prostheses, and it is in this sense that the term will be used throughout this book.

Why are dentures necessary?

Before studying in detail the methods, techniques and theories employed in and related to dental prosthetics, it is necessary to have clearly in mind the purpose which is being served. It is pertinent, therefore, to commence a book of this nature by asking and answering the question: 'Why do we make dentures?'

In order to answer this question the functions of the teeth must be understood. These are threefold:

1. To divide the food finely so that a large surface area is available for the action of the digestive juices.
2. To assist the tongue and lips to form some of the sounds of speech.
3. The teeth form an important feature of the face, and by supporting the lips and cheeks enable these structures to perform their functions of manipulating food and expressing emotion.

The teeth are also mutually interdependent; premature loss of any tooth may cause a collapse of the dental arch and movement of individual teeth with loss of interproximal contacts, thus giving rise to food-packing and gingival damage. Function is necessary:

1. To minimize the risk of caries by preventing food stagnation.
2. To preserve the health of the soft tissues by the massaging action of the passage of food.
3. To prevent tilting, rotation or over-eruption of a tooth which may occur if it is unopposed or in malocclusion.

Prior to the comparatively modern development of highly refined foods the loss of natural teeth often resulted in severe malnutrition but, nowadays, it is quite possible to live a perfectly healthy life with no teeth at all. In spite of this, total loss of teeth is an unpleasant state for the following reasons:

1. It places limitations on the diet and all hard and fibrous foods require to be finely divided or else digestive troubles may result.
2. It produces a certain sibilance in the speech because those consonant stops requiring the presence of the teeth cannot be made efficiently.
3. It results in a prematurely aged appearance due to the loss of support and consequent falling in of the lips and cheeks, and the fact that the jaws can be overclosed produces a bunching up of the soft tissues around the mouth and close approximation of the chin and nose.

4. It can produce loss of confidence and even psychological disturbances from the mutilated appearance.

The results of edentation so far mentioned apply generally; there are other disadvantages applying individually. For instance: wind instrument players and singers are quite unable to perform; clergymen cannot preach; actors and photographers' models cannot follow their employment; and the pipe smoker loses half the enjoyment of his pipe if he cannot hold it between his teeth.

To the majority of people, therefore, the loss of the teeth is a matter of great concern, and their replacement by artificial substitutes is vital to the continuance of normal life.

What are the differences between natural teeth and artificial dentures?

The essential difference between natural and artificial teeth is that the former are firmly rooted in the bone of the jaws and in consequence they can incise, tear and finely grind food of any character because the lower teeth can move across the upper teeth with a powerful shearing action. Artificial dentures, on the other hand, merely rest on the alveolar ridges and are held there by weak forces. In addition, they are subject to powerful displacing forces so their efficiency as a masticatory apparatus is limited. This efficiency can vary within wide limits depending on the shape and size of the edentulous jaws, the type of mucosa covering these jaws, the mental attitude of the patient to the dentures, his ability to learn to use them, and the skill of the operator. These factors are discussed at length in Chapter 2.

Aesthetically, artificial teeth can be indistinguishable from natural teeth and in many cases they can enhance the appearance if the natural teeth were hypoplastic, grossly carious or unpleasantly irregular. The speech of artificial denture wearers should be normal once the tongue and lips have adapted themselves to the dentures. Other functions such as singing, or musical instrument playing, can be made possible by modifying the dentures in various ways.

The main limitations of artificial dentures, therefore, are that they lack stability, and the masticatory force which can be applied by them is limited by this fact and also by the pressure which the edentulous ridges will tolerate. In other respects they can closely rival natural teeth.

What are the displacing forces causing instability?

The most powerful displacing forces are the muscles surrounding the oral cavity, and the tongue. One of the functions of the lips, cheeks and tongue is to receive and manipulate the food and pass it backwards and forwards between the teeth until it has been reduced to a sufficiently fine state for it to be formed into a bolus and swallowed. These movements are powerful, and unless the dentures are very firmly seated (which can be the case only if they have been properly designed and made by a careful and exact technique) and until the wearer has become skilful in manipulating them, they are liable to be moved about with the food. In addition, every time the mouth is opened the muscles of the cheeks tense and if the lower denture is over-extended at the edges it will be raised. Also during speech the tongue tends to tip and in certain cases eject the lower denture unless it is properly designed.

Other displacing forces requiring to be reduced by careful technique and design are:

1. The interference and locking of the cusps of the teeth as the lower move across the upper in chewing. This interference, which can also occur at times other than when eating, tends to displace both dentures from their seating.
2. Viscous and sticky foods tend to unite the dentures and displace them.
3. Gravity will tend to unseat the upper denture.

What are the retaining forces available to counteract displacement?

These can be divided into two classes: positive physical forces; acquired muscular control by the denture wearer.

Physical forces

Adhesion and cohesion

Adhesion is defined as the force of attraction existing between dissimilar bodies in close contact. This force acts most powerfully at right angles to the surface, and is proportional to the area of the surfaces in contact. Cohesion is the force of attraction existing between similar bodies in close contact.

An example of adhesion is afforded by two microscope slides with a very thin film of water between them. The force required to separate the slides, provided it is applied at right angles, will be great but if it is applied at a lesser angle the slides immediately commence to slip over one another and separate easily. The force of adhesion acts from one surface of the film of water to one glass slide and from the other surface of the film to the other glass slide. Within the film of water the force of cohesion unites the molecules, and the thinner the film the more powerful is this force.

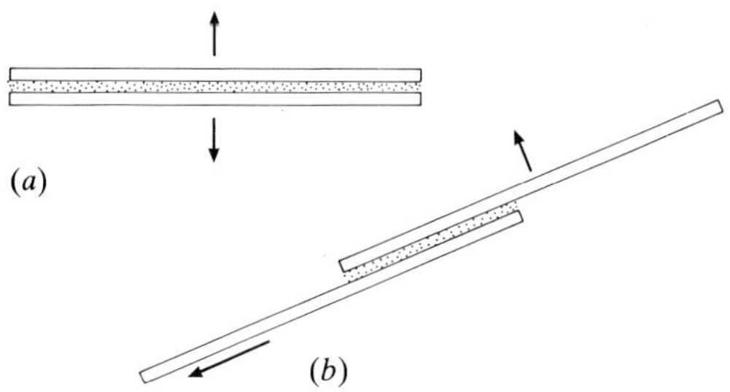

Figure 1.1 (*a*) The large flat surface of a microscope slide provides excellent adhesion when resisting vertical separation. (*b*) A sliding force allows easy separation

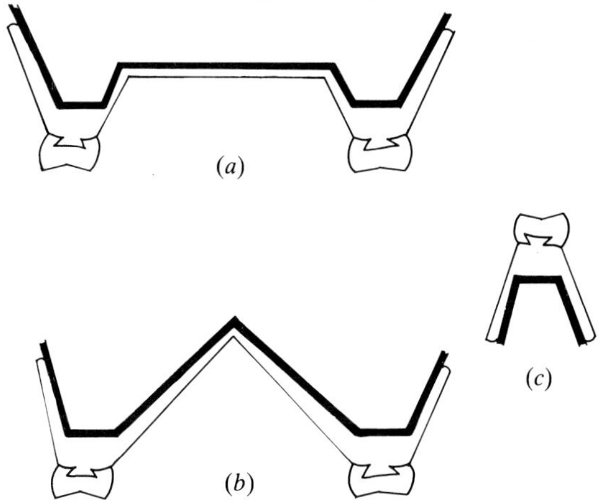

Figure 1.2 (*a*)A flat palate will provide good surface adhesion. (*b*) A V-shaped palate allows sliding and therefore retention by adhesion is reduced. (*c*) A lower denture provides a very small surface for effective adhesion

A denture base is made accurately to fit the oral mucosa on which it rests, and intervening between the two surfaces is saliva. The similarity to the microscope slide analogy is therefore obvious. Thus adhesion may or may not play an important part in retaining a denture in place depending on the shape of the mouth, its surface area, the closeness of apposition of the denture to the tissues and the direction of the displacing forces. The accompanying diagrams should make this clear (Figures 1.1 and 1.2).

Adhesion is by far the greater of these two forces as can be shown by placing a dry slide on a moist one and then forcible separating them; both will be found to be wet, proving that the force holding the molecules of water together is less than that holding the water to the glass.

A complete lower denture covers a very small surface area compared with an upper, and its adhesion is correspondingly less.

The viscosity of the saliva is of importance in the phenomenon of cohesion. Saliva which is more viscous than normal i.e. it contains a larger percentage of mucin, prevents the denture and tissues coming into sufficiently close contact because it increases the thickness of the saliva film and this reduces the cohesive force.

Atmospheric pressure

The periphery of a complete denture should bed slightly into the soft tissues in the sulci and except for the posterior edge of the upper denture, will be covered by the lips and cheeks, i.e. 'wrapped up', in the surrounding soft tissues.

When an upper denture is inserted air is expelled from between it and the mucosa and provided the fit of the periphery to the tissues is good no air can enter because this edge-fit provides an efficient seal (Figure 1.3). This means that the pressure acting on the fitting surface of the denture is less than that acting on the polished surface which, of course, is atmospheric pressure. The difference between these two pressures provides a positive force to maintain the denture in place. Furthermore, if the denture tends to move out of contact with the tissues and provided the seal at the periphery is not broken, the pressure under the denture will tend to fall still further and the atmospheric force will increase.

Undercut area

It is sometimes possible to insert a denture in one direction into an undercut area and thus obtain a purely mechanical resistance to displacement (Figure 1.4).

Acquired muscular control

Dentures are always foreign bodies in the mouth and when fitted for the first time most muscular actions tend to expel them. Gradually, however, the wearer learns to differentiate between the food and the dentures and, at first consciously but later subconsciously, to control and stabilize them with the tongue and cheeks. The tongue, by resting on top of the lower denture and pressing it downwards and forwards, can control its tendency to rise, and

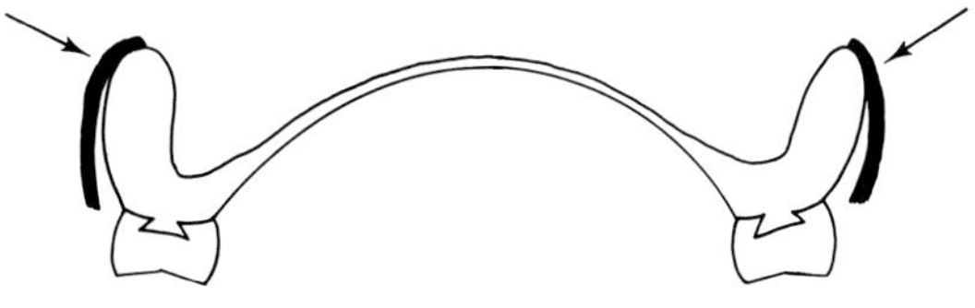

Figure 1.3 Arrows indicate tissues sealing the edges of the denture and so preventing ingress of air

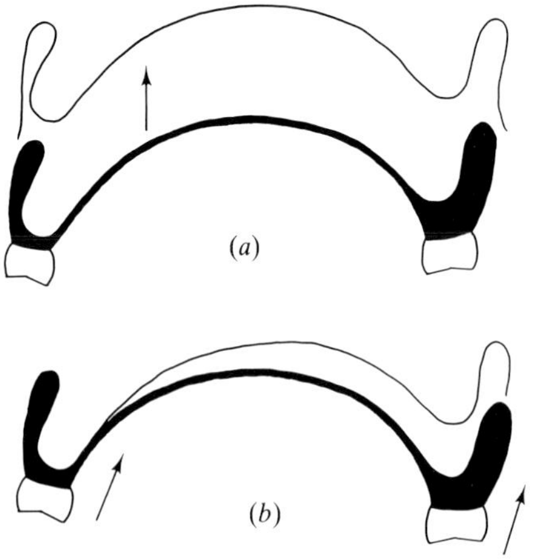

Figure 1.4 (*a*) If the denture is inserted directly upwards it will not go into place. (*b*) If the denture is inserted from the right side, the flange of the denture will go into place and the opposite side may be rotated upwards. The right side of the denture will be retained by the undercut, once in place. Note that the left flange is broader because there has been more alveolar resorption on that side

also counterbalance to a large degree unstabilizing masticatory forces. The tongue can also be unconsciously trained to prevent the back edge of the upper denture dropping while the front teeth are incising.

The muscular cheeks can be trained, again unconsciously, to press downwards on the buccal flanges of the lower denture, while still carrying out their function of placing food between the teeth.

If full use is to be made of muscular control of dentures, their design must follow certain guides which are fully explained in the following chapters.

Why are there so many techniques?

The novice in prosthetics may become bewildered by the plethora of techniques that exists for achieving the same result. For example, there are many techniques for making impressions of the mouth, and for determining the relationship between the upper and lower jaws. Different types of articulator and a large number of posterior tooth forms add to the complexity. The list could be greatly extended, but the examples given serve to draw attention to the fact.

Furthermore, individual operators select and practise a limited number of techniques while regarding the others with indifference or disagreement. The explanation for this state of affairs is briefly as follows.

Prosthodontics is a mixture of science and art and, although there are many rules, the major part of the subject follows guides laid down by practitioners who have developed their skills by their own clinical experience and research. Such practitioners have given rise to what may be termed 'schools of thought', and pupils who have learned from them have continued their methods.

In addition, mouth conditions of individuals vary within wide limits, some presenting with jaw formations which make the fitting and subsequent function of dentures a comparatively simple matter, while in others difficulties of retention and occlusal relationship and other factors require that special techniques be used to make use of every small advantage presented if the dentures are to have any chance of success.

In an attempt to achieve this, many techniques with similar aims have been evolved, and none of them has been of such outstanding merit as to displace the others entirely. Closely bound up with this is the fact that all these techniques require the development of a high degree of skill by the prosthodontist who practises them, and if one technique is producing good results in the hands of one practitioner he is likely to advocate its use and continue to practise it to the exclusion of others.

Finally, in certain aspects of prosthetics, agreement has not been reached on how and why certain phenomena and functions occur and, as in other branches of science, conflicting theories exist, each with its own followers.

For example, in the field of occlusion of the teeth, many clinicians have related the movements of the mandible to the guidance it receives from both the temporomandibular joints and the slope of the tooth surfaces in contact during movement, while others have evolved the theory that the movements of the mandible follow the segment of a sphere, the centre of which is located near the glabella. Articulators and posterior teeth have been designed to enable dentures to be made conforming to the principles of these theories, and as both apparently produce satisfactory results, both have their adherents.

Speed and economy have also had a powerful effect on the development of techniques because the cost of dentures bears a very definite relationship to the time spent on their construction, and simple quick methods have a wide appeal in spite of the fact that they frequently produce dentures which are very inferior in comparison to those which are made by more elaborate and time-consuming techniques.

The only general guide to be followed by the student of prosthetics is to learn to anticipate the difficulties which a given case will present, study any technique which is designed to overcome the difficulties, and select for his practice the one which appeals to him most and produces in his hands the best result.

Chapter 2

Applied anatomy

This section indicates how a knowledge of the structure and function of the tissues in the immediate vicinity of the dentures can be used to determine their logical design and provides reasons for, and answers to, some of the difficulties which are encountered in complete denture prosthetics.

The mouth only represents a true cavity when opened to receive food or during the formation of certain sounds of speech. At other times it is filled almost completely by the tongue and edentulous alveolar ridges.

Figure 2.1 shows the appearance of an open edentulous mouth with the tongue depressed.

Oral mucosa and tissue compression

The varying thickness of the mucosa and submucosa covering the bones forming the palate and alveolar ridges results in the forces which are applied to the denture during clenching and mastication being transmitted unevenly to these supporting structures. In addition to this varying thickness, there are differences in the structure of the fibrous elements of the corium.

Soft tissue is compressed when a force is applied to it because some of the fluids (blood and lymph) which it contains are temporarily shifted. The amount of fluid which a soft tissue contains is dependent both on its thickness and the density of its elements.

Figures 2.2 and 2.3 show that the thinnest and densest layer of mucosa covers the midline of the hard palate. The next thinnest is over the upper and lower alveolar ridges while the thickest layer covers the blood vessels and the nerves of the lateral aspects of the palate.

It will be apparent that, if an upper denture base accurately fits the mucosa at rest, when the denture is driven upwards during mastication the first resistance offered to it will be by the thin tissues of the centre of the palate. Some of the remaining force will then be dissipated in flexing the denture base on either side of the midline until it has sufficiently compressed the slightly thicker tissues over the alveolar ridges which then transmit the force to the underlying bone. The tissues between the midline of the palate and the alveolar ridges being both thick and vascular will seldom be compressed sufficiently to transmit any appreciable force to the bone.

Such a state of affairs is likely to have two results:

1. The tissues in the midline of the palate may become inflamed.
2. The constant flexing of the denture base may cause its fracture from fatigue.

Means of overcoming these results of uneven soft tissue distribution are discussed in Chapter 5.

Abnormally thick mucosa

It is not uncommon for the mucosa over the alveolar ridges to form soft tissue which is thick and flabby in some areas. This may result from:

1. Excessive load being applied to an edentulous ridge, particularly in a lateral or anteroposterior direction. A common example of this is the occlusion of natural lower anterior teeth against a complete upper denture which frequently results in severe resorption of the alveolar bone. The soft tissue covering the resorbed anterior alveolar ridge is mainly composed of bunched rugae from the palatal mucosa and submucosa (Figure 2.4). Other areas of the mouth may undergo similar changes if subjected to excessive loads.

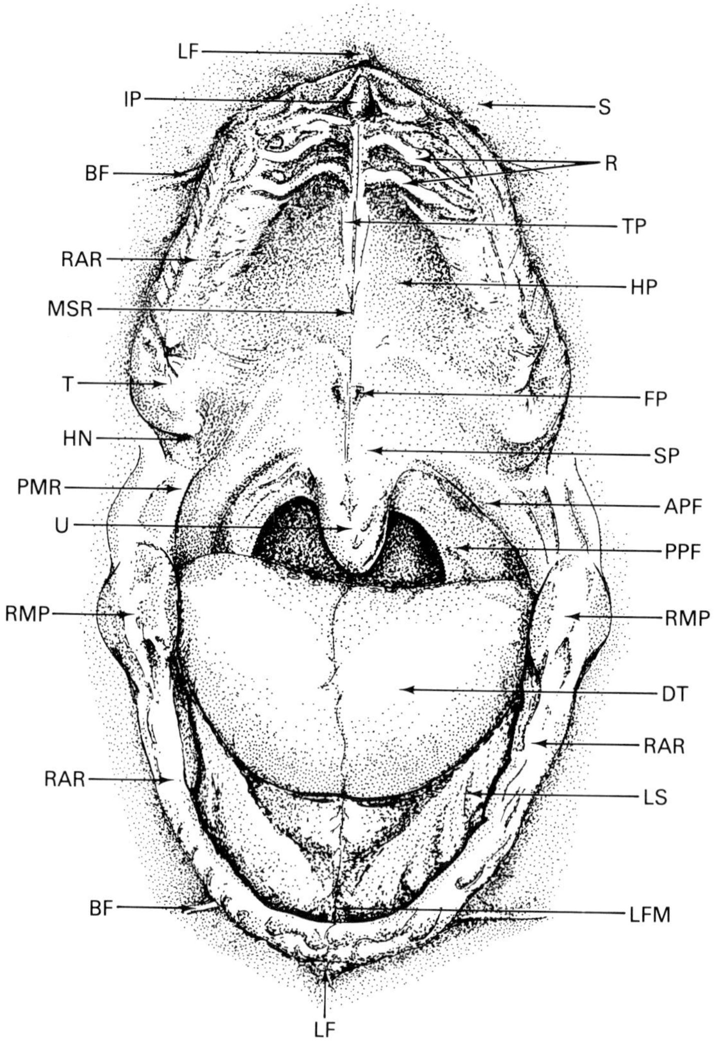

Figure 2.1 The open edentulous mouth with the tongue depressed illustrating the structures which are visible: S, sulcus; R, rugae; TP, torus palati; HP, hard palate; FP, fovea palati; SP, soft palate; APF, anterior pillar of the fauces; PPF, posterior pillar of the fauces; RMP, retromolar (pear-shaped) pad; DT, dorsum of the tongue; RAR, residual alveolar ridge; LS, lingual sulcus; LFM, lingual frenum (mandible); LF, labial frenum; BF, buccal frenum; U, uvula; PMR, pterygomandibular raphe; HN, hamular (or pterygomaxillary) notch; T. tuberosity; MSR, median sagittal raphe; IP, incisive papilla

2. Various forms of hyperplasia may occur from resorption of the alveolar ridges and excessive loads. Such lesions may be found as papillary hyperplasia in the centre of the palate or near the periphery of dentures as fibrous hyperplasia caused by pressure and denture movement (Figure 2.5).
3. Advanced periodontal disease results in loss of supporting alveolar bone and, after extraction of the teeth, the excess gingival tissue may lead to a thick and frequently flabby mucosal covering of the resultant edentulous ridges (Figure 2.6).

The correct manner of dealing with these types of mucosa is discussed in Chapters 4 and 5.

Tissue compression and peripheral seal

Attention has already been drawn to the fact that an important factor in the retention of complete dentures is atmospheric pressure (see Chapter 1). To be effective this requires a good seal to be maintained at the periphery of the denture.

Those parts of the denture periphery which terminate in the sulci may form an adequate seal by virtue of the fact that the mucosa is reflected over to cover them completely, thus preventing the ingress of air. Posteriorly, however, the periphery lacks this natural seal and it is necessary to ensure that these edges sink slightly into the tissues. In order to achieve this, these edges must be placed over very compressible tissue. In the upper jaw such tissue is found in the region of the junction of the hard and soft palates and the correct area to place the posterior edge of the upper denture is just on the soft palate but not so far back that it encroaches on the movable tissue (Figure 2.3 and 2.7). The junction of the hard and soft palates is sometimes delineated by a faint transverse groove and the

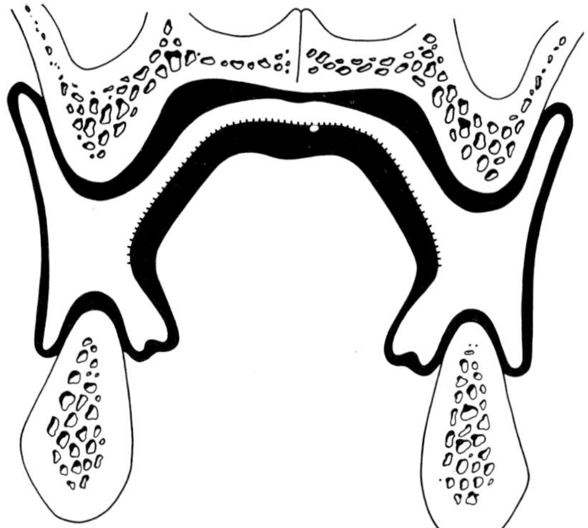

Figure 2.2 This coronal diagram through the first molar region illustrates the varying thickness of the mucosa covering the oral structures

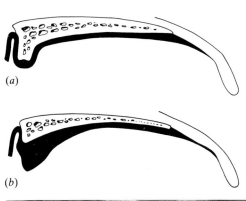

(*a*)

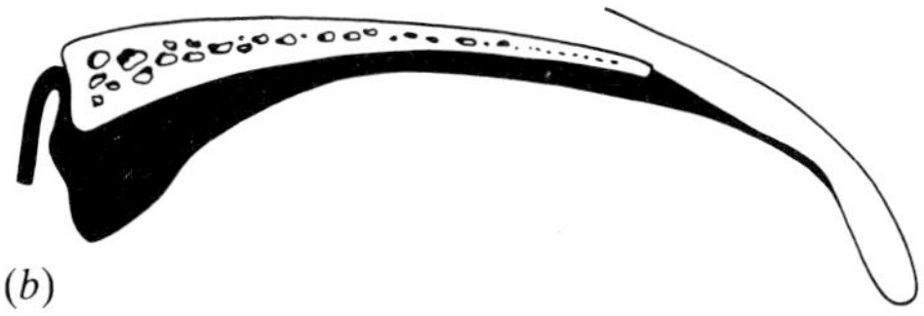

(*b*)

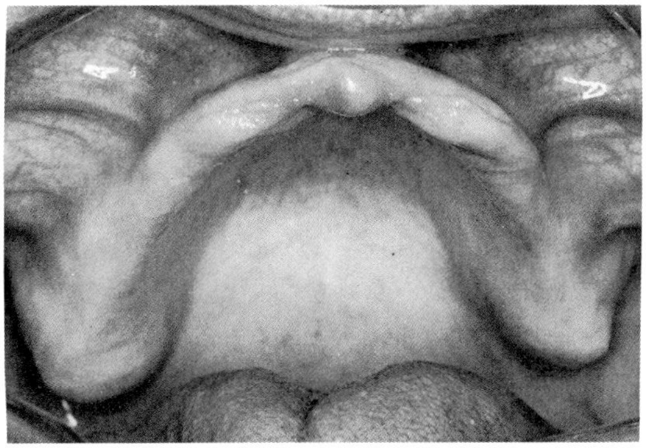

(*c*)

Figure 2.4 (*a*) Sagittal diagram showing normal thickness of mucosa covering alveolar ridge and palate.
(*b*) Resorption of alveolar bone and bunching forwards of the rugal area of mucosa. (*c*) Clinical view of (*b*). Note the rugae lying on the crest of the ridge and the forward position of the incisive papilla

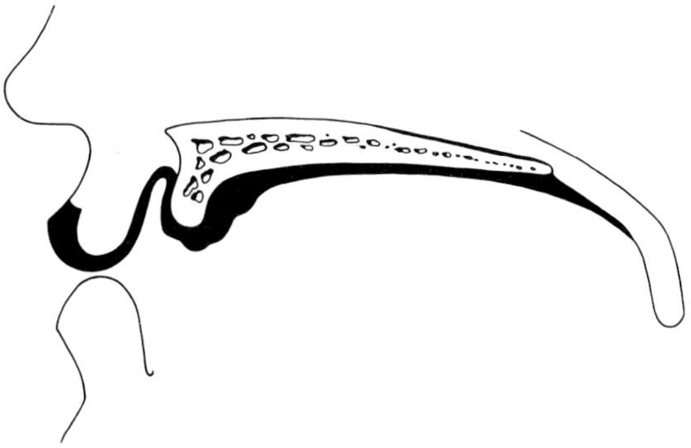

Figure 2.3 Midline sagittal diagram illustrating varying thickness of mucosa overlying hard palate

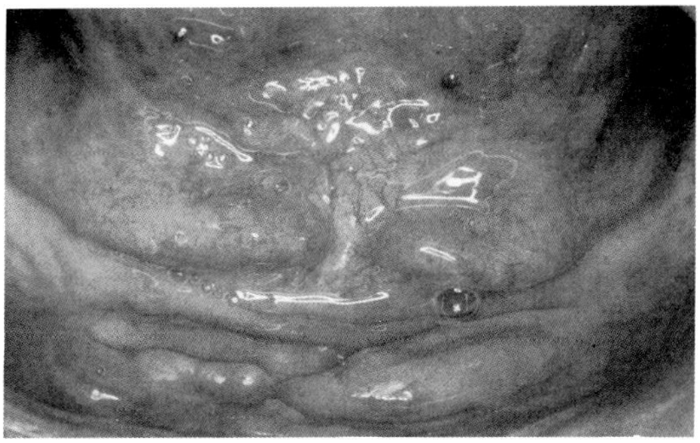

Figure 2.5 Denture-induced hyperplasia of the mandibular labial sulcus

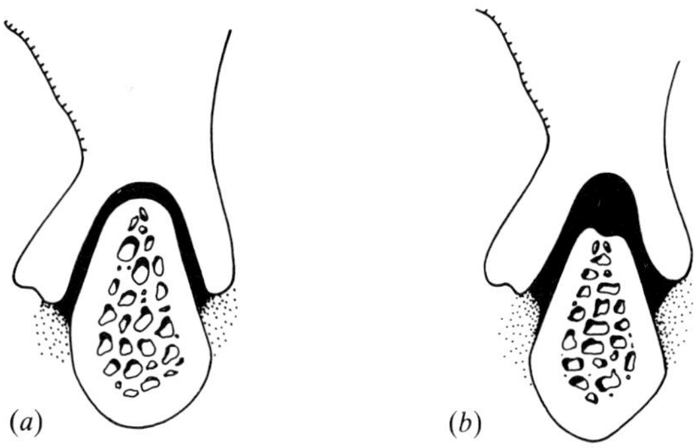

(*a*) (*b*)

Figure 2.6 (*a*) Coronal diagram showing normal thickness of mucosa covering lower alveolar ridge. (*b*) Hyperplasia of mucosa and resorption of alveolar bone resulting from advanced periodontal disease

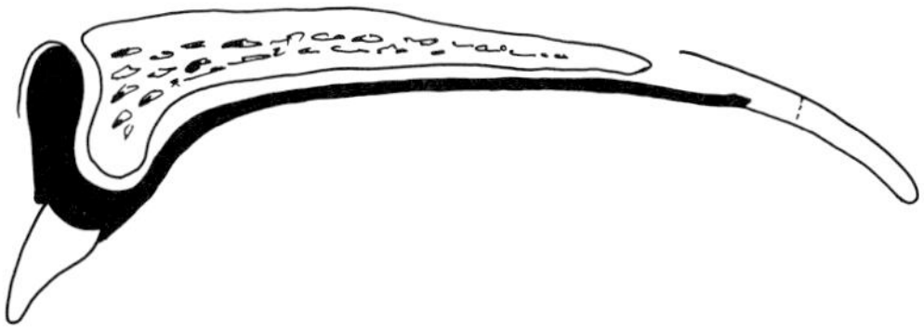

Figure 2.7 Correct placing of the posterior border of the upper denture just on to the non-movable part of the soft palate. The dotted line indicates the vibrating line, the point behind which movement of the soft palate occurs

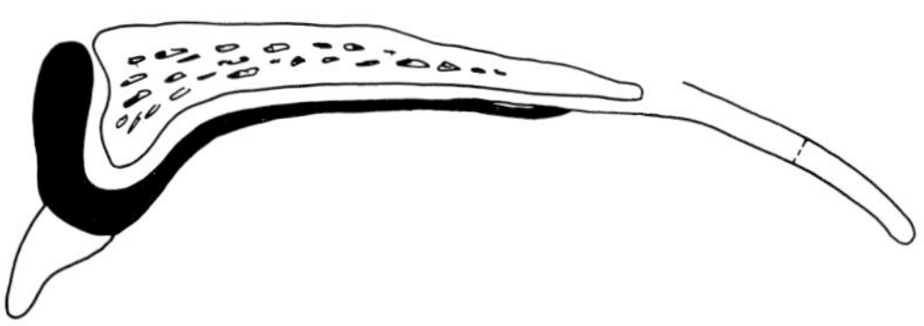

Figure 2.8 Incorrect placing of the posterior border of the upper denture. The effect is magnified to illustrate what occurs

fovea palati. If the posterior edge of the upper denture is placed on the hard palate the mucosa covering the bone is too thin to allow the edge to sink into it sufficiently to provide an adequate seal without causing ulceration (Figure 2.8).

In the lower jaw compressible tissue is found in the retromolar pads and the posterior edges of the lower denture should be placed so as to cross these structures (Figure 2.9).

The detailed methods of placing the postdams on the dentures are dealt with in Chapter 6.

Alveolar ridges

It must be remembered that edentulous alveolar ridges are not natural structures. They are what is left of a bone after disease and surgery have affected it. The alveolar ridges vary greatly in size and shape and their ultimate form is dependent on the following factors:

1. Developmental structure: the individual variation in bone size and its degree of calcification is great.
2. The size of the natural teeth: the teeth, like the bones, show wide individual variation in size. Large teeth are usually supported by bulky ridges, small teeth by narrow ones.
3. The amount of bone lost prior to the extraction of the teeth: periodontal disease is a chronic inflammation of the supporting structures of the teeth and results in destruction of the alveolar process. If the natural teeth are retained until gross alveolar loss has occurred the resultant alveolar ridges will be narrow and shallow.
4. The amount of alveolar process removed during the extraction of the teeth: during extraction with forceps the buccal alveolar plate is sometimes fractured and removed with the tooth. The commonest sites for this occurrence are the upper and lower canine and first molar regions. When teeth are removed by surgical dissection some alveolar process is always destroyed.
5. Rate and degree of resorption: during the first six weeks after the extraction of the teeth the rate of resorption is rapid. During the second six weeks it is fast but begins to slow down. At the end of three months, on average, the immediate post-extraction resorption is complete and thereafter it continues throughout life at an ever decreasing pace (see Chapter 3 for individual variations).
6. The effect of previous dentures: ill-fitting dentures, or dentures occluding with isolated groups of natural teeth, may cause rapid resorption of the alveolar process in the areas where they cause excessive load or lateral stress.

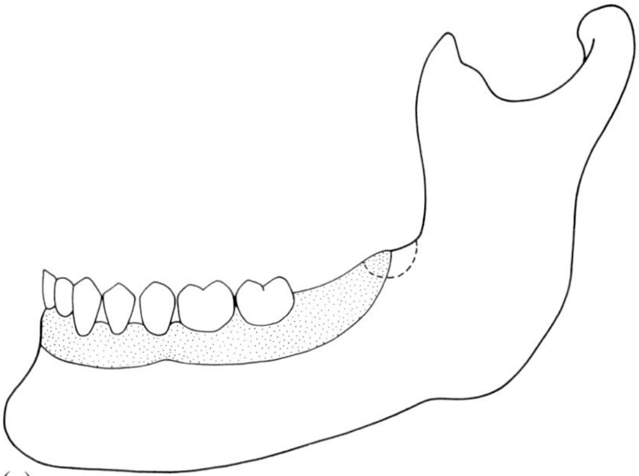

(*a*)

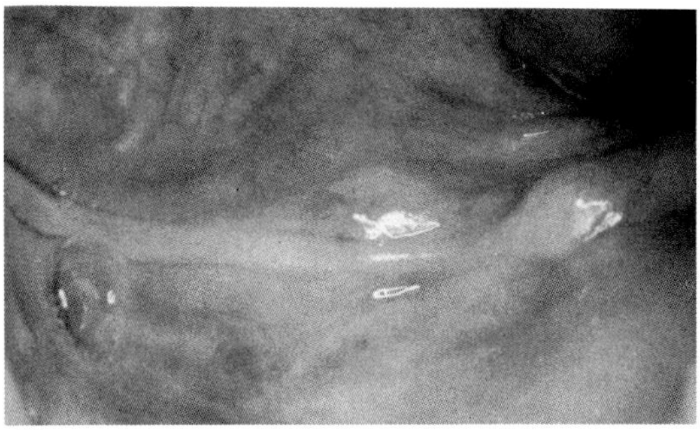

(*b*)

Figure 2.9 The distal edge of the lower denture should cross the retromolar pad. In (*a*) the retromolar pad is indicated by the dotted line and in (*b*) as the prominent pear-shaped elevation at the posterior end of the residual alveolar ridge

Types of alveolar ridges and palate formation and their significance

Maxillary denture-bearing area

1. Well-developed but not abnormally thick ridges and a palate with a moderate vault (Figure 2.10). This is a favourable formation because:
   (a) the centre of the palate presents an almost flat horizontal area and this will aid adhesion;
   (b) the roomy sulcus allows for the development of a good peripheral seal;
   (c) the well-developed ridges resist lateral and antero-posterior movement of the denture.

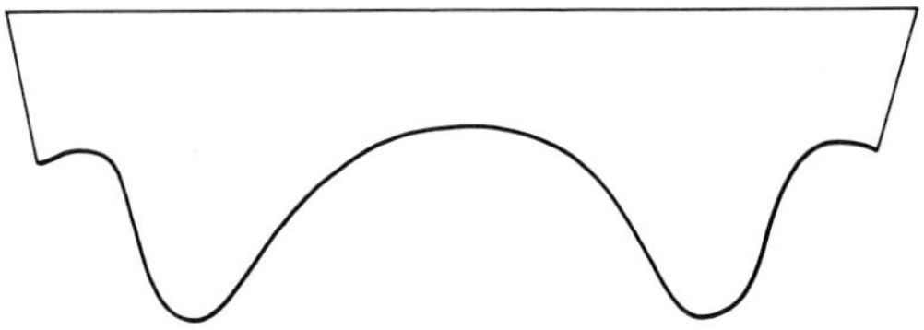

Figure 2.10 Well-developed ridges; palate of moderate depth

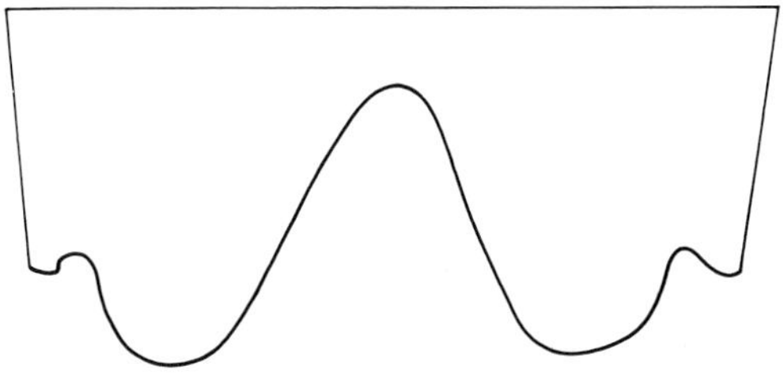

Figure 2.11 High v-shaped palate and well-developed ridges

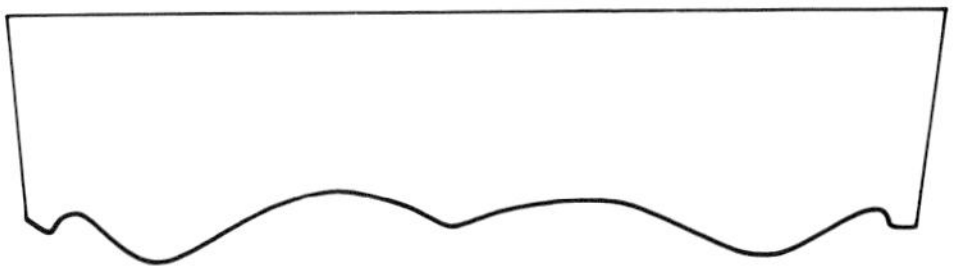

Figure 2.12 Flat palate with small ridges and shallow sulci

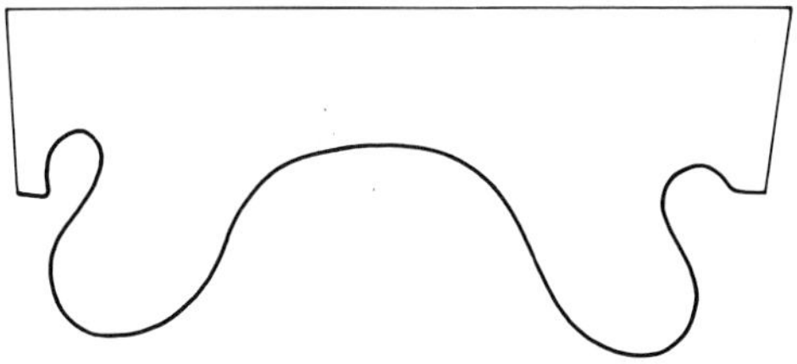

Figure 2.13 Well-developed ridges with buccal undercut areas

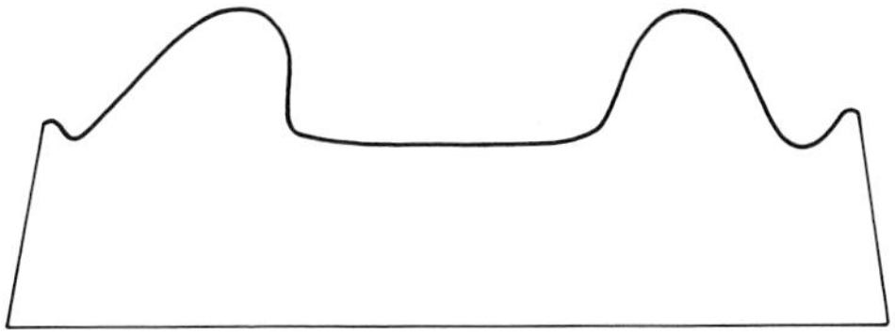

Figure 2.14 Broad and well-developed alveolar ridges

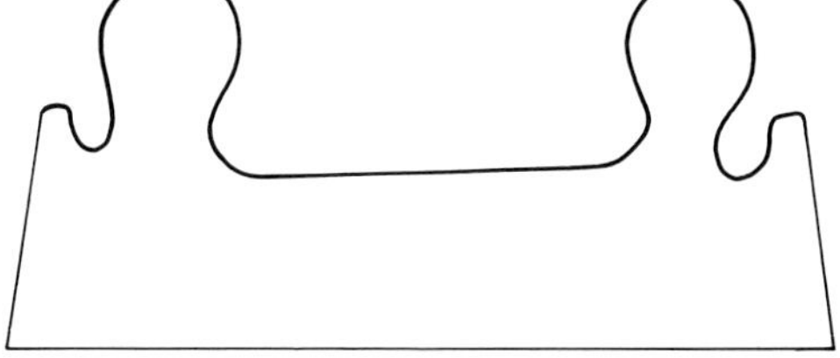

Figure 2.15 Mandibular alveolar ridges with undercut areas

2. High V-shaped palate usually associated with thick bulky ridges (Figure 2.11). This may be an unfavourable formation because the forces of adhesion and cohesion are not at right angles to the surface when counteracting the normal displacing forces of gravity and so peripheral seal is essential.
3. Flat palate with small ridges and shallow sulci (Figure 2.12). This may be an unfavourable formation because:
   (a) the ill-developed or resorbed ridges do not resist lateral and anteroposterior movement of the denture;
   (b) the sulci being shallow do not form a good peripheral seal unless the width of the denture periphery is adequate.
4. Ridges exhibiting undercut areas (Figure 2.13). These are unfavourable because frequently the flanges of the denture need to be trimmed in order to be able to insert it and this may reduce the effectiveness of the peripheral seal.

Mandibular denture-bearing area

1. Broad and well-developed ridges (Figure 2.14). This is a favourable formation because:
   (a) It provides a large area on which to rest the denture and prevents lateral and antero-posterior movement.
   (b) The surface presented for adhesion is as large as it can ever be in a lower jaw.
   (c) The lingual, labial and buccal sulci are satisfactory for developing a close peripheral seal.
2. Ridges exhibiting undercut areas (Figure 2.15) are unfavourable because:
   (a) If the denture is not eased away from the undercuts pain and soreness will result and, if it is eased, food will lodge under the denture.
   (b) The easing of the periphery will reduce the surface area of mucosal contact and will spoil the peripheral seal.
3. Well-developed but narrow or knife-like ridges (Figure 2.16) are unfavourable because:
   (a) The pressure of the denture during clenching and mastication on the sharp ridge will cause pain.
   (b) Adhesive and cohesive forces are negligible.

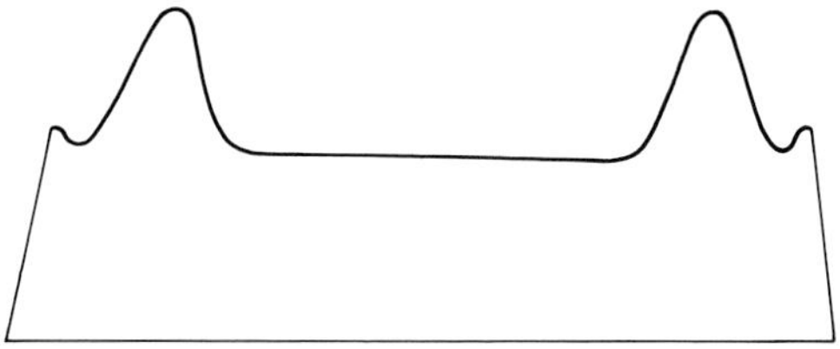

Figure 2.16 Well-developed mandibular knife-like ridges

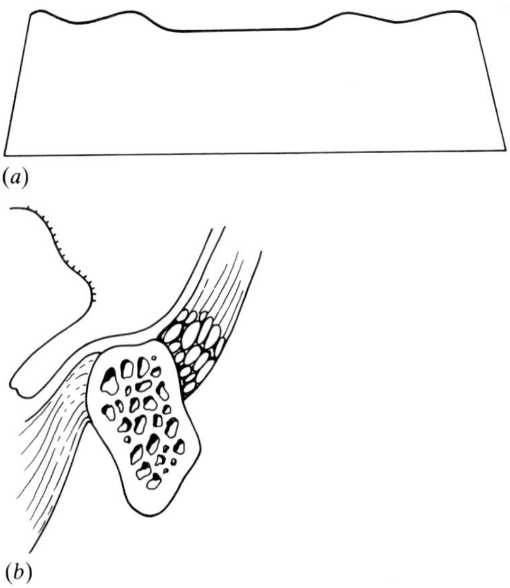

Figure 2.17 (*a*) Illustrates a flat lower ridge in coronal section. (*b*) Illustrates the closeness of the attachments of the buccinator and mylohyoid muscles to a flat ridge

4. Flat and atrophic ridges (Figure 2.17). These are unfavourable because no resistance is offered to anteroposterior or lateral movements. In addition, such ridges are frequently found to have resorbed to the level of the attachments of the mylohyoid, genioglossus and buccinator muscles and, if the denture base is made sufficiently narrow not to encroach on these structures, its area is too small for the denture to function correctly. If the area is increased to encroach on the muscles they may move the dentures when they contract.

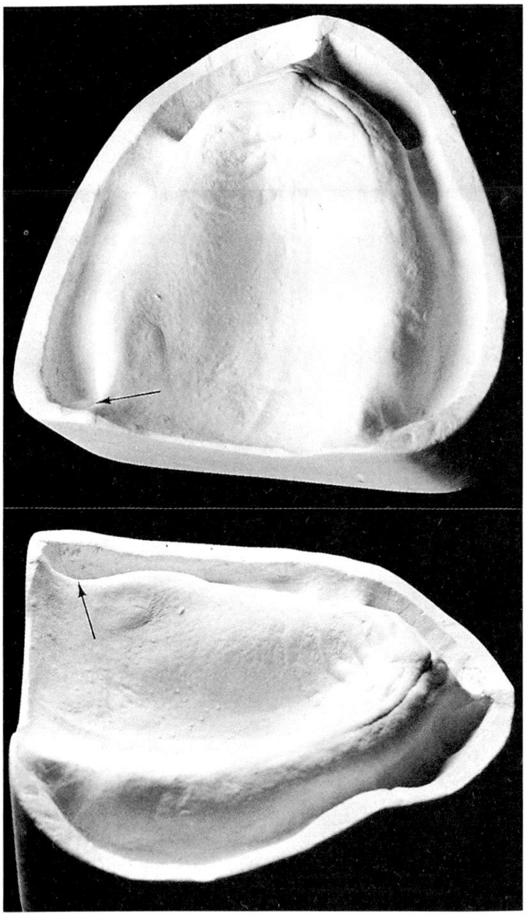

Figure 2.18 Arrows indicate the position to which the posterior border of the upper denture should be carried in the hamular notch

Tuberosities

Large maxillary tuberosities bounded by deep sulci offer very satisfactory resistance to the lateral movement of the denture.

Tuberosities sometimes exhibit buccal undercut areas. If only one tuberosity is undercut this can sometimes be utilized to retain the denture on that side by slipping the distobuccal flange up over the bulge first and then raising the other side of the denture (see Figure 1.4). Tuberosities exhibiting gross undercuts may require surgical treatment (see Chapter 4).

Hamular notch

The tissues in the hamular notch (pterygomaxillary notch) are easily compressed and the postdam line of the upper denture should be carried into this region to ensure an adequate peripheral seal (Figure 2.18).

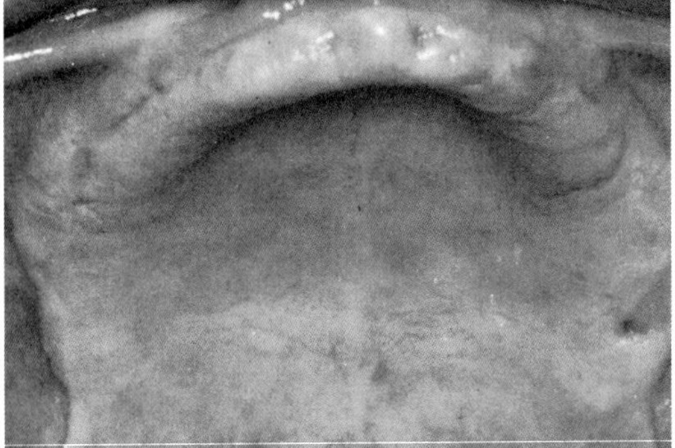

Figure 2.19 Gross alveolar resorption with absence of tuberosities and a prominent pterygomandivular raphe on each side

In cases showing gross alveolar resorption, the hamular notch flattens and the buccinator fibres in the region may become very prominent. Care should be taken in such cases that the posterior edge of the upper denture is not carried too far back on to the pterygomandibular raphe (Figure 2.19).

Hard palate

If a torus palati is present in the midline and very prominent it may increase the difficulties of obtaining a stable upper denture for the reasons given in the section on mucosal compressibility. Steps must be taken to obtain adequate relief for it (Figure 2.20) by using special impression techniques, mechanical relief or, as a last resort, by its surgical excision.

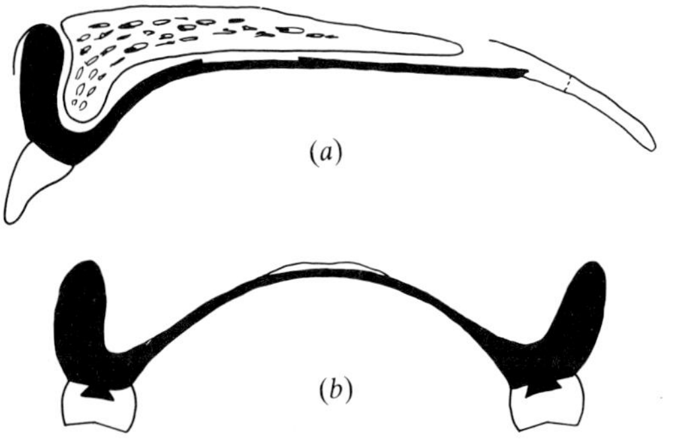

Figure 2.20 Illustrates in sagittal and coronal diagrams how the fitting surface of a denture is relieved to prevent it rocking on a prominent torus palati

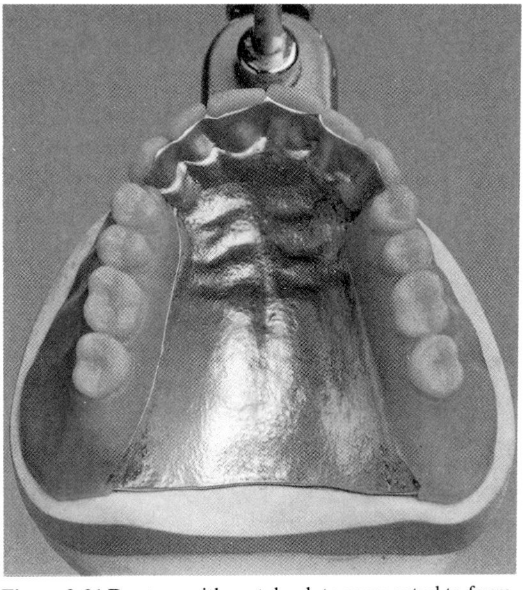

Figure 2.21 Denture with metal palate corrugated to form artificial rugae

Rugae

These are said to be associated with the sense of taste and the function of speech. They assist the tongue to absorb, via its papillae, the fluids containing the four primary flavours. They also enable the tongue to form a perfect seal when it is pressed against the palate in making the linguopalatal consonant stops of speech (Chapter 10).

When a smooth, thick, artificial denture palate covers these elevations of the mucosa, difficulty is sometimes experienced with both taste and speech. The high degree of adaptability of the normal individual usually results in rapid adjustment to these problems, but the copying of rugae on the palatal surface of a denture, or especially by using the corrugation of a thin metal palate, may help to reduce the disability (Figure 2.21). In some cases, however, these artificial rugae cause interference with speech, particularly if they are made too prominent.

Palatal vessels and nerves

Dentures made when using certain compression impression techniques may bring pressure to bear on the foramina through which the blood vessels pass. Relief of the anterior and posterior palatine foramina should be ensured in such cases either by using the correct impression technique or by foiling the cast surface in the area of the foramina.

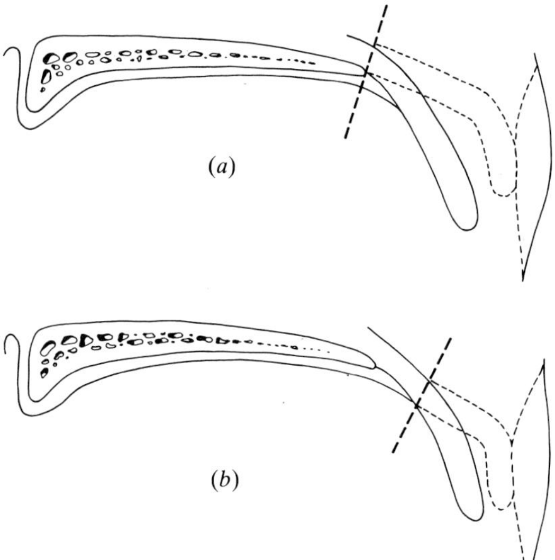

Figure 2.22 Sagittal diagrams illustrating variations in the position of the vibrating line of the soft palate (marked by broken line). (*a*) Movement occurs at the junction of the hard and soft palates. (*b*) Movement occurs some distance behind the junction

Soft palate

Attention has already been drawn to the correct placing of the posterior edge of the upper denture on to the non-movable tissue of the soft palate. Patients may be broadly divided into two classes with regard to this non-mobile area:

1. Those whose palates exhibit movement at the junction of the hard and soft palates.
2. Those whose soft palates move some distance behind the junction (Figure 2.22).

The correct manner of assessing the area in which to place the posterior edge of the upper denture is discussed in Chapter 6.

Anterior pillars of the fauces

The palatoglossal arch follows the movements of the tongue. When the tongue is protruded or moved sideways the arch is pulled forwards. If the posterolingual edge of the lower denture is extended so far backwards that it prevents this forward movement of the arch, either pain may result or the denture may dislodge.

The forward position of the palatoglossal arch, therefore, determines the position to be occupied by the posterolingual edge of the lower denture (Figure 2.23).

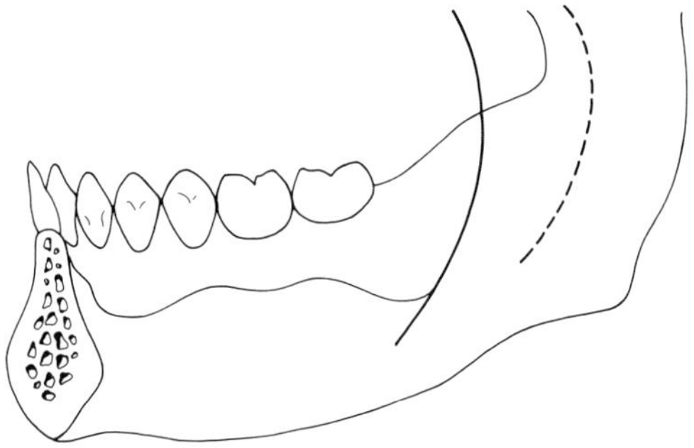

Figure 2.23 Diagram illustrating the positions of the palatoglossal arch. The dotted line indicates its position when the tongue is at rest, and the thick black line its position when the tongue is protruded

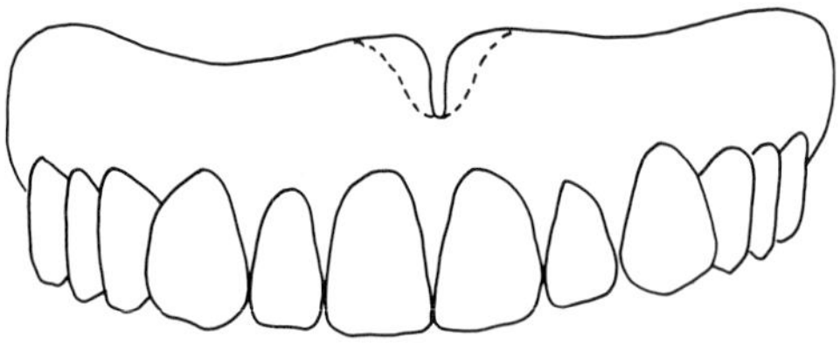

Figure 2.24 The method of shaping the periphery to allow for the labial frenum. The continuous line illustrates the correct contour, the dotted line the incorrect, because the latter shape breaks the peripheral seal

Pterygomandibular raphe

Originating from the hamular process it is in close proximity to that part of the distal edge of the upper denture lying in the hamular notch. If this distal edge is over-extended it will impinge on the fold of soft tissue which is elevated when the mouth is opened and the pterygomandibular raphe becomes tense. This either causes inflammation, reported by the patient as soreness of the throat or, if over-extension is gross, the back of the denture will be flipped downwards each time the mouth is opened, causing the denture to drop.

Frena

These move with the muscles of the lips, cheeks and tongue during speech, mastication and all muscle activity. The peripheries of the dentures must be designed to allow for these movements, but such allowance must not be excessive otherwise the peripheral seal will be broken. The correct and incorrect method of allowing for frena is illustrated in Figure 2.24. Over-developed frena, or those which are attached too high on the alveolar ridge, may be removed surgically. In mouths exhibiting very poor retention, the removal of all the frena increases the peripheral seal.

Sulcus

The depth of the sulcus is dependent on the height of the alveolar ridge, the mobility and tension of the surrounding muscles and the areolar mucosa lining the area. Over-extension of the denture, in height or width, in the sulcus will cause instability or soreness, as will any roughness of the denture periphery. The mucogingival line forms the junction between the attached and reflected mucosa (Figure 2.25).

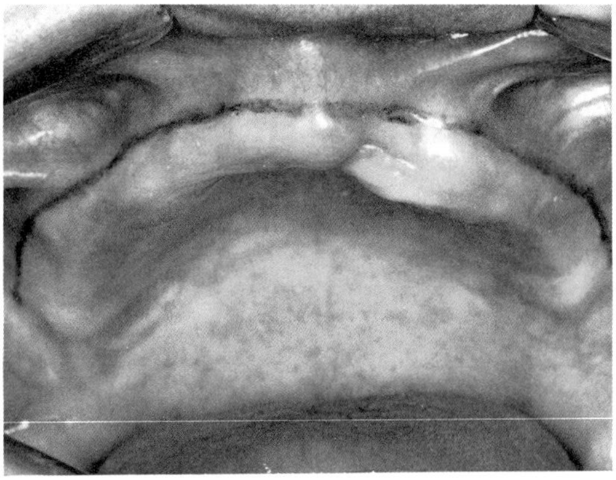

Figure 2.25 The mucogingival line, marked here with indelible pencil, forms the junction between attached and reflected mucosa

Peripheral outline and form of the dentures

The lower denture

Tracing the periphery of the lower denture, commencing with the distobuccal aspect, the outline necessary to conform to the associated muscles is as follows.

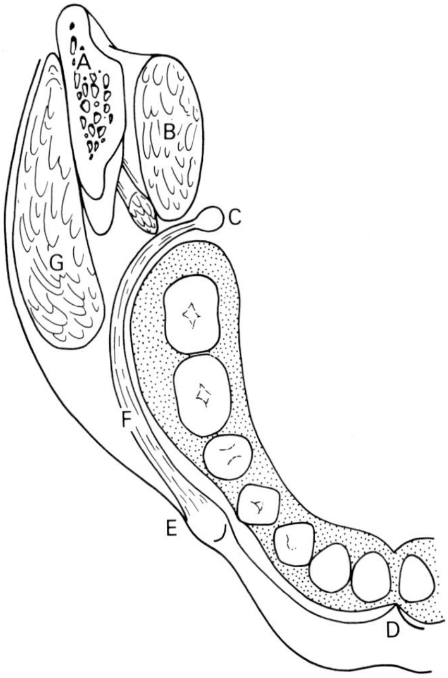

Figure 2.26 A, mandibular ramus; B, medial pterygoid muscle; C, pterygomandibular raphe; D, labial frenum; E, modiolus; F, buccinator muscle; G, masseter muscle

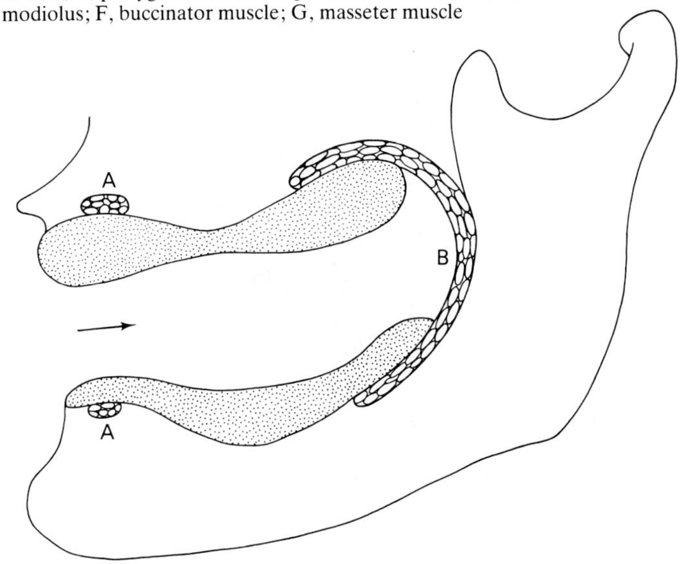

Figure 2.27 (*a*) Incisive muscles; (*b*) buccinator muscle. The arrow indicates the area of action of the modiolus

The periphery runs downwards and outwards from the retromolar pad to the first molar region following the attachment of the buccinator muscle as it sweeps outward from its origin along the pterygomandibular raphe (Figures 2.26 and 2.27). The periphery forms an almost straight edge because the buccinator is flattened by the contracting masseter muscle. For this reason, this part of the periphery is sometimes known as the masseteric plane.

In the region of the molars the lower fibres of the buccinator are attached to bone in a C-shaped curve while the middle fibres bowstring across from the corner of the mouth. In this region the polished buccal surface of the denture is convex looking outwards and upwards in order that the buccinator muscle, as it contracts, forces the cheek inwards to press the denture downwards (Figure 2.28). From this point the periphery runs forwards and sweeps medially to avoid encroachment on the modiolus situated in the premolar region (Figures 2.26, 2.27 and 2.29). This decussation of facial muscles is pulled inwards and backwards and presses hard against the teeth in order to provide a fixed base from which the orbicularis oris can contract. The lower denture requires to be made narrow in this region in order that the pressure of the modiolus may be taken by the upper denture which, due to its greater retention and resistance to lateral movement, is far better able to withstand it.

From this point the periphery curves outwards and downwards again but it must not be carried too deeply in the canine region else contraction of the incisive muscle (incisivus labii inferioris) will force the denture upwards. A balance must be struck

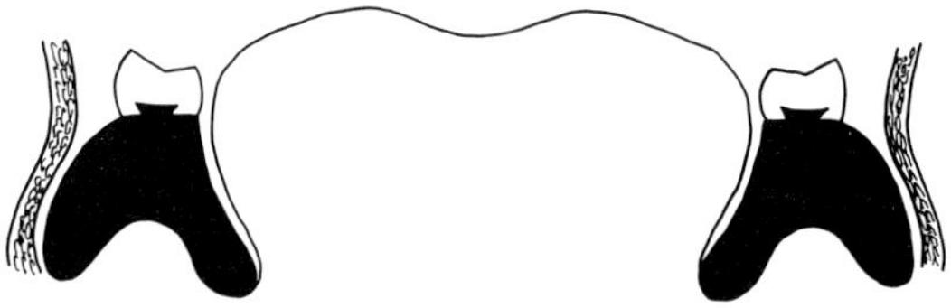

Figure 2.28 Illustrating the correct curvature of the buccal flange of a lower denture in order that the buccinator muscle may assist in the control of the denture

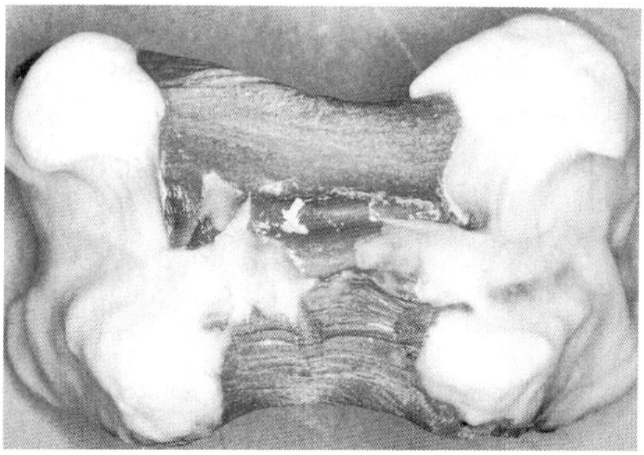

Figure 2.29 Moulding of alginate in the region of the modiolus on each side during the pursing forwards of the lips of a patient

between the incisive muscle, which aids in the attachment of the orbicularis oris to the surface of the alveolar process, and the depressor anguli oris which, when contracting, deepens the sulcus. Over-extension of the periphery in the incisor region will cause lifting of the denture when the mentalis muscle (levator labii inferioris) contracts. In the midline the periphery is shaped to allow room for the labial frenum.

Lingually, commencing at the crest of the ridge in the retromolar area, the periphery runs downwards and backwards, its direction being dictated by the most forward position assumed by the palatoglossus muscle (see Figure 2.23). The depth to which it descends depends on the degree of resorption of the alveolar ridge and the laxity of the soft tissues. If there is little alveolar ridge the lingual pouch in this region is shallow. The periphery follows the curve of the palatoglossal arch. The palatoglossus muscle forms the anterior pillar of the fauces. The palatoglossus arises from the lower surface of the palatal aponeurosis, descends to the lateral surface of the tongue where its fibres interlace with the transverse fibres of the tongue. When the tongue is protruded or moved to one side, the mucosa overlying the palatoglossus becomes taut. When both palatoglossus muscles contract, as in swallowing, they pull the tongue and soft palate together to close the isthmus of the fauces and this action squeezes against the lingual flange of the denture.

The superior constrictor originates from the hamulus, pterygomandibular raphe and distal end of the mylohyoid ridge and, in the lingual part of the muscle, forms a foundation for the mucosa of the floor of the mouth and side of tongue in this region. For these reasons the posterolingual edge of the lower denture must be shaped by the activity of this important muscle. The tissues enveloping the periphery in this region rise to their highest position during swallowing and thus limit the depth of the denture which must not interfere with this movement. This position can be felt by placing a finger in the lingual pouch (also known as the retromylohyoid fossa) and asking the patient to swallow.

From here the periphery rises slightly to cross the narrow posterior edge of the mylohyoid muscle which sometimes is sufficiently well defined to produce a definite notch in the periphery in this region (Figures 2.30 and 2.31). From this point forwards the periphery flattens over the body of the sublingual gland which lies immediately underneath

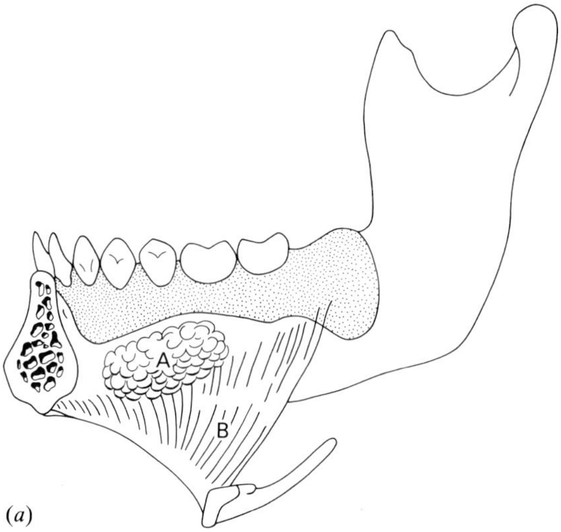

(*a*)

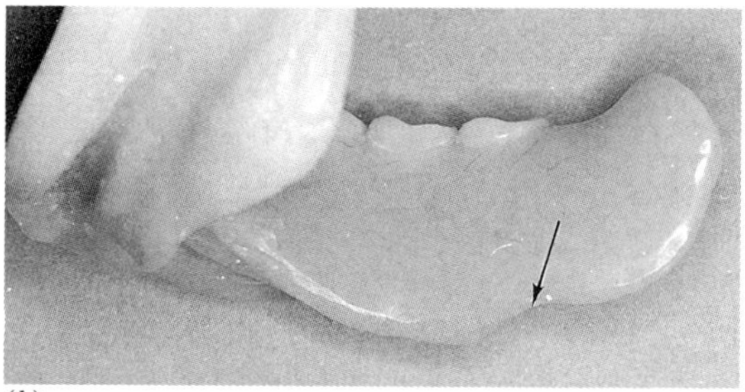

(*b*)

Figure 2.30 (*a*) Illustrating the outline of the lingual flange of the lower denture in relation to the structures in contact with it. A, sublingual gland; B, mylohyoid muscle.
(*b*) Photograph shows notch (arrowed) produced by the posterior edge of the mylohyoid muscle

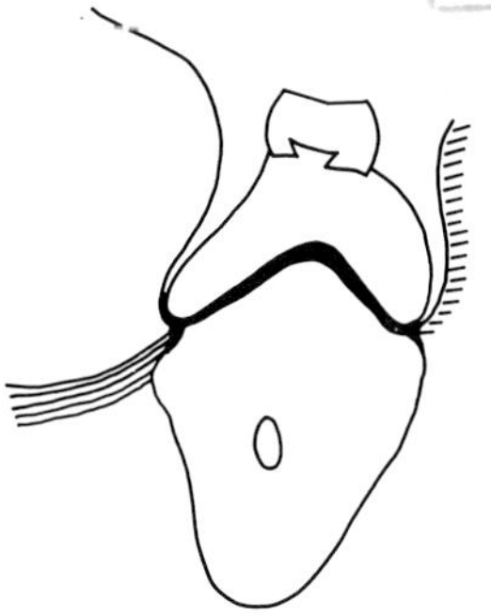

Figure 2.31 Diagram through second molar region of a lower denture, illustrating the relation of the lingual flange to the mylohyoid muscle

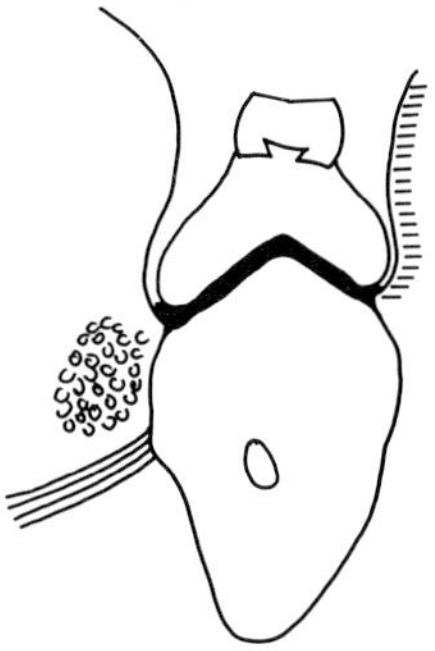

Figure 2.32 Diagram through the first molar region of a lower denture, illustrating the relation of the lingual flange to the tongue, the sublingual gland and the mylohyoid muscle

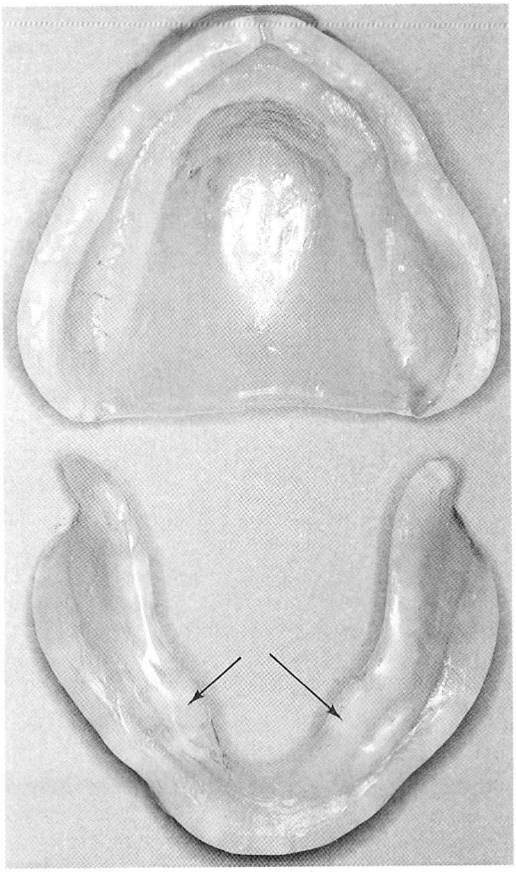

Figure 2.33 Lower denture showing typical S-shaped lingual periphery. Arrows indicate anterior lingual planes

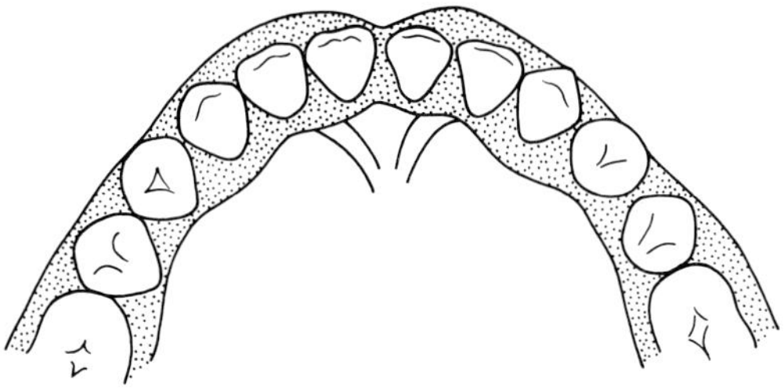

Figure 2.34 Lingual frenum in relation to the lingual flange of the lower denture

the mucosa forming the floor of the mouth (Figures 2.30 and 2.32). Looking from above, the horizontal periphery turns slightly medially to form the anterior lingual plane (Figure 2.33). When it reaches the first premolar region it descends again for a short distance and then rises to clear the lingual frenum which sometimes presents a very broad attachment to the mandible (Figure 2.34). In cases where the anterior ridge is flat the periphery extends distally to butt against the genial tubercles, particularly when these are prominent.

The polished lingual surface of the lower denture from the occlusal surface slopes downwards and inwards, except in the first molar region where it is more vertical to provide for the wide middle third of the tongue. The posterior surface hollows out slightly to accommodate the tongue (Figure 2.32).

The upper denture

The periphery of the upper denture commencing with the posterior border is as follows.

The posterior edge should sink slightly into the non-movable tissues of the soft palate following a line from the hamular notch of one side to that of the other close to the fovea palati (Figure 2.35). The posterior border then traverses the hamular notch and rises up into the sulcus (the tuberosity vestibular space) on the buccal side of the tuberosity (Figure 2.35). The height to which it rises is determined by the attachment of the buccinator in this region as that muscle sweeps backwards to its attachment to the hamulus. The space is also defined distally by

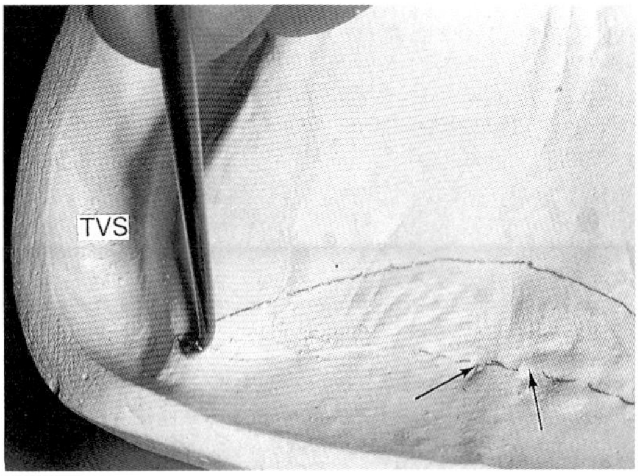

Figure 2.35 Posterior surface of a maxillary cast showing preparation of postdam. Arrows indicate the fovea palati. TVS; tuberosity vestibular space

the mandibular coronoid process and buccally by the contracting masseter muscle. From this point it commences to descend following the buccinator attachment, the lowest point of this descent being at the root of the zygoma. The zygoma having been cleared, the periphery rises again as the sulcus is influenced by levator anguli oris, but the height to which it is made should not be excessive else contraction of the upper incisive muscle (incisivus labii superioris) may displace the denture. Finally the periphery is shaped to clear the labial frenum (Figure 2.24).

The polished buccal surface of the upper denture should be hollowed slightly with the concavity looking downwards and outwards so that contraction of the buccinator muscle may press the denture upwards (Figure 2.36). The orbicularis oris muscle when contracting to press the lips against the teeth does not affect the upper denture as much as it does the lower because of the greater stability of the former. Therefore, the upper anterior teeth should be placed sufficiently far forward in most cases to suit the aesthetic requirements of the case, together with sufficient width of the labial flange to restore the lips to their correct relationship.

Impressions and stock trays

Trays used for making impressions should have a similar outline to that described for dentures. One of the faults found in stock or standard trays is that they are over-extended and this is particularly the case with the distobuccal region of lower trays.

Over-extended trays lead to over-extended impressions and this means that the muscles surrounding the oral cavity will be forcefully pushed out of the way. Dentures made to such over-extended impressions will be displaced by the muscles returning to their normal positions (Figure 2.37).

Particular attention should be paid to the posterolingual flanges of the lower tray because if these are over-extended they will displace the floor of the mouth in that region and the palatoglossus muscles downwards and backwards. On the other hand, if the flanges are short the lateral borders of the tongue will get under the tray and spoil the impression (Figure 2.38).

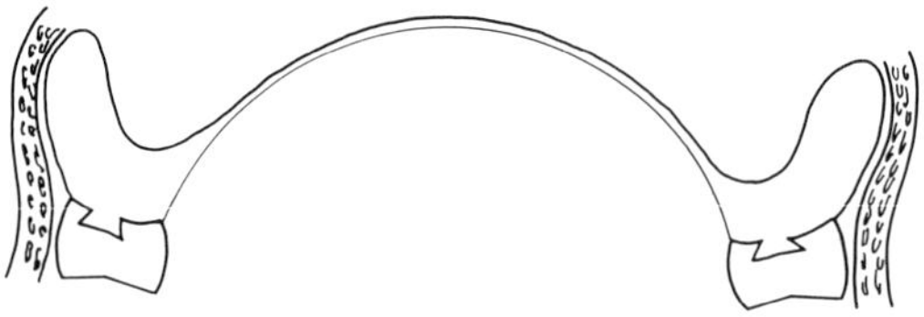

Figure 2.36 Correct contouring of polished buccal surface of upper denture

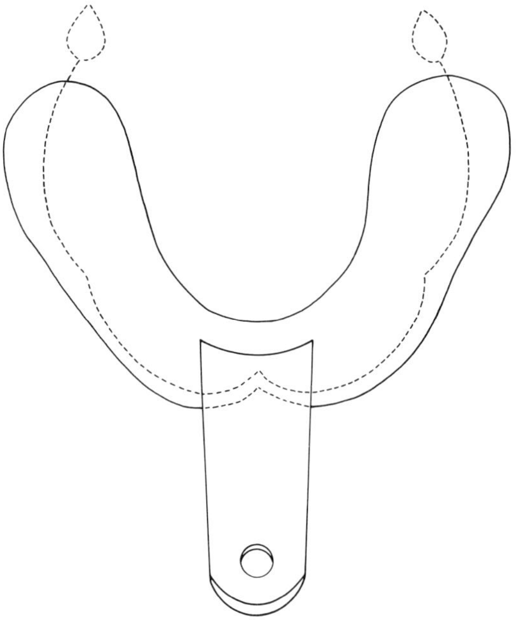

Figure 2.37 Over-extended buccal flanges of a stock tray with insufficient length to include the retromolar pads

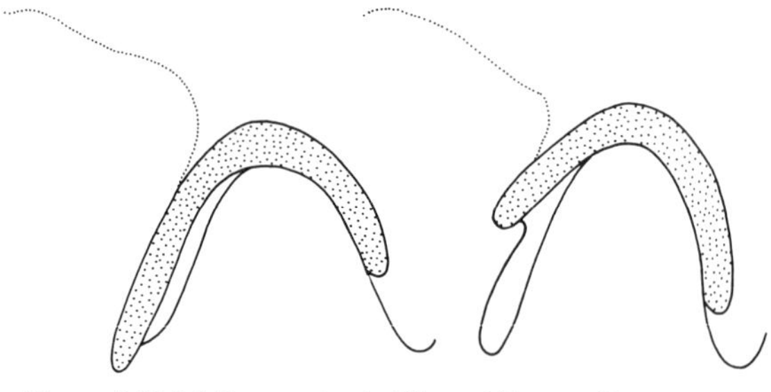

Figure 2.38 (*a*) Over-extended lingual flange of lower tray distorting the floor of the mouth. (*b*) Short lingual flange of a lower tray trapping the tongue beneath its edge

In upper stock or standard trays the posterior edge often curves forward and so the impression fails to record the postdam region at the junction of the soft and hard palate. The anterior flanges, if they are too deep, will displace the labial sulcus upwards.

It should be noted that the shape and size of impression trays have a profound effect on the shape and size of the finished denture, no matter what particular technique is being used.

The tongue

Rest position of the tongue

The dorsum rests against the roof of the mouth and the tip of the tongue rests in contact with the lingual surfaces of the lower incisor teeth.

The lateral borders lie against the lingual borders of the posterior teeth and protrude slightly into the free-way space between the occlusal surfaces of the upper and lower teeth.

Posteriorly the soft palate rests on the dorsum of the tongue during normal nasal breathing.

When the teeth are extracted the tongue spreads laterally and the lips and cheeks fall in to meet it so filling between them the space left by the teeth, sometimes termed the neutral zone or zone of minimal conflict.

Functions of the tongue

Excluding taste, these are twofold. It controls the food during mastication and swallowing. It controls and directs, with the aid of the lips, teeth and palate the vibrating air stream from the larynx to form the sounds of articulate speech.

During mastication the tongue performs as follows. As the piece of food is being incised the tip of the tongue controls and steadies it. In the case of food which does not require incising the tongue is protruded slightly and its centre depressed to form a shallow concavity into which the food is placed.

Next the food is quickly transferred backwards along the depressed surface of the tongue by a series of muscular waves until it has reached a level with the teeth by which it is to be chewed. Hard food is placed further back than soft or fibrous food, an advantage because the mandible is a lever of the third class and the farther back the food is placed the shorter is the arm of the lever.

The middle of the tongue now rises and forces the food laterally between the occlusal surfaces of the teeth which have parted to receive it. The lateral borders of the tongue at this time are on a level with the occlusal surfaces of the lower teeth and pressed hard against their lingual aspects to prevent the food passing downwards between the teeth and the tongue into the lingual sulcus.

The teeth occlude, dividing the food, some of which is squeezed out, some lingually and some buccally. The tongue depresses in the centre gradually to receive the food as it is forced lingually by the occluding teeth and then returns it to them again as they separate. The cheek controls and replaces the food displaced buccally.

This cycle, smoothly continuous, proceeds until the food has been adequately divided and insalivated. The tongue then collects the food and forms it into a bolus which it holds in its central depression. A series of waves travelling posteriorly along the tongue then passes the food backwards. As the bolus reaches the back of the tongue the soft palate rises and the tongue and the palate holding the bolus between them pass it into the pharynx whence it is directed over the epiglottis into the oesophagus.

Finally the tongue scavenges the sulci with its tip to clear the mouth of fragments of food which have escaped the formation of the bolus.

From the foregoing it will be realized that the tongue is a powerful factor mitigating against the stability of the lower denture because of its power and latitude of movement. Care must be taken, therefore, to design dentures so that they impede the movements of the tongue as little as possible and, to gain this end, attention must be paid to the following:

1. The teeth must never be set inside the alveolar ridge or they will cramp the tongue causing movement of the dentures and irritation to the patient (Figure 2.39).
2. The lower denture should present lingual flanges to the tongue which slope slightly inwards from above downwards (see Figure 2.32). In no circumstances should the lingual cusps of the posterior teeth overhang the tongue (Figure 2.40). In other words, no concavities should be presented to the tongue into which its lateral borders can expand and so lift the denture.

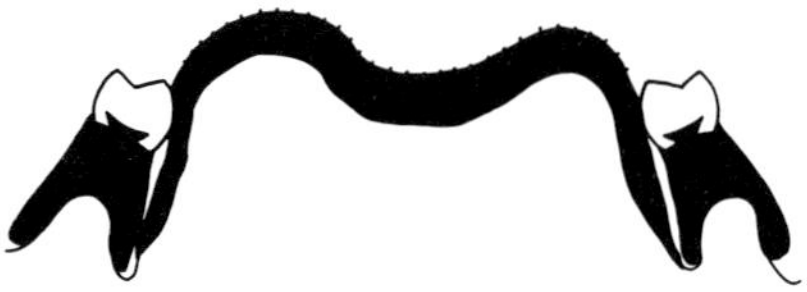

Figure 2.39 The tongue cramped

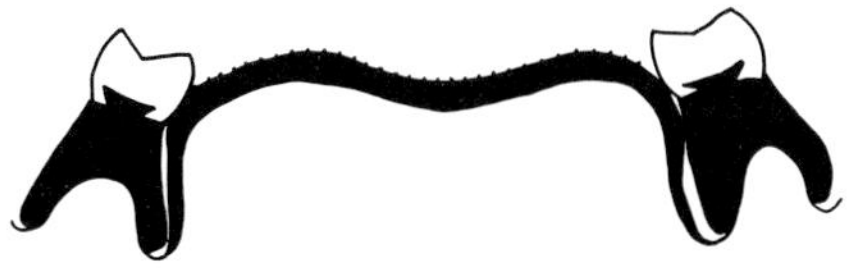

Figure 2.40 Lingual cusps overhanging the tongue

3. The palate of the upper denture should be as thin as is commensurate with the strength of the material used in its construction.
4. The occlusal plane of the lower denture should be kept low, thus allowing the lateral borders of the tongue to rest upon the occlusal surfaces of the teeth when the mouth is opened to receive food and so prevent the lower denture from rising (Figure 2.41).

The tongue as a controlling influence

Observation of people who wear complete dentures satisfactorily, discloses that the tongue is used very largely to control the dentures. It acts in the following ways:

1. The dorsum is pressed against the back of the upper denture to prevent it dropping when incising (Figure 2.42).
2. The tip is pressed forwards and downwards against the anterior lingual surface of the lower denture when the lower lip tends to force the denture backwards (Figure 2.42).
3. The lateral borders of the tongue rest on the occlusal surface of the lower denture when opening the mouth.

Such control takes time for wearers of new dentures to master, and a small percentage never learn at all.

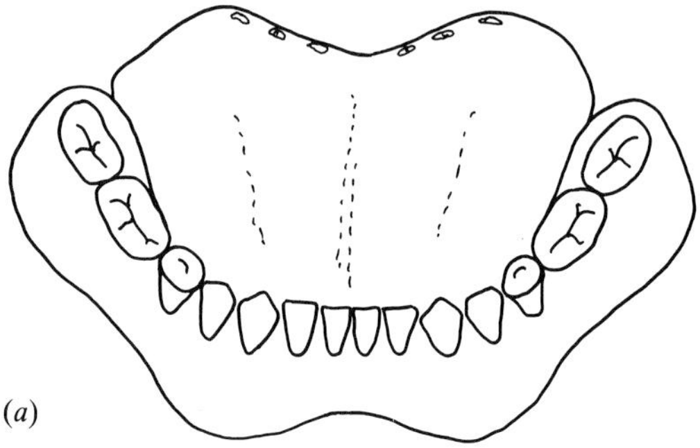
(*a*)

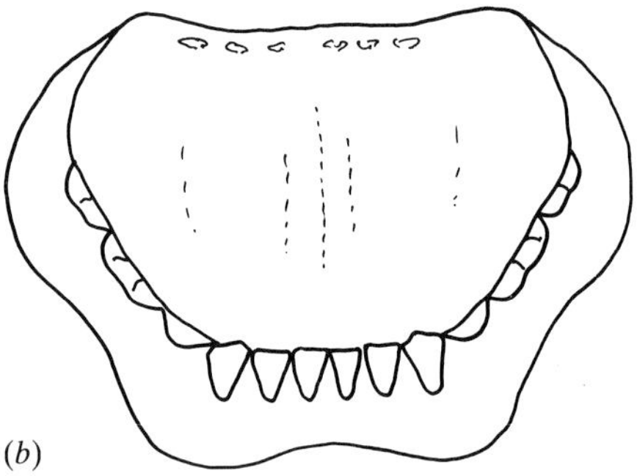
(*b*)

Figure 2.41 (*a*) High occlusal plane preventing the tongue resting on the occlusal surface. (*b*) Low occlusal plane allows the tongue to rest on the occlusal surface

Attention to the design discussed earlier in this section gives patients a better chance of learning this control.

It should be noted that when a person with natural teeth opens his mouth the tongue is reflexly retracted to guard the oropharyngeal isthmus. This reflex often persists in some patients with complete dentures and is often referred to as a low tongue position. These patients require a conscious effort to train the tongue movement forward on opening the mouth.

The tongue in retching and nausea

Anything held on the anterior two-thirds of the tongue is under complete control and can be manipulated by the tongue at will and if necessary ejected from the mouth altogether. Once it has passed on to the pharyngeal part of the tongue, however, this ease of control is lost and, if it is required to eject a foreign body, a convulsion contraction of the muscles forming the pharyngeal sphincter, termed retching or gagging, must occur, and the foreign body is then forcefully expelled.

The retching reflex is stimulated and controlled by nerve endings situated in the soft palate, pharynx and pharyngeal part of the tongue. Retching may occur during impressions and when new dentures are first inserted. From experience, it would appear that the contact of the impression material or the posterior edge of the upper denture with the pharyngeal aspect of the tongue is the chief cause. Methods of making impressions without causing retching are discussed in Chapter 5.

The thickness of the posterior edge of the upper denture, rather than the position it occupies is the cause of the retching. A thick square edge irritates the pharyngeal surface of the tongue constantly when it is in its rest position and so initiates the retching reflex. A thin posterior edge, properly sealed so as to sink into the compressible tissues of the palate, will not irritate the tongue (Figure 2.43).

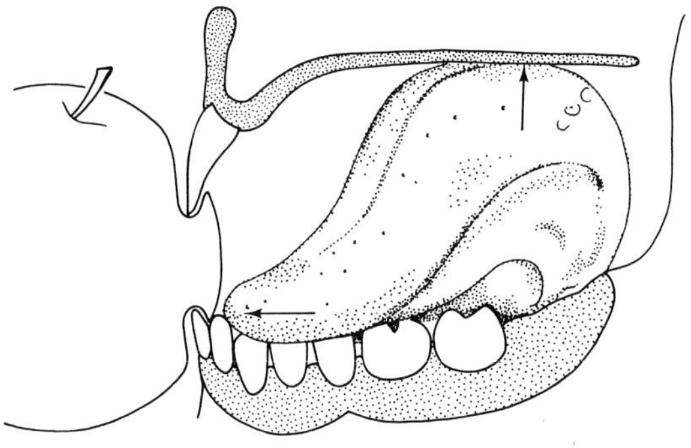

Figure 2.42 Illustrating tongue control when incising an apple. Arrows indicate tongue pressure

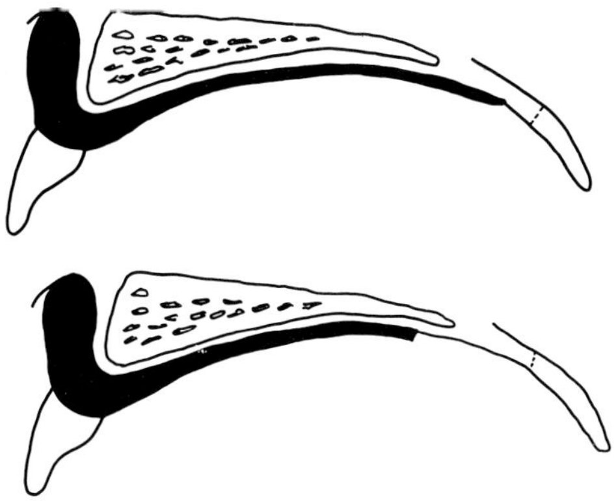

Figure 2.43 (*a*) Showing posterior edge of upper denture correctly postdammed. (*b*) Thick square edge of upper denture incorrectly postdammed

Light or intermittent pressure is another cause of nausea and a further reason for making an adequate postdam in this area.

The rationale of prescribing the sucking of sweets or candy for patients showing a tendency to retch when dentures are first fitted is that the act of sucking and the swallowing induced by the increased flow of saliva keeps the tongue occupied and prevents it resting against the back of the new denture before it has learned to tolerate it.

Wearing dentures during sleep is to be recommended during the learning period for a very similar reason because tolerance is gained by the tongue during the night. If the dentures are removed before going to bed the tolerance gained during the day is lost and the early morning is a time when many people are especially susceptible to nausea or retching.

Temporomandibular joint

When the natural teeth are in normal occlusion with the cusps interdigitating in the opposing fossae the anterosuperior aspect of the head of the mandibular condyle is located with the meniscus in that part of the glenoid fossa formed by the squamous temporal bone (Figure 2.44). When the mouth is opened, or the jaw protruded or moved laterally, the condyle and meniscus travel down the anterior surface of the fossa and, in the widest position of opening, rest just short of the crest of the articular eminence (Figure 2.45).

Muscles of mastication

The muscles of mastication when contracting are capable of applying a force of over 100 kg between opposing natural molar teeth. This is very greatly

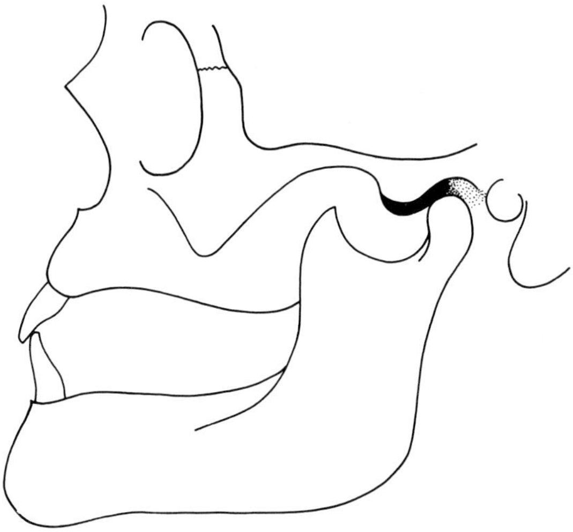

Figure 2.44 The relation of the head of the condyle to the fossa when the mouth is closed

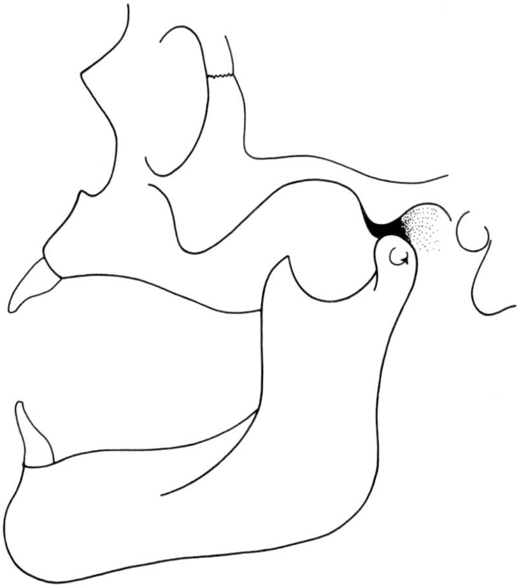

Figure 2.45 The relation of the head of the condyle to the fossa when the mouth is open

reduced when complete dentures are fitted because the mucosa cannot withstand such pressure, a figure of 25 kg never having been recorded.

The mandible, the temporomandibular joints and the muscles of mastication together constitute a double lever of the third class (Figure 2.46). The muscles which apply the powerful closing force to the mandible are the temporalis and the masseter and it is obvious that the farther back in the mouth a piece of food is placed (i.e. the nearer to the insertions of these muscles) the greater the power that can be brought to bear on it.

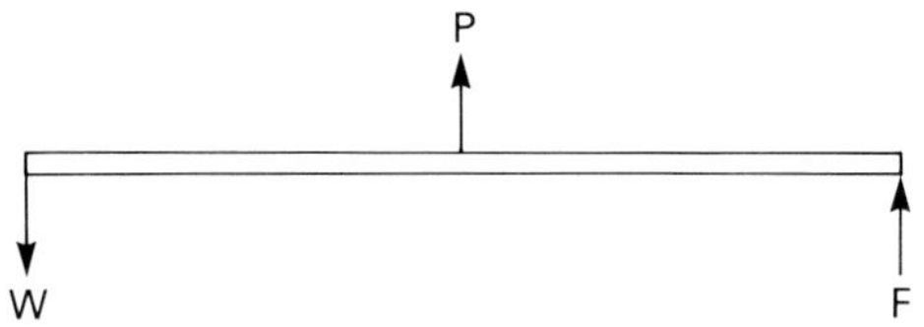

Figure 2.46 A double lever of the third class: W = weight; P = power; F = fulcrum

Muscular power and vertical dimension

The precise control and coordination existing between the muscles of mastication enables them to apply their power to a piece of food and yet bring the teeth into occlusion after its division with such fine precision that no jarring occurs. They are enabled to do this because the position of the teeth and jaws in space at any moment is accurately transmitted to centres in the brain by nerve endings in muscle, mucosa, tongue and periodontal membrane. Such delicate control is only possible, however, if the occlusal surface of the teeth, in their relation to the jaws and muscles, is not suddenly altered. We are all familiar with the sudden alteration of this smooth chewing cycle when normal jaw closure is interrupted by a piece of grit or bone on the occlusal surface of a tooth when eating. The premature contact against the unyielding grit is so powerful that it causes shock and discomfort and occasionally fractures the tooth on which the impact was made.

From this it will be obvious that if dentures are fitted which increase vertical dimension too much the premature occlusion of the teeth which occurs will be so great as to cause both discomfort and damage to the underlying tissues. It may be stated here that one of the commonest causes of failure of dentures results from the fact that they are constructed to an excessively increased vertical dimension.

It is claimed by some that the resorption of the alveolar ridges resulting from the force of occlusion which occurs from an excessive vertical dimension soon reduces the distance between the jaws and restores equilibrium. It is doubtful, however, whether many patients would tolerate such a method of reducing their vertical dimension and, even if they did, the denture bases would no longer fit the new form of the resorbed ridges.

On the other hand, it should be noted that the muscles of mastication develop their greatest power within a short range of the normal vertical dimension, and if this dimension is reduced to a distance less than normal, then loss of power may occur.

In certain patients who present with difficulties in the supporting tissues, or who have worn the same dentures for a very long time, advantage may be taken of this power loss associated with closure of the vertical dimension to reduce the forces applied to new, replacement dentures. Such closure of the vertical dimension, however, should be carried out with care and a full realization of the other disadvantages which may accrue. These are discussed elsewhere in this book.

Muscle tone and antagonism

In a normal mouth with natural teeth the elevator, depressor, protruder and retractor groups of muscles balance one another and so control the movement of the mandible with great precision.

For example, in protrusion the lateral pterygoid muscles draw the head of the condyle and disc forwards, the medial pterygoid muscles produce a strong component force pulling the angle of the mandible forwards, the superficial fibres of the masseter, and to a lesser extend the anterior fibres of the temporalis, bring a forward traction on the mandible. When posterior teeth are present the forward pull of these muscle fibres is accurately balanced by the gradual relaxation of the posterior fibres of the temporalis and some of the deep fibres of the masseter. In retrusion the reverse action occurs.

When the posterior teeth are lost and mastication is performed entirely on the anterior teeth, or when a long period of edentation precedes the delivery of complete dentures, abnormal habits of chewing with the mandible forward are acquired which results in the delicate balance between the protruding and retruding groups of muscles being temporarily lost, the protruding group becoming dominant due to excessive use.

In such cases difficulty may be anticipated when registering the anteroposterior occlusal relationship, and great insistence must be placed on complete muscular relaxation and a very gentle, controlled closing movement to eliminate the dominance of the protruding group of muscle fibres.

Freeway space

When the mandible is at rest it is supported by the elevator group of muscle fibres which are not fully relaxed but are in a condition of partial contraction or tonus which is sufficient to balance the tonus of the depressor muscles of the mandible and gravity.

The position which the mandible assumes at rest is probably constant for each individual and normally when it is in this position the occlusal surfaces of the maxillary and mandibular teeth are separated by about 2–4 mm. This space between the occlusal surfaces of the teeth is termed the freeway space or interocclusal clearance and is important in gauging the vertical dimension of occlusion when making dentures for patients who have lost teeth. This is discussed in Chapter 6.

The lip muscles

The orbicularis oris closes the lips and, when contracting, its lateral insertions into the modioli are fixed by the contraction of the quadratus labii superioris and inferioris, zygomaticus, triangularis, and buccinator muscles. The incisal muscles also fix it to the sulci of the alveolar ridges.

During such function there is considerable inward pressure on the labial surfaces of the teeth and the labial sulci are reduced in depth. The upper denture, due to its better stability, can usually withstand such pressure provided its labial flanges have been designed correctly. The lower denture, however, particularly in cases presenting poorly formed alveolar ridges, is likely to be raised from the ridge in front and pushed backwards. Experienced denture wearers counteract this pressure of the lip by a forward pressure of the tongue but assistance can often be given to the tongue by carrying the heels of the lower denture up the ascending rami of the mandible in such cases. These distal extensions of the lower denture are often referred to as posterior stops.

The elevator and depressor muscle groups antagonize the orbicularis oris, and one another, thus opening the lips and producing facial expression. It must be remembered, if intentionally reducing the vertical dimension, that the origins of the elevator and depressor groups of muscles will be moved closer together, leading to a bunching up of the muscles with consequent loss of tone. This causes drooping of the mouth, puckering and wrinkling of the skin of the lips and face and a flattening of the philtrum giving an aged and even a bad-tempered appearance. Some of this effect can be mitigated by restoring the labial flange of the upper denture to its correct width (Figure 2.47) thus causing the muscles of the lips to follow nearly their original course from origin to insertion and so restore their tone. It is always best, however, to combine this with the correct vertical dimension wherever possible.

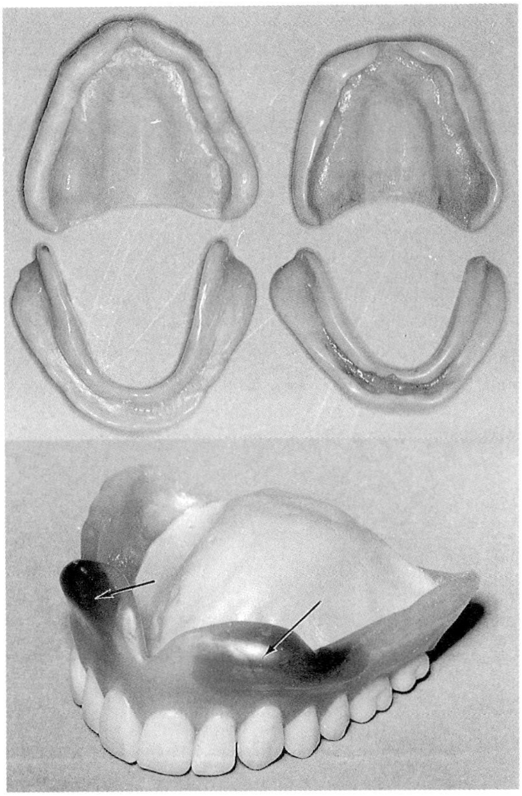

(*a*)

(*b*)

Figure 2.47 (*a*) Old and new dentures for the same patient showing, on the left, the correct design of peripheral width restoring the labial musculature. (*b*) The wrong approach. A 'plumped' denture with wax added (arrowed) produces a very unnatural lip form

Mandibular movements of mastication

The natural teeth are embedded in bone to which they are attached by means of the fibrous periodontal membrane, whose resilience may here be disregarded. The bones comprising the upper jaw move only with the skull and so may be regarded as a fixed base while the lower jaw, which is attached to the skull by the two very mobile temporomandibular joints, is capable of many complicated movements. It is these movements together with those of the surrounding muscles which are of such importance to the prosthodontist.

The temporomandibular joint is unique because some muscle fibres are attached to the interarticular disc which is thus moved during function in its relation to the bones which lie on either side of it (see Figure 2.45). The fact that the disc itself moves has a pronounced and peculiar effect on the movements of the mandible which is unable, except within very strict limits, to move with a pure hinge rotation; it is bound to move forwards when moving downwards.

The normal relationship of the anterior teeth in most Caucasians is with the uppers slightly anterior to the lowers and overlapping them by 1–4 mm, a fact which must be borne in mind when considering normal mandibular movement. The projection in the horizontal plane is termed the overjet and that in the vertical plane the overlap (Figure 2.48).

Now consider what happens when a piece of food is bitten off, chewed and swallowed (Figure 2.49).

First movement: the opening movement

The first movement of the mandible, which is confined to the inferior articular cavity of the joint,

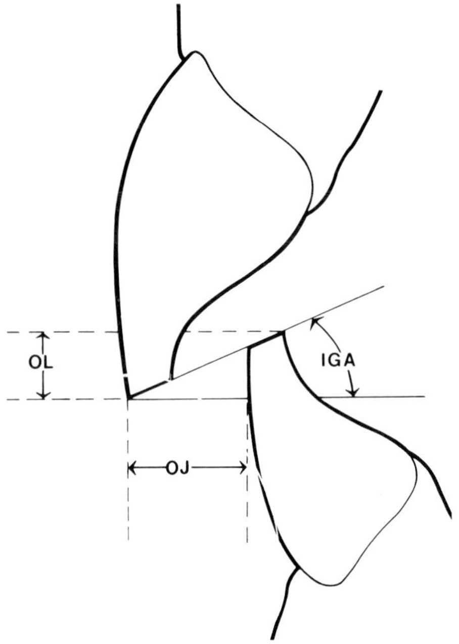

Figure 2.48 The relationship of the incisors in the sagittal plane: OL, vertical overlap; OJ, horizontal overjet; IGA, incisal guidance angle

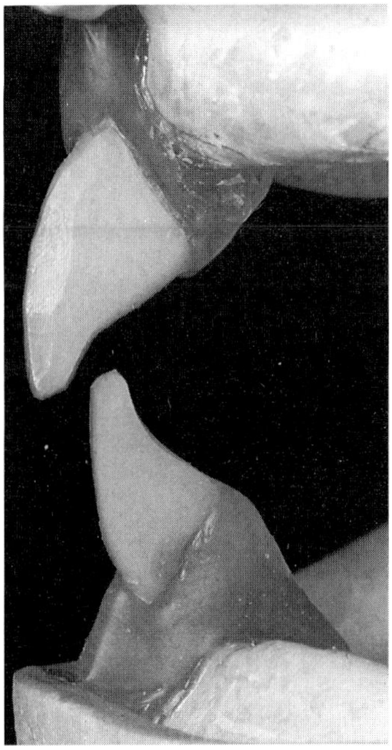

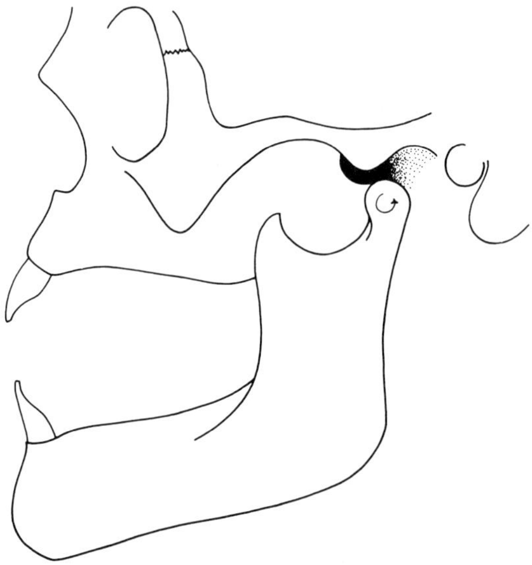

Figure 2.49 Opening and incising movements of the mandible. Opening movement: condyles rotate and move forwards to bring incisors into vertical relationship

is a pure rotation of each condylar head against a stationary disc. It is mainly produced by gravity and the contraction of the anterior belly of the digastric muscle, but the jaw is prevented from dropping too suddenly by the gradual relaxation of the temporalis and masseter muscles. From this point the mandible commences to move forwards by the contraction of the lateral and medial pterygoid muscles, the condylar heads and discs moving downwards and forwards along the anterior surface of each glenoid fossa, this movement occurring in the superior articular cavity. The condyle heads are still able to rotate in relation to the discs, thus controlling the vertical relationship of the teeth though not the anteroposterior.

Second movement: the closing movement

When the upper and lower anterior teeth have parted sufficiently, the food to be bitten off is placed between these teeth and the reverse movement back to intercuspal position takes place, beginning with some degree of approximation of the incisal edges depending on the resistance offered by the food (Figure 2.50). This is brought about by the contraction of the masseter and medial pterygoid muscles and results in a crushing rather than a cutting action.

Third movement: the shearing movement

The final return of the teeth to intercuspal position is the result of further contraction of these muscles and by the posterior fibres of the temporalis accompanied by gradual relaxation of the pterygoid muscles. This muscular synergy returns the condyle

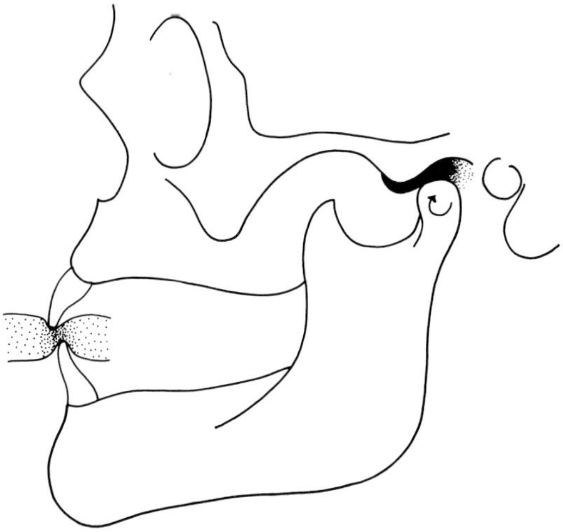

Figure 2.50 Food is interposed between front teeth and the condyles rotate upwards and backwards

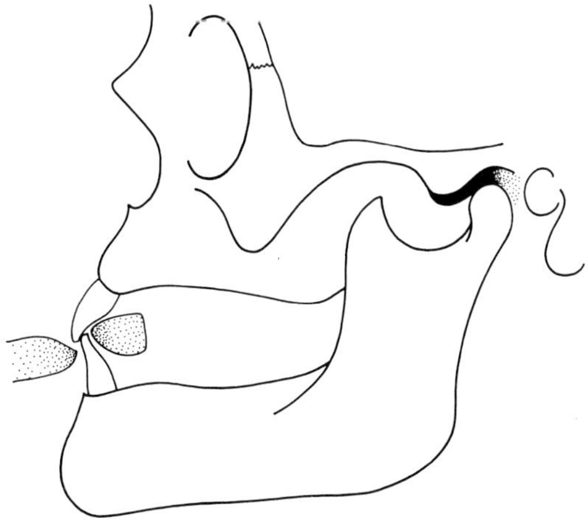

Figure 2.51 Teeth meet and lower incisors slide with shearing action up palatal inclines of upper incisors until heads of condyles are physiologically retruded in glenoid fossae

heads and discs to the rest position in the glenoid fossae at the same time producing a shearing action between the incisal edges of the teeth (Figure 2.51).

These movements have been described as though of equal degree on both sides but, of course, this is not so and invariably one side moves more than the other thus producing a lateral movement which increases the shearing action of the cutting edges of the teeth. It must also be remembered that there is great individual variation in mandibular movement and only the general movements are described here.

Fourth movement: the lateral movement and chewing

The morsel of food in the mouth must be broken up and insalivated before being swallowed and the posterior teeth are used for this purpose. The food is placed between the occlusal surfaces by the tongue and is held there by the lateral pressure of the tongue on the one side and the cheek on the other.

The first few movements are usually those of simple opening and closing which reduce the food to small pieces before the actual chewing begins. Chewing movements approximately conform to the following pattern which is, of course, smoothly continuous although described in stages. There is also much greater individual variation in these lateral movements than in the incisive ones just described, owing to the prevalence of malposition of the teeth, abnormal occlusal relationships and cuspal interference found in human dentitions.

Chewing food begins with an opening movement and the placing of the food on the occlusal surfaces of the posterior teeth on one side, called the working side. There is then a lateral rotation of the

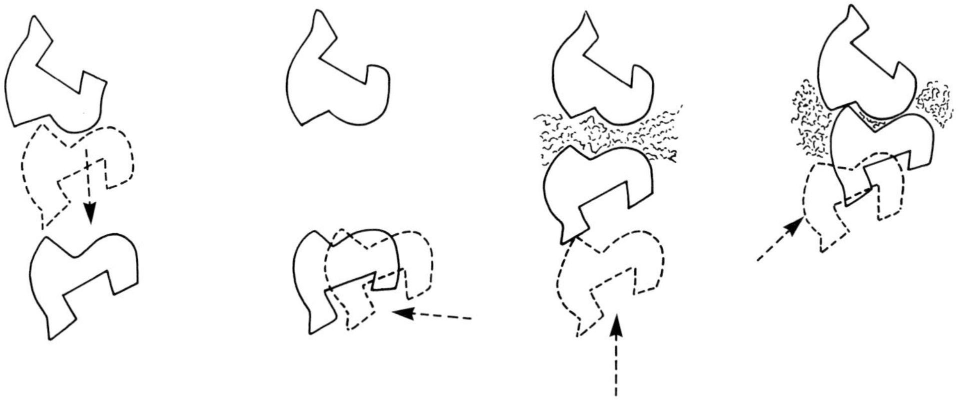

Figure 2.52 The chewing cycle (see text)

mandible towards the working side which is brought about by the orbiting condylar head and disc of the opposite side being pulled downwards, forwards and medially towards the articular eminence by the lateral pterygoid muscle. At the same time the condylar head on the working side rotates about a vertical axis and moves slightly backwards and laterally by contraction of the masseter and temporalis, thus causing a slight but definite lateral shift of the whole mandible. This movement is called the Bennett movement. The amount of Bennett movement (lateral side shift) is less if the medial wall of the glenoid fossa is close to the orbiting condyle or if the temporomandibular ligament on the rotating condyle is tight.

The mandible now moves upwards in this lateral position until considerable resistance is encountered or until the opposing cusps, having penetrated the food, come into contact with each other. The final movement is the upward and medial return towards intercuspal position and it is during this last small movement that the cutting and tearing of tough fibres and the crushing and grinding of hard particles takes place between the approximating cusps (Figure 2.52).

Chapter 3

Taking a history and examining the mouth

Success in complete denture prosthetics depends on four factors:

1. The patient's attitude to dentures and his or her ability and willingness to learn to use them.
2. The condition of the mouth.
3. The skill of the clinician who must acquire all the information he can in order to anticipate difficulties which may arise and to select the technique best suited to overcome them. He must be in a position to warn a patient of expected difficulties, not only to gain cooperation and later perseverance, but also to save himself from possible recrimination when dentures, constructed for abnormal conditions, do not appear to the patient to be as comfortable or efficient as those of his relations or friends. Finally, though of the greatest importance, he should be able to recognize medical problems, oral and general pathology and the oral symptoms of general systemic diseases since he will often see the patient before a medical practitioner has been consulted.
4. The technical assistance available, as without skilled dental technicians and good laboratory service, success in clinical treatment is extremely difficult.

History taking and examination of the mouth will be described separately but this is only for convenience as it must be realized that in practice they are inseparable. For the same reason the patient's mental attitude will be discussed when describing history taking. The usual method in medicine and dentistry of describing the information obtained about a patient is to say that it is made up of signs and symptoms, a sign being a fact which the investigator finds for himself while a symptom is something which is told him by the patient.

Taking a history

This will be described under separate headings merely for convenience but frequently runs concurrently with the examination of the mouth. It should be directed towards discovering those aspects of the case which cannot be observed, augmenting, where necessary, those which can.

Patient's attitude to dentures

Although it is true that nearly all edentulous people who consult a dental surgeon want to have dentures, it must not be assumed that they are all equally willing to play their part in making such dentures successful. An attitude of mind will have been formed by the patient's own past experience of dentures, if any, or from his observation of friends or relatives who wear dentures. If, prior to being rendered edentulous, a partial denture has been worn with comfort and efficiency, the same will be expected of complete dentures. It should be explained to such patients that, although partial denture experience is helpful in relation to complete dentures, the latter require a considerably greater degree of control because they are not, as were the partial dentures, retained or supported by the natural teeth. If this difference in the two types of denture is not explained, the initial difficulty experienced in learning to use the complete dentures compared with the partial dentures may cause the patient much disappointment, and he may condemn the dentures as being faulty, not knowing that some perseverance is necessary.

If complete dentures are already being worn and they have been comfortable and efficient, the same will be expected of the new dentures. If the old complete dentures were troublesome, the attitude may be either expectance of better results with the new dentures or pessimism that nothing better can be hoped for. If no previous denture experience exists, friends or relatives may have coloured the patient's mind with their own attitudes.

In such cases the efficient control and use of complete dentures depends to a very large extent on the formation of new habits, and a new pattern of muscular movement. This demands time and some patience on the part of the wearer. Many complete denture troubles and problems can be traced to the fact that no preparation of the patient's mind preceded the fitting of the dentures. If a leg is amputated the patient anticipates a long learning period before he can walk confidently with its artificial substitute, and he never expects to be able to walk as well with it as he did with his natural leg. In addition he is taught to use the artificial limb and this learning period may extend over several months. It is necessary, therefore, that the correct attitude to complete dentures be instilled into the patient's mind. This cannot be done in a few minutes as the patient is being shown out of the surgery at the final visit; it should be a gradual process spread over all the visits necessary to construct the dentures, and should be related to the attitude already existing in the patient's mind.

The patient should be told what to expect when he commences to wear the dentures; how long the period of learning is likely to be; how considerable perseverance will be required before any degree of skill is attained in their use. This prognosis will bear a very definite relationship to what is discovered during the history taking and mouth examination.

Existence of old dentures

Most patients volunteer information about the existence of old dentures even if it is not already obvious, but every edentulous patient who does not mention old dentures of his own accord should be questioned concerning them. Questions are directed to elicit information regarding the length of time dentures have been worn; how many sets have been made since the teeth were extracted; the success of the existing or old dentures and the attitude of the patient to their appearance.

All this information is important because if the existing dentures have been satisfactory and only the passage of time has made them ill-fitting, any gross alteration of the new dentures may mean their failure. A person who has worn comfortable and efficient dentures has developed a complete control of them which is entirely reflex and is dependent on a subtle appreciation by the tongue, cheeks and lips of the shape and position of the polished surfaces of the dentures, the height of the occlusal plane and exactly when the teeth will make contact. If any of these is altered grossly or suddenly, the established reflexes are upset and conscious control of the dentures must again be exercised. With an experienced denture wearer such control is a thing of the past, and if it can be dispensed with by copying certain aspects of the old dentures success with the new denture is assured. If, on the other hand, certain alterations in the new dentures are essential, e.g. altering the occlusal plane for reasons of appearance or restoring the vertical height to correct an over-closure, then this must be explained to the patient and he must be told that conscious control of the new dentures will be required until new reflex habits are formed.

Information regarding the loss of the natural teeth

If the teeth were not extracted by the dental surgeon who is constructing the dentures, information regarding their extraction should always be sought. A history of difficult extractions should be followed by a radiographic examination of the jaws to verify the absence of retained roots or other pathology.

Questioning should be directed to eliciting the general order in which the teeth were lost. For example, if all the posterior teeth were extracted some years before the anterior ones and no partial dentures were worn in the meantime, then a habit of eating with the anterior teeth will have been formed which, if persisted in, will have a pronounced unstabilizing effect on complete dentures.

A similar condition will exist in patients who have been edentulous for a considerable length of time and have not worn dentures because they are only able to approximate their jaws in the anterior region and consequently forward travel of the mandible is necessary all the time during eating.

When there is a history of abnormal mandibular function or movement, then difficulty can be anticipated when registering the anteroposterior occlusal relationship.

The patient's age

In general, though there are many exceptions, increasing age decreases the readiness to form new habits. The muscular efficiency is often impaired. Thus the elderly patient will require a longer learning period than the younger person when dentures are fitted for the first time. Impaired muscular efficiency of old age may demand special clinical techniques.

The patient's occupation

This will frequently have a bearing on the design of the dentures and the technique used when making impressions, for example:

1. With most professional men and women, and many others whose occupation entails intimate contact with their fellows, appearance and retention are often more important than efficiency;
2. Public speakers and singers require not only perfect retention but also particular attention to palatal shape and thickness because of the importance of these in phonation;
3. Wind instrument players often require a special modification of the shape and position of the anterior teeth.

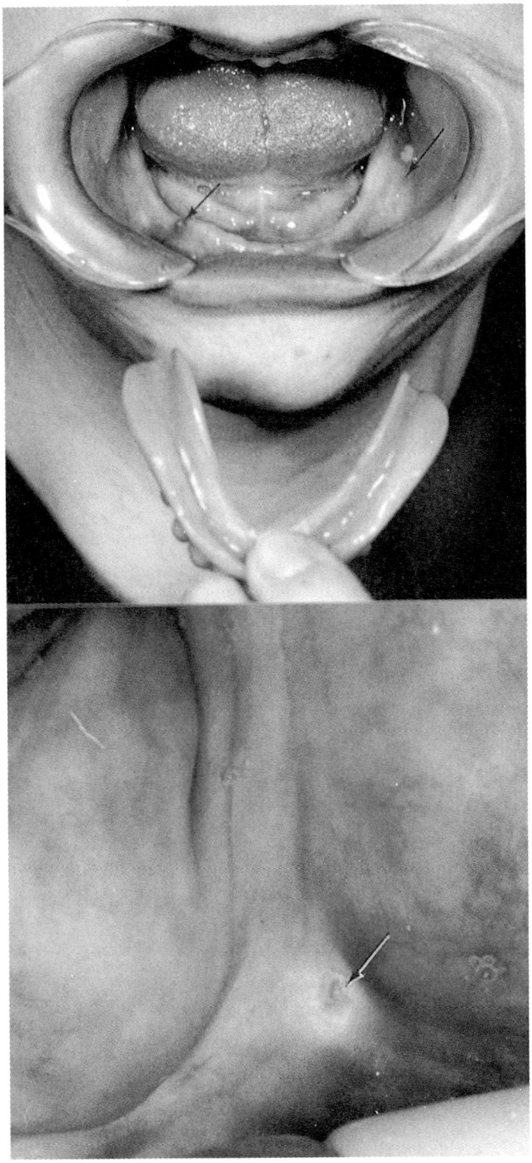

Figure 3.1 Traumatic ulcers (arrowed) caused by faults in the flanges of dentures, together with oclusal errors

The patient's attitude to appearance

This is often a matter of supreme importance to a patient and where this is the case the operator must be prepared to devote extra time and care to this part of denture construction, often to the extent of making individual teeth.

The oral examination will be described under three headings: visual examination, digital examination, X-ray examination.

Visual examination

Colour of the mucosa

Any variation from the normal must be investigated, and though whitish patches or spots of hyperkeratosis are not uncommon, the most usual variation found is an increased redness due to the inflammation caused by mechanical, chemical or bacteriological irritation.

Common prosthetic causes of irritation

Over-extension of the periphery of the denture

This is frequently seen as a bright red area which may break down to an ulceration if the irritation is continued (Figure 3.1). It may be due to over-extension of the periphery of new dentures or to the altered position of existing dentures due to alveolar resorption, the latter being usually confined to the lower denture as there is no appreciable resorption of the hard palate. When seen in the upper denture it is caused by tilting. In some cases this irritation, if continued over a long period of time, will cause a proliferation of the mucosa which is visible as a ridge, flap or series of flaps (Figures 3.2 and 3.3).

Dirty, ill-fitting dentures

The movement of an ill-fitting denture may itself cause inflammation, this being much more likely to occur if the denture is also dirty and consequently harbouring fermenting foodstuffs and bacteria, or deposits of salivary calculus and plaque. The

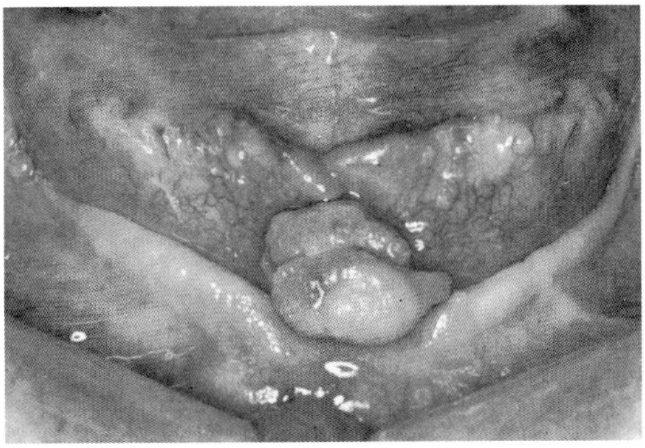

Figure 3.2 Denture-induced hyperplasia caused by over-extension of lingual flange of lower denture (male age 82)

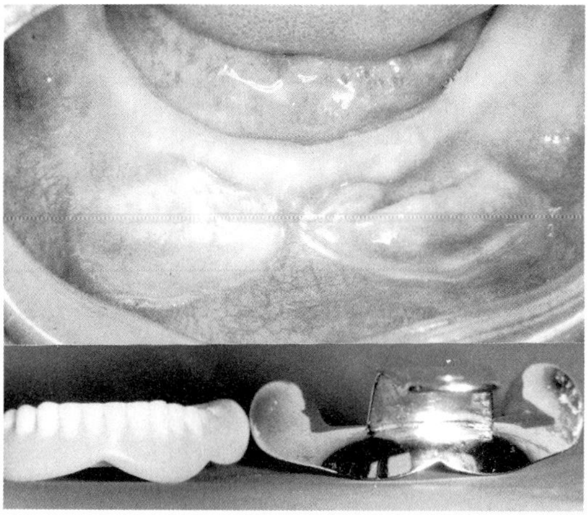

Figure 3.3 Labial peripheral damage caused by lower denture. It should be noted that the peripheral contour of the denture is similar to that of the stock tray. In other words, faults in the impression have been responsible for the eventual oral damage

inflammation usually appears as an ill-defined red area which varies with the extent of mucosa most constantly in contact with the denture.

Continuous wearing of a denture

A denture which is worn continuously day and night may cause a chronic inflammation of the underlying mucosa. This is particularly likely if the denture is not kept clean. In the case of an upper denture a granular or papillary type of hyperplasia of the palatal mucosa may develop and this is of diagnostic value in spotting the continuous denture wearer. A similar condition of palatal inflammation sometimes develops in individuals whose dentures move excessively although they do not wear them at night.

Faulty occlusion of the denture

Inflammation may be found on the crest of the alveolar ridge if the occlusion is too heavy in one particular spot (fault in retruded contact position) or on the sides of the ridge if there is a lateral drag caused by cuspal interference (fault in eccentric occlusal balance). This condition is often seen in an edentulous upper denture-bearing area in the incisor region when the natural lower anterior teeth are still present and faulty habits of mastication on the anterior teeth have been acquired with resultant tipping of the upper denture and consequent trauma.

Rubber suction discs

These are removable rubber discs attached by means of a metal stud to the palatal surface of an upper denture. The development of an area of

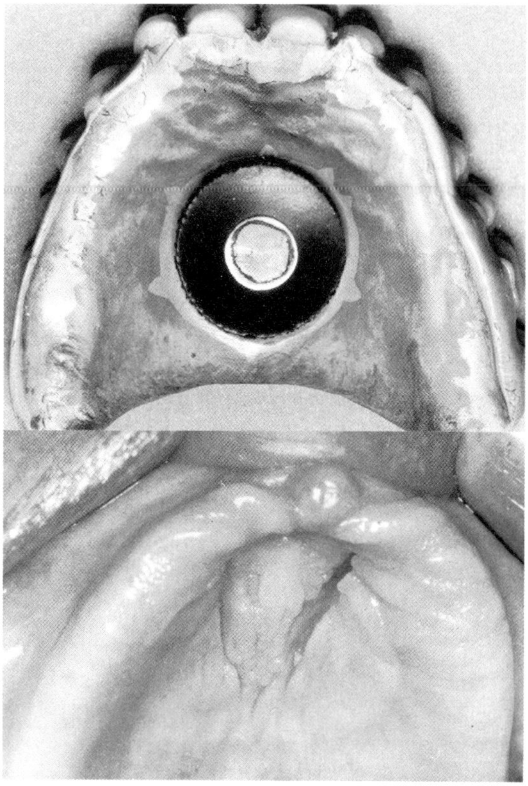

Figure 3.4 Rubber suction disc and palatal damage caused by prolonged use of a denture with a suction disc (different patients)

decreased pressure within the disc aids the retention of a denture but is seldom seen nowadays (Figure 3.4).

They can cause chronic inflammation of the mucosa with resultant hyperplasia. This is due to the softness of the rubber and the fact that it perishes rapidly, and so the area of contact with the tissues is constantly altering. Their use cannot be condemned too strongly.

Traumatic injury

The edentulous mouth frequently sustains trifling injuries to the mucosa from sharp pieces of food such as crusts or small bones which lie underneath the dentures. Occasionally these injuries become infected.

Small spicules of alveolar bone

Sharp edges of tooth sockets not yet rounded by resorption, or which should have been removed at the time of extraction, frequently cause irritation of the mucosa overlying them (Figure 3.5). Small pieces of bone fractured during the extraction of teeth and in the process of being exfoliated may cause inflammation.

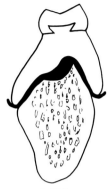

Figure 3.5 Mucosa pressed against sharp edge of tooth socket by the denture

Denture stomatitis

This is usually an expression of oral candidiasis and is often symptomless. It is sometimes termed 'denture sore mouth' because it looks painful or sore, but seldom is, and so this term is not appropriate. It usually affects the upper denture-bearing area which appears oedematous and inflamed. *Candida albicans,* a yeast-like fungus, is implicated in the aetiology.

Other causes of colour variation

These are most frequently a sign of some general systemic disease or disturbance for which reference should be made to the patient's physician, and the only safe rule to follow is never to proceed with prosthodontic treatment until the cause of the colour variation has been diagnosed.

Size and shape of the arches and alveolar ridges

The part played by these in the retention and stabilizing of the dentures has already been described in Chapter 2, and during the visual examination the clinican should decide whether they are sufficiently abnormal either to require some special technique of denture construction or surgical intervention.

The relationship of the upper and lower edentulous ridges should be noted and this can easily be done by asking the patient to close his jaws on to the operator's first and second fingers. If the lips are then parted at the side the jaw relationship can be seen at the approximate vertical separation which will exist when dentures are fitted. Abnormal jaw relationship in different cases may be maxillary or mandibular protrusion, maxillary or mandibular retrusion, or varying combinations of these (Figure 3.6).

It is important to gain some knowledge of the jaw relationship at an early stage so that possible difficulties may be foreseen, the rims of the record blocks constructed in their correct positions and the setting and occlusion of the teeth related to the individual case. These matters are discussed in Chapter 6.

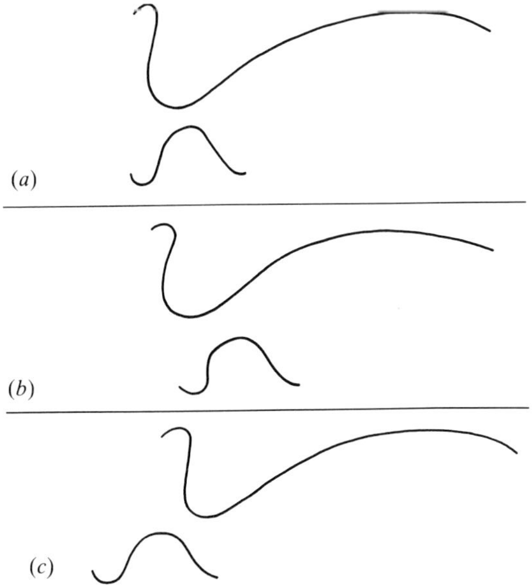

Figure 3.6 Line diagram showing jaw relationships in sagittal section: (*a*) normal; (*b*) inferior retrusion; (*c*) inferior protrusion

Shape of the hard palate

When considered in conjunction with the alveolar ridges, the clinician is able to judge with considerable accuracy any unusual difficulties the patient is likely to experience in the retention or stability of his dentures and should inform him of these at this early stage (see Chapter 2 for details).

Depth of the sulci

Whenever a very shallow and broad sulcus is encountered a careful impression technique will be required in order to obtain an adequate peripheral seal and so utilize physical forces to the full as an aid to retention (see Chapter 2 for details).

Interference factors

The size of the tongue, tightness of the lips and any abnormal muscular or frenal attachments must be noted as they may influence the design of the future dentures and the type and position of the artificial teeth used (see Chapter 2 for details).

Unextracted roots

These may be seen flush with, or protruding above, the surrounding mucosa (Figure 3.7) with or without

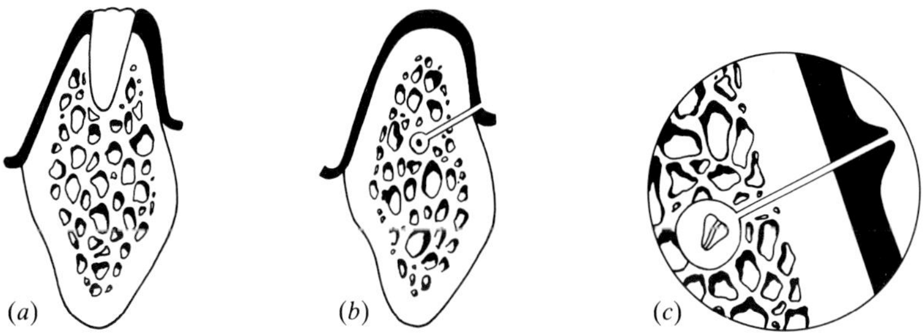

Figure 3.7 (*a*) Root visible on surface. (*b*) Buried root with sinus communicating with buccal sulcus. (*c*) Enlarged view of sinus

an obvious area of inflammation round them. They may be loose or firm, and it is always wise to take a radiograph to confirm the extent of the remnant. Rarely should a denture be made covering an unextracted root, but in the exceptional cases where it must occur, e.g. where, for medical reasons, further surgery is contraindicated, the denture should be relieved over it to avoid irritation of the area.

Sinuses

An infected area in the bone, such as surrounds the retained apex of a tooth, usually communicates with the surface through a channel known as a sinus (Figure 3.7).

The appearance in the mouth is usually that of a very small nipple-shaped elevation with a hole in its centre, most commonly found on the buccal side of the ridge. Dry the area with an air syringe. Pressure with the finger, above in the maxilla and below in the mandible, directed towards the opening will cause the extrusion of a droplet of pus or serum in most cases; this is usually diagnostic and should be followed by a radiograph to locate the position and extent of the infected area (do not use a swab on the area before applying finger pressure as the pus will be absorbed by the swab without being seen).

Unilateral swellings

Any abnormal swellings in the mouth must be investigated and diagnosed, and when found only on one side they are much more likely to be pathological than when they are bilateral.

Digital examination

Before starting to explore the mouth with the finger tips the patient should be asked to indicate immediately if any pain is felt and the cause of such pain must be found. Any area which is painful to the pressure of a soft finger is unlikely to tolerate the pressure of a hard denture (Figure 3.8).

Firmness of the ridges

This is most conveniently tested by placing a finger on each side of the ridge and applying alternate lateral pressure. Ridges vary in firmness. The normal is composed of bone covered with a thin layer of pale-pink mucosa. Others may appear the same but the bone is resorbed and the mucosa is thickened and contains much fibrous tissue which is displaced by lateral pressure.

Flabby, displaceable ridges may be encountered in any part of the upper or lower jaws, but probably the most common position is in the upper anterior region. The history in these cases is almost invariably one of loss of all the natural teeth except

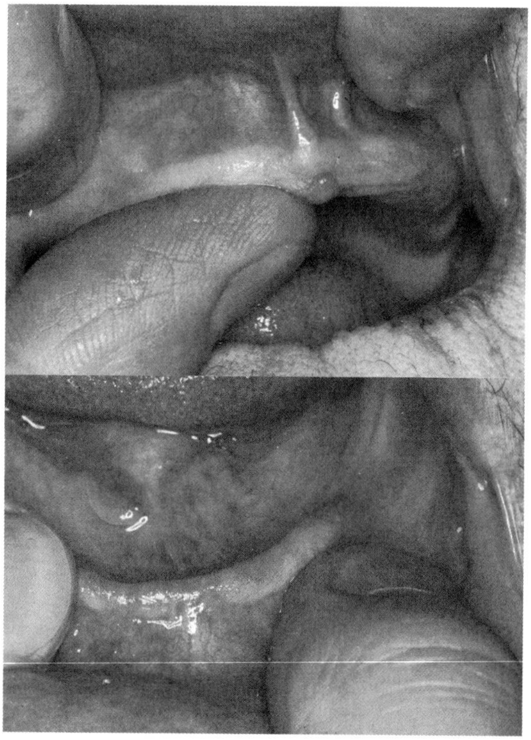

Figure 3.8 Finger palpation of the ridges is an essential part of the clinical examination

the lower anteriors. Later, owing to the failure to wear a partial lower denture or to the wearing of an inefficient denture, the patient acquires the habit of eating entirely on the anterior teeth with resultant excessive loads on the upper complete denture which leads to rapid resorption of the anterior alveolar ridge and the forward massage of the palatal rugae and mucosa (Figure 2.4).

Irregularities of the alveolar ridge

The general size and shape of the ridges will be noted during the visual examination, but palpation will be necessary to determine irregularities of the underlying bone. The information sought is quite apart from that discussed later under the heading of 'hard and soft areas' and is directed at determining the shape and regularity of the underlying hard tissues. Alveolar resorption is never uniform and hard nodules, sharp edges, spikes and irregularities are frequently felt with pain on pressure over these areas a common feature (Figures 3.9 and 3.10).

Radiographs are usually essential before the clinician decides whether surgical correction is needed, or whether the irregularities will reduce in time in the course of normal resorption, or whether relief of the denture alone will be satisfactory.

Variations of mucosa

The ideal mucosa to support complete dentures should be:

1. Firmly bound down to the underlying bone by union with the periosteum which will thus prevent the denture and mucosa moving together in relation to the bone.
2. Slightly compressible thus allowing the denture to settle comfortably into place because the mucosa will adjust itself slightly to the fitting surface of the denture. This will increase the retention by adhesion and cohesion because the film of saliva between the denture and the mucosa will be very thin. It will also allow maximum retention from atmospheric pressure because the denture, bedding slightly into the tissue, will prevent air leaks. In addition, such mucosa will act as a cushion to the normal stresses of clenching and mastication and prevent the development of sore spots and painful areas from pressure between the underlying bone and the denture base.
3. An even thickness, a condition never realized because in a normal mouth the mucosa on the

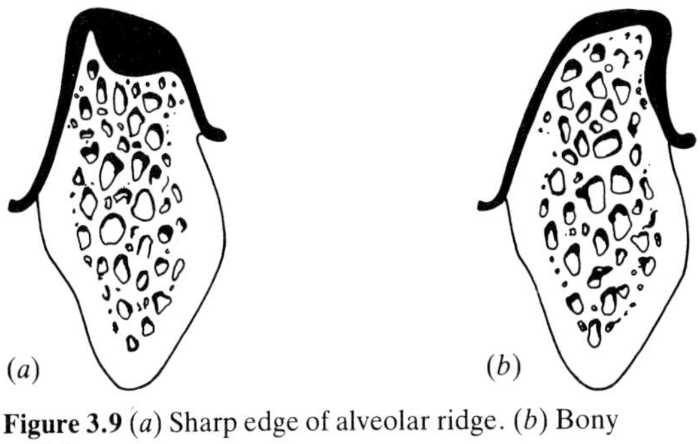

(*a*) (*b*)

Figure 3.9 (*a*) Sharp edge of alveolar ridge. (*b*) Bony nodule.

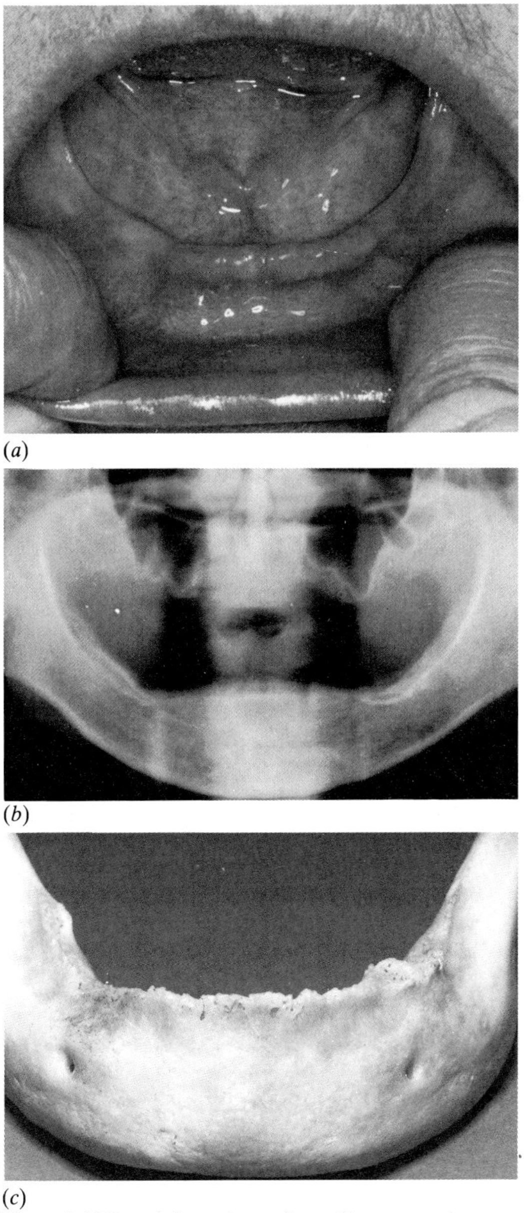

Figure 3.10 Rough irregular surface of lower anterior alveolar ridge. (*a*) Clinical view. Finger palpation of ridge caused pain. (*b*) Radiograph showing bony irregularity. (*c*) Dried mandible with rough alveolar ridge

crest of the ridges covers scar tissue resulting from the extraction of the teeth and this varies in amount. In the midline of the palate the mucosa is thinner than elsewhere. The sides of the vault of the palate are traversed by the anterior palatine, nasopalatine and greater palatine vessels and nerves and these are protected by a layer of submucosa and fat (see Figure 2.2). The tissue of the retromolar pad is often much thicker and more compressible than any other lower ridge tissue although the anterior part of the pad, arising as it does from the extraction site of the mandibular third molar, is usually firm and unyielding (the distal end of the lower denture-bearing area is often known as the pear-shaped pad or area).

Where the differences in compressibility of the mucosa are not great, or of large extent, they will be found to be clinically unimportant, but where the reverse conditions are present there may be a need for special impression techniques or alterations in normal denture construction.

Thin mucosa covering a well-defined torus palati and flanked by thick, compressible mucosa may result in a denture which rocks during function. This is likely to irritate the thin mucosa or cause discomfort and possibly lead to fracture of the denture due to the repeated flexure the base is required to undergo during mastication (Figure 3.11).

Maxillary tuberosities

These may be found on visual examination to be bulbous and to have a definite undercut area above them, but only by palpation can it be determined whether the bulbous portion is composed of hard or soft tissue and whether the denture can be inserted into the undercut area or not (Figure 3.12). If the tuberosity is much undercut and covered with only a thin layer of mucosa, then surgical removal of part of it may be necessary. Surgery may also be required if the tuberosity is fibrous and sufficiently large that it invades the denture space.

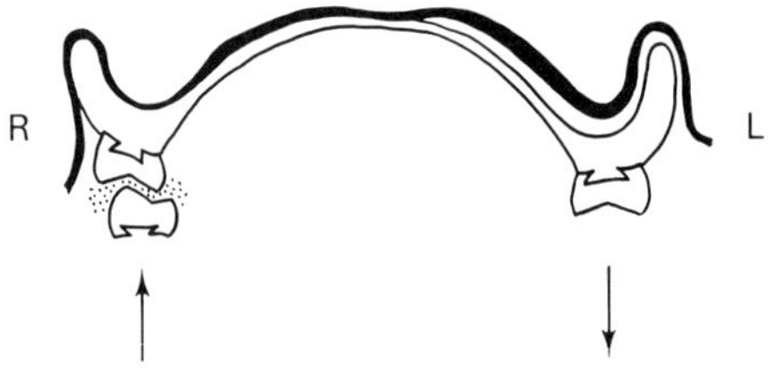

Figure 3.11 The biting force on the right side compresses the mucosa covering the alveolar ridge and causes the denture to rock on the midline torus and drop from its seating on the left side

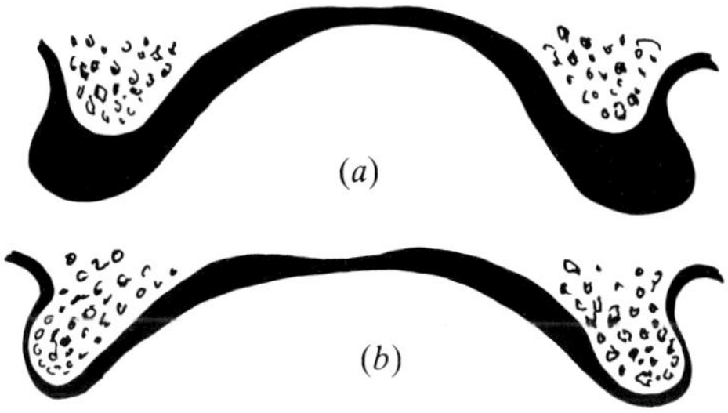

Figure 3.12 (*a*) A buccal undercut formed by soft tissue. (*b*) A buccal undercut formed by bone

Mylohyoid ridges

It is only in the neighbourhood of the second or third molars that the mylohyoid ridges have any prosthetic significance, but in this region it is sometimes possible to carry the denture into the undercut area below and behind the ridge. In the majority of cases these ridges are felt to be pronounced and sharp which is a contraindication for extending the denture over them, unless the denture is relieved, but where they feel ill-defined and rounded a lingual extension is usually successful (Figure 3.13). If the mylohyoid ridges are sharp and painful on finger palpation, and particularly if it is felt important to extend the denture below the ridge, then surgical reduction and smoothing the bone is a most useful and relatively simple operation.

Lingual pouch

This is the area bounded medially by the tongue, laterally by the mandible, posteriorly by the palatoglossus muscle and anteriorly by the posterior 3 mm of the mylohyoid muscle. The extent of the pouch with the tongue at rest, with the tongue protruded sufficiently to lick the lips, and during the act of swallowing, should be noted. This is most

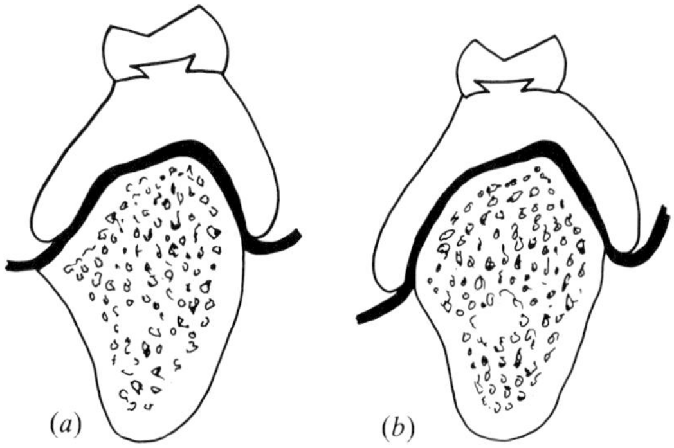

Figure 3.13 (*a*) Sharp mylohyoid ridge with lingual flange of denture finished above the ridge. (*b*) Rounded mylohyoid ridge which may allow the lingual flange of the denture to be carried beneath the ridge

conveniently done by gently inserting the index finger into the pouch and asking the patient to perform the above actions when the alterations in the extent of the pouch can be felt. If a pouch persists during tongue movement and swallowing then the lingual flange of the denture can probably be carried into this area which will assist in the stability of the lower denture. It is worth noting, however, that the mucosa covering the medial aspect of the mandible in this region is often tender to pressure and care must be taken when extending the flange into the pouch.

Painful areas

This is not a separate examination in itself and pain on pressure may be encountered during any of the digital examinations already mentioned. The whole of the denture-bearing mucosa should be palpated and any painful areas must be diagnosed and treated before successful dentures can be constructed.

Radiographic examination

Ideally full mouth intra-oral radiographs should be made of every edentulous patient prior to starting denture construction, otherwise a certain number of pathological or abnormal conditions will pass unrecognized, as for example buried roots and unerupted teeth. When it is considered that this routine is uneconomic or too time-consuming, radiographs should still be taken to confirm or assist in diagnosis in the following findings:

1. Buried roots
2. Sinuses
3. Unilateral swellings
4. Rough alveolar ridges
5. Areas painful to pressure

The information given in this chapter is listed in Table 3.1 for easy reference.

Table 3.1 Summary of information required when taking a history and examining the mouth of an edentulous patient

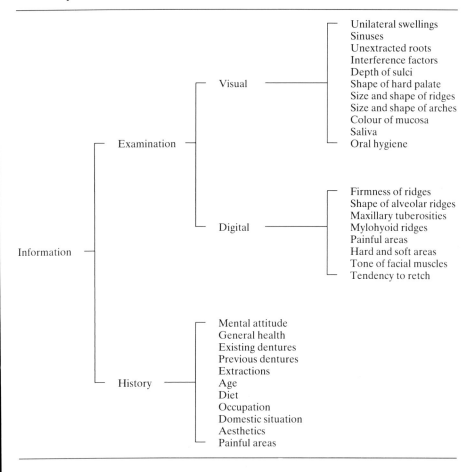

- Information
  - Examination
    - Visual
      - Unilateral swellings
      - Sinuses
      - Unextracted roots
      - Interference factors
      - Depth of sulci
      - Shape of hard palate
      - Size and shape of ridges
      - Size and shape of arches
      - Colour of mucosa
      - Saliva
      - Oral hygiene
    - Digital
      - Firmness of ridges
      - Shape of alveolar ridges
      - Maxillary tuberosities
      - Mylohyoid ridges
      - Painful areas
      - Hard and soft areas
      - Tone of facial muscles
      - Tendency to retch
  - History
    - Mental attitude
    - General health
    - Existing dentures
    - Previous dentures
    - Extractions
    - Age
    - Diet
    - Occupation
    - Domestic situation
    - Aesthetics
    - Painful areas

Chapter 4

Surgical preparation of the mouth

The object of surgical preparation

The object of surgical preparation of an edentulous mouth is to render the denture-bearing area as satisfactory as possible from the aspect of health, comfort and shape. Only rarely is this beyond the scope of the average dental surgeon.

In a large number of cases small alterations could be made to a mouth which might benefit the patient slightly or make things a little easier for the prosthetist, but it must never be forgotten that even the most minor surgery involves cutting living tissue and is rightly feared by nearly everyone, and so should never be lightly undertaken. A very safe rule is never to advise surgical interference unless convinced that the benefits resulting from it will outweigh the risks and discomforts.

Conditions requiring surgery

The following findings, all of which are frequently met, are well within the scope of a dental surgeon:

Hard tissues
1. Buried roots
2. Unerupted teeth
3. Dental cysts
4. Ridge irregularities:
   (a) Feather-edged ridge
   (b) Knife-edged ridge
   (c) Unresorbed areas and bone nodules
   (d) Torus, maxillary or mandibular
   (e) Undercut areas
   (f) Mylohyoid ridge
   (g) Prominent tuberosities

Soft tissues
1. Prominent frena
2. Denture-induced hyperplasia
3. Flabby, fibrous ridge

The first three conditions in the above list, being of general dental application rather than purely prosthetic, will not be mentioned further except to stress that they should almost invariably be dealt with before denture construction is begun.

General surgical principles

Before outlining the techniques of individual operations a few general principles are given.

1. Asepsis must be observed. Since it is quite impossible to sterilize the oral cavity it is perhaps not immediately apparent why sterility on the part of the operator is so essential. Every healthy animal has acquired a high degree of immunity to the bacteria normally present in its mouth. If a dog injures itself it licks the wound and although its saliva is teeming with bacteria the wound rarely becomes septic, but if the same dog were to bite a man and he did nothing about cleansing the injury it would almost certainly turn septic. So, although a sterile field for operations in the mouth is impossible, every care must be taken to prevent the introduction of foreign organisms.
2. Incisions through the mucoperiosteum must be made with firmness and precision otherwise reflection without tearing is impossible.
3. Incisions should err on the side of being too long rather than too short; one extra suture is of no consequence to the patient, while a little extra vision or space is frequently of great assistance to the operator. In addition, a flap which is well

reflected is in less danger of being traumatized during the operation.
4. When operating under local anaesthesia it should be remembered that bone cutting with a hammer and chisel causes much more jarring and discomfort to the patient than cutting with burs. Burs, on the other hand, tend to create more bony debris and good irrigation is essential.
5. Decide beforehand, as far as possible, what is to be done and be sufficiently radical; results will not be obtained by reflecting the mucoperiosteum and then just scratching the bone.
6. If there is any doubt whether a flap will stay in place, suture it. A suture is painlessly inserted under anaesthesia and can be painlessly removed a few days later.

Bony conditions requiring surgery

By far the largest numbers of edentulous mouths which require some surgical preparation for the reception of dentures are those in which there is an abnormal condition of the bony ridges and, while the general technique of operating remains the same, the surgeon should differentiate between the various conditions before starting to operate: slight variations in technique will be needed for the different conditions.

Feather-edged ridge

This can usually be detected on palpation as a thin, irregular, sharp edge painful to pressure. It is due to irregular alveolar resorption and frequently found following the extraction of teeth in patients with a history of advanced chronic periodontal disease. The radiographic appearance is of a very irregular alveolar crest with no clearly defined outline, the bone appearing unusually radiolucent (Figure 4.1).

On exposing the bone exactly the same picture is seen: it is found to be cancellous in type with no suggestion of a cortical layer. The alveolar crest presents innumerable spicules and irregularities which cut very easily with a hand-held chisel.

Knife-edged ridge

On palpation the ridge is felt to be thin buccolingually, sharp but smooth and, like the feather edge, painful on pressure. Found only in the mandible it appears to be due to resorption which is greater buccolingually than vertically. Radiographs show a thin ridge with an irregular, palisade-like formation caused by loss of buccal cortical plate with some persistence of interdental septae. The appearance of the exposed bone confirms this (Figure 4.2).

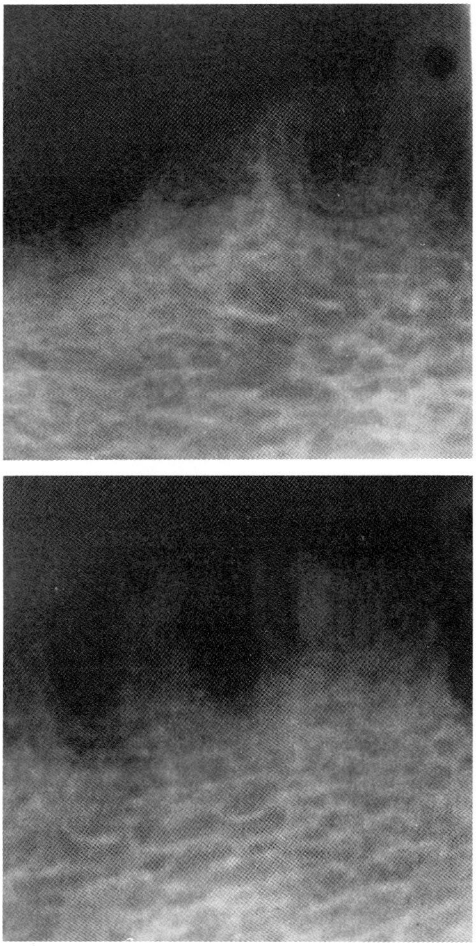

Figure 4.1 Intra-oral radiographs of feather-edged ridge showing surface irregularity. The overlying mucosa is painful on palpation

Unresorbed bony areas

These can usually be felt as smooth, rounded, hard lumps under the mucosa and, although usually symptomless, it is usually best to consider surgical reduction as they often interfere with the design of new dentures or are frequently a source of pain from pressure from new dentures. Radiographically they show as small roundish areas of increased density.

On exposure the nodules are easily seen as raised lumps of smooth, hard, cortical bone.

Alveolectomy

This is the term given to the operation for the removal of alveolar bone (Figure 4.3) and is equally applicable to the removal of a small nodule or the excision of bone from the entire alveolar ridges of

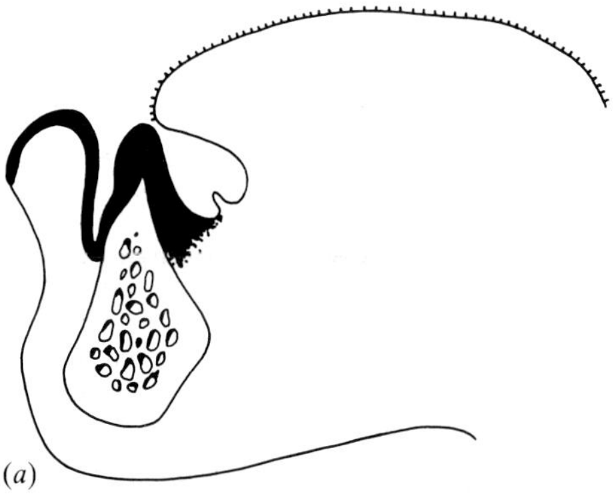

(*a*)

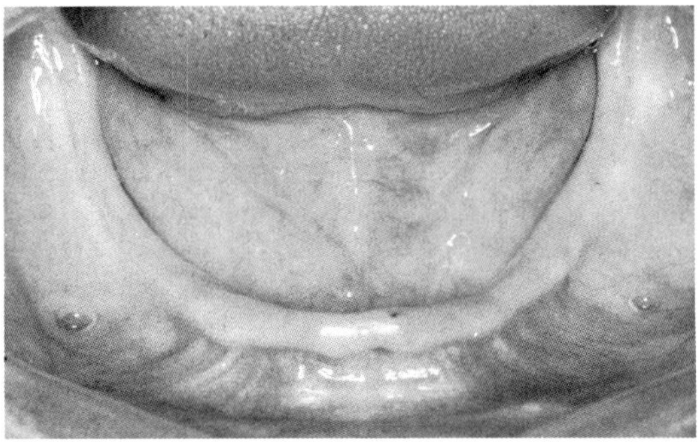

(*b*)

Figure 4.2 (*a*) Sagittal diagram showing knife-edged ridge in lower anterior region. (*b*) Clinical view of typical knife-edged ridge which is very often painful on palpation

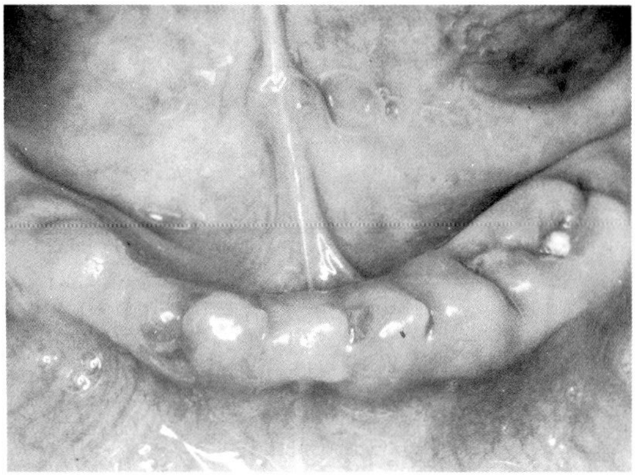

Figure 4.3 Lower incisor region two weeks after extraction of teeth showing careless preparation of alveolar bone for a complete denture. Alveolar surgery was required before prosthetic treatment could be started

both jaws. Local anaesthesia is usually used for the operation as it is more convenient in a dental surgery and is generally preferred by patients.

The incision

An incision is made just below the crest of the alveolus on the buccal side, and care must be taken that all fibres of the mucoperiosteum are severed. This is not always easy if the underlying bone is rough and irregular.

Further incisions at each end of this transverse cut will be needed on the labial or buccal surfaces but carried no deeper into the sulci than is absolutely necessary because the tissues in this area are looser and more vascular than elsewhere and their trauma will result in greater postoperative swelling and haematomata. On the lingual or palatal surfaces further incisions are rarely necessary as the soft tissues here may be reflected towards the inner side of the ridge.

Reflection of tissues

The next step is the reflection of the mucoperiosteum with a periosteal elevator, and is often the only difficult part of an otherwise simple operation. The soft tissues are very adherent to the bone and if thin, great care must be taken not to tear them: this is not easy as often considerable force is required particularly when starting to lever up the flap. This reflection is continued until all the bone to be removed is fully exposed.

Removal of bone

The alveolus is now trimmed to the desired shape and size. Some clinicians prefer to use bone burs for trimming the alveolar ridge but good irrigation and suction are necessary to keep the field clear of blood, saliva and debris. Others prefer chisels held in the hand as these create less debris and, of course, are less noisy for the patient.

When sufficient bone has been removed it is necessary to smooth the surface with bone files. The smoothness or otherwise of the bone can easily be ascertained by running the tip of the gloved finger over the area, having first replaced the mucoperiosteal flap. This last point is very important for these reasons:

1. There is less likelihood of introducing infection.
2. Exposed cancellous bone always feels rough.
3. Clinicians are accustomed to judging the shape and smoothness of bone through an intervening layer of mucosa.

When satisfied with the feel of the bone, the debris caused by filing should be irrigated and the flaps replaced. These flaps will now be found to overlap, and they must be trimmed until their edges just approximate without tension. If too much tissue is removed there will be a gap between the edges which must epithelialize over and healing will be retarded, while if too little is cut away, a thick fibrous band will be left which may well make the later wearing of a denture very difficult.

Suturing

The operation is completed by suturing the flaps in place, sufficient sutures being used to make it impossible for the tongue to catch against or lift a flap. The object of sutures is only to hold the flap in place and must never be pulled tight nor should they be placed too near an edge in case they pull out. If a denture is available it may be inserted, as it will protect the wound from the inquisitiveness of the tongue and so allow healing in the minimum length of time. The denture may be lined with tissue conditioner or black gutta percha, either of which compresses the area of the flap and makes the denture more comfortable.

Postoperative procedure

The patient should be seen 24 h later to make sure that there is no undue swelling or pain. The tissue conditioner or gutta percha may be modified and the patient instructed not to remove the denture except for cleaning. Four to seven days later the sutures may be removed.

No attempt has been made to describe the quantity of bone which should be removed and this omission is deliberate since every case differs and each must be treated according to its individual needs. The general principle is never to operate if the same results can be obtained within a reasonable time by alveolar resorption, but where surgery is necessary the object of an alveolectomy is to shape the bone so that it will form the best possible painless base to support a denture.

Removal of bone nodules

The commonest variation of the above technique occurs when dealing with small nodules of bone. It is often impossible to remove these nodules with rongeurs which tend to slip over the hard, convex surfaces without sufficient grip to cut; when this does occur recourse must be had to a bone bur. The nodules are also very easily removed by hammer and sharp chisel, a suitable method when operating under a general anaesthetic.

Large torus, maxillary or mandibular

There is usually a raised, bony ridge running down the centre of the hard palate from the anterior palatine foramen to the posterior border, or any part of this distance, which is known as a torus palati. Sometimes this ridge is very pronounced and covered with only a thin layer of mucosa (Figure 4.4).

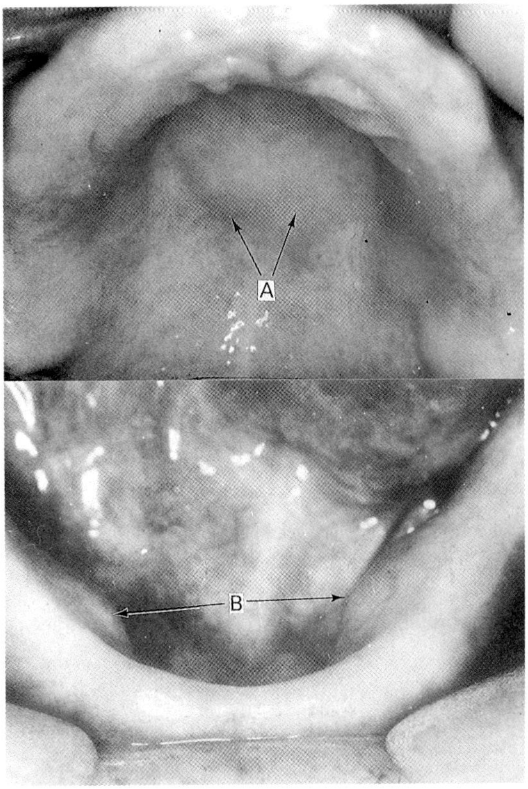

Figure 4.4 Torus palati (*a*) and torus mandibularis (*b*)

There may be two eminences on the lingual aspect of the mandible, one on either side of the midline and usually in the premolar region, each of which is called a torus mandibularis.

These conditions do not inconvenience the patient until he is obliged to wear dentures, when pressure may cause considerable pain.

The best treatment for these cases, unless they are very pronounced, is to leave them alone and to relieve the dentures so that under no conditions can they exert any pressure on the torus.

If it is decided to reduce the tori surgically it will be found after reflection of the mucosa that they present a hard, smooth, cortical layer of bone which it is almost impossible to remove with ronguers. A bone bur or chisel is the best instrument to use, followed by bone files.

It should be stressed that the genial tubercles, which lie immediately on either side of the midline on the lingual side of the mandible, must not be mistaken for a torus mandibularis. When there has been considerable resorption of the mandible the genial tubercles are often prominent above the general level (Figure 4.5) and are a considerable handicap to the prosthetist because the mucosa overlying the area is thin and the denture tends to

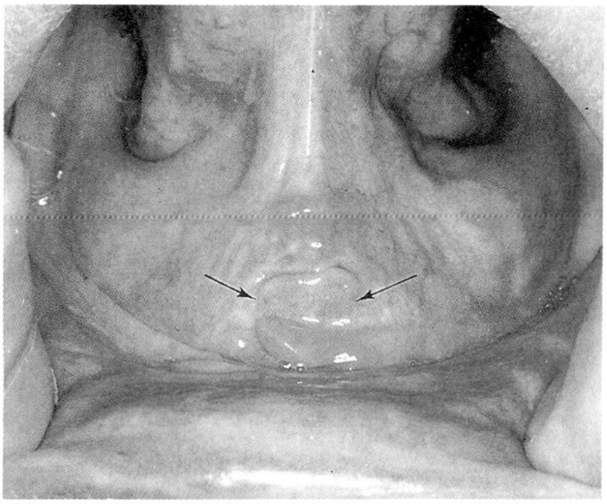

Figure 4.5 Prominent genial tubercles and denture-induced hyperplasia caused by the lower denture rocking over the area

rock over the tubercles as a fulcrum with discomfort to the patient. On the other hand, they serve as an excellent buttress to resist backward movement if the denture is extended correctly in the area. For this reason, and also because the genioglossus muscle is attached, they should not be removed by surgery. In general, the mucosa over surgically-removed tori or genial tubercles is liable to be tender to load for a considerable time and serves as a poor supporting tissue for a denture.

Undercut areas

When these are too deep to permit the entry of a denture they should generally be removed or reduced, and the only guidance is the judgement of the operator as to whether retention of the denture will be satisfactory if the undercut is left and the periphery of the denture adjusted to permit its insertion. The most common positions requiring surgical interference are buccal to the maxillary tuberosities and the lower incisor region, either lingually, labially, or both.

Mylohyoid ridge

When the mylohyoid ridge is sharp (Figure 4.6) and the mucosa overlying it is painful to pressure the ridge may be surgically removed or smoothed to allow the distal lingual flange of a denture to extend correctly without hurting the patient. The incision is made along the crest of the alveolar ridge and reflected lingually. The mylohyoid ridge may either be removed with a chisel or smoothed with a bone bur. This relatively simple operation produces very good results from the prosthetic point of view but take care not to damage the lingual nerve and remember that the mucosa over the area may be painful weeks after operation.

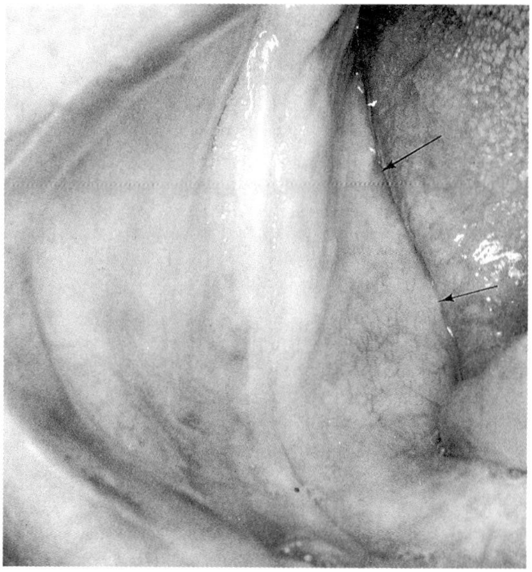

Figure 4.6 Right mylohyoid ridge

Prominent maxillary tuberosities

The operation for eliminating an undercut in the region of the maxillary tuberosities, and to create vertical space, in no way differs from other forms of alveolectomy, except in the first incision which is best made in the form of a semicircle extending along the alveolar crest below the bone to be removed and sweeping mesially to the required height in the sulcus (Figure 4.7).

An incision of this shape will make the reflection of the mucoperiosteum considerably easier, and in cases where it is only necessary to remove a small amount of bone it may obviate the necessity of suturing as the small semicircular flap will be held in place by the pressure of the cheek. In all cases when the removal of bone is contemplated it is wise to take a radiograph preoperatively to ascertain the size and proximity of the maxillary antrum, and to eliminate the presence of an unerupted third molar.

Soft tissues requiring surgery

There are a number of soft tissue problems which may require surgical intervention to improve the retention or support of dentures. In the examination of the patient it is important to be sure of the actual benefits the patient will gain by surgery. Remember that many soft tissue abnormalities have arisen under conditions of load and so the mucosa is well suited to pressure from a denture. After surgery, while the healed area may appear to be satisfactory, the tissue surface may be much less suited to accepting load and denture pressure.

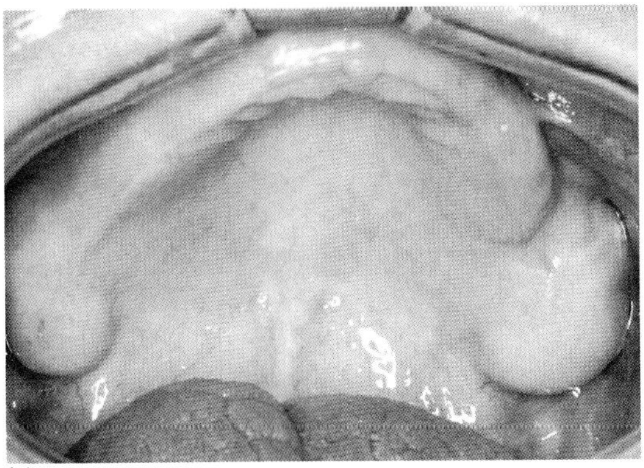

(*a*)

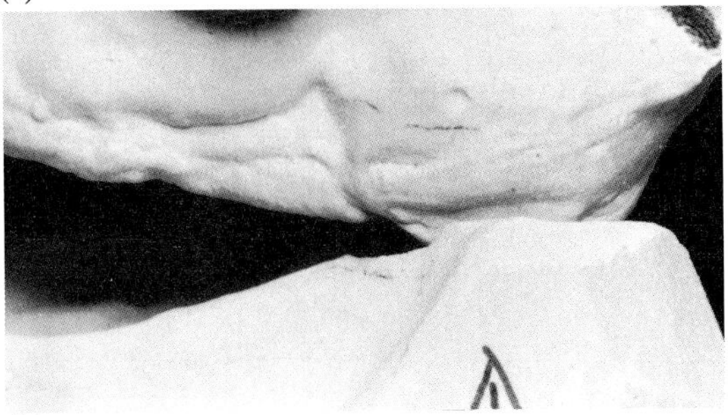

(*b*)

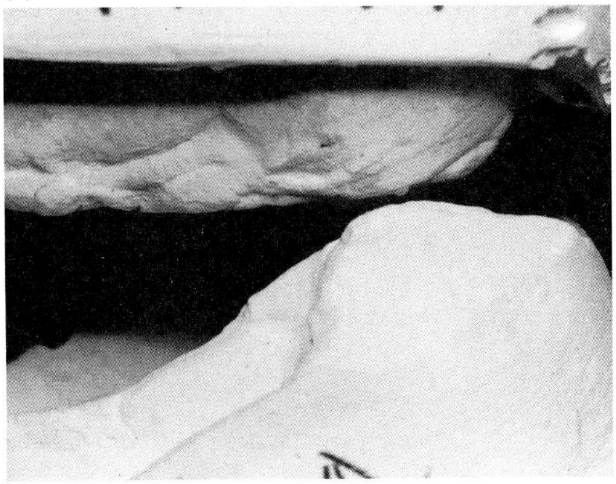

(*c*)

Figure 4.7 (*a*) Prominent bony maxillary tuberosities. (*b*) Preoperative casts mounted on articulator to provide an indication of the amount of bone to be removed at the time of surgery. (*c*) Postoperative casts mounted showing the interalveolar space gained by surgery

Interfering frena

Frenal attachments rarely require excision as it is nearly always possible to design the denture to accommodate them, but cases do occur where, unless removed, they make the satisfactory design of a denture impossible.

The operation of frenectomy is a simple one, the denture being used to keep the cut surfaces apart and so prevent their re-uniting. The impression, from which the denture is constructed, must be taken in a free-flowing material so that the position of the easily displaced frenum is accurately recorded. When the denture is ready for finishing the frenal attachment on the cast is cut away and the sulcus trimmed to the desired depth, the flange of the denture waxed into this sulcus, and the denture processed (Figure 4.8).

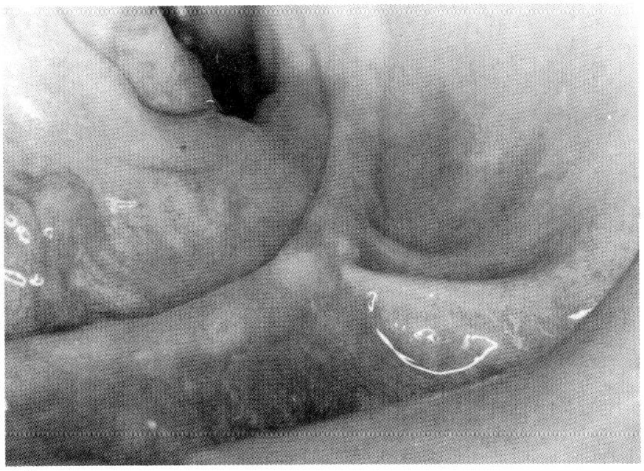

(*a*)

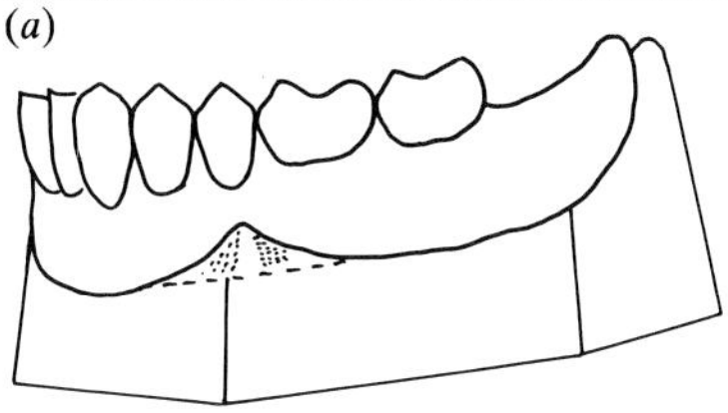

(*b*)

Figure 4.8 (*a*) Buccal frenum, lower left region, showing attachment at mucogingival junction. (*b*) Side view of the frenum showing the depth to which the cast is trimmed prior to finishing the denture

Technique of frenectomy

The operation consists of anaesthetizing and then excising the frenum with scalpel or scissors to the same depth as was previously done on the cast. As soon as the bleeding is controlled, the denture is inserted and the patient instructed that it must not be removed, except for cleaning, until the cut surfaces have completely epithelialized over. The patient should be seen occasionally during this period so that any soreness arising from the wearing of the new denture can be dealt with, as under no conditions may it be left out for more than a few minutes at a time.

Denture-induced hyperplasia

These benign overgrowths of mucosa are usually associated with old dentures where alveolar resorption has resulted in a gradual shift in position of the denture leading to chronic irritation of the sulci from the now over-extending denture flange. These hyperplasias are often multiple, one flap having grown and then become enclosed under the denture either because of the looseness of fit or because the patient finds it more comfortable in this position. A second flap forms and is in turn enclosed, and so on until in some cases there are six or eight of these overgrowths like leaves of a book (see Figures 3.2, 3.3 and 4.5).

If the irritation caused by the over-extended periphery of the denture is removed, the hyperplastic tissue will slowly reduce in extent. The flange is cut back and the denture lined with tissue conditioner or black gutta percha. The occlusal faults are usually contributing to the shift in position of the denture and so occlusal pivots are useful to eliminate this cause. The patient is encouraged to massage the area with a soft bristle toothbrush. Often no other treatment is required, but frequently these hyperplasias require surgical removal especially if they are of long standing. The operation is simple, the flaps of soft tissue being cut off at their base by scalpel or scissors, but the removal should be conservative since a radical removal will leave a much wider wound which, when sutured, will tend to reduce the sulcus depth considerably. Where the wound is small it can usually quite satisfactorily be left to epithelialize over, but in more extensive cases the edges must be gently drawn together by one or two sutures.

When the denture-induced hyperplasia is well established the sulcus is often non-existent and removal of the hyperplastic tissue is best combined with surgical deepening or widening of the sulcus in order to improve the muscle activity around the denture periphery. This is called vestibuloplasty or sulcoplasty and there are many methods of doing this. The operation is most commonly performed in the labial incisor region of the mandible, but it may be used in atrophic cases in other areas of the mouth. In most techniques the attachment of the muscles entering the sulcus are dissected from the periosteum and sutured at a lower level. The exposed wound may be allowed to heal by secondary epithelialization but, in most cases, a

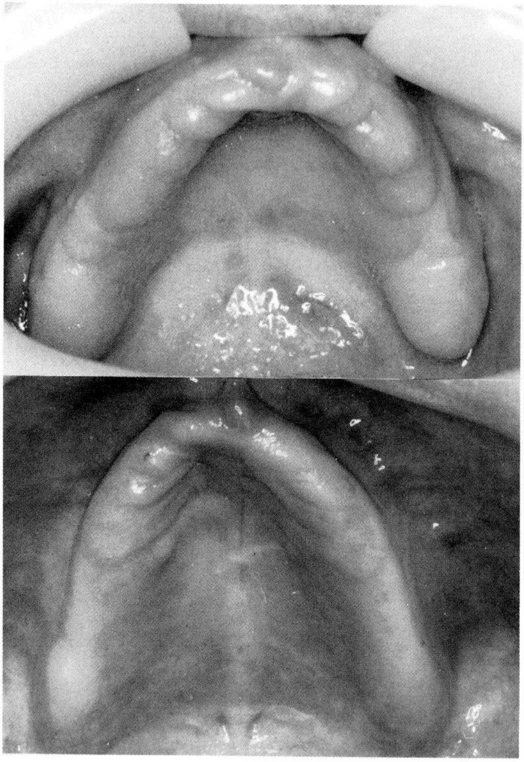

Figure 4.9 Flabby, displaceable maxillary ridges caused by excessive load and prolonged wearing of ill-fitting dentures

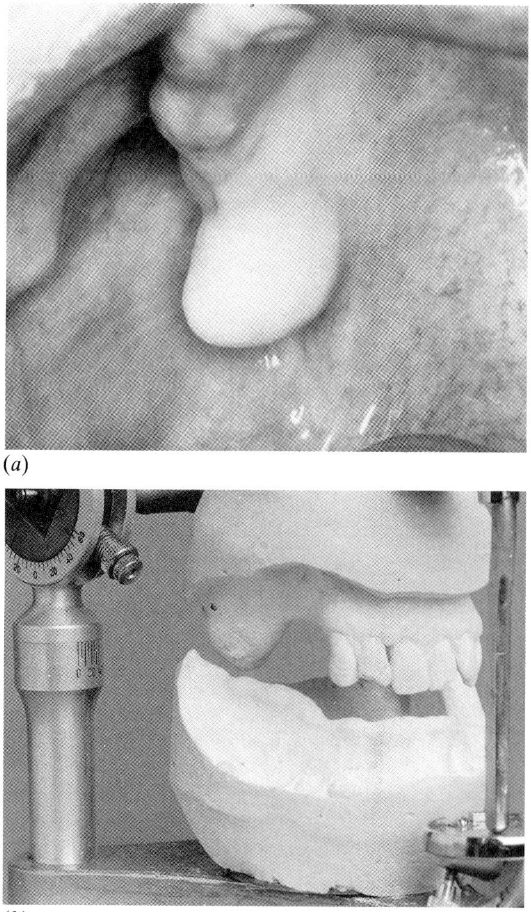

(*a*)

(*b*)

Figure 4.10 (*a*) Fibrous maxillary tuberosity. (*b*) Casts of another case mounted to indicate the amount of tissue to be removed by wedge incision graft of skin, mucosa or dermis is used to effect a more permanent and satisfactory sulcus form.

Flabby, fibrous ridges

A condition is quite frequently encountered where an alveolar ridge which appears normal is found on palpation to lack bony support and to be readily displaceable on pressure. The cause is usually excessive load on the alveolar ridge, often from lateral pressure, which has resulted in bony resorption and thickening of the mucosa and submucosa (Figure 4.9).

It is rarely necessary or even desirable to remove this fibrous tissue, particularly in the maxillary anterior region, as in most cases a flabby ridge is better than no ridge at all, and by using special impression techniques satisfactory dentures can usually be constructed. When, however, it is decided to operate the treatment should be as conservative as possible, the minimum amount of tissue being removed.

The position where it is commonly necessary to remove fibrous tissue is around the maxillary tuberosities where the excess tissue has arisen

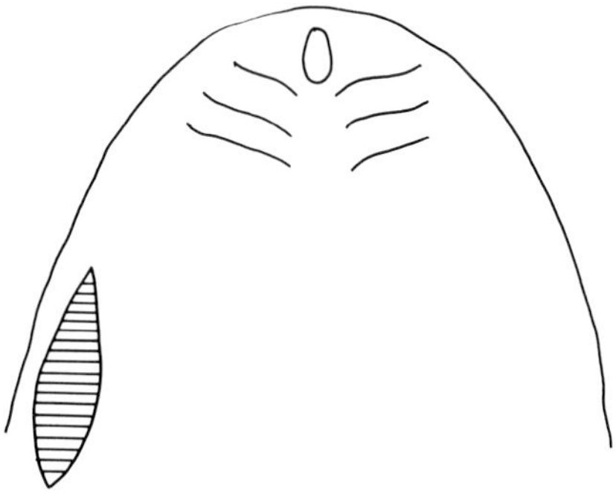

(*a*)

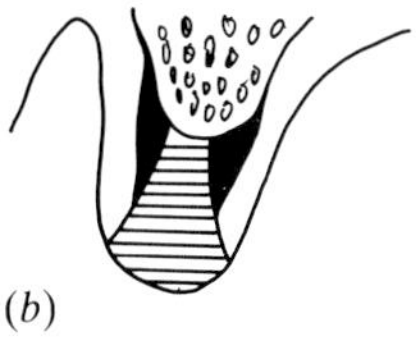

(*b*)

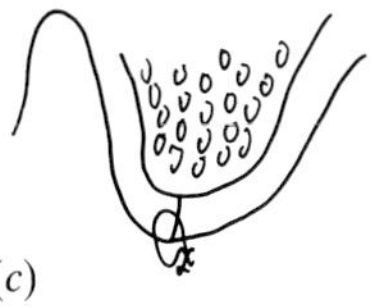

(*c*)

Figure 4.11 Technique of reducing a fibrous tuberosity. (*a*) Occlusal view of first wedge (hatched). (*b*) Anteroposterior view of wedge (hatched). Darker areas represent additional tissue removed (undermining is insufficient). (*c*) Mucosa opposed and sutured

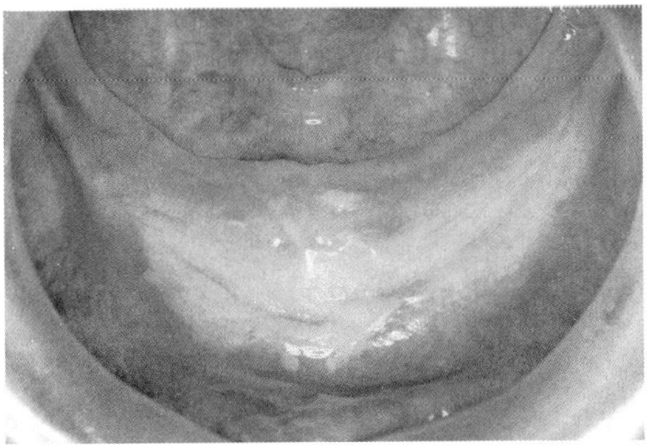

(*a*)

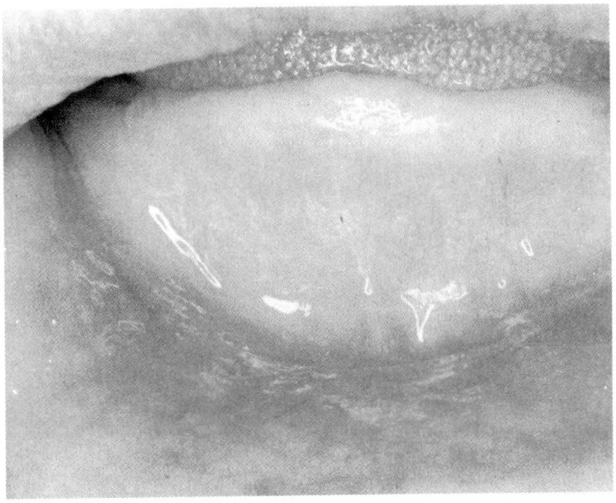

(*b*)

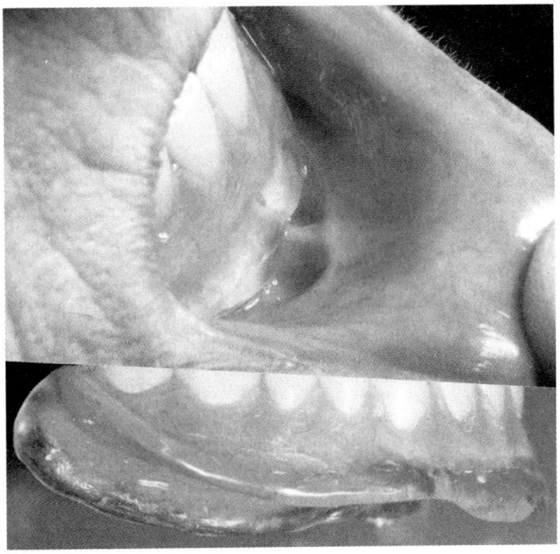

(*c*)

Figure 4.12 Mandibular labial vestibuloplasty. (*a*) With skin transplant. (*b*) With mucosa and muscle repositioned. (*c*) Another case, combined with mylohoid ridge resection, shows the denture extended into the pouch-like vestibuloplasty and posteriorly into the retromylohyoid fossa around a previously over-erupted third molar with chronic periodontal disease. The large tuberosity may be so close to the mandible when the latter is in its normal rest position that satisfactory dentures cannot be made until some of the tissue has been removed (Figure 4.10). The technique of the operation is first to remove a V-shaped wedge from the centre of the ridge. The mucosa on either side of the area occupied by the wedge is then undermined by the removal of fibrous tissue. Finally, the flaps of mucosa so formed are approximated by sutures (Figure 4.11).

Other forms of surgical preparation

More extensive operations such as orthognathic surgery, mandibular resection, epithelial inlays, extensive vestibuloplasty (Figure 4.12) and alveolar ridge augmentation, are outside the scope of the average dental surgeon and consultation with a specialist prosthodontist or an oral surgeon is necessary. Any description of these operations is out of place in a book of this type but they are excellently dealt with in current surgical literature.

Chapter 5

Impressions for complete dentures

In order that a denture may be correctly designed and the necessary technical work carried out accurate casts of the patient's mouth are necessary and various methods by which these may be obtained will be described in this chapter.

While all operators agree that the casts must be an accurate reproduction of the mouth there is considerable difference of opinion over the interpretation of the word *accurate*. The base on which the denture will rest is covered with mucosa which is compressible or displaceable and the shape of this base at rest differs from the shape when resisting the stresses of occlusion and mastication imposed through the denture which it supports. Further, the denture will be surrounded by moving tissues and the question arises, what position should these tissues occupy when making an impression to produce an accurate cast?

Ideally one wishes to obtain from the impressions, casts of those areas of the mouth which will be covered by the dentures, together with the soft tissues which will be in contact with their peripheries at rest and during any normal movements made in speech and mastication. Also the cast should represent the bearing surface as it will be when the denture is functioning during occlusion and mastication, i.e. transmitting pressure.

The area included in the impression is sometimes far greater than can be used, and sometimes much smaller, but it is not possible to design a denture accurately unless the whole area which it should occupy is included in the cast, although, for reasons which have been discussed in Chapter 2, it is not always desirable to finish a denture to this outline. The extent of the impression should be as follows:

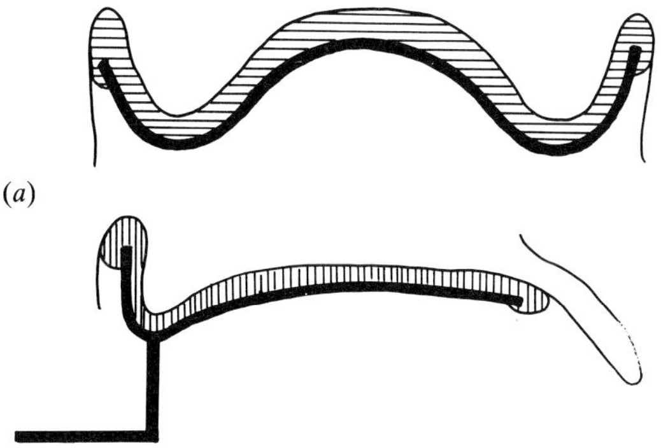
(*a*)

(*b*)

Figure 5.1 (*a*) Coronal and (*b*) sagittal views of the correct extent of an upper impression

The edentulous upper: from the functional depth of the labial sulcus anteriorly to 2 or 3 mm beyond the posterior border of the hard palate, as ascertained by palpation; laterally from the functional depth of the buccal sulcus on one side to the functional depth of the sulcus on the other (Figure 5.1).

The edentulous lower: from the functional depth of the labial sulcus anteriorly to 2 or 3 mm on to the retromolar pad posteriorly; from the functional depth of the buccal sulcus to the functional position of the floor of the mouth lingually on both sides (Figure 5.2). The position of the floor of the mouth depends on the position of the tongue and, as over-extension of the denture is apt to cause ulceration of the mucosa and instability of the denture, it is desirable to make the impression with the floor of the mouth raised to the functional position, which is obtained by protruding the tongue to the extent required to moisten the lips.

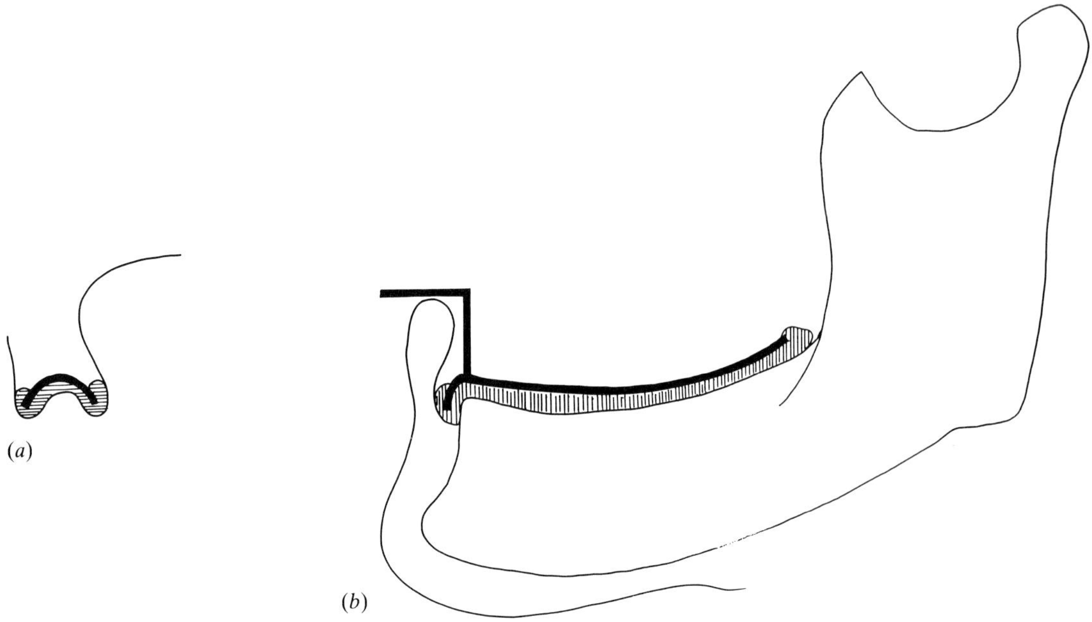

Figure 5.2 (*a*) Coronal and (*b*) sagittal views of the correct extent of a lower impression

The ideal impression material

Many materials have been advocated for impressions and while none is perfect each is usually superior to the others in some respect and, in order to have some means of comparison, it is useful to enumerate the properties which should be possessed by an ideal impression material, which should:

1. Be non-injurious to the tissues, non-poisonous and non-irritant.
2. Be capable of compressing the soft tissues to any desired degree without itself being distorted. This would enable an impression to be made of the tissues in the position they will occupy under occlusal stresses.
3. Be sufficiently fluid on insertion to give accurate surface detail. Closeness of contact is all important if the full advantages of adhesion and cohesion are to be obtained (see Chapter 1).
4. Be able to reproduce accurately any undercuts which are present. This implies that the material shall be either sufficiently elastic to spring out of the undercuts or sufficiently brittle to break easily. If brittle, the material should be capable of easy reassembly.
5. Have a pleasant taste, smell and appearance.
6. Have no dimensional changes either in or out of the mouth at all normal degrees of temperature and humidity. This is necessary in the interests of accuracy.
7. Set or harden at, or near, mouth temperature. If this is not the case then the removal of the impression from the mouth without distorting it will be virtually impossible.
8. Have a setting time under the control of the operator to allow for individual variations of skill and speed.
9. Be capable of having additions made and of reinsertion in the mouth, without distortion. This will allow minor corrections to be made without having to make an entirely new impression.
10. Be reasonably simple to use.
11. Be compatible with all materials in general use for making casts. It is undesirable that the choice of the material for making casts should be governed by the impression material.
12. Be reasonably inexpensive with a good shelf-life.

Before describing any actual techniques of impressions there are a few general considerations, common to all, which must first be described.

The position of the patient and operator

For most prosthetic operations the dental chair is set in the upright position, this being specially important during impressions since one of the fears existing among patients is that of being choked by the material in use. When the patient is seated the chair

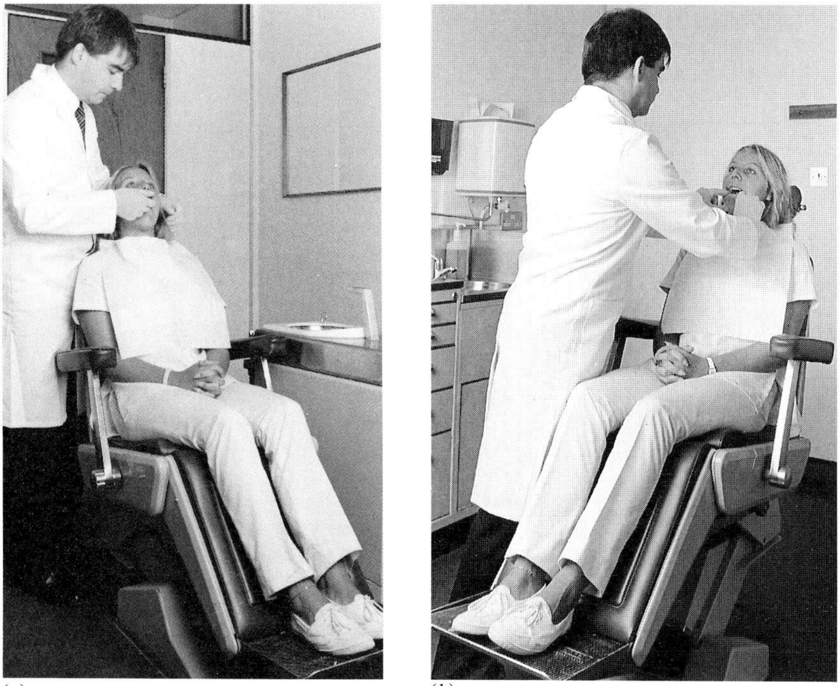

(*a*) (*b*)

Figure 5.3 Illustrating the position of the operator when taking (*a*) upper and (*b*) lower impressions with the dental chair in the upright position

and head rest should be adjusted so that the head and neck are in line with the trunk. If the head is allowed to bend backwards from the neck the supra- and infrahyoid muscles will be tense and difficulty in swallowing will result, and should a fragment of impression material break away from the main impression, it can more easily fall into the throat and possibly cause obstruction in the airway. Apart from the dangers, the patient's comfort must be considered if the operator is to receive the full cooperation required to produce a satisfactory impression.

A suitable covering in the form of a bib or towel should be provided to protect the patient's clothing. A warm, flavoured mouthwash to rinse remaining fragments of impression material should be ready to hand. The patient should be provided with a tissue or small napkin.

The positions of the operator are shown in Figures 5.3 and 5.4.

Impression trays

Impression trays are used as rigid containers for carrying the impression material into the mouth, for maintaining it in position during setting or hardening, and supporting it during removal from the mouth and when pouring the cast.

The dental supply houses manufacture a wide selection of standard or stock impression trays (Figure 5.5), but variations in the sizes and shapes of jaws are such that little hope exists of any one of them fitting an edentulous mouth with the desired accuracy (Figure 5.6). Too much space will exist between the tray and the tissue in some regions while in others the flanges of the tray will impinge on the ridge or sulcus. To produce a satisfactory impression and avoid variations in transmitted pressure there must be a reasonably even thickness of impression material over the entire fitting surface and the flanges of the tray must almost reach the functional position of the sulci and frena and yet not displace them. It is unusual for a stock tray to fulfil these requirements and, therefore, individual trays should be constructed for each patient. The individual tray materials vary according to the type of impression technique selected, the more common being (Figure 5.7):

1. Shellac or a similar thermoplastic material.
2. Acrylic resin, either heat- or cold-cured.
3. Thermo-formed or swaged polymer sheet.
4. Tin–lead alloy, poured into a plaster mould made from a wax pattern, sometimes referred to as the cheoplastic casting process; this type of tray is less common nowadays.

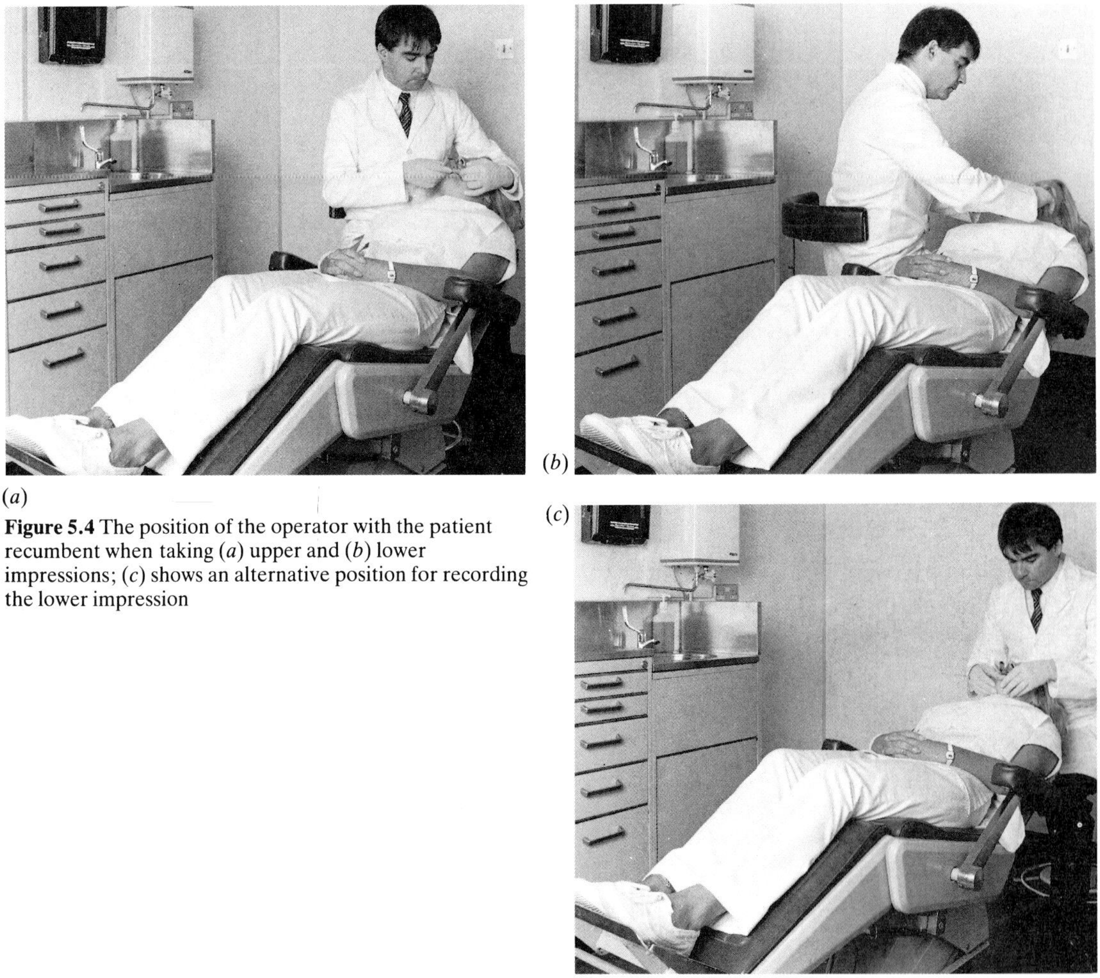

(*a*)

(*b*)

(*c*)

Figure 5.4 The position of the operator with the patient recumbent when taking (*a*) upper and (*b*) lower impressions; (*c*) shows an alternative position for recording the lower impression

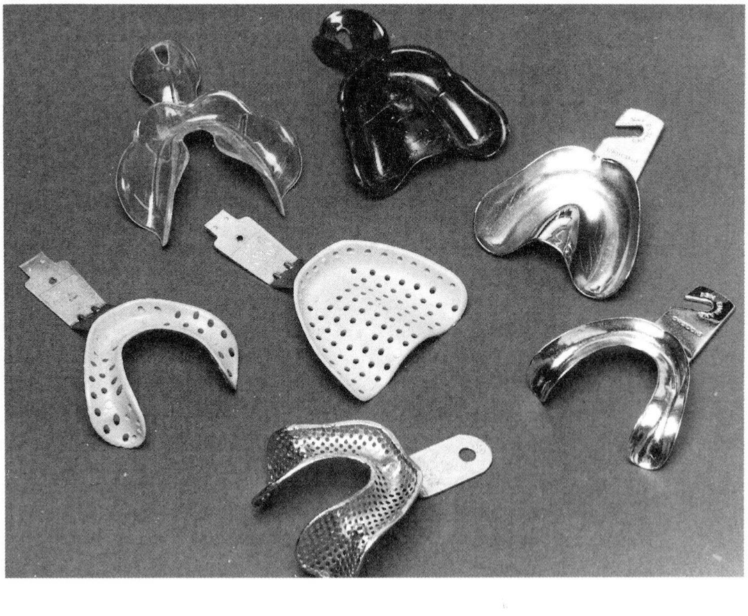

Figure 5.5 Examples of edentulous stock trays. Non-metallic trays are made of polystyrene, polycarbonate or nylon

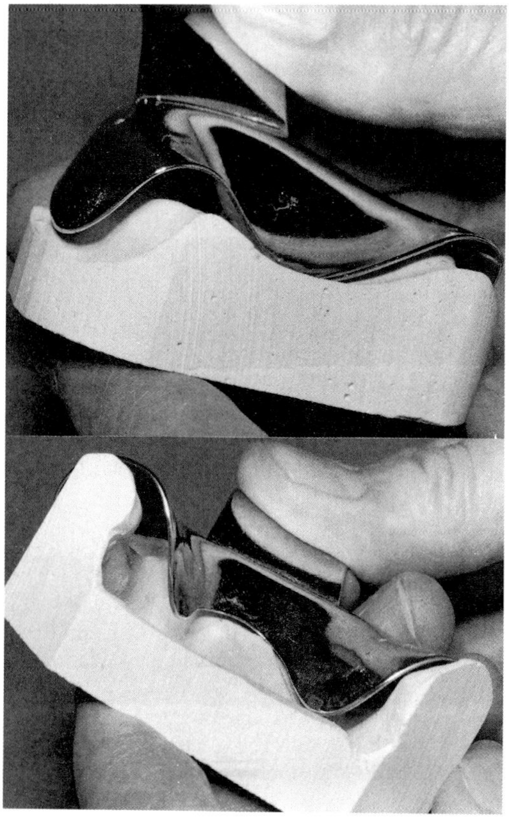

Figure 5.6 The inaccurate fit of metal stock trays. Metal stock trays are made in aluminium, Britannia metal, nickel silver and occasionally in stainless steel. They are usually chromium-plated or nickel-plated

(*a*)

(*b*)

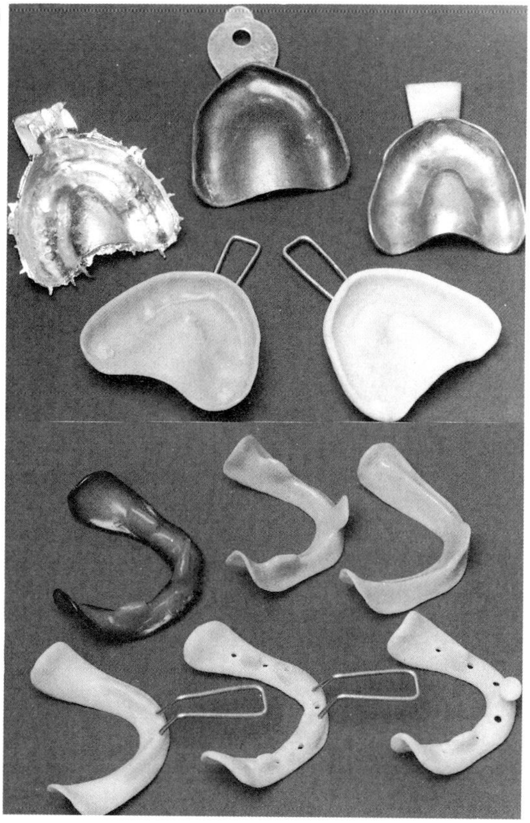

Figure 5.7 Individual trays. (*a*) Maxillary thermoplastic, tin-lead, cold-cure acrylic, heat-cure acrylic (note stops) and tin-lead as it appears from the mould. (*b*) Mandibular: top row, heat-cure acrylic; bottom row, cold-cure acrylic

It will thus be appreciated that for each patient two sets of impressions are usually necessary. The first, the preliminary (or primary) impressions, are made in stock trays from which casts are poured and the second, the master impressions, are made in the individual trays constructed on these casts. It is on casts poured in the second, or master impressions, that the dentures will be constructed.

The preliminary impression

Composition (impression compound)

Since this impression will not be used directly in the construction of the denture but only for making an individual tray for one patient, great accuracy is not required and so it is reasonable to select a technique which is both simple and quick and which gives the patient the minimum of discomfort. For these reasons composition may be chosen as the impression material, but it must be emphasized that this is not a suitable technique for a master impression, although such an impression can be obtained with composition using a special technique as described later in this chapter.

Composition, sometimes called impression compound, is the name given to a class of thermoplastic materials containing various waxes, resins and fillers which soften in hot water and harden at or slightly above mouth temperature. Many proprietary brands are obtainable with optimum working temperatures about 65°C at which temperature they should flow easily. Whichever composition is selected for this impression the manufacturers' instructions regarding its working temperature should be observed.

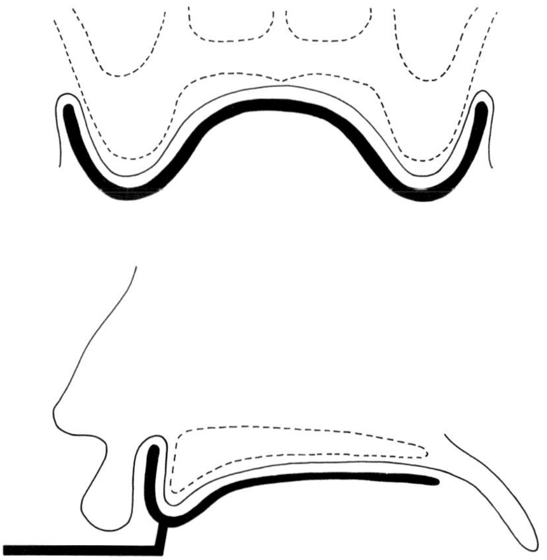

Figure 5.8 (*a*) Coronal and (*b*) sagittal diagrams showing correct extension of an edentulous upper tray

Selection of the stock tray

The alveolar ridges and palate are examined for shape and size, and from a selection of stock trays, suitable upper and lower ones are chosen and tested in the mouth for their approximation to the oral structures.

The upper or maxillary tray

The tray is angled into the mouth and the posterior border raised to make contact with the anterior part of the soft palate. It can then easily be seen if the tray will cover the maxillary tuberosities and allow enough room for the impression material. The tray is then raised anteriorly and the lateral flanges watched for clearance of the alveolar ridges. As the tray is brought up at the front, the upper lip is lifted so that the labial flange can be checked for fit in this region (Figure 5.8). The tray must not be pulled forward during examination for buccal and labial clearance. Sufficient space must exist between the tray and the tissues for the impression material and, in some cases, it may be necessary to bend the metal tray slightly with pliers to provide adequate space or, with plastic trays, to cut and trim the flange to accommodate frena and prevent pressure on bony structures such as the zygomatic process of the maxilla. The tray should be checked to make sure that it does not rock from side to side through making contact with the hard palate and also that the upstand is sufficiently long that the tray handle does not interfere with lip movement.

The lower or mandibular tray

Insert the left heel of the selected tray into the mouth and with the patient's right cheek held outwards rotate the right heel in. Pass it backwards until the distal ends cover the retromolar pads, while at the same time the patient protrudes the tongue slightly to facilitate placing the tray between it and the lingual surfaces of the ridge. Lift the tray anteriorly and slowly lower again observing its approximation to the ridge both lingually and buccally. When satisfied that the selected tray covers the ridge and allows sufficient space for the impression material the flanges are visually checked for over-extension into the labial and buccal sulci. The lingual depth is confirmed by having the patient raise the tip of the tongue to the roof of the mouth. If the tray is not over-extended lingually only slight finger pressure in the premolar regions will be needed to keep it in position. Should the flanges grossly interfere with the frena or sulci they must be trimmed or another tray selected before the impression is made. Finally make sure that there is sufficient flange depth in the region of the posterior lingual pouches. Shortness in these areas can be corrected by adding a little warmed tracing stick composition (of a higher softening point than that to be used for the impression) to the lingual flanges of the dried tray (Figure 5.9). Reinsert the tray into the mouth and ask the patient to protrude the tongue slightly. This will trim the added composition to the functional depth of the pouches by raising the floor of the mouth and drawing forward the palatoglossus muscles. On removing the tray from the mouth

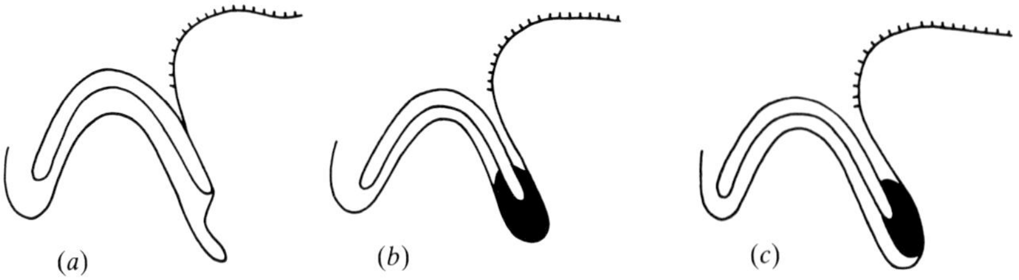

Figure 5.9 Coronal diagrams taken through the second molar region of a lower stock tray showing: (*a*) a short lingual flange trapping the base of the tongue; (*b*) the flange extended with composition; (*c*) the added composition displaced lingually to allow room for the impression material

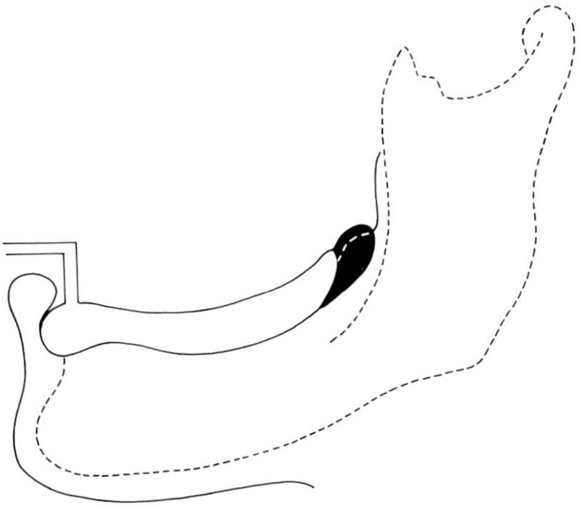

Figure 5.10 Composition added to the distal end of a lower tray to cover the retromolar pad

displace the composition medially to provide space for the impression material and then chill. A short tray can be extended distally in the same way, to cover the retromolar pads (Figure 5.10). Unless sufficient tray extension exists distally and lingually to push the tongue aside, it is likely that when the impression is seated the lateral surfaces of the tongue will be trapped beneath the lingual flanges resulting in an impression which is short in the retromylohyoid fossae.

The sequence of making the impressions

The trays having been selected and necessary adjustments carried out, the next consideration is whether the upper or lower impression should be made first. From the patient's point of view the upper impression usually causes the greater discomfort and anxiety, either through stimulation of the retching reflex or from fear of being choked by the material, but these symptoms are usually absent with the lower impression. Some operators prefer to start with the more troublesome impression first assuring the patient that, although the upper may be a little unpleasant, no such reactions will be experienced with the lower. However, there are some patients who having felt sick once will do so again even with a lower impression, so it is advisable that in most cases the lower impression should be made first. A further reason for this is that a foreign body placed in the mouth produces an increase in the rate of salivation and it is therefore preferable to have the lower impression seated in position before this takes place. If the upper precedes the lower, the operator and the patient may be embarrassed by the accumulation of saliva in the floor of the mouth, the result being a poor or difficult impression.

The lower impression

The selected composition is placed in a water bath, preferably thermostatically controlled to maintain the recommended temperature. After a few minutes the composition is removed from the bath, folded repeatedly from the edges to the centre thus always presenting a smooth surface on one side and replaced as quickly as possible to prevent undue loss of heat. Kneading of the composition incorporates water which acts as a plasticizer and this procedure is repeated until the material has acquired a uniform softness throughout.

When the composition is ready for use the metal lower tray is warmed in a Bunsen flame, the composition formed into a suitable-sized roll and placed in the tray. (If a disposable plastic stock tray is used there is no need to warm it.) It is important to have sufficient bulk extending beyond the flanges so that there is no restriction in flow when pressed into position over the ridge. A trough may be indented in the composition with the finger to simulate the ultimate ridge impression, the surface quickly flamed so that surface detail will be recorded, and tempered by immersing momentarily in the hot water bath to avoid burning the patient. The tray is placed in the mouth and, when the operator is satisfied that it is in position in relation to the ridge and correctly centred, the patient is instructed to raise and slightly protrude the tongue and, as this movement begins, the tray is pressed vertically downwards to seat the impression to the desired depth. Pressure in a backward direction may also be required to counter the forward thrust from the tongue when protruded.

As soon as the impression is seated in position it must be held there firmly but without any increase in pressure. In other words, the maximum pressure must be exerted when the composition is nearest to the optimum working temperature as the farther it drops below that, the less readily will it flow.

The impression obtained so far will reproduce, though not accurately, the denture-bearing surface, but will be over-extended round the periphery and an individual tray constructed from it would require considerable time-consuming adjustment before it could be used for making a master impression. This reduction of the individual tray can be eliminated, or at least very considerably reduced, if the muscles around the periphery are brought into play to mould the preliminary impression and this is done in the following manner.

The tray is held firmly in position while the patient protrudes the tongue. This movement of the tongue draws forward the palatoglossal arches, raises the floor of the mouth and tenses the lingual frenum and thus moulds the composition in the lingual sulcus to the raised position of these structures. The buccal sulci and frena are moulded by manipulating alternate cheeks downwards and outwards, to free any trapped folds of tissue and then pulling gently upwards, inwards and slightly backwards to obtain the approximate functional position.

The impression is now completed and all that remains is to hold it lightly but firmly in place for a further minute, remove, chill thoroughly in cold water and inspect.

Common faults in lower impressions

1. Insufficient depth in the posterior lingual pouch, caused by:
   (a) Flange of the tray short in this region.
   (b) Lack of composition in the tray.
   (c) Too little force used in seating the tray.
   (d) Tongue trapped by the tray flanges because the patient failed to raise the tongue as the tray was seated (Figure 5.11).
   In some cases it is necessary to push the compound into the lingual pouch area with the forefinger just before the tray is finally seated.
2. Insufficient depth in the lingual, labial and buccal sulci, caused by:
   (a) Lack of impression material.
   (b) Not seating the tray with sufficient pressure.
   (c) Material too cold and so failure to flow.
3. The presence of a smooth hollow in the buccal distal periphery, caused by: the cheek not being released from beneath the composition border during functional trimming (Figure 5.11).
4. Edge of the tray showing through the impression, caused by:
   (a) Incorrect centring of the tray before seating.
   (b) In the anterior lingual region, the forward thrust of the tongue not being countered by sufficient backward pressure on the tray.
   (c) Use of too large or too small a tray for the mouth or failure to trim the flanges adequately.
5. An asymmetrical impression, caused by:
   (a) More composition on one side of the tray than the other.
   (b) Failure to centre the tray in the mouth.

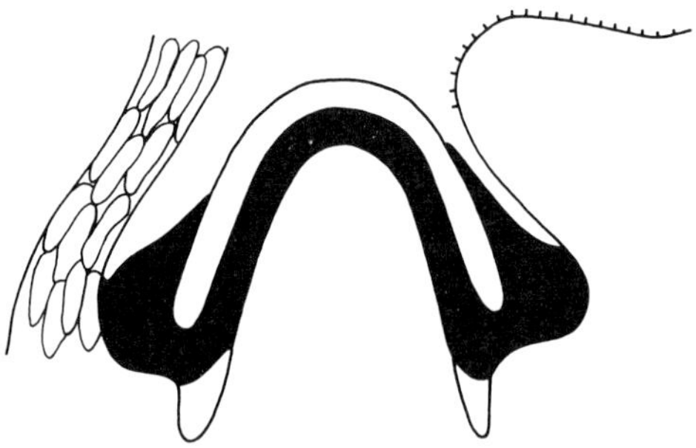

Figure 5.11 Showing how tongue and cheek may be trapped under impression material if correct trimming movements are omitted

Corrections to faults 1 and 2 may be made by adding small softened pieces of composition to the imperfect areas and then reseating and remoulding the impression. The error due to cheek folds, 3, should be corrected by reheating the impression in that area and readapting, while faults numbers 4 and 5 usually require an entirely new impression.

When adding composition to an impression the latter should first be thoroughly chilled and dried and the area requiring correction flamed sufficiently to make it sticky. A piece of the softened material is then taken, lightly flamed and attached to the main impression and moulded to the approximate shape required. Its surface is again flamed and then passed through the hot water bath before being reseated in the mouth. Only the area to be readapted should be heated, the remainder being kept as cool as possible to avoid distortion on reinsertion. Another way of correcting faults is to use tracing stick which is softened in a flame and applied to the warm composition, then tempered in hot water.

The upper impression

The composition is softened and prepared in the way already described for the lower impression. When ready it is formed into a ball and placed in the centre of the palate of the warmed tray. It is then moulded outwards to the periphery until the whole tray is filled, leaving a smooth, uncreased surface indented to form a trough for the ridge and slightly raised in the middle for the palatal vault. Sufficient composition must be moulded along the periphery to enable the depth of the buccal and labial sulci to be reached without having to force the tray upwards too far. This is because excessive pressure together with an abundance of composition in the palatal region will cause it to flow backwards so far over the soft palate that retching and vomiting may result.

Figure 5.12 illustrates the manner in which the composition flows to fill the palate and buccal sulci. It will be seen that the palatal area receives composition from two directions, while the sulci are filled from only one.

Once the composition has been adapted to the tray the surface is lightly flamed, tempered in the water bath, inserted in the mouth and centred under the ridge. Keeping the tray handle in line with the

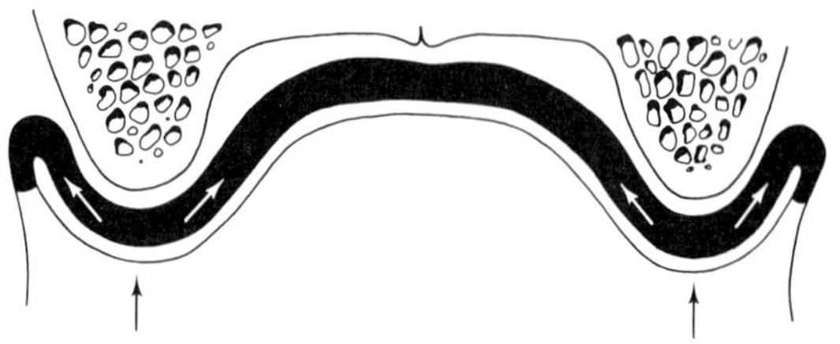

Figure 5.12 Arrows indicate the flow of composition to fill the palate and the sulci of an upper impression

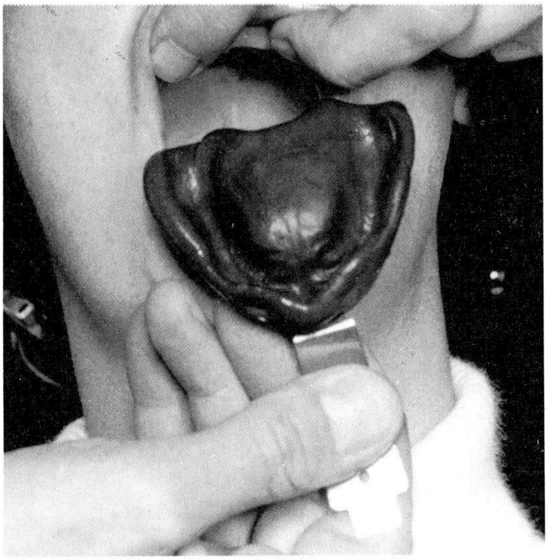

Figure 5.13 Removal and examination of upper compound impression

median sagittal plane of the face ensures correct centring. Firm upward pressure now seats the impression in place ready for the peripheral moulding. Alternate cheeks are gently pulled upwards and outwards, and then downwards and inwards and slightly backwards: the first movements release any trapped air or folds of tissue, while the other three movements simulate the function of the cheek when drawn in to aid the placing of food over the occlusal surfaces of the teeth, and to clear the sulci of debris. The labial trimming can similarly be carried out by manipulations by the operator or the patient can be asked to purse up the lips as tightly as possible, then to retract them forcibly and finally to try to push the impression down with pressure of the upper lip. During these manoeuvres the tray is firmly held in position and for a further minute before being removed, chilled and inspected (Figure 5.13).

In order to avoid cross-infection between the clinical area and the laboratory, the impressions may be immersed in a 1 in 20 aqueous solution of chlorhexidine gluconate before delivery to the laboratory.

Common faults in upper impressions

1. A crevice or deficiency in the midline of the palatal vault caused by:
   (a) Insufficient composition in the palatal area when filling the tray.
   (b) Insufficient pressure.
   (c) Composition too cold so that its flow was impaired.
   (d) Trapped air.
2. Excess composition extending well beyond the posterior palatal border of the tray, caused by:
   (a) Excessive or prolonged pressure when seating the tray.
   (b) Too much composition in the palatal area when filling the tray.

   Composition which is unsupported by the tray will fall away from the palate by its own weight dragging some of the supported composition with it and producing an inaccurate impression. Upward pressure on the tray should cease when the impression material is approximately 1 cm beyond the posterior border of the tray.
3. An impression short in one or more regions of the sulci, especially around the tuberosities or the labial sulcus, caused by:
   (a) Insufficient material in the tray.
   (b) Failure to mould the peripheral composition in this region when filling the tray to ensure that it will slip up between the cheek and the tuberosity or the lip and the alveolar ridge.
   (c) Failure to pull the upper lip outwards and upwards sufficiently to allow the composition to flow into the labial sulcus.
   (d) Insufficient pressure.
   (e) Composition too cold.
4. Tray flange showing through the composition, caused by:
   (a) Poorly selected or adapted tray.
   (b) Incorrect centring of the tray.

   Most deficiencies can be corrected by the addition of small amounts of composition, as described for the lower impression, but if the tray has been wrongly positioned or is too small it is better to remake the impression than to attempt adjustments.
5. Excess composition in the labial sulcus, caused by:
   (a) Failure to locate the tray under the ridge.
   (b) Too much composition in the front of the tray.

Warning: be sure that composition does not burn the patient. Check the tray temperature against the back of the hand before inserting in the mouth and, whenever composition has been softened in a flame, it must be immersed for a moment in hot water before being put in the mouth otherwise a serious burn will result.

Alginate (irreversible hydrocolloid)

Alginate is a better choice of material for preliminary impressions of edentulous patients for the following reasons:

1. It produces a good surface detail because of its rheological properties. During the working time there are no viscosity changes.

2. It produces a reliable representation of the surrounding anatomical structures and muscle activity.
3. Provided the stock trays are properly prepared the resultant impression will be more symmetrical and less liable to include areas of distortion and over-extension which are common criticisms of composition.
4. It is sufficiently elastic to be withdrawn over undercuts without becoming permanently deformed.
5. It is less viscous than composition and so less displacement of soft tissues, such as flabby ridges, tuberosities or retromolar areas, will take place.

All these features will produce better preliminary casts and for this reason more acccurate and useful individual impression trays.

Constituents

The active ingredient is sodium alginate which when mixed with water produces a colloidal sol. If calcium ions are now added the sodium alginate is transformed into calcium alginate, which forms a gel, so setting occurs. If sodium alginate and calcium sulphate (a source of Ca ions) are mixed with water, gelation takes place so rapidly that no time is allowed for conforming the material to the impression tray and inserting it in the mouth. A controlling agent is therefore added in the form of trisodium phosphate. This substance has a greater affinity for Ca ions than has sodium alginate and is transformed into calcium phosphate and, therefore, so long as any of it remains unchanged, it will delay the formation of calcium alginate. The set may thus be delayed for as long as required by the addition of the appropriate quantity of trisodium phosphate which is decided by the manufacturer.

The setting time is usually delayed 1.5 min, which is ample time in which to mix, conform to the tray, and insert in the mouth.

Method of using alginate

Several varieties of alginate impression material are available with slightly different methods of proportioning the water and powder. The manufacturer's instructions applying to the brand being used should be strictly adhered to because the reactions of alginate materials are sensitive to small variations in the powder/water ratio and the temperature of the water. The powder container should be thoroughly shaken to ensure dispersion of the constituents. This produces a cloud of material, but dustless alginates are now produced by manufacturers by coating the powder with a dihydric alcohol.

A rubber bowl and curved metal spatula should be used for mixing so that the powder and liquid can be thoroughly incorporated by a firm rotary motion of the spatula against the side of the bowl. Thorough and speedy mixing is essential so that the trisodium phosphate is evenly dispersed throughout the mass and the mixing time should be that stated by the manufacturer.

Impression trays

The same type of stock metal or disposable plastic (nylon or polystyrene) tray described for impression compound is suitable for alginate. The difference, however, lies in the necessity, in almost every case, to modify or adapt the tray with additions of impression compound before the alginate is used. This is partly because stock trays only approximate to the wide variations in edentulous mouth shapes and sizes, and partly because during gelation the tray can easily meander forwards or sideways to produce an asymmetric impression or the edge of the tray can cut through the setting alginate because of its low viscosity before gelation occurs.

The alginates, unlike composition, will not adhere to the tray of their own accord; fixation may be effected by one of the following methods:

1. Perforated trays will produce a mechanical union as the alginate flows through the holes. In some of the more free-flowing alginates the material continues to flow through the perforations until gelation occurs and this produces a dimpling effect on the resultant cast surface. This is particularly liable to occur if too much pressure is used to hold the tray in place or if the size of the perforations is too large. If, on the other hand, the perforations are too small or too far apart the mechanical locking effect is insufficient to retain the set alginate. It should also be realized that perforations do not retain the material around the periphery, an important area of any impression. For this reason, it is usually best to use an adhesive (see below) around the tray edges of a perforated tray.
2. Adhesives consisting of polyamide in isopropyl alcohol which may be either painted or sprayed on the tray surface immediately before loading the alginate.
3. Sticky wax may be melted on to the surface of a metal tray immediately before the alginate is placed in it.
4. Wisps of cotton-wool may be secured to the tray with sticky wax or sandarac varnish and will become incorporated into the alginate as it sets.

Attachment of the alginate to the tray is essential because if it pulls away a distorted impression will result which may easily pass unnoticed since the detail of the surface will remain unchanged.

Modifying the stock trays

The purpose of alginate preliminary impressions is to extend slightly beyond the limits of the denture-bearing area so that on the preliminary casts the individual trays can be designed and made with the correct outline form. For this reason the stock trays usually require modification. After the upper tray has been selected, take a piece of softened composition about the size of a walnut and tease it along the peripheral edge of the tray, including the posterior edge, and then insert the tray in the mouth. Take care to keep the handle in line with the median sagittal plane of the head and as the tray is held lightly in place pull the lip and cheeks around the rim of composition. Remove the tray before the composition has fully hardened and push the composition a few millimetres buccally in order to make space for the alginate. The composition at the posterior edge should cover the pterygomaxillary notches and extend on to the soft palate. Check that the modified tray is reasonably symmetrical.

The same technique can be used for lower trays, but in those cases where there has been much resorption and the alveolar ridge is flat, or even non-existent, it is better to fill the tray entirely with composition and record an overall impression. This has the benefit of pushing aside the floor of the mouth and cheeks which tend to become trapped by the edge of a tray unless it is first improved with composition. Remove the tray before the composition has hardened and adapt the material with the fingers, partly to make space for the alginate and partly to make the modified tray symmetrical. Very often the composition extends too far buccally in the molar region on one side or is slightly short in one lingual pouch or over the genial tubercles and if these obvious errors are not corrected at this early stage they are likely to persist through later stages of the denture construction.

Making alginate impressions

The technique of inserting and seating the impression material in the mouth is almost identical with that used for impression compound.

With regard to the upper impression, however, one point requires emphasizing. It is most important to ensure that the minimum quantity of alginate flows past the posterior edge of the tray. A mass of material in this region, unsupported by the tray, will pull away from the palate under the influence of its own weight, giving rise to warpage and strains which will affect the impression further forward. For this reason some operators favour raising the back of the tray first so that the composition forms an effective seal with the palate and prevents the backward flow of the alginate.

Once an alginate impression is in place it must be kept perfectly still for 2–3 min, the time required for gelation. It is essential to keep the tray still because as heat accelerates the gelation of the alginate, that part of the impression in contact with the mucosa will set before that in contact with the tray and, if the unset portion is moved in relation to the already set portion, internal stresses will be induced in the material. These stresses will be released on removal of the impression from the mouth and cause warpage.

As an alginate impression requires to be kept in the mouth for some time, a saliva ejector should be available otherwise the volume of saliva collecting in the floor of the mouth may cause the patient distress.

Removal of the impression

An alginate impression when set develops a very effective seal and so before trying to remove it from the mouth, this seal should be freed by running the

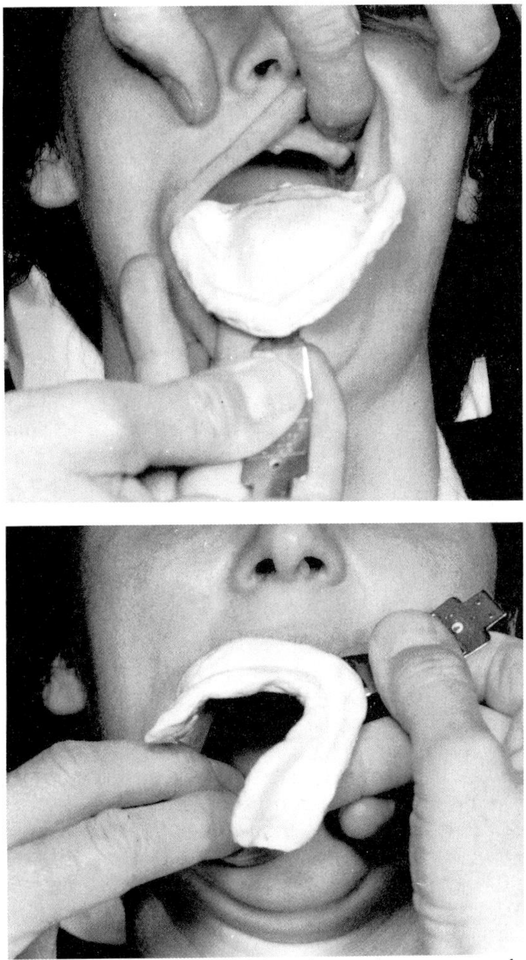

Figure 5.14 Inspection of alginate impressions on removal from mouth

finger round the periphery. Remove with a firm movement to ensure the best elastic behaviour. A long continuous pull will frequently cause the alginate to tear or pull away from the tray. Immediately after removal from the mouth the impression should be washed under the cold tap to remove saliva and placed in the humidor or wrapped in a damp gauze (Figure 5.14).

A humidor is a vessel with an airtight lid containing a little water and a shelf on which impressions may be placed out of actual contact with the water but in a moist atmosphere. The reason for using a humidor or gauze is that alginate rapidly loses water if left exposed to the normal atmosphere and shrinks as a result. Another frequent cause of distortion of alginate impressions is that they are left standing on the bench, the whole weight of the impression and tray being taken by the back edge or heels of the impression. They should always be suspended by their handles or supported in a cradle (Figure 5.15).

Pouring alginate impressions

The impressions should be poured as soon as possible after they have been made. The reasons for this are that:

1. Even in the humidor an impression tends to undergo alteration in water content and changes shape as a result, either by syneresis (separation of liquid from a gel) or imbibition (water absorption).
2. Stresses are induced in the material when the impression is being made, as it is physically impossible to hold an impression perfectly still in the mouth of the patient, and these are released slowly. The sooner it is poured, the fewer will be the stresses released. There is also less likelihood of the impression becoming warped. Thirty minutes is the maximum time which should elapse between making the impression and pouring it.

The technique of pouring is similar to that used for any other preliminary impression and no separating medium is needed. The one point to watch is that no force, sufficient to distort the alginate, is used. For example, if the mound of plaster or stone on the bench is allowed to become too stiff before inverting the impression into it, it will be necessary to use force to seat the impression, and the alginate will be distorted. It should also be ensured that the flanges of the impression are never forced into contact with the bench.

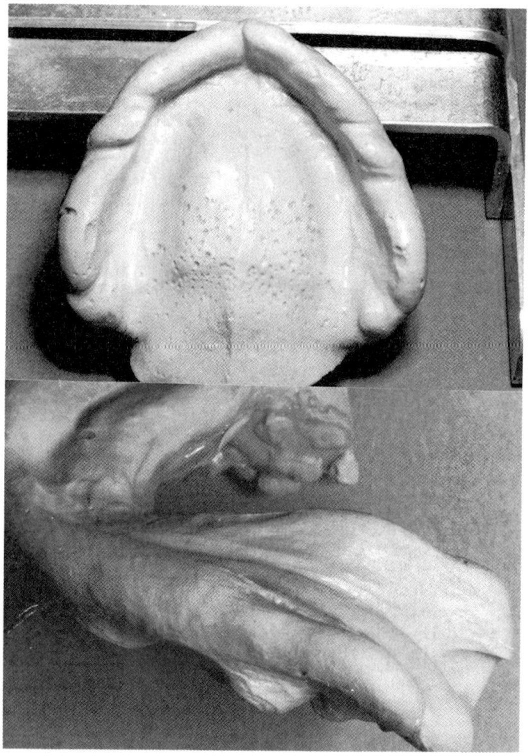

Figure 5.15 Upper and lower alginate impressions supported in cradles prior to covering with a damp gauze (note the surface of the upper affected by secretion of palatal glands)

The master impression

Four groups of impression materials are available for obtaining the master casts. The impression techniques advocated for these materials are innumerable, though often differing only in minor details, so a selection will be described to cover sufficient general techniques suitable for any mouth conditions which are likely to be met with in dental practice.

The materials and their methods of use to be described are:

1. Plaster (with anti-expansion liquid).
2. Zinc oxide–eugenol paste (ZOE or impression paste).
3. Alginate (irreversible hydrocolloid).
4. Elastomers (polysulphides and silicones).

It should be noted that 1 and 2 are non-elastic (sometimes called rigid) while 3 and 4 are elastic.

In addition, there are certain special techniques used for complete denture impressions and these will be described:

1. Composition compression impression.
2. Displaceable maxillary ridge.
3. Displaceable mandibular ridge.
4. Denture space impression.
5. Biometric impression trays.

Impression plaster

The two properties of dental plaster which render it unsuitable for use as an impression material are the length of time it takes to set (about 15 min) and the fact that it expands on setting. Fortunately both these faults can be remedied easily.

Heat will shorten the setting time of plaster but will not lessen its setting expansion. The salts of most metals will also reduce the setting time of plaster and many of them also reduce the setting expansion. The addition of 4% potassium sulphate to the water with which the plaster is mixed will make its setting expansion clinically negligible but, at the same time, will reduce its setting time to about 1 min. If borax is also added to the water the setting time is increased and, by varying the quantity of borax in the solution, mixes of plaster can be obtained which set from 1 min to some hours. Addition of 0.4% borax to the potassium sulphate solution will give a setting time of about 3 min, which is a convenient time for most operators, but which can be shortened or lengthened as desired by adding less or more borax.

Thus, if the following solution, which is usually referred to as an anti-expansion solution, is used in the correct proportions with plaster a constant setting time will result and so a consistent technique can be developed.

Potassium sulphate	4 g	4%
Borax	0.4 g	0.4%
Alizarin red (colouring)	0.04 g	0.04%
Water to	100 ml	

50 g of plaster to 30 ml of solution
Setting time 3 min.

This setting time of 3 min is only approximate as variations occur with different batches of plaster.

Special plasters

Special plasters are obtainable for impressions which contain potassium sulphate and borax in the solid form and so have only to be mixed with water. Another type contains starch which makes a very smooth mix with the added advantage that it is slightly sticky and so will adhere to the tray even when in a thin wafer; such impressions can be readily removed from the cast by boiling water which causes the starch granules to swell and so disintegrate the whole impression.

Mixing plaster for impressions

The setting time of plaster is constant under constant conditions, but vigorous spatulation will delay the initial setting though having little effect on the final setting time. This is because spatulation prevents the quickly growing crystals of gypsum which develop from centres of crystallization from joining up until crystal growth has reached such a stage that set is imminent.

The correct technique for mixing plaster for impressions is to place about 20 ml of anti-expansion solution in a dry bowl, quickly sift plaster and allow it to stand for 30 s without disturbance other than to flick any dry plaster on to the solution. At the end of half a minute it will be found that the plaster is moistened throughout and one or two gentle stirs with a spatula will render the mass homogeneous. This quantity will result in more plaster than will be necessary for even the largest edentulous jaw and obviously any smaller quantity can be made with the same results provided that the plaster/solution ratio is the same.

Individual trays

These may be constructed of any one of the materials already mentioned, although the best is cold-cure acrylic because it is rigid and will not be affected by the exothermic reaction of setting plaster. The handle on each must be positioned so as to clear the lip and avoid its distortion. The vertical distance from the sulcus to the handle is, on average, about 2 cm and this means that in those cases where there has been much resorption, the handle upstand must be made long enough for the handle to exit through the oral commissure. In full ridges the upstand is correspondingly shorter. The clearance between the tray and the cast should be about 2.5 mm which is attained by using a spacer of two thicknesses of base-plate wax or synthetic asbestos between the cast and the tray when constructing the latter. The lower tray should have a finger stand on each side in the first molar region (Figure 5.16).

Checking and trimming the trays for plaster impressions

The upper tray

If the individual tray is loaded with a fluid material like plaster and the tray inserted, the chances of

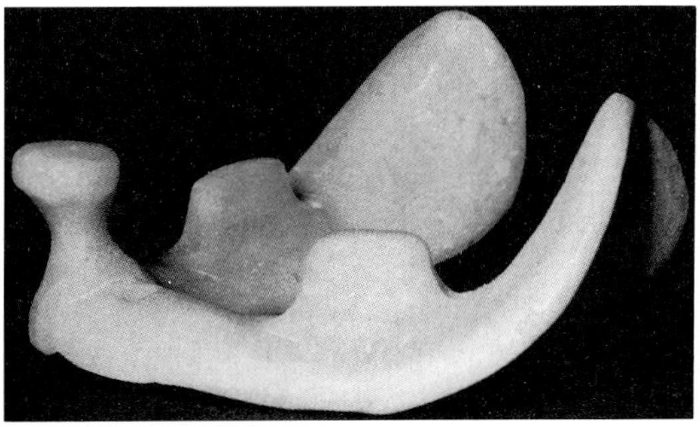

Figure 5.16 Cold-cure acrylic tray suitable for lower plaster impression. Note the finger stands in the molar regions and the button-shaped handle

locating the tray in its correct position are small. There is also the problem of the fluid plaster merely dribbling over the edge of the tray in the sulcus to result in a periphery of indeterminate form. Some clinicians attempt to avoid these problems by using a thicker mix of plaster but then the peripheral form is liable to be over-extended as the sulcus tissues distort under pressure from the excessively viscous mix.

For these reasons it is essential to check the tray in the mouth and then add tracing stick (impression compound) in a particular sequence before introducing the plaster.

With the tray held in contact against the palate the cheek should be pulled outwards and the sulcus examined. If the cheek forms a V-shape with the edge of the tray then the tray is over-extended and should be cut away in this area. The tray is the correct height if the curve of the sulcus can be seen above the tray edge with the tray held in contact with the ridge and palate. In the postdam region the tray should extend on to the soft palate about 5 mm beyond the fovea palati.

Tracing stick is now added to the tray in various regions. A small piece about the size of a pea is placed on the anterior palatal vault and the tray, tempered in hot water, is seated in the mouth to locate its vertical position. The thickness of this location stop should be the same thickness as the spacer wax which was used in the laboratory, i.e. about 2.5 mm. Remove the tray and chill it. Tracing stick is then added to the postdam region, tempered through hot water and located in the mouth so that the compound passes through the hamular notches on both sides and contacts the soft palate. This stretches the tissue of the soft palate beyond the distal border of the denture and therefore ensures a good postdam seal, but the compound in the hamular notches should be sufficiently soft not to displace the tissue, otherwise the denture will cause discomfort in these regions. This completes the tripod vertical location of the tray.

A buccal trim is now added to the tray, the function of which is to restore the cheeks and the lips to the positions that they occupied before the natural teeth were lost. When the buccal trim is properly made with tracing stick the correct width of the sulcus is indicated and the impression plaster will then record the height of the sulcus appropriate to that width. Tracing stick should be added in about three sections round the buccal side of the tray and it is usually better to start with the patient's left side. Compound is added level with the tray edge, tempered in warm water and the tray located in position on its stop. The compound for the buccal trim should not be too soft (consistency of putty is best) and the best way to trim it is to ask the patient to close on your fingers which are placed between the tray and the lower ridge. This has the effect of contracting the masseter which moulds the compound. Remove from the mouth, chill and repeat the process on the patient's right side. The buccal trim is completed by adding tracing stick to the anterior part of the tray and then the empty tray should be retentive because of the buccal seal. The lip at the horizontal level of the buccal trim should be restored to its dentate form (Figure 5.17).

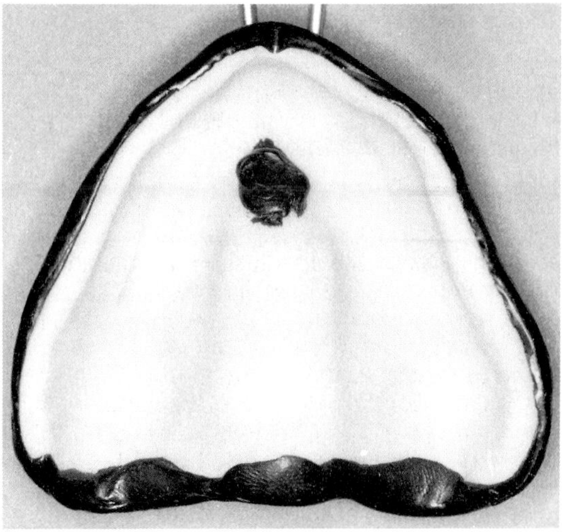

Figure 5.17 Maxillary individual tray prepared for plaster impression. Note the completed ring of tracing stick to ensure that the empty tray, at this stage, is retentive.

The lower tray

The object of a lower plaster impression is to record as accurately as possible the lower part of the denture space which may be defined as the space in the edentulous mouth formerly occupied by the tissues since lost. It is difficult to accomplish this with an individual tray without modifying it because the tongue, lip and cheeks collapse over the tray and narrow the sulcus so that the impression is then a record of an abnormal situation.

Make sure the handle of the tray does not interfere with the lip in any way and, if it does, cut off the part of the handle which comes between the lips to leave only the upstand. The tray is laid into position and with the index fingers on the premolar regions ask the patient to open his mouth. If the tray is felt to rise when this is done it is probably over-extended buccally and should be cut back. After the buccal flange is correct ask the patient to push against the upstand with his tongue and if the tray rises the lingual flange is over-extended and should be reduced.

Tracing stick is now added to the lower tray but in a different way than to the upper. Place a small piece of tracing stick on the tray in the region of each pear-shaped pad and over the crest of the ridge in the midline, temper in hot water and insert the tray in the mouth. This will locate the same position of the tray in the mouth as it was on the preliminary cast. Tracing stick is then added to the distolingual flange on one side from the distal part of the sublingual gland to join up with the already added compound. Temper and insert in the mouth. As soon as the tray is seated the tongue is brought forward to touch the upstand of the tray. This will mould the compound in the lingual pouch or retromylohyoid fossa. This is repeated on the other side. Tracing stick is now added in the molar region but only on the superior surface of the tray. The purpose of this is to form a vertical wall against which the buccinator will act as it sweeps round to the pterygomandibular raphe. The shape of the tracing stick is determined by having the patient contract the masseter. Repeat on the other side. Add a similar wall of compound in front of the upstand to determine the activity of the lower lip. This completes the preparation of the lower tray.

Using impression plaster

The lower impression

It is usually best to trim and modify both trays in the order stated, i.e. upper first, so that when the lower tray has been modified and adjusted the operator can then complete the lower plaster impression before the upper. Raise the dental chair slightly and adjust the headrest with the head tilted backwards so that the mandibular body is horizontal when the mouth is open.

The mix of plaster is adjusted so that it is slightly thicker than for an upper impression for these reasons:

1. The tray is inverted to enter the mouth and the plaster must not fall out the tray.
2. The saliva may affect the plaster surface and a quick set is desirable.
3. The object in the lower is to record more space than in the upper.

The tray is overfilled with the mix so that all the tracing stick additions are covered with plaster. The patient should rinse to clear the mouth of saliva just before the plaster is inserted. Angle the tray into the mouth and position it over the lower ridge as the first two fingers and thumb of the left hand spread the lower lip and hold it outwards. Locate the tray as the patient protrudes the tongue to touch the upstand of the handle. Wrap the cheeks and lip around the tray. Place the index fingers on the finger stands and be sure that the lower lip is not distorted during the setting of the plaster. After set, broach the peripheral seal by retracting the lip, angle the impression out and retrieve any fragments with dressing tweezers. Allow the patient to rinse.

When the tray is in the mouth the excess plaster sweeps up around it and therefore produces a good impression of the denture space and surrounding muscle activity as well as the periphery. It is in this respect that plaster is a very good material for lower master impressions.

The upper impression

The clinician works from the side and slightly behind the patient so the patient's head must be at a convenient height. The maxilla is parallel to the horizontal. Immediately before recording the impression the postdam may be marked in the mouth with indelible pencil across the vibrating line between the hard and soft palates. Insert a saliva ejector which helps to avoid smudging the pencil mark.

A bubble-free mix of plaster is made and poured into the prepared tray. Wipe the buccal surface with plaster as this will encourage the plaster to flow into the sulcus. Remove the saliva ejector, lay the tray on the lower lip and grasp the upper lip with the thumb on the outside and the first and second fingers on the inside. As these two fingers slip backwards the whole of the labial and buccal sulcus is exposed to view and at the same time the tray is elevated towards the postdam region. This action prevents any plaster flooding on to the soft palate. As soon as the back of the tray contacts mucosa, the front of the tray is lifted up to cover the anterior ridge. The plaster should sweep into the buccal and labial sulcus without trapping any air as the fingers are gradually eased forwards but still in control of the lip. This is important as air and saliva may be trapped around the labial frenum and a final lip movement is necessary to avoid this. In the last stages, the tray is puddled (see below) into position to place it on to its location stop anteriorly and the postdam tracing stick posteriorly. Allow the lips to collapse around the tray while the tray is held in place with one finger in the centre of the palate. If the patient feels nauseated the head should be cradled forwards in the clinician's left arm and the patient instructed to breathe through the nose. Allow the excess saliva to dribble out the mouth.

The buccal seal is broken by pulling the lip and cheeks upwards as the tray is slowly wriggled out of the mouth. Plaster tends to absorb saliva and this may cause difficulty in removal of the impression. If this occurs spray a little water around the periphery to wet the tissues.

Inspect the mouth for any fragments and allow the patient to rinse. Fractured pieces may be united with molten modelling wax added on the buccal side which will cause only minimal interruption in the periphery. Sticky wax is not advised as it is too bulky and tends to pull away surface plaster. Fill any blowholes with modelling wax provided the peripheral plaster surrounding the crater is sufficiently well defined to judge the contour. If the deficiency is greater, a new impression is probably the best treatment. A successful upper impression can be recognized if the plaster has washed across the buccal and labial tracing stick without over-extending the sulcus in a buccal direction. The location stop and postdam tracing stick may be seen through the plaster. In this way the impression plaster has determined the height of the sulcus appropriate to the width already decided by the buccal trim. This method takes the guesswork out of impression making. If, on the other hand, the buccal tracing stick cannot be seen, or if the impression is obviously asymmetric, then the plaster has distorted the peripheral tissues and rendered the impression useless. The set plaster can be easily chipped out for the impression to be made again. Remember that when you examine a master impression it should be identical to the finished denture you are making for the patient (Figure 5.18).

Instead of tracing stick compound for the buccal trim some clinicans use carding wax but this has the fault that the exothermic heat of the setting plaster distorts the wax. Others use silicone putty, but in general these materials have the wrong consistency for developing a buccal trim and are not recommended.

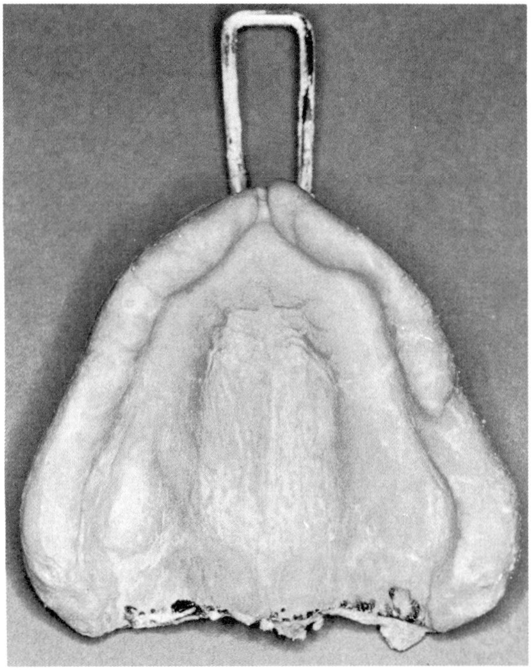

(*a*)

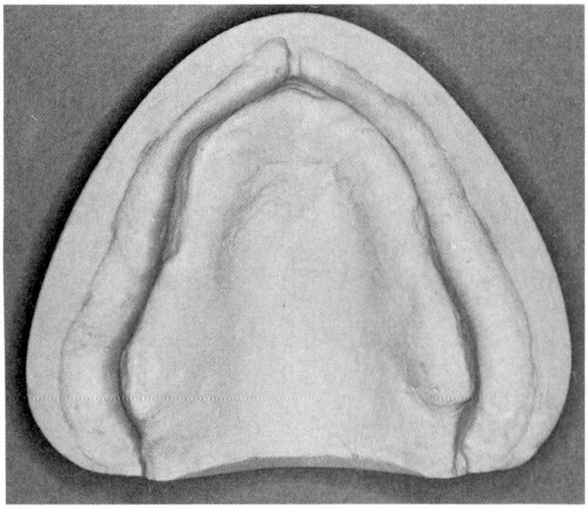

(*b*)

Figure 5.18 (*a*) Maxillary plaster impression and (*b*) cast poured from it. Note that the buccal surface of the periphery restores the lip and cheeks to their pre-extraction form (same case as *Figures 5.17* and *2.47a*)

Puddling of plaster

In the above description of the plaster impression technique the term 'puddling' has been used. This action plays an important part in the use of this material for impressions. A comparison with wet sand will clarify what is meant. Firm pressure on a mound of wet sand will first express the water and then, if continued, cause the sand to break away still leaving the hand uncovered. If instead of using firm direct pressure, however, the hand is wriggled and puddled into the mass with a gentle vibratory movement the wet sand will flow round and over it without any tendency to break away. Plaster impressions should always be treated as if they were composed of wet sand.

Failures with plaster impressions

Failures are due usually to one, or a combination of, the following:

1. Using an individual tray of the wrong design.
2. Failure to reduce the depth of the flanges of the tray.
3. Adapting tracing stick wrongly.
4. Insufficient plaster in the tray.
5. Too much plaster in the tray.
6. Slowness on the part of the operator allowing the plaster to set before the tray is adequately seated in place.
7. Incorrect centring resulting in an asymmetric impression.
8. Not puddling the tray into position, resulting in failure to seat the tray properly.
9. Failure to observe the extrusion of sufficient plaster beyond the back edge of the upper tray.
10. Direct pressure instead of puddling when seating the impression, and delayed peripheral trimming, result in faults and deficiencies on the edges of the impression.

11. Inclusion of part of the surrounding soft tissues such as the cheek or tongue.
12. Trapped bubbles of air. These usually result from failure to expose the sulcus as the tray is being seated. In mouths which exhibit a lot of mucus bubbles in the sulci, a better impression will be secured if the patient washes the mouth or if these bubbles are wiped away with a gauze napkin just prior to inserting the impression.

Plaster as an impression material gives exact reproduction of the denture-bearing surface at rest, with excellent surface detail. However, since it is semi-liquid when introduced into the mouth, very little compression of the soft tissue takes place and for this reason it is not the most suitable material for a patient presenting with varying thicknesses of mucosa covering the denture-bearing surface. In other words, because of its accuracy and reproducible peripheral form (if the buccal trim is correctly applied) it is an excellent material for good retention but it is less suited where there are problems of support.

Zinc oxide–eugenol paste (ZOE or impression paste)

This paste is basically a mixture of zinc oxide, white powdered resin, eugenol or oil of cloves, natural oils and fillers. It is smooth, flows readily, and is very sticky until it has set, which takes 2–3 min in the mouth. Because of its stickiness this material is admirably suited for wash impressions. Such impressions, as their name implies, are very thin and are made in individual trays with minimal clearance on the preliminary cast.

The individual tray must be very carefully adapted to the mouth, particular attention being paid to ensure that the paste is everywhere carried to the full functional depth of the sulci.

The proprietary brands of paste are mostly supplied in two tubes, one containing basically zinc oxide and the other basically eugenol. For the lower impression about 6 cm and for the upper 8 cm of each are squeezed on to the mixing pad, thoroughly spatulated, and evenly distributed over the surface of the carefully dried tray.

Before starting to mix the paste the patient's lips and neighbouring skin should be lightly covered with face-cream or petroleum jelly to prevent the paste adhering to these dry surfaces should it touch them during the insertion of the tray. Many operators wear disposable rubber gloves. Should some zinc oxide paste inadvertently touch a patient's or operator's dry skin, it can readily be removed by a napkin moistened with orange oil or chloroform.

Owing to its more sluggish flow, and smaller bulk, it cannot be puddled into place like plaster, but as soon as the tray has been centred in the mouth, it should be seated by a firm constant pressure which should be maintained for a short time before peripheral trimming is carried out.

Some patients may complain of a burning sensation with this material due to the slight irritation caused by the oil of cloves or eugenol. Impression pastes are available which are eugenol-free, the eugenol being replaced by carboxylic acid.

Muscle-trimmed lower impression

This type of impression requires careful attention to detail and is therefore rather a time-consuming procedure, but it is one that is justified by the results obtained. It is chiefly used in those cases where the lower ridge is very poorly defined, and where the factors of muscle balance and tongue control are adverse. The results obtained with this technique are due to the functional adaptation and meticulous care in covering the maximum possible area.

It is an advantage if the preliminary impression is made in alginate as there is then less likelihood of the individual tray being grossly over-extended or asymmetric. Mark on the cast made from the preliminary impression the approximate functional position of the periphery and construct a close-fitting tray in either cold-cure or heat-cure acrylic to this outline. A spacer of only 0.5 mm is desirable. A small vertical handle should be fitted in the approximate position and angulation of the lower incisors, so designed as not to interfere with the movement of the tongue and lips. A finger stand should be made on each side (Figure 5.16).

The steps in making the impression are as follows:

1. Examine the mouth to discover the position occupied by the buccal sulcus in function by gentle manipulation of the cheek (Figure 5.19). Towards the back of the mouth note that the contraction of the buccinator and masseter muscles almost completely obliterates the sulcus. This is because the buccinator sweeps across the ridge to gain its attachment to the pterygomandibular raphe (Figure 5.20).

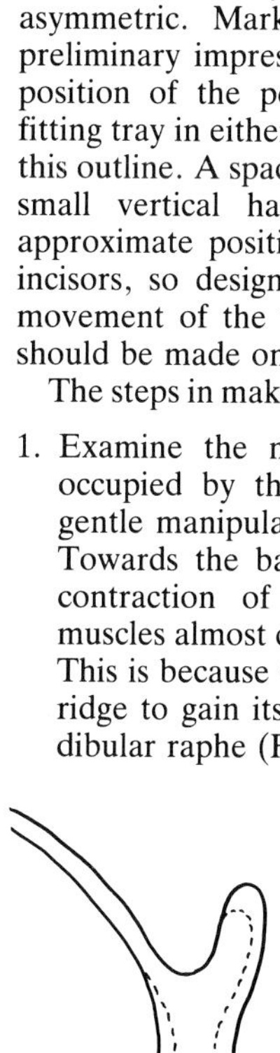

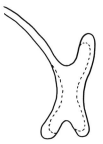

Figure 5.19 Position of sulci. Continuous line illustrates their relaxed position; dotted line their approximate functional position

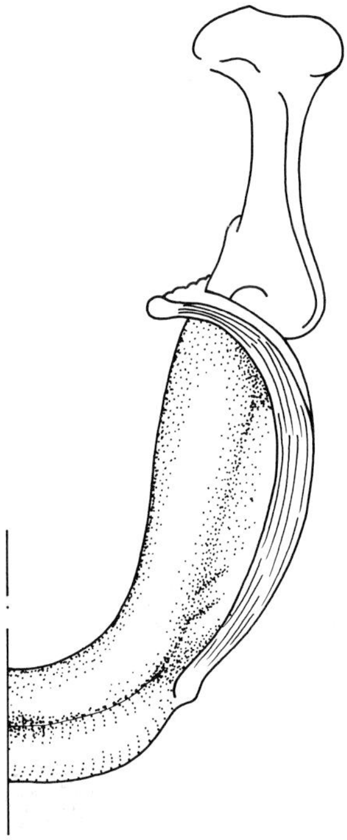

Figure 5.20 Diagram illustrating how the buccinator muscle crosses the alveolar ridge at the back of the mouth to gain its insertion into the pterygomandibular raphe

2. Cut back the buccal periphery of the tray so that it is about 2 mm short of the position occupied by the buccal sulcus in function (Figure 5.21).
3. Examine the position occupied by the labial sulcus in function by gently pulling up the lip and cut back the tray just short of this position.
4. Cut the distolingual aspect of the tray so that it is just short of the position occupied by the palatoglossus muscle when the tongue is protruded to touch the lips (Figure 5.22). This is most easily accomplished by placing the tray in position in the mouth and laying the finger in the posterior lingual pouch over the tray; ask the patient to protrude the tongue and it can be felt whether the palatoglossus muscle comes into contact with the tray. Trim until the muscle just fails to reach the tray.

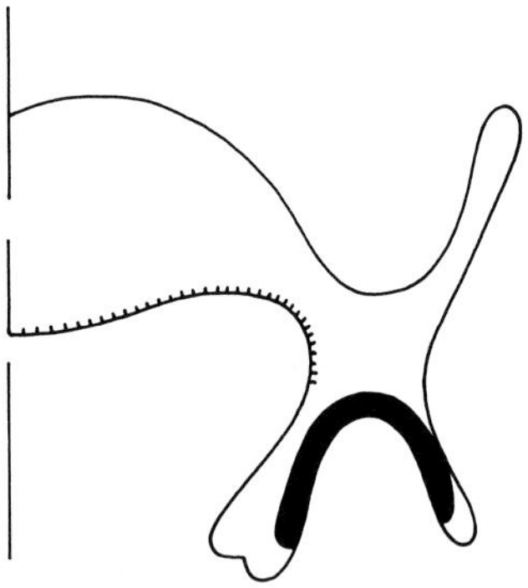

Figure 5.21 Correctly trimmed tray 2 mm short of the functional positions of the sulci

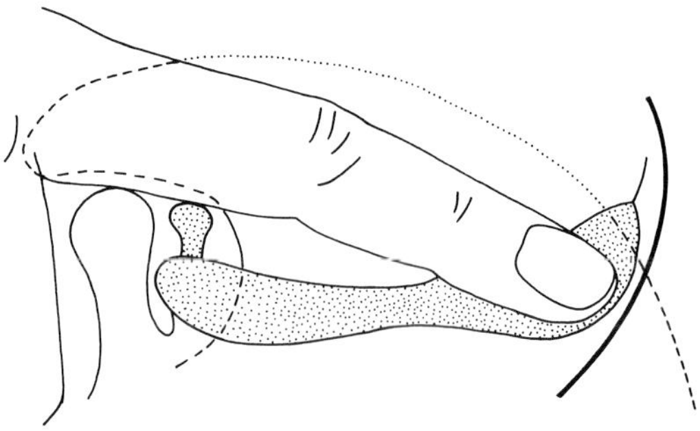

Figure 5.22 The thick curved line represents the position of the palatoglossal arch when the tongue (shown by dotted line) is protruded. The tray as illustrated is correctly trimmed and the position of the palpating finger shown

5. To examine the functional position of the floor of the mouth ask the patient to place the tip of the tongue against the handle of the tray. In the majority of cases the whole floor of the mouth will rise up and overlap the ridge and it will appear as if no lingual sulcus exists; this appearance, however, is usually false. The structures in the floor of the mouth immediately under the mucosa consist, for the most part, of the sublingual salivary gland, from about the first molar region forwards, and the deep part of the submandibular salivary gland further back. As these glands are pulled upwards by the action of the tongue they overlap the ridge and mask the sulcus (Figure 5.23).

   The most satisfactory way to trim the tray to the functional position of the lingual sulcus is to place the index fingers on top of the tray. If the tray is too deep the lingual tissues will exert an upward pressure, the degree of which can be judged by the force required to keep the tray in contact with the alveolar ridge. Cutting back the tray should be continued until only the slightest finger pressure is needed to hold the tray in position. A little practice is needed to gain this sense of touch trimming, but by running the finger along the top of the tray while the patient keeps the tongue forwards, it will soon be learnt where adjustment is required.
6. Trim the tray posteriorly so that it crosses the middle of the retromolar pads. This is very important because the excellent retention exhibited by the final denture cannot be obtained without a perfect peripheral seal being effected in the retromolar area and this can only be attained on the compressible tissue that comprises the distal part of the pads.

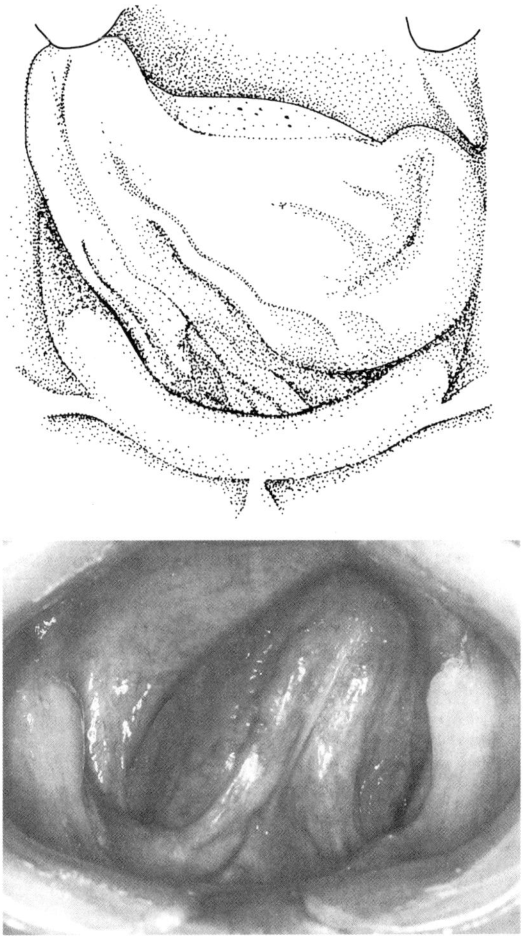

Figure 5.23 Illustrating how the structures of the floor of the mouth rise and overlap the ridge when the tongue is raised

7. Trim the tray so that it is clear of the frenum of the tongue both when it is protruded and when the tip of the tongue is in contact with the palate.

The correct shape of the tray is essential to the success of this type of impression. When the tray has been satisfactorily trimmed, the next procedure is to adapt the entire periphery to the functional positions of the various sulci; this is done by tracing on to the periphery of the tray a low fusing composition and while this is soft placing the tray in the mouth. This softened composition is then moulded by the movement of the various sulci and adapts itself closely to their functional positions.

The technique of adapting the periphery

The periphery of the tray which is now everywhere short of the functional sulcus is adapted by a technique known as muscle-trimming or border moulding.

Apparatus required: Bunsen, pin-point flame, bowl of water (temperature 65°C), bowl of cold water and tracing stick (a pencil-shaped stick of composition usually coloured to differentiate it from ordinary impression composition).

1. Soften the end of the tracing stick in the Bunsen. Commencing at the distal aspect of the left buccal periphery, 'paint' the trimmed tray with the tracing stick for a distance of about 3 cm. The softened composition will adhere to the periphery of the tray. The procedure of 'painting' the composition to the periphery of the tray is termed tracing.
2. Brush the composition with the pin-point flame to soften it uniformly as it will have started to harden while it was being traced, temper it in the bowl of hot water and quickly place the tray in the mouth. It is most important to remember that whenever composition is heated with a flame it must always be immersed for a few seconds in hot water to equalize the temperature, otherwise the patient's mouth may be seriously burned.

   Using one hand to hold the tray in place and support the jaw, mould the softened periphery to the correct form by carrying out functional movements of the cheek with the other hand, or by asking the patient to suck the cheeks gently inwards. This operation will adapt the composition into close intimacy with that part of the buccal sulcus adjacent to it.
3. Remove the tray from the mouth, and place it in the bowl of cold water for a few moments to chill. Remove the tray from the water to examine the composition, which if correctly adapted, should show a smooth, matt, rolled, everted edge (Figure 5.24).

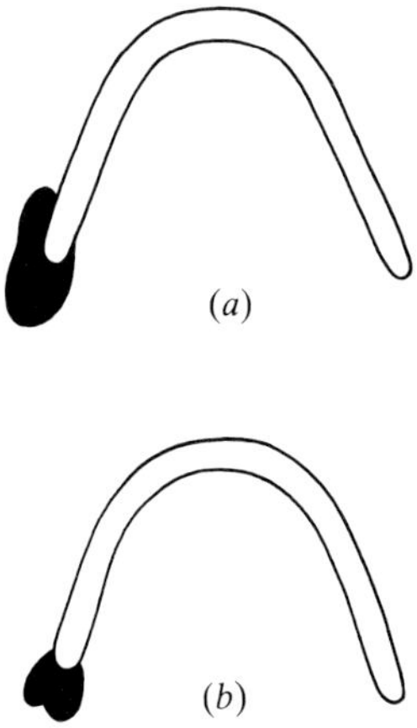

Figure 5.24 Section through lower tray showing traced periphery. (*a*) Composition smooth, rolled and everted. (*b*) Composition rough and not everted

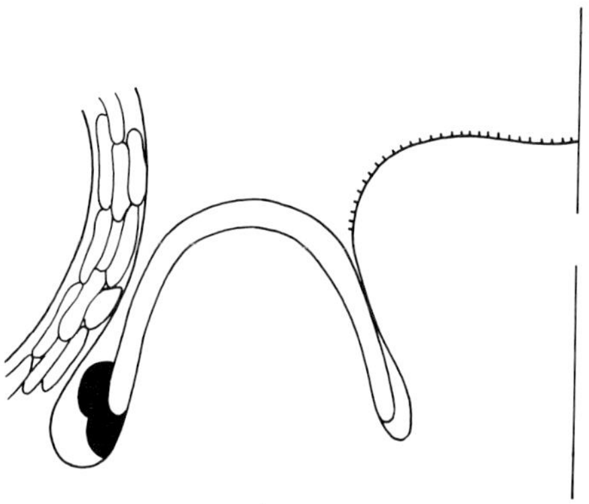

Figure 5.25 Illustrating how the error shown in *Figure 5.24 (b)* occurs

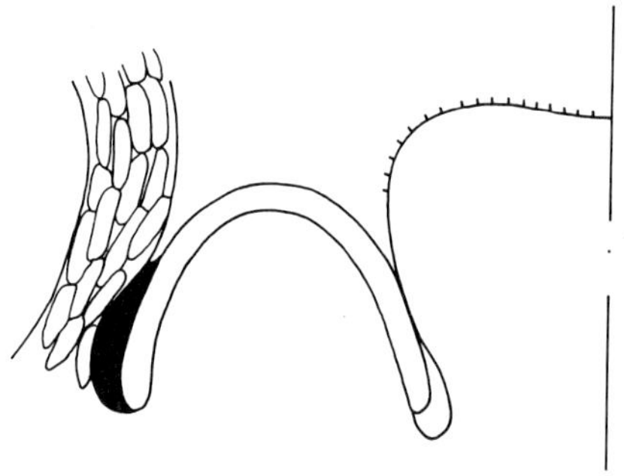

Figure 5.26 Tray over-extended, composition completely everted

If it does not appear everted, looks rough or is shiny instead of matt there was not sufficient composition present to fill the sulcus in its functional position (Figures 5.24 and 5.25).

To correct this error, dry the original composition with gauze and add to it by tracing on another layer and readapt to the sulcus. If the tray has not been trimmed sufficiently short of the functional position of the sulcus the composition will be everted completely and the edge of the tray will show through (Figure 5.26). In this case the tray must be trimmed further.

4. Adapt the whole of the buccal and labial periphery, working in sections of about 3 cm at a time. Pay particular attention to the adaptation around the frenal attachments.
5. When the buccal and labial border is complete, commence the lingual tracing, starting with the distal border adjacent to the left palatoglossus muscle. Trace on the composition, flame, dip in hot water and place the tray in the mouth taking care not to distort the composition against the side of the tongue as the tray goes into place. Hold the tray in place with the fingers in each premolar region while at the same time asking the patient to place the tip of the tongue against the tray handle. This action pulls forward the palatoglossal arches and conforms the composition to its correct shape.
6. Continue the lingual tracing, section by section, trimming with the tip of the tongue in the forward position, because in addition to pulling the palatoglossus muscle forwards, this action also raises the floor of the mouth.

   The lateral aspect of a correctly trimmed lingual periphery is shown in Figure 2.30. The notch discernible in the region of the second molar is made by the mylohyoid muscle which, in this region, is just a thin slip merging with the posterior aspect of the mylohyoid ridge.

   The most satisfactory way to trim the lingual periphery is to work forward from the left palatoglossus muscle to the region of the left canine; then forward from the right palatoglossus muscle to the right canine, leaving the area of the lingual frenum to be trimmed last.
7. When adapting the anterolingual periphery, instruct the patient first to protrude the tongue and then roll it back and touch the palate with its tip (Figure 5.27).
8. The final areas to be adapted are over the retromolar pads. Trace both these areas together by applying composition into the fitting surface, and then place the tray in the mouth and hold it with a firm pressure for about 30 s. If the tracing of the entire periphery has been carried out correctly the tray should resist removal and come away with a definite sucking sound.

Retention tests of trimmed tray

Tests for retention and methods of correcting faults are as follows:

1. Protrude the tongue. The tray should remain in place but if it lifts soften the tracing in the palatoglossal areas and readapt.

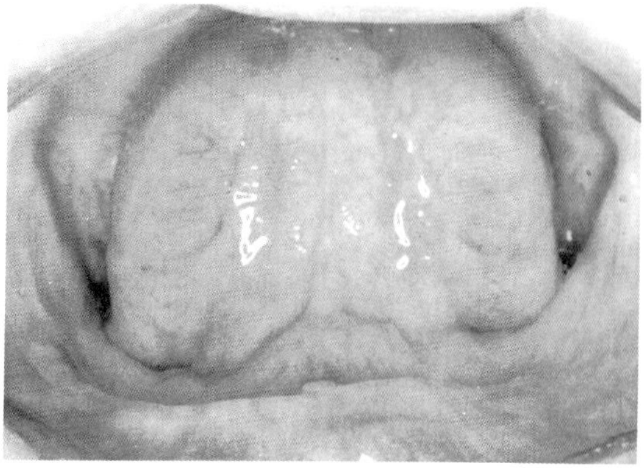

Figure 5.27 Roll the tongue back and touch the palate with its tip

2. Move the tongue in a lateral direction. The tray should remain in place but if it lifts, the lingual extension is too deep on the contralateral side. Soften the tracing on the side which lifts and readapt.
3. Roll the tongue back to touch the palate. The tray should remain in place but if it lifts the lingual extension anteriorly is too deep, and should be softened and readapted.
4. Open the mouth. If the tray lifts, soften and readapt the buccal and labial peripheries.
5. Grasp the handle and exert a vertical upward pull. Resistance should be felt, but if the tray comes away easily, tracing stick should be added to the lingual periphery in the premolar regions and readapted.
6. Exert forward pressure on the distal aspect of the handle. The tray should resist and only come free with a sucking sound. If there is no resistance add composition over the retromolar areas and readapt.

Completing the lower impression

Having carefully adapted the periphery by muscle-trimming there still remains to be obtained the detailed impression of the peripheral and fitting surfaces. This is most satisfactorily done by using an impression paste. Squeeze 6 cm of each paste on to a mixing pad and mix until the colour is uniform. (Some manufacturers supply a liquid thinner of natural oils to make the paste less viscous if this is thought desirable.)

Spread a thin layer over the dry tray, including all the tracing stick, place the tray in the mouth and seat firmly. Instruct the patient to bring the tongue forwards as the operator works the cheeks and lip around the buccal and labial peripheries. Hold the tray in place for at least 2 min and then ask the patient to rinse his mouth with cold water. Remove the impression and place in a bowl of cold water, fitting surface upwards, supported by a submerged gauze square to prevent its edges being spoiled by contact with the bowl.

Examine the periphery of the completed impression. It may be found that areas of tracing stick show through the paste, while in other areas the paste has covered the composition and corrected the slight inaccuracies of adaptation. The surface of the paste impression should appear smooth and duplicate the surface details. Faults in a paste impression are easily corrected by drying the inaccurate area, spreading over it a thin layer of freshly mixed paste, and re-seating. The completed impression may be placed in the mouth and tested, when it should be practically impossible for the patient to dislodge it by any of the usual movements of the tongue, cheeks or lips.

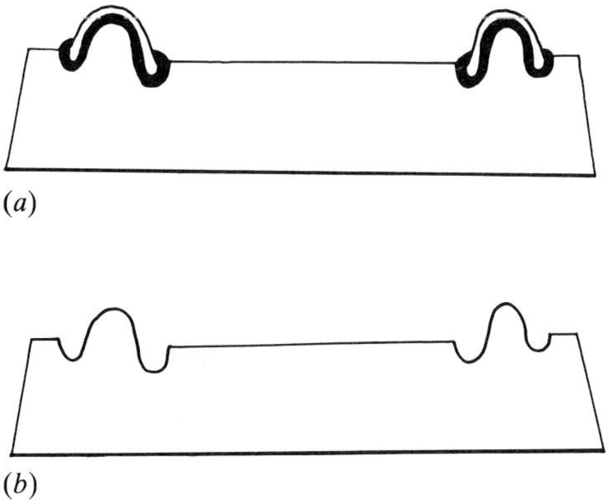

Figure 5.28 (*a*) Stone cast poured with impression in place. (*b*) Cast after impression has been removed. Note how the peripheries of the impression have been reproduced on the cast

Pouring the impression

In pouring the impression the dental stone is brought up the external surfaces of the flanges to a height of 3 mm in order that the peripheral contour, including its actual breadth, is suitably recorded and finally reproduced in the finished denture (Figure 5.28). The best way of ensuring this is to box the impression and vibrate the vacuum-mixed stone into it. It will be appreciated that the clinical stage for this impression is detailed and exacting and producing an accurate cast is equally important.

Muscle-trimmed upper impression

The technique just described for muscle-trimming or border moulding of lower impressions can also be used in upper impressions and there are no essential differences in technique.

On the preliminary upper cast one is more likely to find undercuts than in the lower cast and these should be blocked out with wax before laying down a spacer of 0.5 mm thickness otherwise the impression paste may be distorted at the final stage.

In addition to buccal and labial muscle-trimming an upper tray should be postdammed. The technique for postdamming is to add a tracing of composition along the fitting surface of the posterior palatal border, joining the buccal tracings round the tuberosities. This composition is then softened in the usual way, and the tray inserted and held firmly in place. The patient is instructed to swallow several times in order to mould the tracing in the hamular notches to its functional position.

It should be understood that the technique of muscle-trimming is entirely different from the buccal trim already described for upper plaster impressions in which the aim is to determine the width of the pre-extraction sulcus by means of a relatively stiff addition of tracing stick. With the sulcus held out at this width a fluid impression material, such as plaster, is able to determine the height of the sulcus appropriate to the particular width. Plaster is particularly applicable to this principle, not only because it can be made in a very fluid mix which sets quickly, but also because it is hydrophilic and possesses a degree of 'body' to fill the empty sulcus space. This property of being hydrophilic means that the material is compatible with the wet surface of an edentulous sulcus, often made wetter by the extra salivation during impressions, and in contradistinction to hydrophobic materials like polysulphide and silicone rubber which will be discussed later.

Muscle-trimming, unlike the technique of buccal trim, attempts to define the three-dimensional form of the peripheral sulcus by functional means at one time and it is likely that at any one point along the periphery the tracing stick may be narrow and deep or broad and shallow, the final form depending on the amount and viscosity of the tracing stick, the degree of muscle-trimming by the patient or operator, and so on. There is, therefore, an element of chance in the final product and so time and great care must be spent in the clinical procedure and reliance must be placed on the final testing of the muscle-trimmed tray before applying the impression paste. It will be obvious that the muscle-trimmed periphery is likely to be narrower and higher, in general, than the buccal trim which will produce a broader and shallower periphery on the finished denture.

The technique of buccal trim (as described for plaster impressions) can also be used with impression paste as long as it is appreciated that the space between the edge of the trimmed tray and the height of the sulcus is sufficiently small that the impression paste can fill it without slumping. Impression paste is essentially a wash material and cannot be used as a space-filler in the same way that plaster can. Therefore, if impression paste is being used as the final wash material along with a buccal trim, rather than a muscle-trimmed periphery, a very fine judgement must be applied to the height of the periphery before adding the paste, if errors are to be avoided in the master impression.

Alginate (irreversible hydrocolloid)

The use of this material for preliminary impressions has already been described and only the points related to its use for recording master impressions will be mentioned.

Individual trays, with a space of at least 2 mm on the preliminary casts, should be made of a rigid material, preferably cold-cure acrylic, although thermo-formed polymer sheet or metal-filled shellac may be used.

It is essential, as in all individual trays, to check the depth of the tray flanges at the start and cut back over-extensions with a suitable rotary bur. Location stops of tracing stick should be used as any pressure on the setting alginate due to movement of the tray will result in stresses within the material which will distort the impression after removal from the mouth.

The periphery of each tray should be adapted with tracing stick rather than wax or silicone putty, neither of which is compatible with the surface texture of alginate.

On the upper tray the best form of tracing stick addition is that described for ZOE impressions. The muscle-trimming need not be so exact, however, and should be kept slightly short of the functional depth and width of the sulcus because alginate is a much more viscous material than impression paste and over-extensions should be avoided. For the same reason the rheological properties of the selected alginate are important and a viscous material, which might be suitable for partial dentures, should not be used.

A postdam is essential. If any alginate creeps beyond the back of the tray during insertion the excess can be swept away with a curved spatula before gelation starts, otherwise this unsupported excess will cause stresses within the rest of the impression.

The most effective method of retaining the alginate to the tray is to use a polyamide adhesive and it should be painted not only on the fitting surface of the tray but also on the buccal side of the tracing stick to hold the alginate as it turns over the periphery. Failure to do this will result in minute tears which may not be seen but which will result in impression inaccuracies.

On the lower tray the best form of tracing stick addition is that described for lower plaster impressions as these additions aid the repositioning of the surrounding muscles and indirectly, therefore, the shape and form of the buccal and lingual sulcus. For the lower impression a slightly more viscous alginate may be used because, like a plaster impression technique, there is more space to fill but it should always be remembered that the areolar tissue of the sulcus is very liable to be distorted by a stiff material. It is not surprising, therefore, that alginate impressions are often over-extended and frequently asymmetric such that they have to be discarded.

It is in the pouring of the impressions to produce the master casts that alginate is particularly vulnerable because the material, being elastic, is easily distorted. It is theoretically possible to box alginate impressions but in practice it is difficult as the material cannot be allowed to dry and is not conducive to normal boxing methods. Alginate can also be distorted if it is handled too much. It is usually better, therefore, to pour alginate impres-

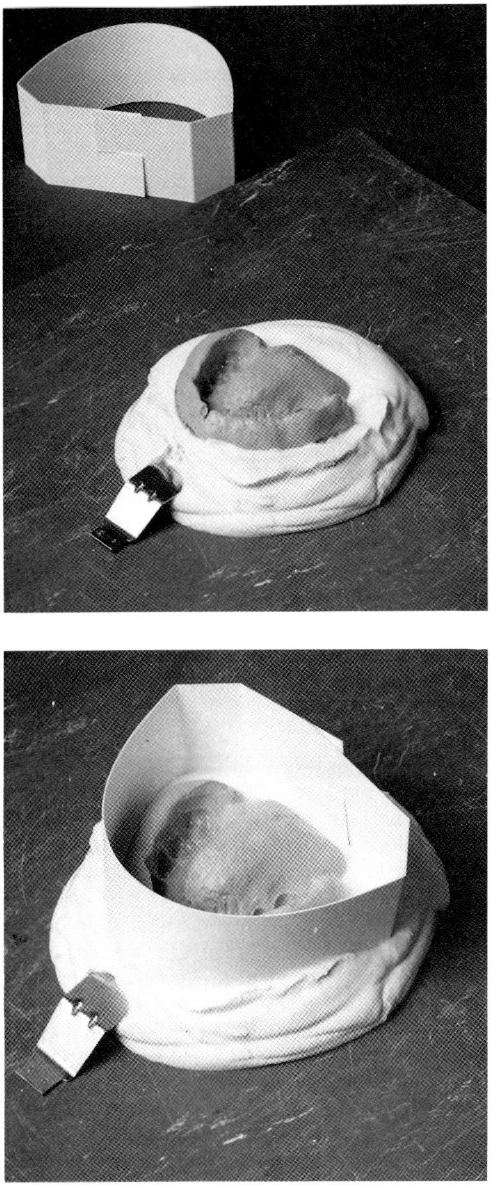

Figure 5.29 A method of boxing an alginate impression (see text)

sions in two stages: dental stone is vibrated into the impression sufficient to cover the alginate while the impression is still cradled and, when set, this stone is based either with a second mix of stone or dental plaster. If boxing is considered essential the impression is laid into a mix of plaster and surrounded by a paper former. When set the plaster is coated with a separating agent and poured in dental stone (Figure 5.29).

Elastomers (polysulphides and silicones)

There are many similarities in the use of these materials to the ones already described and only points of difference will be mentioned.

Polysulphides

These are also known as rubber-base materials or thiokol rubbers. They consist of two pastes: a base paste, containing polysulphide and filler (usually titanium dioxide), and an activator paste, containing lead dioxide, sulphur and oil.

Equal ropes of each paste are spatulated to produce a homogeneous mix which, by polymerization and cross-linkage, forms an elastic solid in a few minutes. Polysulphides are produced in various degrees of viscosity and normally for master impressions for complete dentures the medium-bodied is used (Figure 5.30).

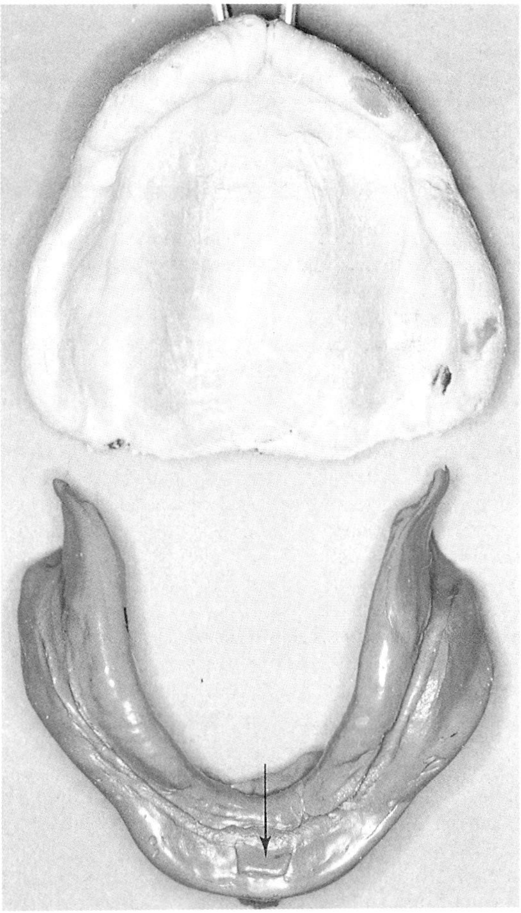

Figure 5.30 Master impressions. Upper plaster; lower polysulphide (medium-bodied). Arrow indicates location stop (tracing stick) penetrating the elastomer

Preparation of individual trays, made with a spacer thickness of a sheet of modelling wax (1.3 mm), is similar to that for alginate impressions. Because of the relatively long setting time in the mouth, and because the setting is a polymerization process, it is desirable that location stops are prepared on each tray with tracing stick so that there is minimum movement of the tray. Retention of the material to the tray is by a rubber adhesive which should be applied, in advance of mixing the pastes, not only on the fitting surface but also to the peripheral surfaces to prevent separation from the tray. Polysulphide is a hydrophobic material and behaves badly in a wet edentulous mouth in the sense that it tends to track away from the impression tray over the mucus-covered mucosa. In an upper impression the material can slump away from the sulcus depth to give rise to inaccuracies. This fault can be partly rectified by using a heavy-bodied grade but then the viscosity of this is such that it causes inaccuracy in the sulcus by displacing the tissue.

Polysulphide is useful where undercuts exist because of its elastic properties and good tear strength. The impression should be removed quickly from undercuts to ensure the best elastic behaviour of the material.

Silicones

These consist of two components: a base, comprising a silicone polymer and a filler which by variation in its content can produce varying viscosities of the base (i.e. putty, paste or wash) and a reactor, comprising a cross-linking agent and an activator. (If the reactor contains a filler then it is produced in the form of a paste.)

The material sets by a cross-linking reaction, in some products as a condensation-curing (with by-products such as alcohol or hydrogen), in others as an addition-curing with no by-products. There is a very wide range of these materials but the usual method of use in complete denture impressions is as follows.

An individual tray is made of a rigid material such as cold-cure acrylic with a fairly large spacer of 3 mm. The periphery is checked in the mouth for possible inaccuracies or over-extensions and cut or modified accordingly. No further additions are made to the tray before applying the silicone impression material, usually in two stages. First, a putty is applied over the whole surface of the tray, rather like using impression compound, and the tray placed in the mouth. Lips and cheeks are activated to muscle-trim the periphery and the material allowed to set to a flexible dough. Secondly, the putty is dried and coated with a mix of silicone in the form of a wash which bonds chemically and which provides the final accuracy and fine surface detail.

Other silicones are dispensed as pastes and, in the form of medium viscosity materials, may be used in a one-stage technique like the polysulphides.

These elastic materials are useful where undercuts exist and they are dimensionally accurate. They have drawbacks in that they are hydrophobic and the varying degrees of viscosity are difficult to handle, particularly in an edentulous mouth with its wide spectrum of tissue properties from mucoperiosteum, tightly bound-down, to loosely woven areolar tissue in the sulcus. For these reasons, the putty silicones can cause distortions and displacements of tissue which cannot readily be rectified by the hydrophobic, low viscosity silicone washes.

Special impression techniques

There are a number of special impression techniques that are useful in dealing with particular clinical circumstances:

1. Composition compression impression.
2. Displaceable maxillary ridge.
3. Unemployed mandibular ridge.
4. Denture space impression.
5. Biometric impression trays.

Composition compression impression

There are often considerable differences in density and thickness of the mucosa in different parts of the denture-bearing area, usually, though by no means always, more marked in the upper than in the lower. The following technique, which has a number of slight variations, is designed to take an impression of these tissues under pressure so that, under the stresses of mastication, the pressure transmitted through the entire mucosa to the underlying bone is approximately equal over its whole surface. Unfortunately, this ideal can never be attained since pressure can only be evenly transmitted to the bone when all the mucosa is fully compressed and this state may not be achieved by the operator when taking the impression. Further, as masticatory stress is variable, this will result in variable compressibility of the mucosa and uneven pressure on the supporting bone. Nevertheless, this type of impression results in a denture which has excellent support, requires no relieving and, since the periphery is functionally adapted, possesses adequate retention.

Composition (impression compound) with its high viscosity, is the only material suitable for this technique and by varying its degree of softness, and thereby its rate of flow, the amount of compression obtainable can be controlled within reasonable limits. A compression impression which has been thoroughly chilled, its surface heated and the impression reseated can exert far greater compression than one in which the composition is equally softened throughout its entire mass.

A composition should be selected which softens at a temperature around 65°C, flows readily when softened, can be flamed without burning or blistering and which sets hard at mouth temperature. It is a help, and a considerable time saver, to have a thermostatically controlled water bath set at the optimum temperature for the material being used. A bowl of iced water to chill the impression will save chairside time, but cold tap water can be used equally well except that it takes longer.

The individual tray

An individual tray is always required for this technique and it should be made in the following way.

Preliminary impressions are recorded with a low-viscosity alginate or plaster to obtain mucostatic impressions and casts with good surface detail. Individual trays are made in cold-cure acrylic with a spacer between the cast and the tray of 3 mm. The periphery of the trays is made to the level of the mucogingival line, i.e. well short of the mucobuccal fold. The maxillary tray extends about 5 mm on to the soft palate and straight across from one hamular notch to the other; the mandibular tray finishes a few millimetres on to the pear-shaped pad. Each tray must be rigid and to ensure this the spine may be reinforced with an addition of acrylic or wire. A vertical handle in the midline, projecting at an angle of the incisor teeth, completes the design.

Cover the whole tray with an even thickness of new composition; composition which has been used even once is quite useless for this purpose as many of the more volatile constituents will have been lost, thus altering its working properties, raising its softening point, and decreasing its ability to flow. Cover the surface of the composition with petroleum jelly and make an impression of the cast, making sure the material flows into the mucobuccal fold. Tease the compound around the tray edge and chill the whole in cold water. Cut off any obvious excess with a knife.

The impression

Besides bowls of hot and cold water, a small pin-point flame will be required. Only the upper impression will be described as the technique for the lower is similar.

Soften the surface of the composition lining the tray by immersing in hot water. As soon as the composition has become uniformly soft, it is seated in the mouth with only gentle pressure, and no precautions are taken against distorting the surrounding soft tissues by over-extension as this will be corrected at a later stage. The impression should be held in place until it has hardened which usually takes about 2 min. It is then withdrawn and immediately placed in the bowl of cold water, being left there until it is thoroughly hard right through. Composition is a very poor thermal conductor and if cold tap water is being used, it should be chilled for at least as long as was spent in heating; this applies to every occasion when heat is applied.

The impression is now dried, the whole surface heated rapidly with a small flame until glossy, dipped for a moment in hot water, seated in the mouth and pressure applied. The reasons for each step mentioned are as follows:

1. It is dried as otherwise it will be unevenly heated and softened.
2. Rapid heating of the surface will leave the remainder of the composition hard so that pressure can be applied without distorting it.
3. Flamed composition, like hot sealing-wax, will stick and burn so every time a flame is used the impression must be dipped into hot water before being inserted in the mouth (this process is often referred to as 'tempering').

The pressure in the upper must be directed upwards, and a more evenly balanced pressure is obtained by pressing with one finger in the centre of the palate than one finger of each hand on either side. This is because right-handed people unconsciously tend to press harder with the right hand, and this would make for uneven compression. If both hands are used, however, uneven pressure may be checked by reference to the patient, and if the pressure appeared to him to be less on one side than the other, then the whole of this step must be repeated with greater care.

Remove the impression when hard and place at once in cold water; this cooling immediately on removal from the mouth must be carried out throughout the whole technique, as the residual heat in the deeper layers will cause distortion, even during handling.

So far, an impression has been obtained which, under an upward and backward load of unknown quantity, will bear equally on hard and soft areas, but which is somewhat over-extended and has no peripheral seal.

The peripheral borders are now trimmed with a sharp knife until they are approximately 3 mm short of the functional position of the sulci and frena, and the width is also reduced to about 3 mm by removing part of the rolled border in contact with the cheeks and lip. Particular attention must be paid to this stage of the technique as any composition that impinges on the sulci or frena will result in the finished denture being dislodged by muscular activity.

Once this trimming of the impression is completed, the periphery is rebuilt and adapted section by section, using a low-fusing tracing composition in stick form. Begin at the distal end of one buccal

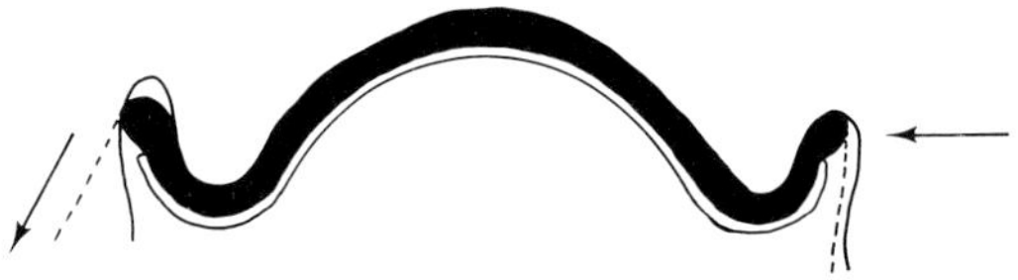

Figure 5.31 Right side of diagram illustrates the direction in which pressure must be applied to keep the composition in contact with the tissues when functional trimming is being carried out. Left side illustrates what occurs if the cheek is merely pulled outwards and downwards

border, dry, add tracing composition for 2–3 cm, flame, temper, insert and mould for the functional position. Details of trimming for the functional position have already been given in previous techniques, but emphasis must be laid on the fact that some pressure must be maintained to keep the soft composition in contact with the mucosa of the ridge so that excess composition will be rolled to the correct position and not pulled away (Figure 5.31).

Repeat the procedure until the whole periphery from tuberosity to tuberosity has been re-adapted and, after each section has been trimmed, place the impression in cold water until it is thoroughly hard.

The posterior palatal border still remains to be adapted and this is done as follows.

The vibrating line of the soft palate is first located, usually by asking the patient to open his mouth widely and say a prolonged 'ah', when the movement of the palate is easily seen. This line may be marked in the mouth with an indelible pencil. Dry the impression, add a tracing on the fitting surface on the vibrating line, flame, temper, place in the mouth and hold in the centre of the palate with a firm pressure. Chill thoroughly after removal.

There remain two areas which so far have received no attention, the hamular notches, and it is here that the final seal is produced. Place a tracing in both these areas and, after the usual routine, seat the impression firmly in position and ask the patient to swallow several times which will trim the soft tissues in these regions.

The impression should now be complete and it should be impossible for the patient to dislodge it by any normal movement of the lips and cheeks.

Tests for retention

1. Upward and outward pressure in the incisor region. If the impression can be dislodged without great difficulty the posterior border requires further postdamming.
2. Upward and outward pressure in the premolar regions. If the impression falls, then further peripheral seal is required on the opposite side, usually around the tuberosity. Sometimes a difficult air leak can be spotted by seeing a small collection of bubbles at one spot on the periphery and this must be corrected in the usual way.
3. Pulling down the upper lip. Over-extension in the labial sulcus is common and if this test dislodges the impression the labial periphery must be readapted.

   At some point during the impression the seal will become sufficiently good to make removal of the impression difficult, and this can be overcome by asking the patient to close the lips and blow out the cheeks, thus forcing air under the impression and allowing it to drop.

Difficulties

The commonest cause of failure with this technique is impatience on the part of the operator at the time spent in chilling the impression but, unless it is thoroughly hardened after each insertion in the mouth, warpage will occur and the only remedy for this warpage is to start the impression over again from the very first step as there are no short cuts.

Refining the impression

With a very careful clinical technique the surface detail of the composition, and the junction between the tracing stick and composition, is sufficiently good to pour the master cast. In many cases, however, an impression paste wash is desirable to refine the surface before pouring the impression. It must be emphasized that the technique has been designed to obtain uniform compression of tissues, so, for this reason, the final wash must be as thin as possible, otherwise all the clinical effort will be wasted. The only satisfactory material for this wash is one of the eugenol-free impression pastes in which the eugenol has been replaced by carboxylic acid. This material can be further improved for the technique by reducing its already low viscosity by the addition of a few drops of thinning liquid, composed of natural oils such as light mineral, linseed or olive oil. During the setting of this wash pressure must be maintained on the tray otherwise compression will be lost. The importance of using a rigid tray in this technique must be obvious. When the paste wash has set the impression is removed and chilled. In a successful result the composition should show through the wash signifying that the latter is sufficiently thin and that compression has been maintained.

Note on closed mouth impression technique

Variations on the compression impressions just described are used in conjunction with occlusion rims in the closed mouth technique in which the master impressions and jaw relation record are made simultaneously under functional conditions of occlusal loading. This technique is discussed in Chapter 6.

Note on mucostatics

A number of clinicians adopt a different point of view about impressions and believe that a mucostatic technique is better than mucocompressive.

A mucostatic denture base is one that maintains a constant relation to the supporting tissue and to obtain this the impression is recorded without distortion of the mucosa. As the retention of the base depends entirely on surface forces of adhesion and cohesion, a minimum film of saliva is necessary. For these reasons the patient is often pre-medicated with atropine to reduce salivary flow so that the surface of the impression, made in low-viscosity impression paste, is in very close and intimate contact with the mucosa.

Advocates of this view believe that mucosa behaves as a liquid so that pressure on it is transmitted in all directions. In this sense the mucosa cannot be compressed, only distorted or displaced, and a mucostatic base is as firm on soft tissue as it is on bone when vertical load is applied.

In order to maintain the mucostatic theme, the denture base is finished without encroaching on muscle tissue and so the periphery is much shallower and thinner than with other techniques. An impression, based on the theory of mucostatics, should follow the same outline. The small periphery does not prevent lateral movement of the denture and so, on the lower denture, a shallow lingual flange is used to resist this displacement. This arrangement has been likened to the flange on the inside of a railway truck wheel. On the upper denture the flange, made short of muscle activity, also offers little resistance to lateral or anteroposterior displacement but, in this denture, physical retention from surface forces is said to suffice.

Displaceable maxillary ridge

A relatively common finding in the upper jaw is an anterior ridge which is displaceable, often described as flabby. It is often seen in cases where the natural lower anterior teeth have occluded against a complete upper denture without adequate restoration of the posterior occlusion. Consequently, the anterior excessive load causes bony resorption and a massaging forwards of the anterior palatal mucosa of the rugal area. These cases often show the incisive papilla lying towards the front of the flabby ridge and the bunched pairs of palatal rugae on the crest of the ridge (Figure 5.32). Such tissue has developed under conditions of load and causes little discomfort but the problem is one of deficient support as the present denture, and any future denture, always shifts on the unfavourable foundation. In many cases, the displaceable ridge extends backwards and sometimes even involves the tuberosities.

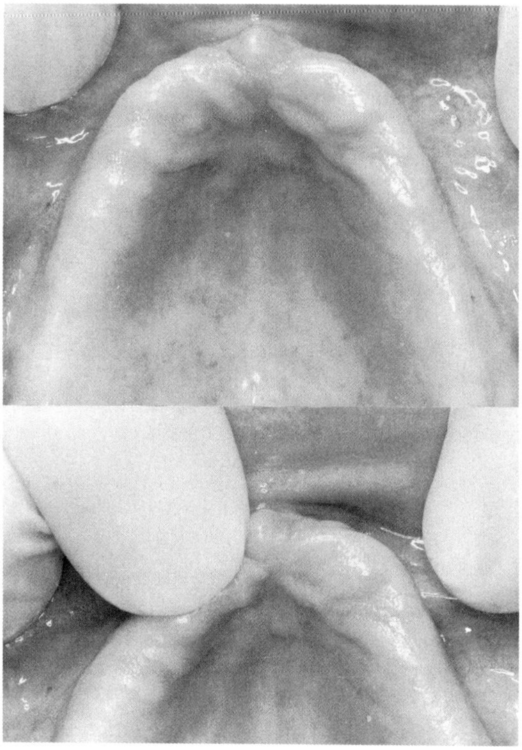

Figure 5.32 Maxillary anterior displaceable (flabby) ridge

Impression techniques

Mucocompression without displacement

This is a two-stage technique designed to compress the flabby tissue so that the compression throughout the whole of the maxillary denture-bearing area is as uniform as possible.

The preliminary impression is made with plaster in a fluid mix with anti-expansion solution. Before using the plaster the periphery and postdam of the stock tray should be rimmed with impression compound or tracing stick to ensure a more accurate adaptation. The plaster should be puddled in the mouth to avoid displacing the ridge. Pour the impression and make a cold-cure acrylic tray.

The second stage is to check the extension of the individual tray in the mouth and modify it in depth where necessary. A composition impression is made from the cast and chilled in water. The periphery is adapted with a knife and tracing stick which is also added on the postdam region to complete the border seal. At this stage the impression should have adequate retention with the upper lip repositioned to its approximate pre-extraction form. The flabby area is outlined in the mouth with indelible pencil, the impression re-inserted and then removed to show the outline on the impression surface. With a small pipette flame the surface surrounding the

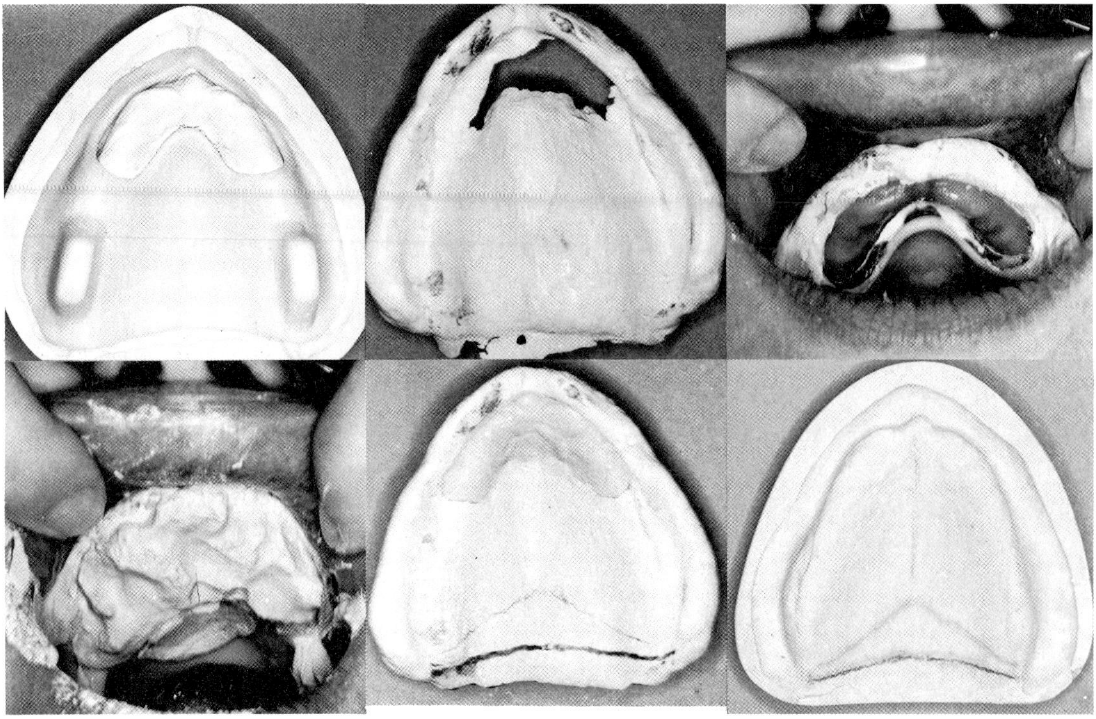

Figure 5.33 Open-window impression technique for maxillary displaceable ridge (see text)

flabby area is softened leaving the compound overlying the flabby area hard. The impression is tempered through water at 65–70°C and inserted quickly into the mouth. Load should be applied in a vertical direction to compress the flabby tissue without displacing it. This procedure may have to be repeated once or twice until the impression withstands an upward dislodging force. The impression is dried and completed by an impression paste wash, using one of the eugenol-free impression pastes with a drop or two of thinner to reduce the viscosity. The impression is kept under heavy load during the setting of the paste to maintain the compression of the flabby tissue. If the impression has been made properly the compound should show through the very thin wash in the flabby ridge area. The postdam area is marked with indelible pencil.

Mucostatic, open-window technique (Figure 5.33)

On the preliminary cast an individual tray is made with an opening surrounding the flabby tissue. The periphery of the tray is corrected in the mouth with tracing stick and an impression-paste wash made. When this is set, the tray is removed and excess paste around the opening is trimmed away. Reinsert the tray and apply a mix of impression plaster over the flabby tissue which lies in the window. When the plaster has set remove the whole. This technique avoids distortion of the flabby, displaceable tissue but the resultant support of the denture is less efficient than that obtained by the previous technique. Consequently, the denture is more liable to shift under occlusal load.

Unemployed mandibular ridge

In a patient who has had a complete lower denture for a number of years, alveolar resorption continues. This resorption mainly affects the alveolar ridge which consequently becomes smaller in height and width. The end result is that, over the years, support of the denture becomes progressively transferred to the peripheral parts of the denture-bearing area while the alveolar ridge takes less and less of the load. In this sense the ridge crest becomes 'unemployed'. It often happens in these cases that the alveolar bone resorbs unevenly and at a quicker rate than the soft tissues, with the result that the ridge crest is composed almost entirely of mucosa and connective tissue while the amount of alveolar bone is very small. The lower denture is often fairly comfortable because the changes are gradual and progressive, but on finger palpation the ridge crest is

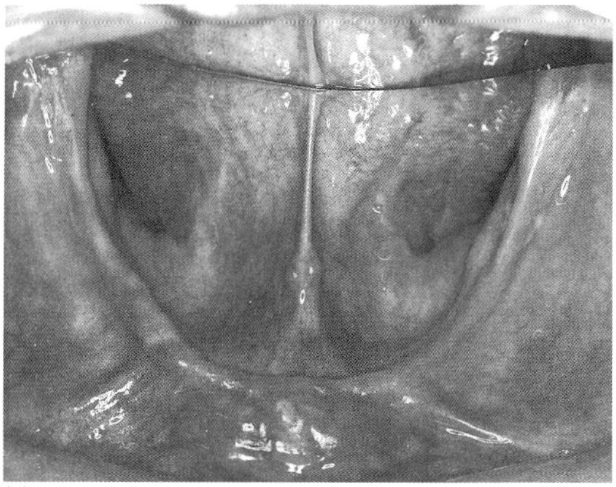

(*a*)

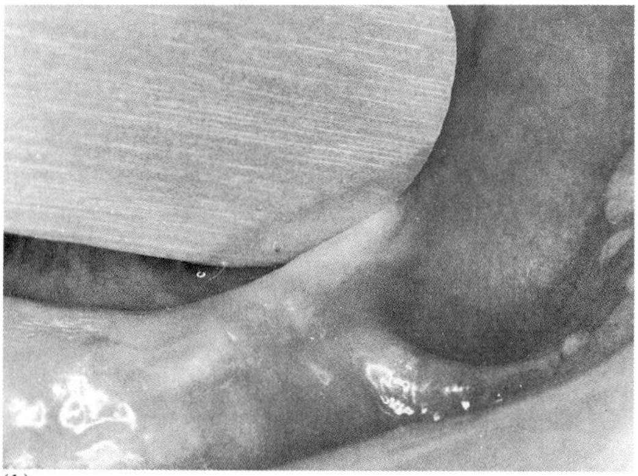

(*b*)

Figure 5.34 Unemployed lower ridge. (*a*) Typical narrow alveolar ridge. (*b*) An unemployed ridge is easily displaced because of the bony resorption

painful although it may not be painful when the denture is in the mouth.

Examination of the mouth usually shows small areas of hyperkeratosis in the peripheral parts of the denture-bearing area because of the load transfer, while the ridge crest is mobile and easily displaced in a buccolingual direction (Figure 5.34). The amount of mobile tissue varies in different patients but, in the extreme case, it may extend from one molar region around to the other, while the degree of mobility also varies and depends on the amount of resorption that has taken place and the time lapse since the denture was made. The problem in this so-called unemployed ridge becomes apparent at the time of making the replacement denture and, if the situation is not recognized, the impression displaces the ridge and places load directly on the crest. Because the crest of the ridge has become unused to accepting any load over the years a denture made from such an impression will have the same detrimental effect (Figure 5.35). The clinical result of this is usually that the patient cannot tolerate the replacement denture in the mouth because of

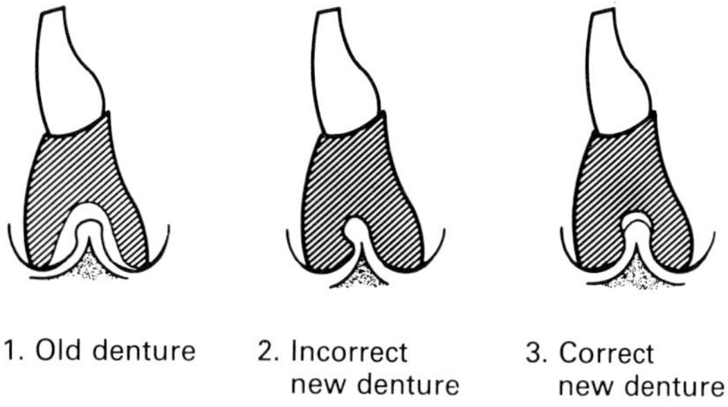

Figure 5.35 Lower unemployed ridge. The object is to design a denture with maximum extension without loading the crest of the residual alveolar ridge

discomfort or pain due to the crest of the ridge experiencing load for the first time for many years. For these reasons the best treatment for this kind of case is given below.

The preliminary impression is recorded in a stock tray with the periphery adapted with compound. The impression material can either be alginate, in the milder cases, or plaster in the more painful and more easily displaced cases. This impression is poured in dental stone and an individual tray made in cold-cure acrylic with a spacer of 2 mm. The part of the tray overlying the ridge crest is perforated with a 2 mm round bur at approximately centimetre intervals. An impression compound impression is taken of the cast with this tray and chilled. This produces a mucostatic impression and when this is placed in the mouth it may cause the patient some discomfort because load is being applied to the crest of the ridge. The periphery of this impression is still inaccurate and so it is trimmed by cutting back the compound and applying tracing stick around the periphery. This is continued until the impression is retentive in the mouth. The compound over the ridge is then cut with a sharp knife or a large slow-running bur until the tray and the holes are exposed. Any rough edges of compound are carefully cleared away and when this impression is placed in the mouth and loaded it should not cause any pain or discomfort. If it does, more compound should be cleared away. The holes in the tray, now exposed, release the peripheral seal and the impression may feel loose. The last stage of the technique is to dry the impression and record the working surface with impression paste under heavy digital pressure to transfer as much of the load as possible to the peripheral parts of the denture-bearing area.

At this last stage the impression paste exudes out of the holes and prevents any load being applied to the unemployed part of the ridge. In a correctly made impression the compound periphery shines

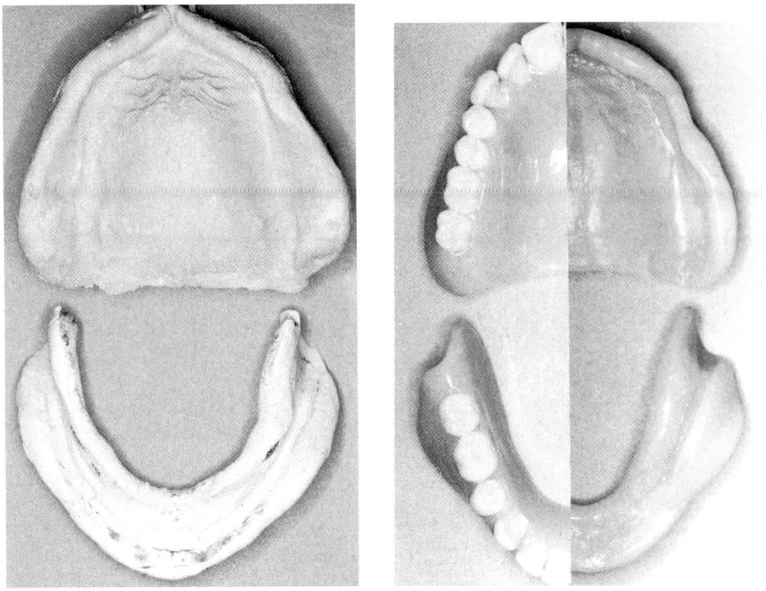

(*a*) (*b*)

Figure 5.36 Lower unemployed ridge. (*a*) The completed impressions and (*b*) the finished dentures for the same case (the upper impression is plaster)

through the very thin impression-paste wash, while the impression paste over the crest of the ridge is fairly thick (Figure 5.36). From this fact one can conclude that the impression recorded is mucostatic over the crest of the ridge and mucocompressive on the peripheral parts. If the denture is made on this cast, it can be inserted without any symptoms of pain or discomfort.

Denture space impression

The denture space is the space in the edentulous mouth previously occupied by the natural teeth and tissues which have been lost. It is sometimes desirable to record this space functionally so that the design and shape of the denture, particularly the lower, is in harmony with the surrounding facial muscles and tongue. It is particularly useful in those patients who have difficulty in controlling a denture or who are sensitive to different shapes in their mouths, often referred to as stereognostic oral sense.

There are a number of different techniques (sometimes known as piezographic) but all rely on using materials that can be moulded by contraction and relaxation of muscle and then gel or set to retain the resultant shape.

1. On a master upper cast make a record block and carve it to restore the upper lip.
2. On a lower cast make an acrylic base with a vertical upstand in the approximate buccolingual position of the teeth.
3. Register the retruded jaw relation (see Chapter 6).
4. Cover the lower base with a visco-elastic material which reacts to repetitive forces over a period of time; tissue conditioners, which gel but do not set, are ideal for this purpose. Alternatives are impression wax and, to a lesser extent, ZOE or alginate.
5. It is best to keep the jaws in the retruded contact position while the patient moves the cheeks, lips and tongue through their full functional range for 5–10 min (Figure 5.37).
6. The resultant impression is poured with buccal and lingual registers or indices and when the acrylic base and impression material are discarded the resultant space is used to fabricate the denture (Figure 5.38).

Biometric impression trays

It can be argued that complete dentures should be designed to restore the lips and cheeks to their pre-extraction form and position. Master impressions should record fitting and peripheral surfaces that will be exactly copied in the finished dentures. Therefore, if individual trays are made to biometric measurements of the average changes which take place after teeth are extracted, then it is likely that such trays will lead to more refined and precise impressions. This is the basis of the design of biometric trays.

Maxillary tray

1. Mark the mucogingival line on the cast and draw another line 3 mm below this (i.e. nearer the mucobuccal fold).

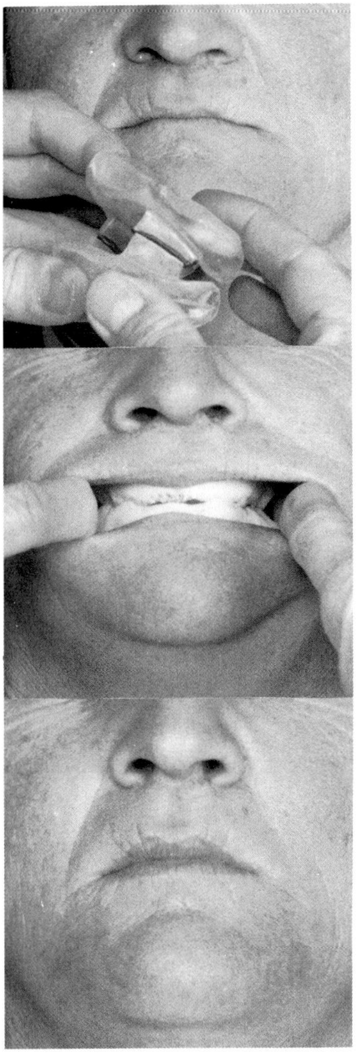

Figure 5.37 Denture space impression. Acrylic bases are coated with tissue conditioner which the patient moulds with the surrounding musculature

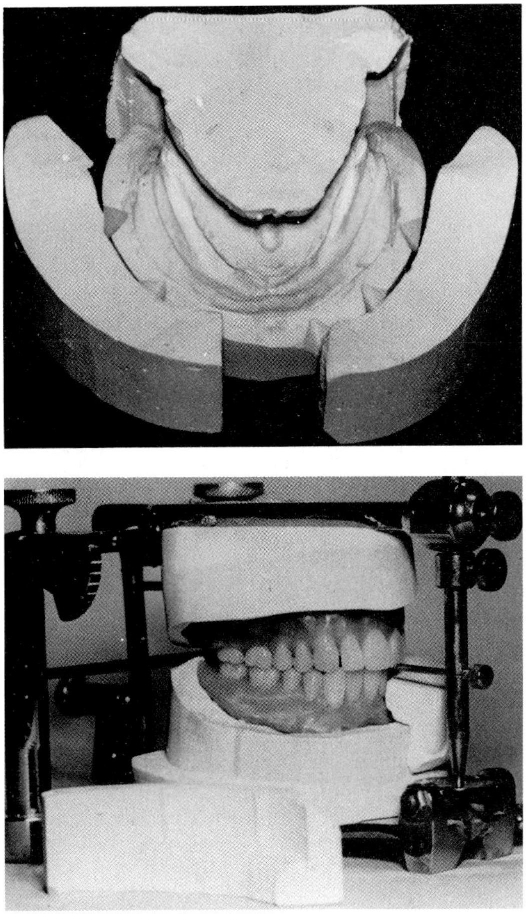

Figure 5.38 Denture space impression. The impression is poured in stone and buccal and lingual registers are keyed around it. The resulting space is filled by the teeth and denture base. (Note the convex/concave shape of the buccal surface of the lower denture as determined by the active buccal musculature)

2. Fill the space between the second line and the mucobuccal fold with wax.
3. From the remnant of the palatal gingival margin mark off in the various regions as follows:
   sagittal incisor 6 mm
   coronal canine 8 mm
   coronal premolar 10 mm
   coronal molar 12 mm.
4. Join the marks to provide the buccal outline of the tray (Figure 5.39)
5. Lay a 0.5 mm spacer.
6. Make a cold-cure acrylic tray.

This tray is checked in the mouth. A localizing stop and postdam are added in tracing stick and the impression completed with impression paste, making sure that the paste flows round the periphery on to the facial surface (Figure 5.40).

Mandibular tray

1. The aim is to construct a tray that holds the lip and cheeks in their pre-extraction position so that the impression material is supported as it flows round the tray edge up against the tissues.
2. A spacer of 0.5 mm is laid on the preliminary cast and the tray constructed in cold-cure acrylic so that it represents as far as possible the finished denture.
3. The molar region is convex buccally.
4. the premolar region is narrower and more concave.

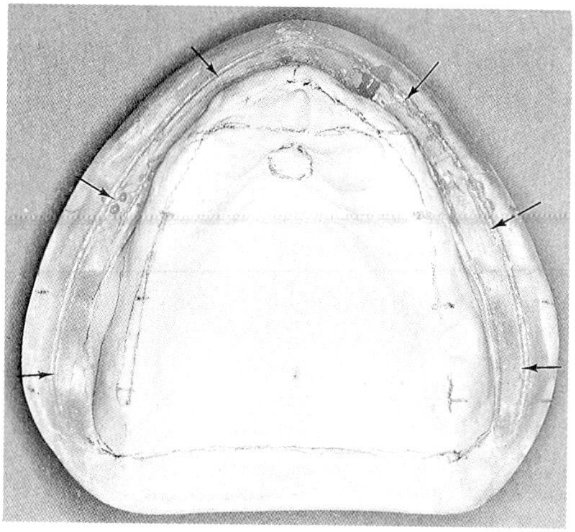

Figure 5.39 Biometric maxillary tray. On the preliminary cast the buccal outline for the tray is marked off on the wax in the sulcus (see text)

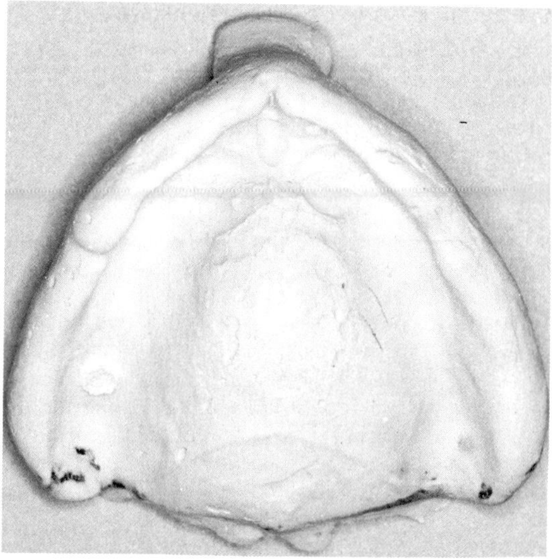

Figure 5.40 Biometric maxillary tray. The completed zinc oxide–eugenol (ZOE) impression

5. The incisor region slopes forward to simulate the natural tooth inclination, this part acting as a handle.
6. Location stops may be used in the mouth particularly if a slow-setting impression material is being used, such as polysulphide rubber which, in a dry mouth, is a good material for this technique. In a wet mouth, impression paste is better. Whichever material is used it should be smeared over the whole of the tray including the buccal, labial and lingual surfaces to obtain an impression of the fitting, peripheral and polished surfaces with the mouth half-open. The lip, cheeks and tongue are supported in their pre-extraction position to ensure the sulcus form is correct while the material sets (Figure 5.41).

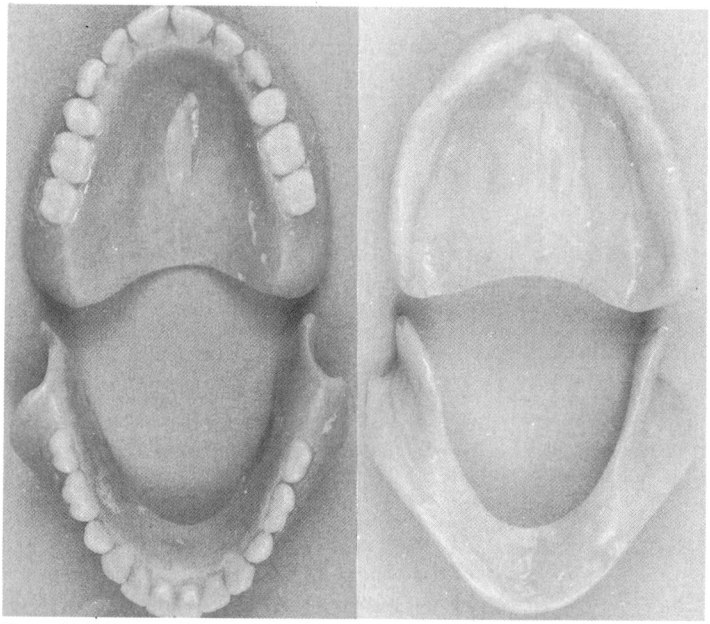

Figure 5.41 Biometric lower tray. Complete lower denture made from impression in a biometric tray. Note the wide base extension, the narrow buccolingual width of the occlusal surface and the proclined position of the lower incisors, all factors defined by the impression technique

General remarks on impressions

Most of the difficulties encountered when making impressions can be traced to the operator's lack of attention to details of technique, and especially the acceptance of a poor stock tray impression with the comment that, 'it will be good enough for making an individual tray'. It is of extreme importance that the preliminary impression records the entire possible denture-bearing surface but, at the same time, does not encroach on the movable muscular tissues.

Individual trays must be carefully checked for possible over-extension and, whatever the material of choice, it is necessary to ensure that sufficient space exists in all regions between the fitting surface of the tray and the tissues to be recorded. A suitable thickness of material is necessary to ensure dimensional accuracy and to avoid contact of mucosa by the tray.

Nausea

A disturbing factor experienced by some patients is the sensitivity of the soft palate and the dorsum of the tongue to foreign bodies; such conditions may produce retching (gagging) and in rare instances actual vomiting. This is a normal reaction to gentle, intermittent stimulation of these parts and many patients are more affected during the selection of a standard tray than during the actual impression with its firmer contact over a more restricted area and its avoidance of the dorsum of the tongue. Unfortunately, with the more difficult cases there is always a psychological factor present as well, probably connected with a fear of choking, but a successful operation can be assured by adopting one or more of the following methods:

1. A firm, sympathetic manner of self-confidence on the operator's part.
2. Assure the patient that no difficulty will be experienced if instructions are followed, and that the discomfort will be minimized as much as possible, being in any case only for a short time.
3. The patient should blow the nose to clear any nasal obstruction and then be encouraged in deep, nasal breathing.
4. Explain to the patient that, as soon as the impression is seated, the head may be brought well forward over the lap and that a bowl will be provided to hold under the chin to catch any saliva that may run out of the mouth; this will reduce the fear of being choked.
5. Carry out the impression technique using as little material as is commensurate with procuring a satisfactory impression; avoid touching the dorsum of the tongue with the back of the tray and seat the impression as quickly as possible.
6. (a) a phenol or thymol mouth-wash, or (b) the application of a surface anaesthetic either in the form of a cream or a spray.

As sensitive patients will experience the same difficulty at each succeeding visit and as the wearing of the finished denture will be difficult, an acrylic base-plate may be made on the preliminary maxillary cast and given to the patient with instructions to practise wearing it for increasingly longer periods each day until it can be worn for at least an hour without discomfort.

Impression materials vary in their nauseating effects, owing partly to their viscosity and hence their control, and partly to their consistency and flavour. Patients dislike plaster even if it is flavoured; the alginates are tolerated slightly better; composition is usually tolerated well, probably owing to its putty-like consistency and its heat; impression paste is tolerated, probably because it is used in small bulk, but the taste and smell of eugenol is not readily accepted; the elastomers are very acceptable apart from the relatively long time in the mouth and the rubbery smell of the polysulphides.

Impressions for bedridden patients

Occasionally the prosthetist is called upon to make impressions for a patient who is confined to bed. The best thing to do if possible is to turn the patient round in bed so that the head board of the bed does not obstruct the operator. The use of hydrocolloid with a relatively high viscosity is indicated as it can be more readily controlled. Lengthy techniques cause undue fatigue and should be avoided, especially as it is often difficult to stabilize the head without a head rest.

Summary of advantages and disadvantages of various impression materials

In conclusion, it is useful to summarize the advantages and disadvantages of the various impression materials which have been discussed.

Composition (impression compound)

Advantages

1. It can be used for compressing soft tissues.
2. It can be added to and re-adapted.
3. It can be used for any technique requiring a close peripheral seal.
4. It can be used in combination with other materials.

5. It is a good space-filler and does not slump.
6. Pouring the impression may be delayed as there are no appreciable dimensional changes.
7. It is cheap.

Disadvantages

1. It distorts easily and should not be used where excessive undercuts exist. It may also be distorted if any pressure is applied to it out of the mouth before it has been chilled.
2. It does not reproduce fine surface detail.
3. As it can be re-softened and used again it tends to be unhygienic because it cannot be sterilized without destroying its properties.
4. It can only give an accurate impression with a long and difficult technique.

Indications for use

1. As a preliminary impression for the construction of individual trays.
2. To modify the fit of stock trays.
3. As a base in wash impression techniques.
4. To obtain peripheral seal.
5. For compression impressions.

Alginate

Advantages

1. It produces excellent surface detail.
2. It is dimensionally accurate if poured within a short time of removal from the mouth.
3. It is elastic and will spring over bulbous areas returning to its correct position when removed from the mouth; this only applies if the undercuts are not too deep.
4. It is hygienic, as fresh material must be used for each impression.
5. It does not lose surface detail in wet mouths.
6. It is relatively inexpensive.
7. There is a wide range with different viscosities for different clinical situations.

Disadvantages

1. It does not readily flow into areas in which the tray does not extend.
2. It cannot be used alone for compressing the tissues.
3. It cannot be added to if faulty.
4. Distortion may occur without it being obvious; it must be held stationary in relation to the tissues throughout its setting period and it must remain adherent to the tray during removal.
5. It is liable to distortion in the laboratory.
6. It is difficult to box in the laboratory.

Indications for use

1. For preliminary impressions.
2. For master impressions in rigid individual trays.
3. Whenever there are undercuts not suitable for rigid materials.

Plaster

Advantages

1. It produces good surface detail.
2. It is dimensionally accurate if used with an anti-expansion solution.
3. The low viscosity, at a particular liquid–plaster ratio, is ideal for peripheral accuracy.
4. It does not distort on removal from the mouth but fractures if deep undercuts exist and may be accurately assembled out of the mouth.
5. The rate of set is under the control of the operator.
6. It is compatible with all materials commonly used for making casts.
7. It is hygienic, as fresh plaster must be used for each impression.
8. It is cheap.

Disadvantages

1. It cannot be used for compressing the tissues.
2. In very wet mouths the surface of the plaster tends to be washed away spoiling the surface detail, especially in lower impressions.
3. It cannot be added to if faulty.
4. Its taste and rough feel when in the mouth induce nausea in some patients.
5. Exothermic heat is disliked by many patients.
6. It requires a separator before pouring in the laboratory and this may cause surface inaccuracy.

Indications for use

1. In all normal mouths when the factors affecting retention are favourable.
2. At a particular viscosity it is useful as a space-filling material in lower impressions.

Impression paste (ZOE)

Advantages

1. It produces excellent surface detail.
2. It is dimensionally accurate as it is only used in a thin layer.
3. It is hygienic, as fresh material must be used for each impression.
4. It does not lose surface detail in wet mouths.
5. It can be added to and re-adapted if faulty.
6. In thin washes it can be used for compressing soft tissues.

7. It reduces nausea to a minimum.
8. It adheres well to a dried surface so that when the minimum of material is used there is little degree of flaking on removal from the mouth.

Disadvantages

1. It cannot be used when more than a slight undercut exists.
2. May slump in thick layers and therefore can only be used as a wash material.
3. Will not produce a satisfactory impression of the periphery unless supported by a very accurate or border-moulded tray.
4. Some patients find the eugenol content unpleasant.

Indications for use

1. As a final wash material when using techniques which have produced a closely adapted periphery.
2. In cases exhibiting pronounced nausea.

Elastomers

Advantages

1. Excellent surface detail.
2. Dimensional accuracy.
3. No separator required before pouring casts.
4. Record undercuts but polysulphides may suffer from permanent deformation on removal.
5. Polysulphides have good tear resistance.
6. Addition silicones have excellent dimensional stability, even in cold sterilizing solutions.
7. Wide range of different viscosities available to match different clinical situations.
8. Low viscosity silicones suitable for wash techniques.
9. Putty silicones are useful as space-filling materials.
10. Pleasant appearance and feel in the mouth

Disadvantages

1. They are hydrophobic and so tend to slip on wet, mucus-covered mucosa.
2. Prolonged setting time, especially polysulphides.
3. Tear resistance of silicones is low.
4. Condensation silicones are dimensionally unstable.
5. Silicone putty can easily distort peripheral tissues.
6. Most expensive of all impression materials.
7. After set, borders cannot be adjusted.
8. Polysulphides have strong odour of rubber.

Indications for use

1. Where there are severe undercuts.
2. In patients exhibiting xerostomia.
3. In patients with lesions of the mucosa, such as pemphigus or lichen planus.
4. For master impressions in rigid individual trays

Relief areas

Owing to the varying thickness of the mucosa on which the denture rests it is frequently necessary to relieve the denture over areas of thin mucosa in order to avoid pain and/or rocking of the denture and the commonest position requiring such relief is the median sagittal raphe of the palate (Figure 5.42). Many technicians empirically relieve the centre of the palate but this leads to unsatisfactory results as the areas needing relief are not uniform in shape, position or in the depth of relief required.

The operator should palpate the denture-bearing area when first examining the mouth and decide which area, if any, will require relieving. Having taken the master impression all areas to be relieved should be marked on the surface with indelible pencil. The depth of the relief is dependent on the compressibility of the mucosa and should be sufficient to prevent the denture from pressing on

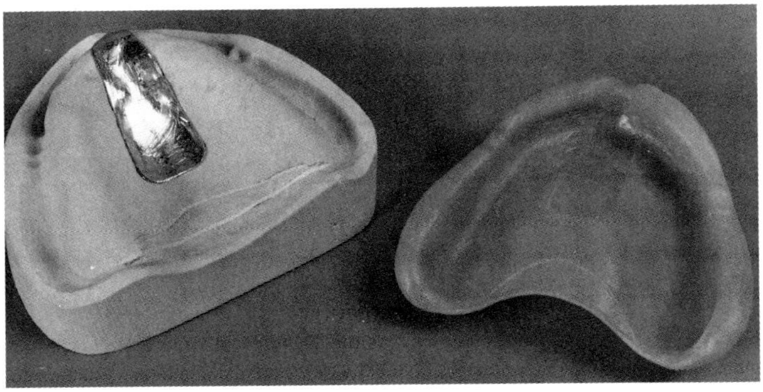

Figure 5.42 Relief of median sagittal region of maxillary denture. Relief should not be used as a routine but only when there is a definite need

the areas of thin mucosal coverage when masticatory loads are imposed. A simple means of conveying the information regarding depth to the technician is to write on the prescription card the number of sheets of metal foil to be used in constructing the relief.

Relief areas on dentures should always merge into the surrounding fitting surface and should never have a clearly defined outline as this can cause mucosal irritation.

Apart from the midline of the palate, other areas that may require relief are the incisive papilla, the maxillary rugae, areas of mucosal damage (such as lichen planus), the buccal surface of prominent tuberosities, mental foramen, crest of lower anterior ridge, prominent genial tubercles and torus mandibularis.

It should be stated, however, that relief should not be used routinely in complete dentures.

Chapter 6

Jaw relation records

The first stage in the construction of complete dentures has been described in the preceding chapter and has resulted in two casts which are accurate reproductions of the denture-bearing area of the patient's mouth. While the natural jaws bear a very definite relation to each other, both at rest and when functioning, the two casts do not. It is the purpose of this chapter to explain how the casts may be related to each other in the exact manner of their natural counterparts.

The maxillo-mandibular relations

There are three relationships of the mandible to the maxilla:

1. With the mandible in its retruded position.
2. With the mandible in its rest position when the teeth are always out of contact (relaxed relation).
3. The dynamic relationship of the jaws during function.

Retruded position

The maxilla is firmly united to the skull and only moves with this structure. The mandible on the other hand is attached to the skull by the two temporomandibular joints and is capable of opening, closing, protrusive, retrusive and lateral movements, and also combinations of any of these. The mandible is prevented from overclosing by the occlusion of the natural teeth, and it is also necessary to retrude the mandible at the conclusion of all functional movements, in order that the cusps may interdigitate. These two facts result in the mandible returning, at the conclusion of every masticatory stroke, to a position in which the cusps of the opposing teeth are in contact, and the heads of the condyles are placed back in the glenoid fossae. This maxillo-mandibular relation is termed the retruded position (Figure 6.1).

Relaxed relation or rest position

When the mandible is not functioning, and provided the subject is not in a state of tension, and is breathing normally through the nose, the muscles and ligaments which are attached to the mandible support it in a relationship to the maxilla which is remarkably constant for any given individual. In this relation the heads of the condyles are retruded in the glenoid fossae and the occlusal surfaces of the teeth are separated by 2–4 mm (Figure 6.2). The term relaxed relation is also commonly used for any relationship of the mandible to the maxilla from this physiological rest position up to but not including contact of the teeth.

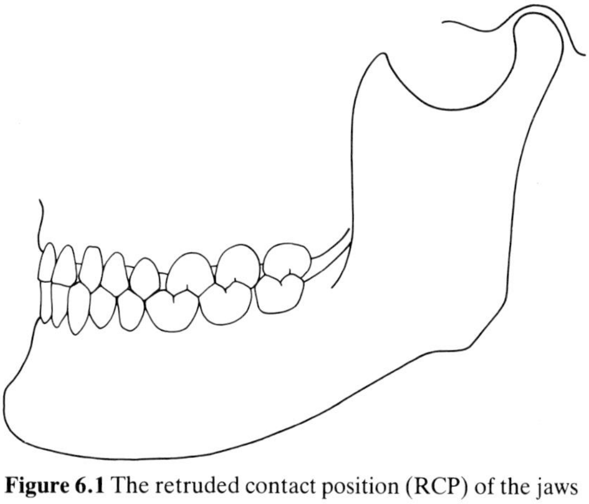

Figure 6.1 The retruded contact position (RCP) of the jaws

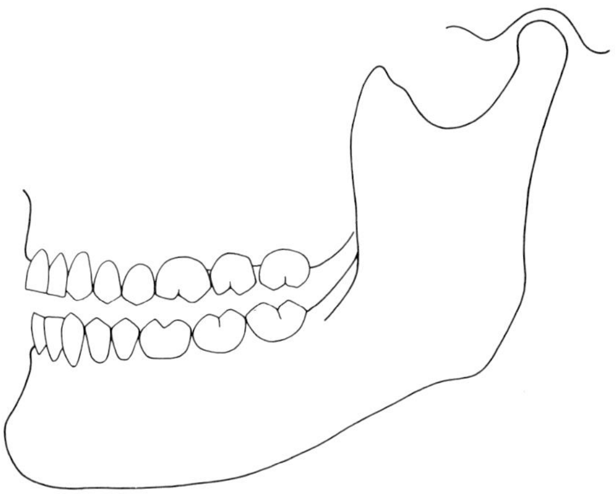

Figure 6.2 The relaxed or rest relation of the jaws

Although the rest position is reasonably reliable for any given patient, it should be remembered that it is influenced and perhaps altered by any of the following factors: head position, loss of teeth, denture or record block in the mouth, physical exercise, tongue and lip posture, respiratory requirements, emotional tension, drug therapy, occlusal characteristics, pain, age, time of day, and therefore a degree of caution must be exercised when relying on exact measurement.

Functional relation

When the mandibular condyles are drawn forwards by the contraction of the lateral pterygoid muscles, they are forced to move downwards because their superior articular surfaces, the articular eminences, are sloped downwards and forwards. When the occlusal surfaces of the teeth make eccentric contact during function, the cusps and incisal edges of the mandibular teeth slide up the cuspal inclines of the maxillary teeth. Thus the mandible follows definite paths dictated by the guidance it receives from the condylar paths posteriorly and the cusp slopes and incisal edges anteriorly.

The edentulous state

When an individual is rendered edentulous all tooth guidance is lost and thus the mandible may close until the mucosa of the lower ridge meets that of the upper. It is no longer necessary for the individual to retrude the mandible at the conclusion of each functional movement, because no cusps require to be interdigitated (Figure 6.3). Finally, the functional paths of the mandible are lost because, although the condylar guidances still exist, the cusp and incisal guides do not.

The relaxed relation tends to remain unchanged because it is dependent on the muscles not teeth. The problem, therefore, which faces the prosthetist is to discover the relations which the mandible bore to the maxilla when the natural teeth were present and relate the casts to each other in a like manner. The teeth may then be set up on the casts with the knowledge that they will occlude correctly when placed in the mouth.

The relations which require to be recorded

These depend on the type of articulator which is to be employed. Plane-line articulators only require the retruded position, while adjustable articulators require that the paths of the condyles and their relationship to the mandible be also recorded.

The difference between these two types of articulator is that the plane-line permits only a hinge movement while the adjustable or moving condyle type copies functional movement (Figures 6.4, and 6.5).

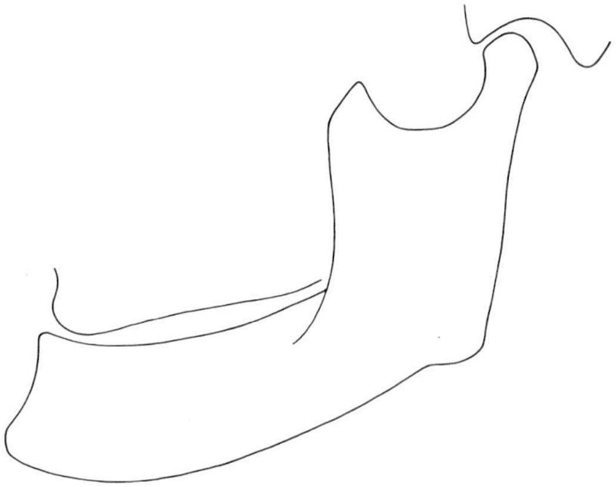

Figure 6.3 Complete loss of tooth guidance for the position of the mandible

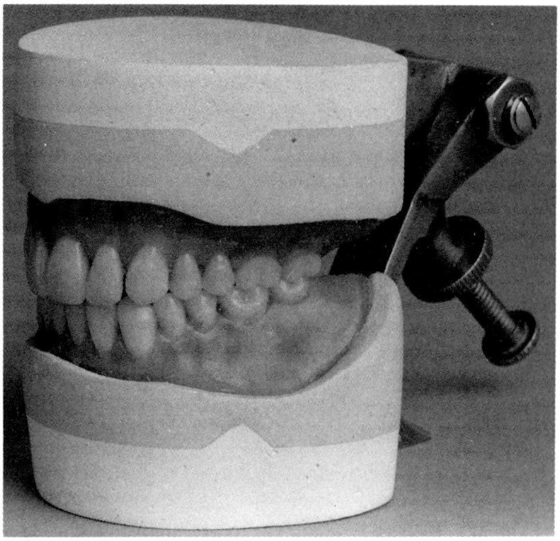

Figure 6.4 A plane-line articulator

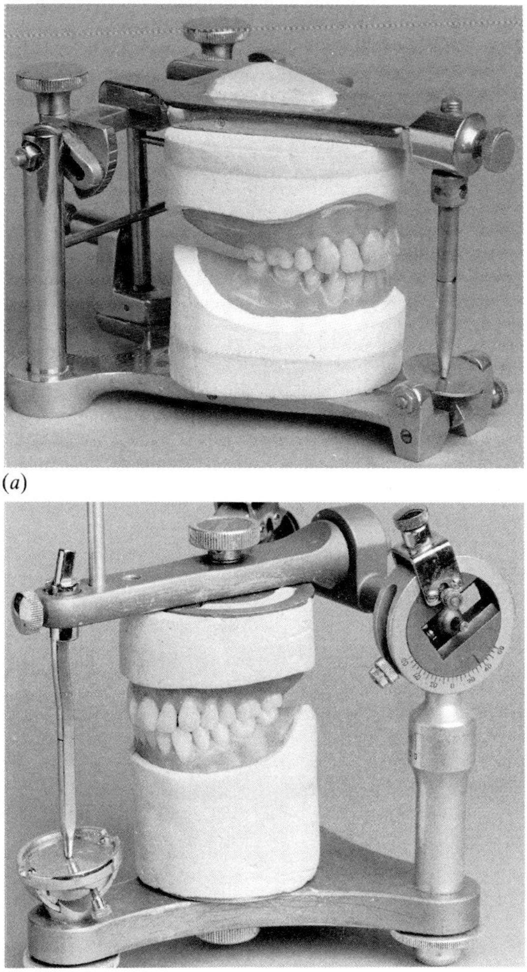

(*a*)

(*b*)

Figure 6.5 Examples of moving condyle (semi-adjustable) articulators. (*a*) Gibling; (*b*) Dentatus

In addition, other facts required by the operator to enable him to construct the dentures are noted, and these will be described together with the technique employed to obtain the retruded position. Some form of simple, intra-oral apparatus is needed to register these various relationships of mandible and maxilla and before describing the technique for obtaining these positions, various types of record blocks used for this purpose will be discussed.

Record blocks

These consist of two parts (Figure 6.6): the base-plate and the occlusal rim

Base-plates

These may be divided into two classes: temporary and permanent.

Temporary base-plates are eventually discarded and replaced by the denture base material, while those of the permanent group will ultimately form part of the finished denture.

Temporary base-plates may be made of: wax, thermoplastic material, swaged polymer, or cold cure acrylic. Permanent bases may be made of cast or swaged metal, or acrylic.

Wax base-plate

This type is used in conjunction with a wax rim, forming an all wax record block, but it is a thoroughly unsuitable material for a base-plate. It softens readily at body temperature resulting in distortion during the record taking, thus preventing the accurate repositioning of the block on the cast, leading to an incorrect occlusal relationship being established on the articulator. It is occasionally used for obtaining an approximate jaw relation record as part of a diagnostic plan or as a guide to another type of record block.

Thermoplastic base-plate

There are a number of proprietary brands available which differ slightly in brittleness, toughness and melting point but all have a considerably higher softening point than wax and thus allow the operator longer time for manipulation in the mouth. They are tougher than wax and, if used in conjunction with composition rims, recordings of mandibular positions can be obtained with a fair degree of accuracy.

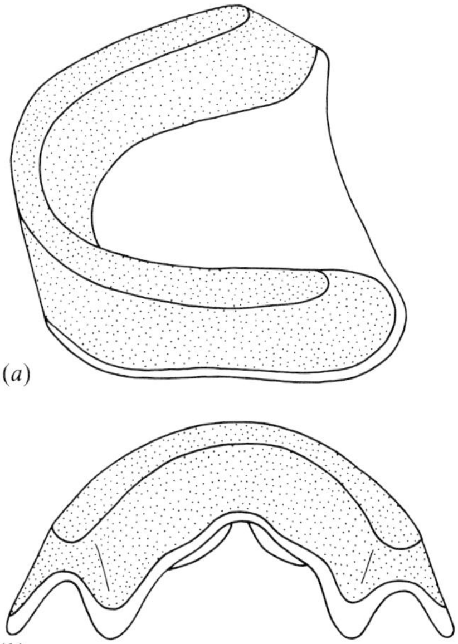

(*a*)

(*b*)

Figure 6.6 Record blocks: (*a*) an upper; (*b*) a lower

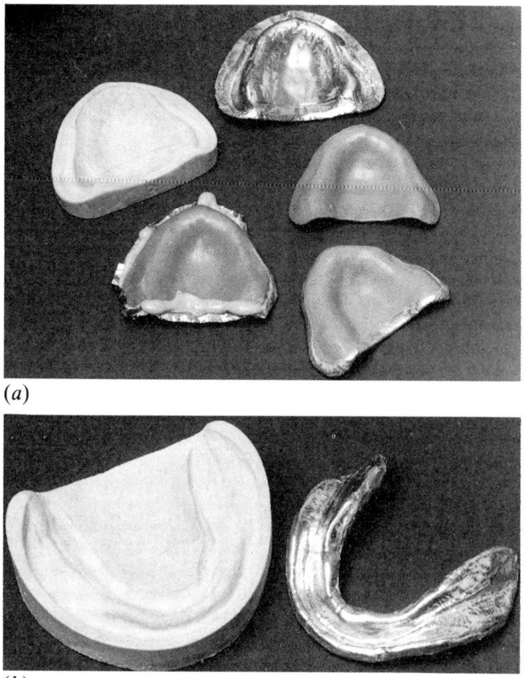

(*a*)

(*b*)

Figure 6.7 Stabilized base-plates for record blocks. (*a*) Stages in making an upper base; (*b*) a finished lower base (see text)

There are two criticisms which may be levelled against them. First, being hard they tend to rub the cast, and secondly they tend to warp slightly at ordinary room temperature because of relief of stresses, particularly if they were not thoroughly softened before being adapted to the cast.

A method of reinforcing a base-plate is to burnish 0.06 mm tin foil over the cast surface, leaving an excess around the sulcus. A mix of zinc oxide-eugenol paste is applied to the foil and the previously shaped thermoplastic base-plate placed in position. Before the paste sets the excess foil is pulled up around the edge to create a well-finished border. This technique, although more time-consuming, produces a rigid and accurate base (Figure 6.7).

Swaged or thermo-formed polymer base-plate

Sheets of polymer are softened by heat and adapted to the cast by direct or vacuum pressure. When cool, the excess is trimmed off to leave a close-fitting rigid base-plate, although in many cases the transverse deflection is high. This means the base can flex in use.

Cold cure acrylic

This material may be purchased in bulk, especially for making base-plates and individual trays.

The powder and liquid are mixed and allowed to form a dough which is then pressed into a thin sheet between two pieces of polished metal or glass protected by cellophane or polythene. This sheet of acrylic is then conformed by hand or by a rubber swager to the plaster cast which has previously had excessive undercuts waxed out and been painted with cold mould seal (sodium alginate), a separator. The base-plate is roughly trimmed to shape with scissors while still soft and the final trimming is done with a bur when the acrylic has polymerized.

Acrylic bases have the advantage of being a close fit and not softening or warping in the mouth.

Cast or swaged metal bases

Such bases will form part of the finished denture and are, therefore, classified as permanent; any type of occlusal rim can be mounted on them according to the requirements of the case.

They are designed to cover the palate in the normal way and usually terminate on the buccal aspect of the crest of the alveolar ridge (Figure 6.8). Buccal and labial flanges are not extended to the full depth of the sulci because of the difficulty of obtaining a good peripheral seal or of easing the finished denture.

They are resistant to the influences of mouth temperature and capable of withstanding the stresses and strains exerted during the trimming and

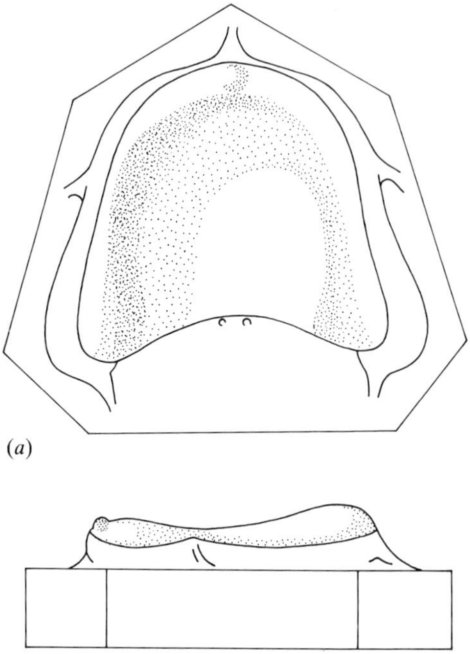

(*a*)

(*b*)

Figure 6.8 The area covered by a metal base. (*a*) From above; (*b*) from the side recording of the occlusal relationship without distortion. The accurate fit of these bases enables the prosthetist to record mandibular movements under the best conditions possible, as displacement of the bases from the alveolar ridges is minimized, and possible error from that source avoided.

Acrylic base (heat cured)

This base has the unique advantage that it enables the retention of the finished denture to be determined at an early stage, when steps can be taken to improve it if it is unsatisfactory. Its only disadvantage is that a second processing to attach the teeth and complete the denture may cause dimensional changes in the base which can be prevented either by attaching the teeth to the base with cold cure acrylic or by using a carefully controlled processing time cycle.

Occlusal rims

Three materials are in general use for the construction of the rims: wax, impression compound, and a mixture of plaster with an abrasive, such as pumice or sand.

Wax rims

Modelling or base-plate wax, composed of beeswax, paraffin wax and harder and tougher waxes like carnauba, is commonly used for making jaw relation records.

Advantages

Quick and simple to use but because of the low thermal conductivity and difficulty of uniform heating, stresses are easily set up in the wax.

Disadvantages of some waxes

1. They distort considerably if kept in the mouth for more than a few minutes without removal and chilling, and so can only be used satisfactorily by a careful operator.
2. Inaccurate for patients who bite hard on the blocks which readily distort under pressure and are slightly resilient.
3. They soften too easily to be used with accuracy for recording lateral and protrusive positions of the mandible in addition to retruded position.

Composition rims

These are suitable for most cases and techniques.

Advantages:

1. They have a sufficiently high softening point for them to be used for any intra-oral records.
2. They are not readily distorted under pressure.

Disadvantages:

Composition takes longer to cut and trim than wax but the chairside time spent on trimming the rims can be very considerably reduced if a 'squash' record is taken at the same time as the impressions. A 'squash' record is an approximate or tentative one taken by placing a roll of softened wax or a T-block on the lower alveolar ridge and requesting the patient to relax and close the jaws slowly. When the operator considers that the jaws are separated by the correct distance, he tells the patient to stop closing. The wax is removed from the mouth and chilled. This does not give an accurate relationship of the jaws but enables the technician to mount the casts on a plane-line articulator in approximately the correct position, and then to construct composition rims of almost the correct vertical height.

The simplest method of trimming a composition rim is to soften the occlusal surface with a pin-point flame, press it against a flat, wet surface, e.g. a glass or porcelain slab, and then cut away the excess which will have been squeezed out sideways before it has hardened.

Plaster and abrasive rims

Such rims are used when mandibular movements are made by the patient grinding the lower rim against the upper until an even gliding contact is produced, so shaping the surface of the rims to correspond with the functionally generated path taken by the mandible in movement.

A description of this technique will be found in Chapter 9.

Recording retruded contact position

Testing the upper record block

It is essential that both the retention and the stability of the blocks are good if accurate results are to be obtained and both must be checked before starting to trim the rims. The terms retention and stability are frequently used in the following pages so, in order to avoid ambiguity, they should be defined precisely.

Retention is the ability of a denture to remain in contact with its supporting mucosa, i.e. the resistance to removal in a direction approximately at right angles to the occlusal plane.

Stability is the ability of a denture to remain stationary in relation to the surrounding musculature and opposing occlusal surface. This is unobtainable with complete dentures owing to the very slight compressibility of even normal mucosa when subjected to masticatory pressure, but a denture is considered to be clinically stable if it remains stationary in relation to its bony support within the bounds of compressibility of normal mucosa. Both these descriptions must remain true during all normal movements of mastication and speech.

Retention

The retention of an accurately adapted base is usually quite good, but it should invariably be checked for over-extension since the movement of the lips, cheeks and frenal attachments will dislodge it if the flanges are too deep.

If the retention is not good and the base is of wax or another thermoplastic material, distortion of the base is at once suspect and the fit of the base on the cast should be carefully inspected. When retention is poor, even with a well-fitting wax or shellac base or any of the other materials, and there is no over-extension of the flanges, then the use of a little gum tragacanth ('denture fixative') to retain the record block is indicated, provided that the operator does not suspect an inaccurate impression or cast as being the cause of the lack of retention.

Stability

This may be tested by alternate finger pressure on the rim on either side of the mouth. If the base tends to rock it may be due to the rim being mounted too far outside the centre of the ridge or to insufficient relief in the centre of the palate. It may also be due to the underlying mucosa being very flabby and displaceable. Whichever is the cause it must be corrected before proceeding.

A word of explanation is required here since the above paragraph apparently contradicts the statements regarding the position to be occupied by the artificial teeth (see Chapter 8). Record blocks are constructed with flat occlusal surfaces and therefore any pressure on them will be almost vertical; in order to resist this pressure they must be partly placed over the centres of the supporting ridges though this may not be the position which the artificial teeth will occupy. Encroachment on the tongue space with resultant instability is of minor importance at this stage as no functional movements will be required.

Trimming the upper record block

When trimming the rim there are four main considerations and they must be taken in the order given.

1. Labial fullness

The lip is normally supported by the alveolar process and teeth which, at this stage, are represented by the base and rim of the record block. Therefore the labial surface must be cut back or added to until a natural and pleasing position of the upper lip is obtained. Note that the upper lip may appear too full because the lower lip, at this stage, is unsupported. The lip line (i.e. a straight line just in contact with the inferior border of the upper lip when relaxed) will be raised if the labial surface of the block is too bulky and will be lowered if the support is inadequate (Figure 6.9).

2. The height of the occlusal rim

The technician will mount the incisor teeth with their incisal edges in the same position as the occlusal surface of the upper record block which must, therefore, be trimmed vertically until it represents the amount of the anterior teeth intended to show below the lip at rest. The average adult

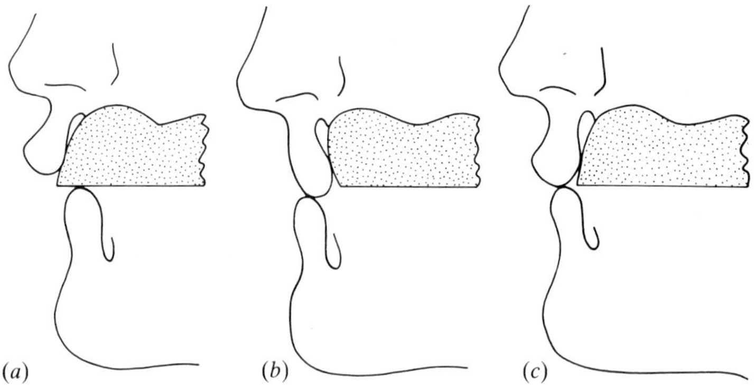

Figure 6.9 Diagram illustrating the effect of the labial bulk of the upper record block on the position of the upper lip and its inferior border. (*a*) Too full; (*b*) not full enough; (*c*) correct

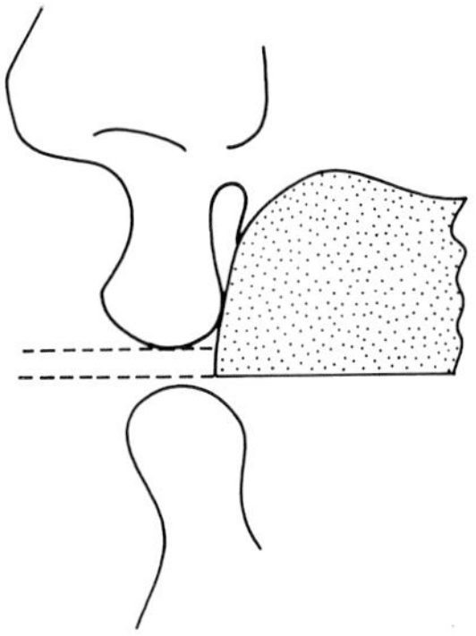

Figure 6.10 Illustrating the amount of the upper occlusal rim which should be visible below the upper lip in the average case (the distance between the dotted lines is 3 mm)

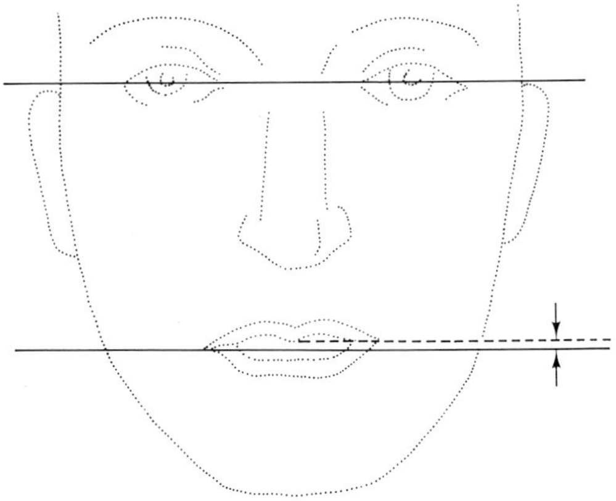

Figure 6.11 Illustrating the plane parallel to which the upper occlusal rim should be trimmed. Space between arrows indicates the amount of rim showing below upper lip (about 3 mm)

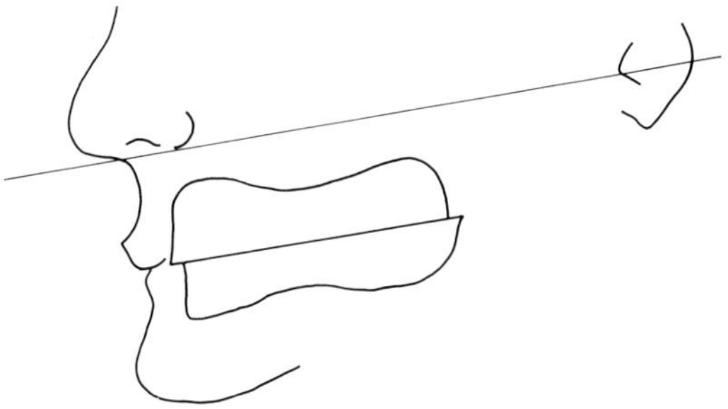

Figure 6.12 Illustrating the imaginary naso-auricular line and the manner in which the rims are trimmed parallel to this line

shows approximately 3 mm of the upper central incisors when the lips are just parted, but there are many variations from this amount which should be accepted as a guide rather than a rule (Figure 6.10). A greater length of tooth than normal may be shown if the patient has:

1. A short upper lip.
2. Superior protrusion.
3. An Angle class II malocclusion of the natural teeth.

and less will be shown:

1. With a long upper lip.
2. In most old people, owing to the attrition of the natural teeth and some loss of tone of the orbicularis oris muscle.

3. The anterior plane

Since the upper anterior teeth are set with their incisal edges in the same position as the occlusal surface of the rim, it is important for the anterior plane of this rim to be trimmed level. If the anterior teeth are set to a plane which drops to one side of the mouth the appearance may be displeasing. Generally the plane to which the anterior teeth should be set, and to which the rim must be trimmed, is parallel to an imaginary line joining the pupils of the eyes or a line at right angles to the median sagittal plane of the face (Figure 6.11). Sometimes the lip line, or even the interpupillary line, will be found to have a distinct drop to one side of the face, in which case the operator will have to locate the anterior plane by aesthetic judgement.

4. The anteroposterior plane

This plane indicates the position of the occlusal surfaces of the posterior teeth and is obtained in conjunction with the anterior plane. The rim is trimmed parallel to the naso-auricular or ala–tragus line (Figure 6.12) (an imaginary line running from the external auditory meatus or tragus of the ear to the lower border of the ala of the nose). It has been found from the study of many cases that the occlusal plane of the natural teeth is usually parallel to this line. It must be remembered that the posterior teeth are set to a slight anteroposterior curve, while the naso-auricular line is straight, and is used as an aid to the technician rather than a fixed position, as is the case of the anterior plane. The occlusal plane is an imaginary flat surface which extends from the mesio-incisal angles of the upper central incisors to the mesiopalatal cusps of the upper first molar teeth. It does not coincide with the occlusal surfaces of the teeth and its main use is as a fixed position to which to refer when describing the position of individual teeth or other structures.

Thus, when the rim has been trimmed to these planes it indicates the place of orientation for setting the artificial teeth, and when this has been done to the satisfaction of the operator, attention is focused on the position occupied by the posterior palatal border of the base.

The position of the posterior palatal border

It will be remembered from the discussion on the retention of complete dentures that an adequate seal must be obtained along this border if the upper denture is to be prevented from tipping when pressure is applied to the palatal surfaces or incisal edges of the anterior teeth. The seal must be situated in the region of compressible tissue just distal to the hard palate, but it must be anterior to the vibrating line (the line from which visible movement of the soft palate takes place). This is of great importance (Figure 6.13). If the back edge of the denture extends posteriorly beyond this vibrating line, the seal will be broken when the soft palate rises during deglutition and speech, and the denture will momentarily become loose and may drop; the patient is also likely to complain of nausea. If the posterior palatal border does not reach this compressible area, retention will be poor because the seal will be inefficient and again the patient may complain of nausea since the edge of the denture

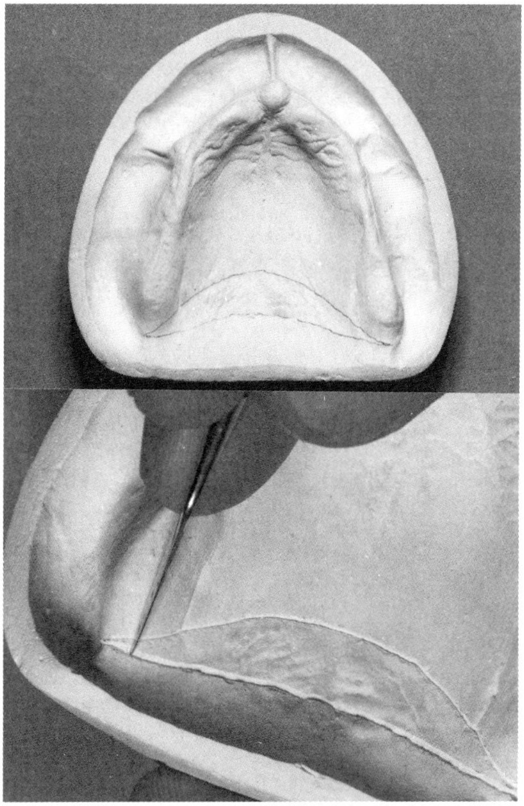

Figure 6.13 Two postdams are marked. The more distal (major postdam) indicates the junction between hard and soft palates. The other (minor postdam) is made more shallow and is intended to act as a barrier to saliva which may be milked across the major postdam and thus affect retention

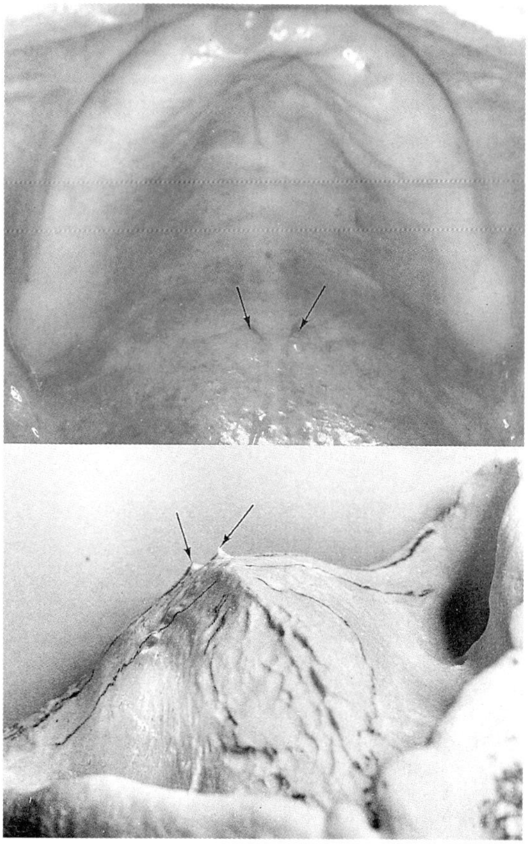

Figure 6.14 Fovea palati (arrowed) on the anterior part of the soft palate. Plaster impression shows the fovea on the distal border (arrowed)

may irritate the posterior third of the tongue as it will not bed into the tissues.

The operator first discovers the position of this vibrating line by asking the patient to say a prolonged 'ah', with the mouth widely opened, and noting the line from which the soft palate moves. For reference it is useful to mark this line on the palate with an indelible pencil. The tissue in front of this line is explored with a blunt instrument and the area of soft compressible tissue noted. In some cases this area may extend for several millimetres before merging with the thinner and denser tissue which commonly covers the hard palate, while in other cases only a small margin between the vibrating line and the less compressible tissue of the hard palate will exist (see Figure 2.22).

Another method of finding the postdam area is to press the blunt surface of a ball-ended instrument gently against the hard palate and gradually work backwards until a compressible area is discovered, then note its relation to the previously marked vibrating line.

The posterior border can be located with great accuracy if it is possible to see the two small pits (fovea palati) one on either side of the midline on the anterior part of the soft palate (Figure 6.14). The fovea are usually, though not invariably, present and are situated just anterior to the vibrating line, thus marking the posterior limit of the denture.

The posterior border of the record block is adjusted by trimming or by adding wax, to coincide with the position which has been selected for postdamming.

The adjustments to the upper block are completed with the marking of certain guide lines of which the first to be mentioned is essential, the other two optional.

Guide lines

1. The centre line or midline

In the normal natural dentition the upper central incisors have their mesial surfaces in contact with an imaginary vertical line which bisects the face and, for aesthetic reasons, it is desirable that the artificial substitutes should occupy the same position. If this centre line is not clearly marked on the labial surface of the upper occlusal rim, the technician has to depend on the position of the incisive papilla or the labial frenum as denoted on the cast, and while these landmarks are usually found in the midline this is not invariable. If, at the trial stage, the midline is found to be incorrect, then both the upper and lower dentures will have to be entirely reset to correct it, a considerable waste of time for patient, clinician and technician.

Few human faces are symmetrical. Therefore there can be no hard and fast rule for determining the centre line, which thus depends upon the artistic judgement of the clinician. The following aids are suggested as a help in deciding where to mark a vertical line on the labial surface of the upper rim:

1. Where it is crossed by an imaginary line from the centre of the brows to the centre of the chin.
2. Immediately below the centre of the philtrum.
3. Immediately below the centre of the labial tubercle.
4. At the bisection of the line from corner to corner of the mouth when the lips are relaxed.
5. Where it is crossed by a line at right angles to the interpupillary line from a point midway between the pupils when the patient is looking directly forwards (Figure 6.15).
6. Midway between the angles of the mouth when the patient is smiling

The accuracy of the centre line marking is best judged from a position directly in front of the patient and a little distance away.

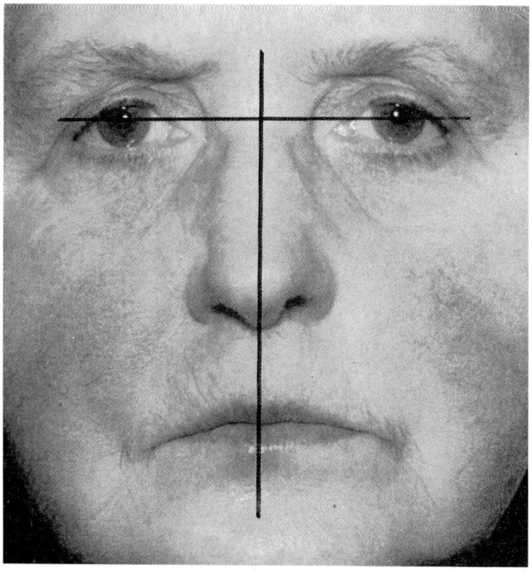

Figure 6.15 Centre line of record block on a point midway between the pupils

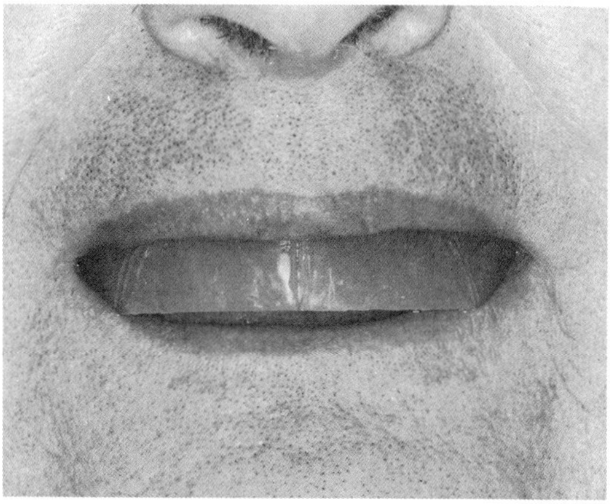

Figure 6.16 Centre line, high lip line and canine lines marked on labial surface of maxillary record block

2. The high lip line

This is a line just in contact with the lower border of the upper lip when it is raised as high as possible unaided, as in smiling or laughing. It is marked on the labial surface of the rim and indicates the amount of the denture which may be seen under normal conditions, and thus assists in determining the length of tooth needed (Figure 6.16). This line was of considerable importance when vulcanite was the only base material available and its unnatural appearance made longer teeth preferable. Polymethyl methacrylate and other present-day denture base materials do not suffer from this disadvantage.

3. The canine lines

These mark the corners of the mouth when the lips are relaxed and are supposed to coincide with the tips of the upper canine teeth but are only accurate to within 3 or 4 mm. These lines give some indication of the width to be taken up by the six anterior teeth from tip to tip of the canines (Figure 6.16).

Trimming the lower record block

Having trimmed and marked the upper block, all that now requires to be done is to trim the lower block so that when it occludes evenly with the upper, the mandible will be separated from the maxilla by the same distance that it was when the natural teeth were in occlusion, or as near to this distance as it is possible to obtain. If the mandible is now made to assume its retruded position with the rims of the blocks in contact, and these are sealed together in this position, then the retruded contact position will have been recorded.

It will be appreciated, therefore, that two dimensions are involved in this jaw relation record:

1. The vertical dimension i.e. the distance by which the jaws are separated with the rims in contact.
2. The horizontal relationship, i.e. the relationship of the mandible to the maxilla in the horizontal plane when the condyles of the mandible are fully retruded in the glenoid fossae.

There are thus two more stages to be completed. The first is to trim the lower block so that it occludes evenly with the upper at the correct vertical height, and the second is to unite the blocks with the mandible retruded.

The block should first be tested for retention and stability as was done for the upper, and if these are unsatisfactory they must be remedied before proceeding.

Next, the occlusal surface of the rim is adjusted so that when it is in even contact all round with the upper rim the jaws are separated by the required distance. In most instances the rim of the lower block will be too high and require to be reduced, but occasionally it may be too low and require building up by the addition of wax or composition.

The vertical dimension

As mentioned at the beginning of this chapter, there is normally a gap of 2–3 mm between the occlusal surfaces of the teeth when the mandible is in the rest position, and this gap is called the freeway space (Figure 6.17). Probably the best technique is to record the rest position with the rims in contact and then remove the thickness of the desired freeway space from the occlusal surface of the lower block (Figure 6.18).

While many clinicians of experience rely solely on their judgment of the patient's appearance for obtaining this vertical dimension, there are a number of indicators available to help the less skilful or less artistic operator, although these are aids and not accurate measurements.

Freeway space measurement

This is probably the most useful measurement, but it must be remembered that it is merely a help and must not be relied on as being accurate. The technique is split up into stages for ease of description.

1. Insert the upper record block.
2. Make a thin horizontal line or pinhead-size mark on the tip of the patient's nose and another on the point of the chin in an area where there is the least movement of the soft tissues. These marks

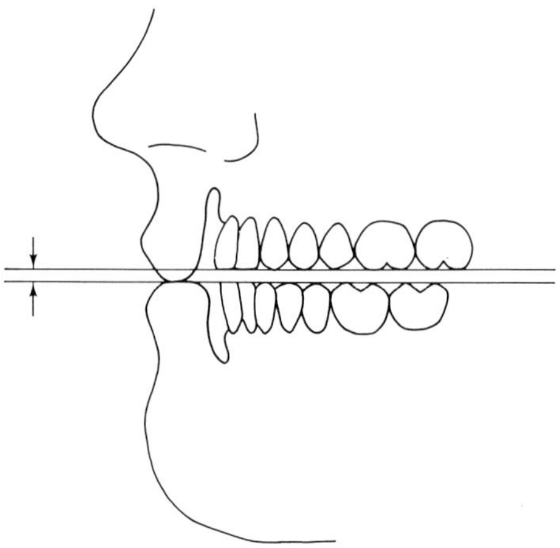

Figure 6.17 Freeway space (interocclusal clearance) is the space between the teeth when the mandible is at rest

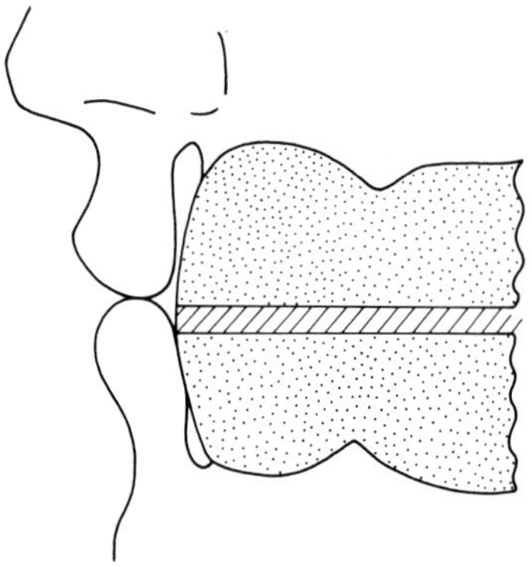

Figure 6.18 Illustrating the rest position of the mandible with the occlusal rims in contact. If the ruled section is removed from the lower rim that amount of freeway space will be provided

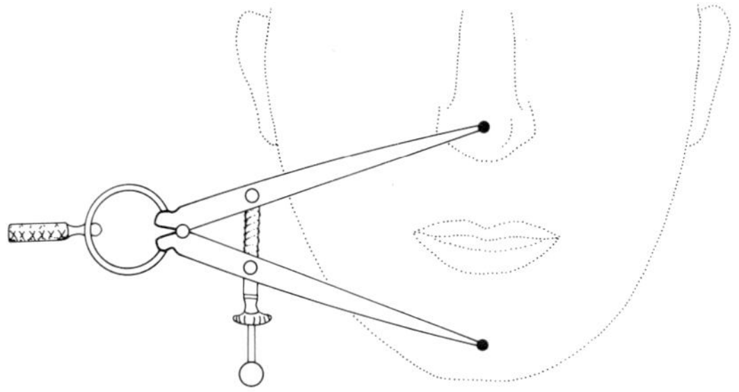

Figure 6.19 Measuring the distance between the marks with dividers with the mandible at rest

should not be made with an indelible pencil as they are too difficult to remove, but felt pen is quite suitable. Alternatively, a piece of adhesive tape may be placed on the nose and chin and the marks made on these.

3. The patient must be comfortably seated in the chair and asked to relax the whole body as completely as possible and allow the jaw to rest in a comfortable position with the lips closed. When this position is achieved, measure the distance between the marks either with a pair of dividers or a millimetre rule (Figure 6.19).
4. Ask the patient to moisten the lips with the tongue and then close them to a comfortable position. Check the measurement previously obtained.
5. Ask the patient to swallow and relax without separating the lips. Again check the measurements.
6. Ask the patient to repeat the letter 'M' several times, finishing in the middle of the last 'M' i.e. not completing the sound by separating the lips. Again check. Any, or all, of these methods of obtaining a relaxed position must be repeated, until two or three constant readings are obtained.
7. Insert the lower record block and adjust the occlusal surface of the lower until it occludes evenly with the upper at the distance between the marks of the constant reading. Such trimming may be facilitated if the surface of the lower block is softened by flaming and the patient asked to close it against the upper.
8. Produce a freeway space by removing a further 2 or 3 mm from the lower record rim.
9. Check the existence of this freeway space by asking the patient to relax with the record blocks in his mouth and with his lips closed. Then ask the patient to close the blocks together, when a slight but definite movement of the chin will take place if there is an adequate freeway space (Figure 6.20). An intelligent patient may be questioned as to whether the blocks are in contact or not when he is relaxed. Errors in this technique are due to the marks having to be made on soft tissue which is always movable and not directly related to movement of the mandible.

Speaking space

The mandible moves vertically and anteroposteriorly during speech so that the lower teeth invade the freeway space. Therefore some patients need more freeway space than others depending on the range of mandibular movement during speech. The closest speaking space is the space between the occlusal surfaces of the teeth when the mandible is elevated to the maximum extent during speech. There should be at least 1 mm of closest speaking space in all complete dentures.

It should be emphasized that the freeway space is a resting measurement while the closest speaking space is a dynamic measurement.

Measurement described by Willis

This is a proportional measurement which is taught in art schools, and while it is true that a drawing made to these dimensions will be pleasing in its

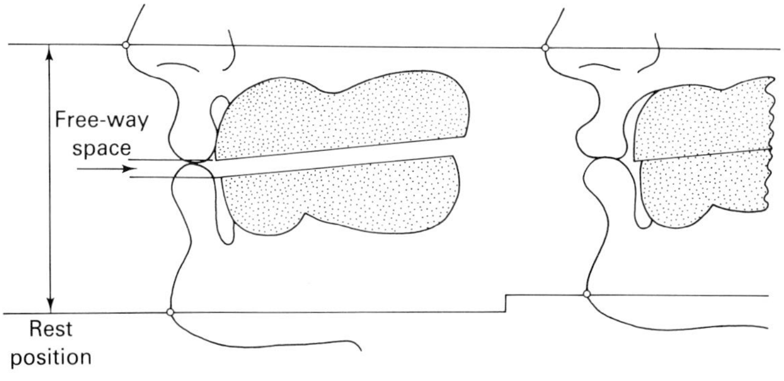

Figure 6.20 The freeway space. The first diagram illustrates the rest position of the mandible showing the rims parted. The second diagram illustrates the small upward movement of the chin which occurs when the rims occlude

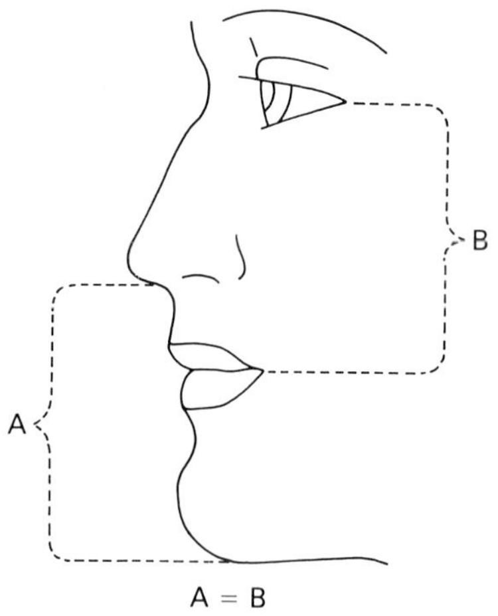

Figure 6.21 Details of facial proportions described by Willis

proportions, there are many individuals whose faces, although not appearing in any way distorted, do not conform to these somewhat ideal limits. It is easy to take these measurements with accuracy on a two-dimensional drawing, but two different clinicians will rarely agree on a patient's measurements to within a few millimetres.

The theory of this measurement is that the distance from the lower border of the septum of the nose to the lower border of the chin is equal to the distance from the outer canthus of the eye to the corner of the relaxed lips with the teeth in occlusion (Figure 6.21).

Another general proportion of the face in assessment of vertical dimension and used as a rough guide is to divide the face into three equal parts:

Hairline to nasion
Nasion to philtrum–columella junction
Philtrum–columella junction to below the chin.

Ridge relationship

An indication of the correct vertical height can be obtained from the parallelism of the upper and lower posterior ridges. Excessive divergence from the parallel, seen when the casts have been mounted on an articulator, indicates that the vertical height is probably wrong and should again be checked.

Incorrect vertical dimension

Up to this point the emphasis has been on the patient's facial appearance, because it is largely by this means that the correct vertical height is judged, but the effects of an incorrect height are greater than merely an unsatisfactory appearance. The degree of error, either of over-opening or of over-closing, necessary to produce any of the following results, cannot be given because a very small deviation from the normal occlusal face height will produce symptoms in one patient, while a greater deviation will be tolerated with comfort by another.

Effects of excessively increasing the vertical dimension

Discomfort

A patient acquires over a period of many years habits which control, automatically and unconsciously, certain muscular movements, among them being those of the tongue and mandible when eating and talking. An example, which can be readily appreciated, of this unconscious control will be found in the act of running up a flight of stairs. The steps being all the same distance apart, one's weight is taken evenly and smoothly on each successive stair without any conscious thought, but if, without one's previous knowledge, one tread is at a different height from the others, a very nasty jar will result. In an exactly similar way, pressure is smoothly and gradually applied between the teeth when eating, but if the vertical height is altered an unpleasant sensation will draw attention to what is normally a purely automatic movement. By altering the vertical height the environment in which these unconscious movements take place has also been altered and, until a new cortical pattern has been established, discomfort will result.

Trauma

The jarring effect of the teeth coming into contact sooner than expected may cause only discomfort, but in most cases it will also cause pain owing to the bruising of the mucosa by these sudden and frequent contacts. Particularly is this so under the lower denture whose area to resist pressure is so much less than the upper (the average maxillary denture-bearing area is 23 cm^2 while the average mandibular area is only 12 cm^2). Easing the fitting surface over sore areas does not cure this trouble; it only destroys the fit in one part and increases the pressure in another.

Loss of freeway space

Loss of the normal space between the occlusal surfaces of the teeth, when the mandible is in the rest position, may have several effects, one of which is nearly always annoyance from the inability to find a comfortable resting position. Other effects may be trauma caused by the constant pressure on the mucosa, and muscular fatigue of any one, or any group, of the muscles of mastication.

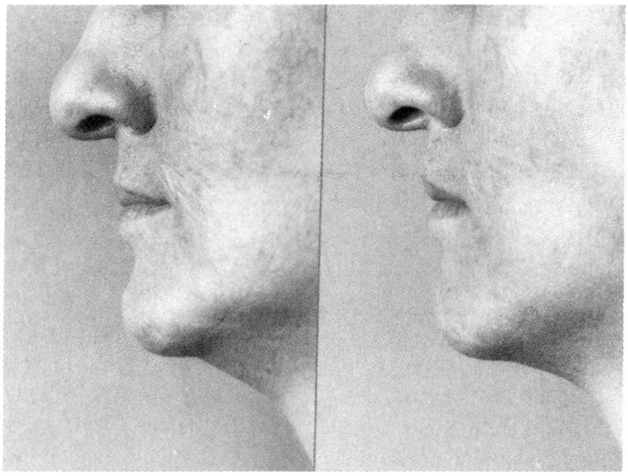

(*a*) (*b*)

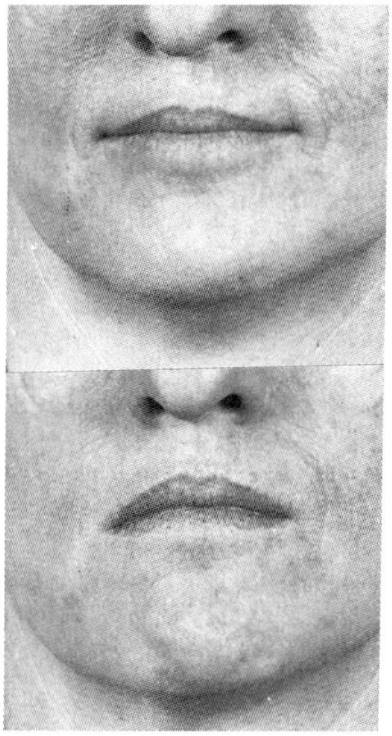

(*a*)

(*b*)

Figure 6.22 Effect on appearance of increasing the vertical dimension of occlusion: (*a*) correct vertical dimension; (*b*) excessive vertical dimension

Clicking teeth

The tongue becomes accustomed to the presence of teeth in certain fixed positions and, during speech, helps to produce sounds without the teeth coming into contact. When, however, these teeth are raised, due to too great a vertical height, opposing cusps frequently meet each other, producing an embarrassing clicking or clattering sound. This same effect is also often produced during eating, but is not so obvious as it is muffled by the food.

Appearance

The result of increasing the vertical dimension must be an elongation of the face, but if it is only slight it will usually pass unnoticed. What will generally be obvious, however, is that at rest the lips are parted, and that closing them together will produce an expression of strain (Figure 6.22).

Effects of excessively reducing the vertical dimension

Inefficiency

This is due to the fact that the pressure which it is possible to exert with the teeth in contact decreases considerably with over-closure because the muscles of mastication are acting from attachments which have been brought closer together.

Cheek biting

In some cases where there is a loss of muscular tone, as well as a reduced vertical height, the flabby cheeks tend to become trapped between the teeth and bitten during mastication. When the over-closure has been deliberate, it is possible to avoid this cheek biting by setting the upper posterior teeth more buccally than normal, thus producing a greater overjet. Cheek biting often occurs because the buccal flange of the denture is too narrow which allows the cheek to fall in (Figure 6.23).

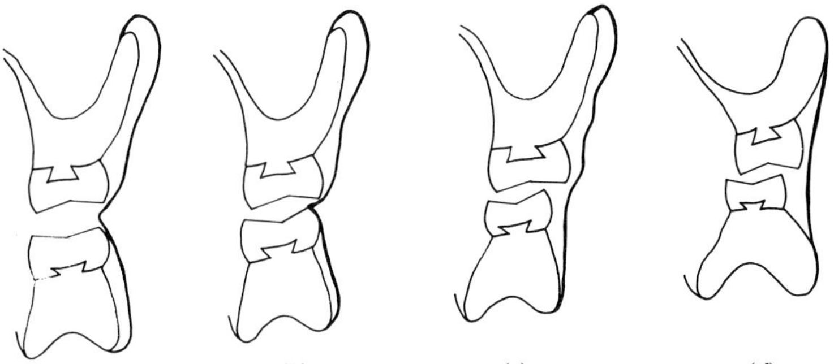

(*a*) (*b*) (*c*) (*d*)

Figure 6.23 Cheek biting. (*a*) How it occurs. (*b*) Small buccal overjet. (*c*) Increased buccal overjet to prevent biting. (*d*) Maxillary buccal flange with correct width holds the cheek in its correct position and avoids biting

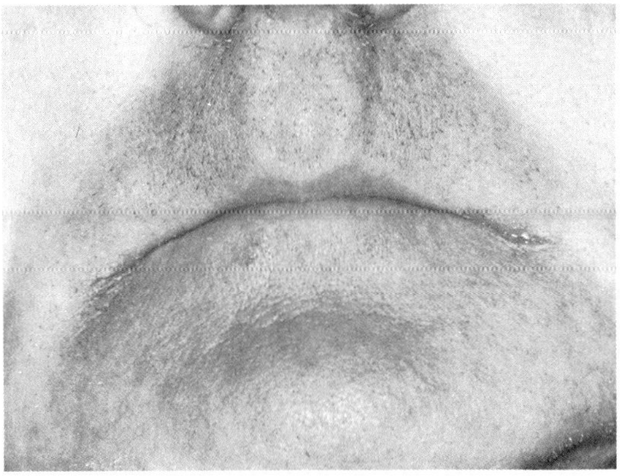

Figure 6.24 Angular cheilitis. Note the involution of the lips and the transitional epithelium, especially towards the corners (patient wearing complete dentures)

Appearance

The general effect of over-closure on facial appearance is of increased age. There is closer approximation of nose to chin, the soft tissues sag and fall in, and the lines on the face are deepened. The greater the degree of over-closure, the more exaggerated are these effects.

Soreness at the corners of the mouth (angular cheilitis)

Over-closure of the vertical height sometimes results in a falling in of the corners of the mouth beyond the vermilion border and the deep folds thus formed become bathed in saliva (Figure 6.24). This area may become infected and sore and is then difficult to cure while it remains moist. Opening the vertical height helps to restore the corners of the mouth to their normal position, but this must be combined with ensuring that the anteroposterior position of the lips is also correct. A deep natural fold is often difficult to eliminate and in no case must the increased vertical height exceed the freeway space.

Pain in the temporomandibular joint

In cases of over-closure of the jaws, pain in the temporomandibular joint may occur. The loss of posterior occlusion subjects the joint to a greater proportion of load and if the meniscus is damaged then clicking or crepitus may be heard on movement. The temporalis and masseter muscles are affected by lack of posterior teeth and may be a source of pain or discomfort as they take on a protective role. In such cases the patient has to protrude the mandible in order to occlude the teeth and the lateral pterygoid muscles become painful, the pain being centred on or anterior to the temporomandibular joints. This relationship between joints, muscles and occlusion is often termed the temporomandibular joint pain dysfunction syndrome.

Pre-extraction records

In practice the dental surgeon will usually either extract the teeth and construct the dentures, or replace existing dentures; it is not often that patients present themselves for treatment without either natural or artificial teeth. Before the patient is edentulous the dentist has the opportunity to record the vertical dimension and the position and shape of the teeth. Methods that may be used to obtain this information are given below.

Willis gauge

When this is used for recording the vertical height before extraction, the arm A (Figure 6.25) is placed in contact with the base of the nose and the arm B is moved along the slide C until it is lightly but firmly touching the lower border of the chin, when it is locked in position by a screw. The distance on the scale C is recorded on the patient's chart.

This is not a very accurate measurement; it depends on the operator always applying exactly the same degree of pressure when the instrument is making contact with the base of the nose and with the undersurface of the chin.

Profile tracing

One of the earliest and simplest methods of obtaining profile records was to adapt a piece of soft lead wire to the contour of the face starting on the

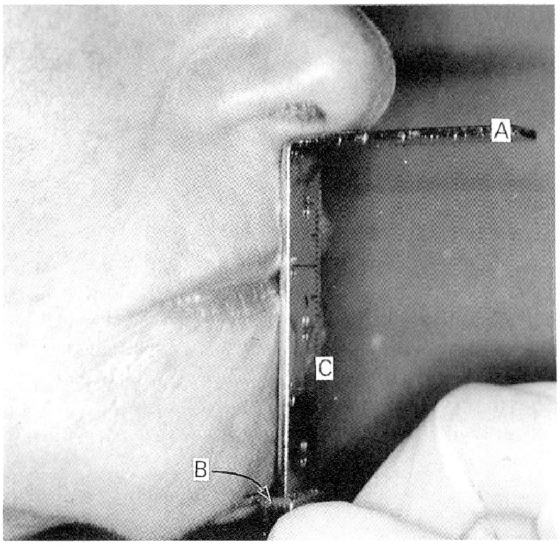

Figure 6.25 A Willis gauge in position on the face. It is improved if the arm B is bent to a curve as this shape fits under the chin more easily

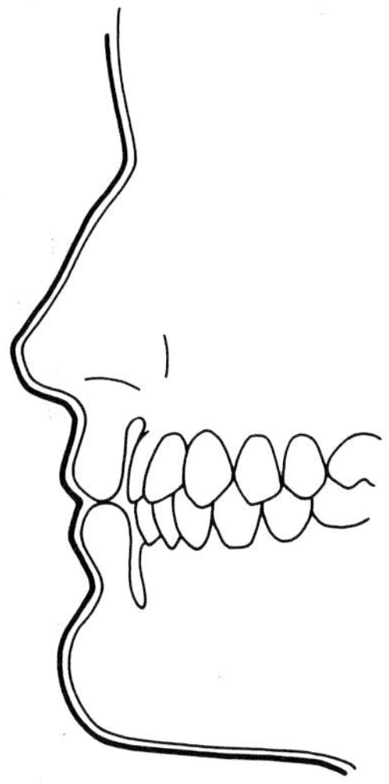

Figure 6.26 Profile tracing (see text)

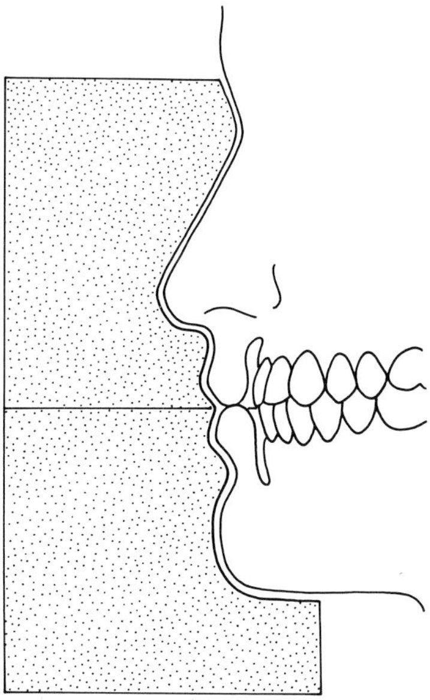

Figure 6.27 Profile template with horizontal line drawn to indicate position of maxillary central incisors

brow, following down the nose and lips and ending just below the chin (Figure 6.26). It was then carefully laid on a piece of stout card, the outline pencilled and the profile cut. This template was then placed on the face to check its accuracy and to mark the position of the upper central incisors (Figure 6.27).

Any further information, such as name, address, date, colour and shape of the teeth could be entered on the template and filed away for future reference.

Nowadays photographs or cephalometric radiographs are used for profile records.

Casts on an articulator

These indicate the amount of vertical and horizontal overlap as well as assisting in the selection of size, shape and position of the teeth to be used for the dentures. Another method is to make impressions immediately prior to the extraction of the teeth, which are then extracted, sterilized, and inserted into the impression. The casts thus obtained contain the natural teeth in their original position, but cannot be used as a record of shade because this changes in time.

The horizontal relationship

Having discussed the vertical dimension, the horizontal relation of the mandible to the maxilla still remains to be found, often referred to as the retruded position or, when teeth or occlusal rims are in contact at an acceptable vertical dimension, the retruded contact position, (RCP).

Many individuals, who have been without teeth for some considerable time, have a tendency to protrude the mandible when asked to close the jaws together, for the simple reason that the crushing of any food taken into the mouth has to be carried out by the approximation of the anterior alveolar ridges as the posterior ridges will not meet. In order to function in this manner the mandible has to be drawn forward which, in the early days of edentation, starts as a conscious act, but as time passes rapidly becomes automatic. Such patients cause difficulty for the clinician when trying to obtain the retruded position of occlusion. Also, many patients manage for a number of years with only the natural anterior teeth standing without wearing dentures to replace the missing posterior teeth and once again an unconscious protrusion of the mandible results.

Both these habit-forming conditions cause difficulty for the clinician when attempting to secure the position of retrusion. Sometimes it is desirable to record the acquired position instead of the true position, and this was discussed in Chapter 3, but it is only the true retruded position which is being considered here.

Stress has purposely been laid on the difficulty to be expected in many cases in obtaining a correct retruded record, because great patience will often be needed as satisfactory dentures cannot be constructed unless the record is correct.

There are many aids to help the prosthetist to obtain the retruded position and where one fails another may well succeed.

Instructions to the patient

Always ask the patient to 'close', never ask him to 'bite'. 'Bite' conveys the impression of incising, and to incise requires some protrusion of the jaw, which

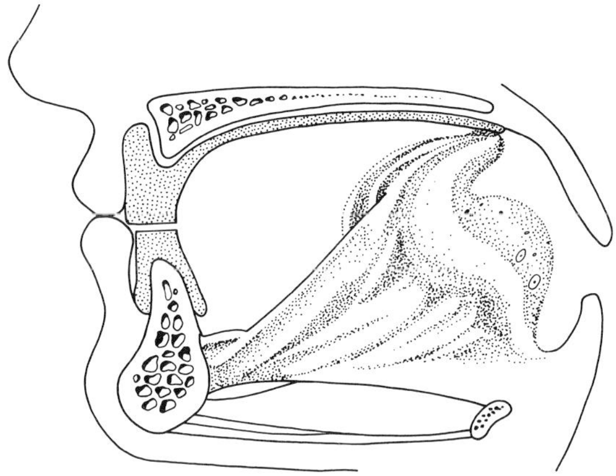

Figure 6.28 Illustrating the position which the tongue should assume when closing the blocks to obtain the retrusive record

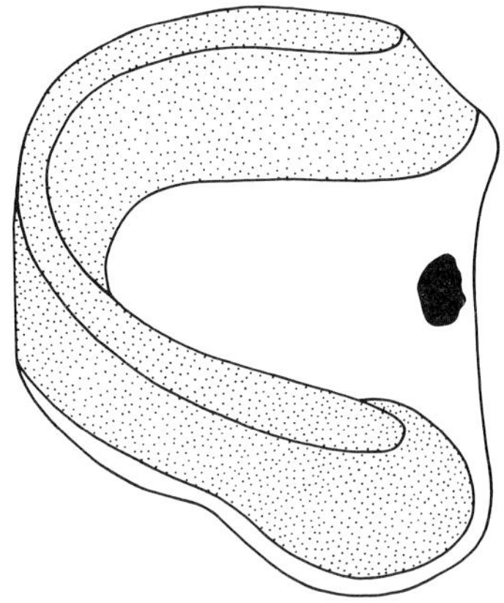

Figure 6.29 Small piece of wax or compound on the maxillary record block is touched by the tongue

is just the reverse of what is required. 'Close on your back teeth', even though the patient has no natural posterior teeth, is a useful instruction.

Tongue retrusion

Ask the patient to place the tip of the tongue as far back on the palate as possible, to keep it there and close the blocks together until they meet (Figure 6.28). Some patients have a tendency to let the tongue move forward and it is often helpful to put a small knob of soft wax near the posterior border of the upper record block (Figure 6.29). The position of the wax should be shown to the patient before the record block is inserted in the mouth and when the block is in place the patient is requested to place the tip of the tongue in contact with the wax and keep it there while he closes. The reason behind this suggestion is that the tongue, when in this position, will exert a muscular pull on the mandible in a backward direction.

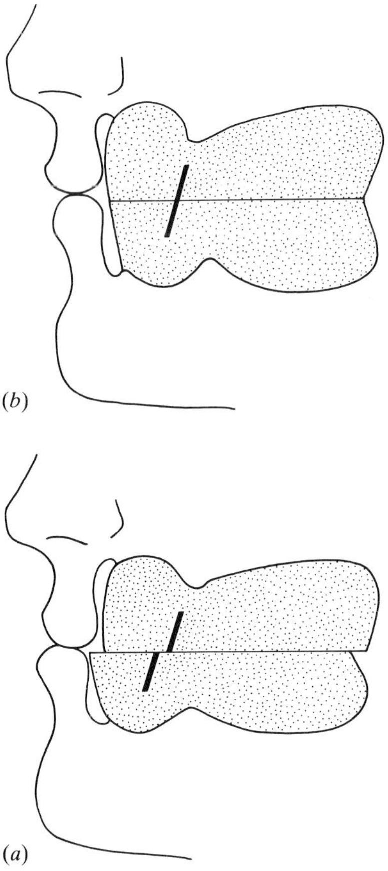

Figure 6.30 The use of guide lines to check the retrusive position of the mandible. (*a*) Line on upper and lower block coincide. (*b*) Lines no longer coincide indicating that the mandible is protruded

As soon as it is considered that the mandible is retruded, two approximately vertical lines should be scored on the buccal aspects of the occlusal rims one on either side in the premolar region. These lines should extend across both rims and are used for checking the retrusion of the mandible when using other aids. It will be obvious that if the mandible is correctly retruded, the lines on the lower block will always coincide with those on the upper when the jaws are closed. If, however, any alteration in the maxillo-mandibular relation occurs, the lines on the lower block will no longer coincide with those on the upper, and this will indicate an altered relationship (Figure 6.30).

Control of mandible

The clinician stands so that he looks directly in front of the patient. The index fingers are placed on the lower occlusal rim so that the tips touch the medial aspect of the ascending ramus. Ask the patient to close on his back teeth and as the rims come together the fingers are moved buccally, all the time stabilizing the blocks and preventing any shift. The finger position tends to induce retrusion. Wire staples on the buccal surface of the lower block serve as useful platforms for the index fingers at the last stage of closure.

Relaxation

If the patient can be persuaded to relax the muscles of the jaw, it will automatically assume the retruded position and this will be greatly assisted by general body relaxation. The patient must be very comfortably seated in the chair and asked to relax as completely as possible preferably with the feet supported on a foot rest. Relaxation depends very largely on the operator, some with a quiet, almost hypnotic manner, find it almost invaribaly successful, while others, because of too brisk a manner, find it useless. When general relaxation is obtained the patient is asked to close the blocks slowly together and the continuity of the vertical lines made previously is checked. If the mandible is now found to be more retruded, fresh lines are made for further checking; if the lines coincide it may be assumed that the position is correct, or further checks as described below may be carried out.

Swallowing

Ask the patient to swallow and conclude the act with the blocks in contact. This is based on the fact that with a natural dentition the teeth are brought into a retruded position during swallowing.

Fatigue

Ask the patient to protrude and retrude the mandible continuously for as long as possible and to finish in a retrusive position with the blocks in contact. The object is to tire the lateral pterygoid muscles so that they will relax when the movement ceases, and so allow the condylar heads to be retruded.

Head position

Lower the head rest and ask the patient to bend the head backwards as far as possible. This will produce a backward pull on the mandible and makes it difficult to protrude, but places the patient in a position in which it is awkward for the clinican to check the relationship of the blocks.

The temporalis muscle check

The anterior fibres of the temporalis muscle only contract on closure of the mandible if it is retruded.

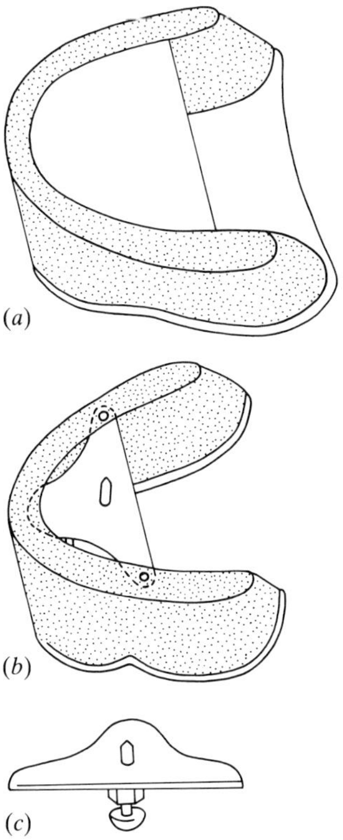

Figure 6.31 Details of intra-oral gothic arch tracing apparatus. (*a*) Upper block with tracing plate inserted. (*b*) Lower block with tracing point and holder inserted. (*c*) Tracing point and holder

Thus if the fingers are placed on the temples and the patient closes the rims firmly the contraction or not of the anterior fibres of the temporalis may be used as an assessment of mandibular retrusion.

The gothic arch tracing

This may be obtained either by intra-oral or extra-oral methods; both make use of the same principle and result in a reliable assessment of RCP. The technique shows the horizontal movement of the mandible in the form of a tracing, made by a pointed attachment fitted to one block on a recording plate fitted to the other (Figures 6.31, and 6.32).

Consider for a moment the lateral movements of the mandible. Starting from the retruded position and moving to the right, the left condyle is drawn forwards down the articular eminence, while the right condyle acts as a pivoting point, and vice versa for the left lateral movement. If a tracing is taken from a given point in the midline of the mouth, two lines result which converge to a sharply pointed apex; if the mandible were then protruded, the

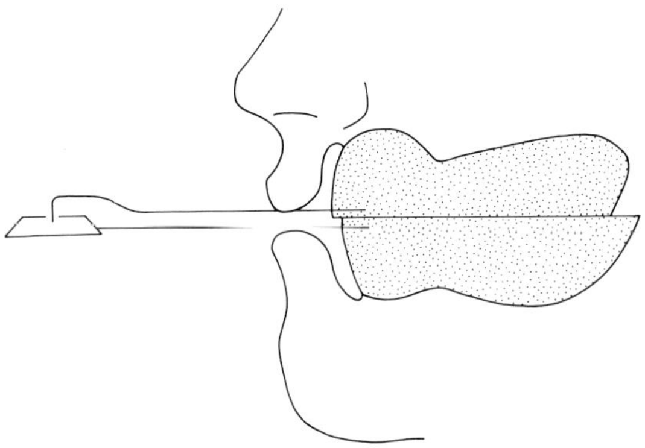

Figure 6.32 Details of extra-oral apparatus, showing tracing stylus attached to the upper block and tracing plate attached to the lower block

tracing would also start and finish at this point, since it indicates the retruded position (Figure 6.33). If this principle is applied, the point at which the tracings intersect and form a sharp, pointed arrow head will be the retruded mandibular position for a given individual.

Tracing devices and technique

The intra-oral device consists of a carrier, through the centre of which is threaded a pointed stylus controlled by a locking nut. After the correct vertical height has been obtained, the carrier is fitted to the lower rim so that the tracing point is placed centrally across a line joining the premolars. The tracing plate is cut from flat sheet metal and inserted parallel to, and just below, the occlusal surface of the upper rim. Place the blocks in the mouth with the stylus adjusted to hold the rims slightly apart. The patient now performs lateral jaw movements, keeping the tracing point in contact with the plate the whole time. When the operator is satisfied that the patient can perform these movements correctly, the upper block is removed and after the tracing plate has been filmed with carding wax the block is replaced in the mouth. Lateral and protrusive movements are again made, the tracings examined, and if a clearly defined arrow head has been recorded the retruded position has been obtained. Drill a small hole through the apex (Figure 6.34) to accommodate the point of the stylus and ask the patient to move the mandible until the point slips into the hole; the blocks should now be in even contact and no longer held apart by the screw. The blocks are united in the mouth with warm wire staples held in suture needle holders or mosquito forceps and inserted (Figure 6.35). Take care not to burn the patient's lips.

Another method of making a tracing is to fix the tracing plate and stylus directly to base plates made of cold-cure acrylic. Obtain the vertical jaw separation by screwing the stylus up and down, locking it at the correct height and then performing the tracing as described above. The base-plates are united in the mouth in the retruded relationship by placing plaster between them which, when set, firmly unites them in the correct relationship. This

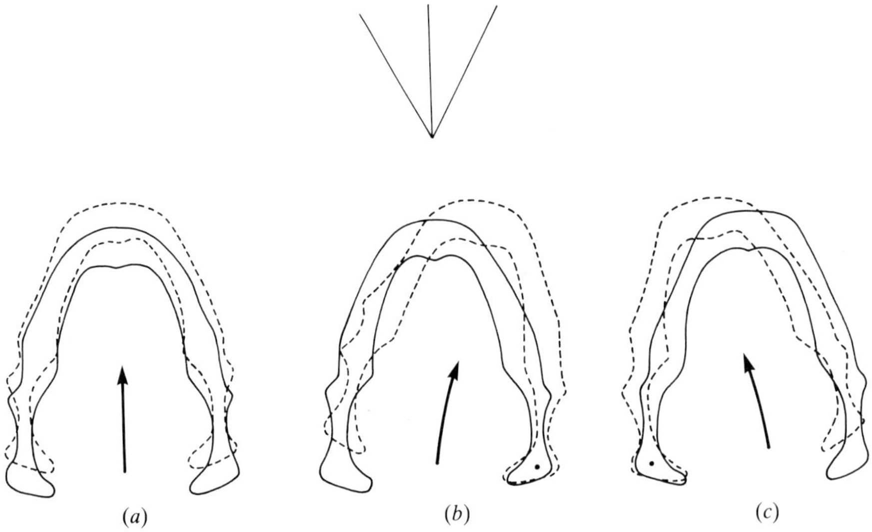

Figure 6.33 Illustrating how a gothic arch tracing is made. The arrow indicates the direction of travel of a stylus attached to a lower block tracing on a plate fixed to the upper block. (*a*) When the mandible is protruded; (*b*) when it is moved to the right; (*c*) when it is moved to the left. Insert shows the form of the completed tracing

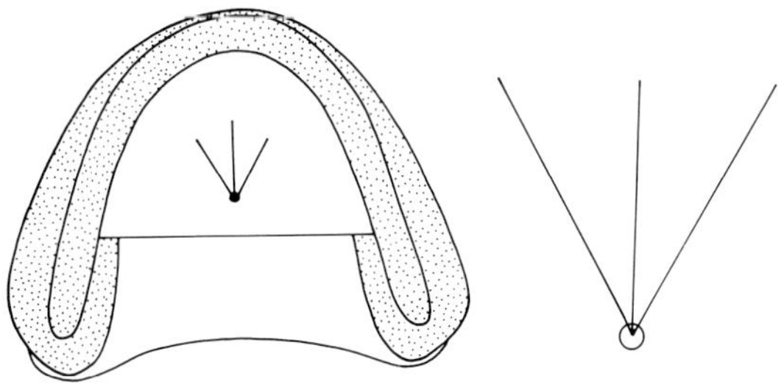

Figure 6.34 Upper block with completed gothic arch tracing and hole bored at apex. Insert shows enlarged view of tracing and hole

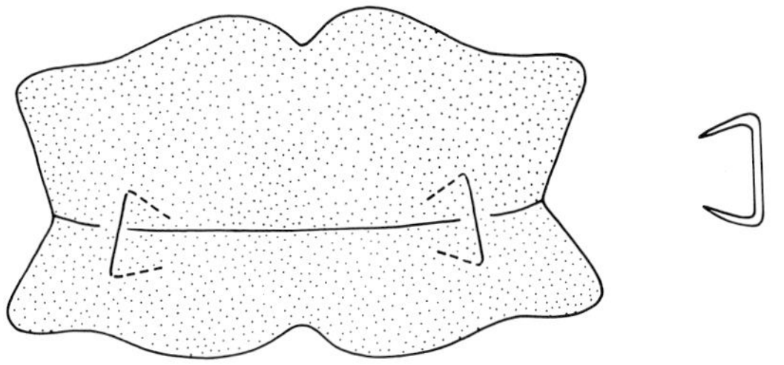

Figure 6.35 Illustrating the method of sealing the record blocks with warmed wire staples

method gives no indication of the incisal or occlusal planes or centre line and, therefore, an additional upper base plate is required to which the selected six upper anterior teeth are attached in the desired position by wax at the chairside. The casts are mounted on the articulator by means of the tracing apparatus and then the upper base carrying the anterior teeth is substituted and the set-up continued by the technician, the upper anterior teeth remaining in place.

In some cases several tracings will have to be taken before the typical arrow head or gothic arch is secured; a rounded apex indicates that the condylar heads are not fully retruded (Figure 6.36).

The extra-oral apparatus is similar to the intra-oral except that the stylus and tracing plate are outside the mouth, being attached to the record blocks by rods which pass between the lips (Figures 6.32 and 6.37).

These techniques are dependent on well-fitting, stable bases. Acrylic undoubtedly gives the most uniformly successful results.

Methods for sealing the record blocks together

Heat

When it is not intended to record more than the retruded position, the blocks can be sealed together in the mouth by means of a hot wax-knife, care being taken that the knife is not hot enough to cause the wax to run. With this method it is sometimes difficult to remove the united blocks from the mouth, but if the patient is asked to open his mouth widely and to push the blocks out with his tongue, no difficulty will be encountered.

Wax wafer

A few V-shaped notches are cut in the occlusal surfaces of the rims (Figure 6.38) care being taken not to obliterate the centre line or check marks. The blocks are placed in the mouth, the lower with two thicknesses of softened wax covering its occlusal surface. The patient is asked to close the blocks together, using whatever method has been found most useful, and as soon as the clinician has checked that the retruded position is correct the patient is asked to close more firmly. The problem with this method is that the wax may not be uniformly soft so, as the patient closes, uneven pressure may cause mandibular deviation or mucosal compression on one side. Because of these common faults plaster is better than wax and is particularly helpful in those cases where the patient tends to slide the jaw forward as he closes. The softness and lack of resistance of the plaster, thus reducing the pressure required to close, often inhibits the desire to protrude the jaw and leads to an even, all-round contact of the blocks.

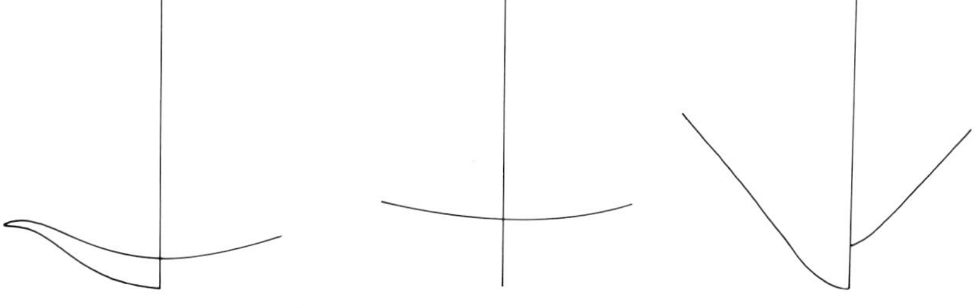

Figure 6.36 Illustrating various tracings which may be obtained. All indicate that the mandibular condyles are not fully retruded

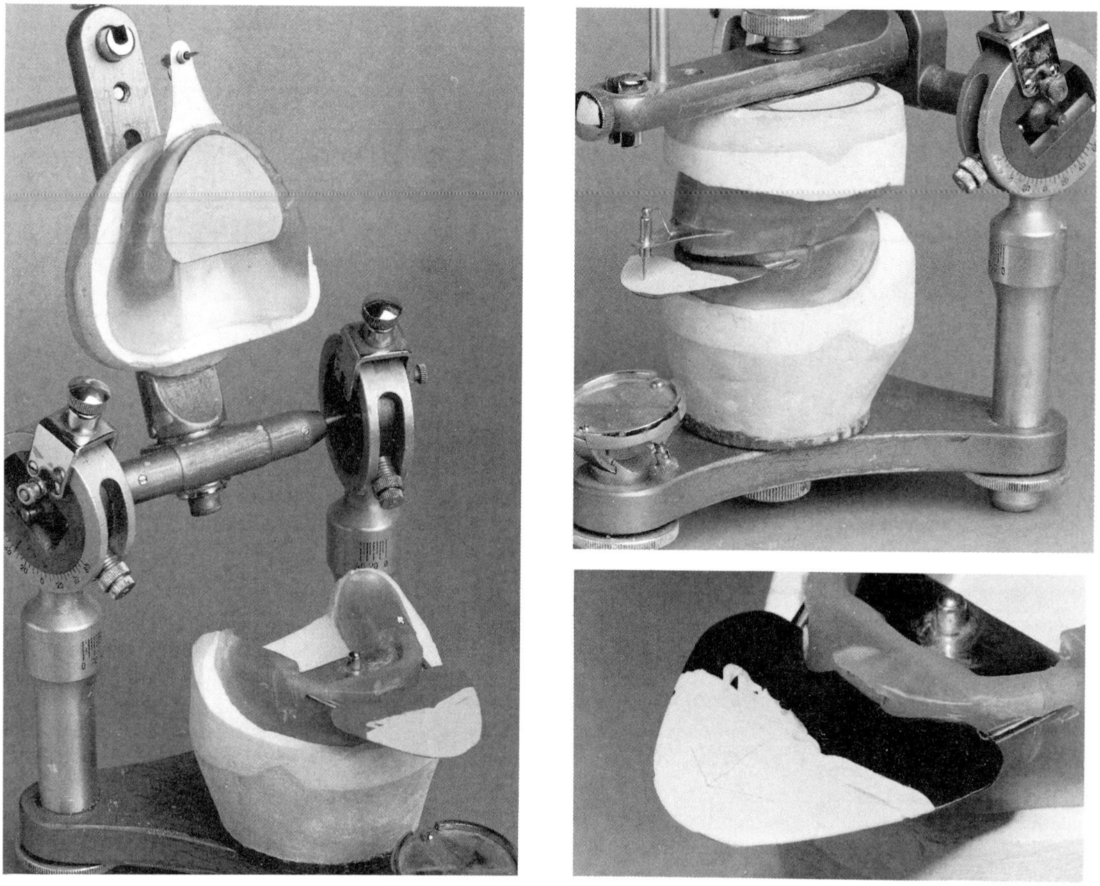

Figure 6.37 Extra-oral tracing apparatus. Casts mounted in retruded contact position following satisfactory gothic arch tracing as seen in close-up of tracing plate

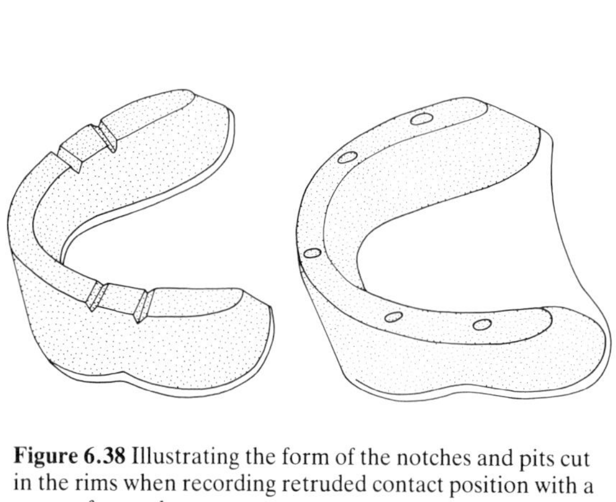

Figure 6.38 Illustrating the form of the notches and pits cut in the rims when recording retruded contact position with a wax wafer or plaster

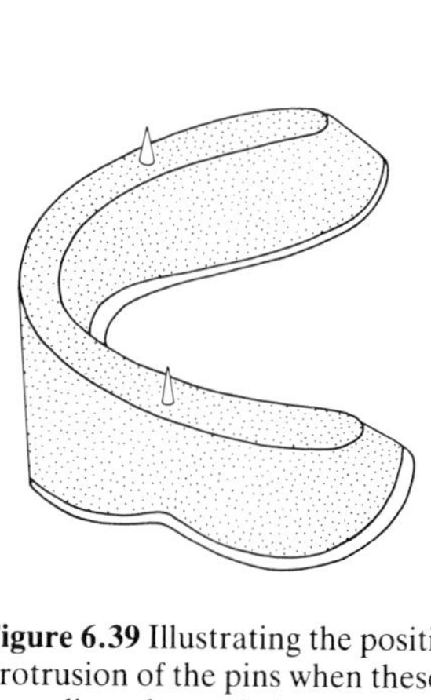

Figure 6.39 Illustrating the position and degree of protrusion of the pins when these are used during the recording of retruded contact position

Pinning

Some patients tend to protrude the mandible when they have brought the record blocks into occlusion, and if a wax wafer is used in these cases it acts as a lubricant between the rims and permits this sliding movement. In such cases the blocks may be fixed by means of pins of stainless steel wire instead of a wax wafer. These are warmed and inserted in each lower premolar area protruding not more than 2 mm above the occlusal surface (Figure 6.39). The lower block is thoroughly chilled to support and retain the pins and the upper rim very slightly softened in the area into which the pins will be forced. As the blocks are inserted and closed together, the pins prevent the sliding movement unless the upper rim has been over-softened.

Common errors in jaw relation records

Errors in occlusion of the finished dentures frequently arise as a result of errors at the record stage other than an incorrect vertical or anteroposterior jaw relation. The commonest of these are:

1. Tilting of the blocks off the ridges as a result of uneven contact.
2. Premature contact of the heels of the record blocks leading to displacement or tilting of the blocks.
3. Contact of the heels of the casts which prevents them being accurately seated in the blocks.
4. Lack of simultaneous all-round contact of the occlusal rims which may be avoided by asking the patient 'which side meets first?'

Chapter 7

The selection of teeth

At the conclusion of registering the jaw relations, the choice of the teeth to be used on the dentures requires to be made. The selection of artificial teeth which are suitable in shape, size and colour is not easy. There are many difficulties even to the experienced clinician, particularly if he lacks artistic appreciation. This tends towards art and less to science and, while the principles which follow will enable any clinician of average artistic ability to select teeth suitable for the average patient, the most pleasing results will always be obtained by those with an aesthetic sense.

Classification of patients

There are three classes of patients who present themselves for complete dentures:

1. Those who still retain most of their upper anterior teeth which, for one reason or another, will soon be extracted. This group is considered under Immediate Dentures (Chapter 26).
2. Those who are already wearing complete dentures. If the dentures have been worn for any length of time it is probable that the patient, and his immediate circle of relations and friends, are satisfied with the appearance of the dentures which may, for this reason, be copied. It is rarely advisable to make very marked alterations in an individual's appearance, and improvements are best restricted to the selection of slightly larger teeth of a slightly darker shade, although modifications can also be made to the denture base design to restore or improve facial appearance.
3. Those who present for the first time already edentulous and who have not yet been supplied with dentures, or who have lost them or who are dissatisfied with the appearance of existing dentures. The selection of suitable teeth for this group will be considered under the headings: shape, size and colour.

Shape

Soon after the introduction of porcelain anterior teeth it was realized that there was some relationship between the shape of the edentulous upper arch and the upper teeth. For example, a V-shaped arch is associated with incisors which are much narrower at the neck than at the incisal edge; a squarish arch with almost parallel-sided incisors; and a round arch with ovoid teeth (Figure 7.1).

Classification of Williams

The classification of Leon Williams, though not scientifically correct, is undoubtedly the simplest and most useful guide yet suggested, with the added advantage that most manufacturers of artificial teeth have adopted it for their products. He claimed that the shape of the upper central incisor bears a definite relationship to the shape of the face. Thus, if one of these teeth were enlarged, and the incisal edge placed above the brows with the neck of the tooth on the chin, then the outline of the tooth would nearly coincide with that of the face (Figure 7.2). He classified the form of the human face, for simplicity, into three types: square, tapering and ovoid, each type merging into the others without any clear line of demarcation. In order to determine to what type an individual belongs the clinician imagines two lines, one on either side of the face, running about 2.5 cm in front of the tragus of the ear

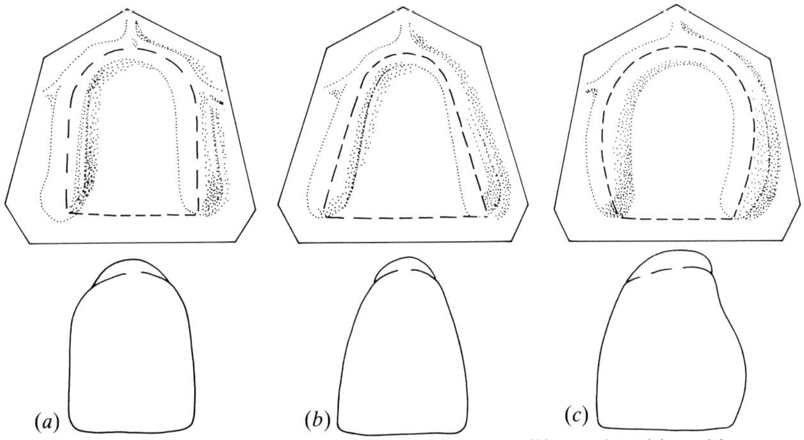

Figure 7.1 Tooth form in relation to arch form: (*a*) square; (*b*) tapering; (*c*) ovoid

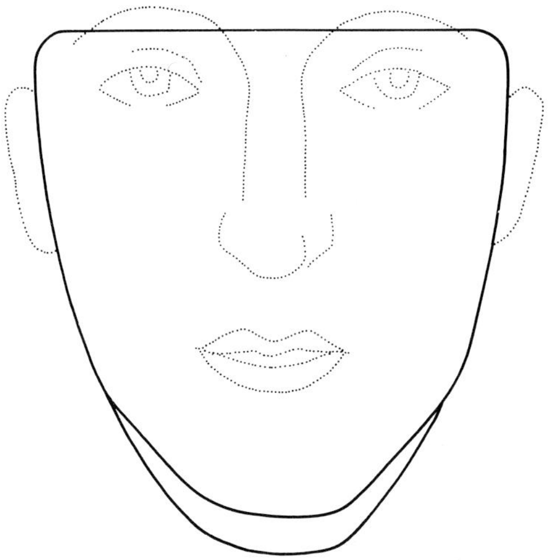

Figure 7.2 The outline of a maxillary central incisor superimposed on a face

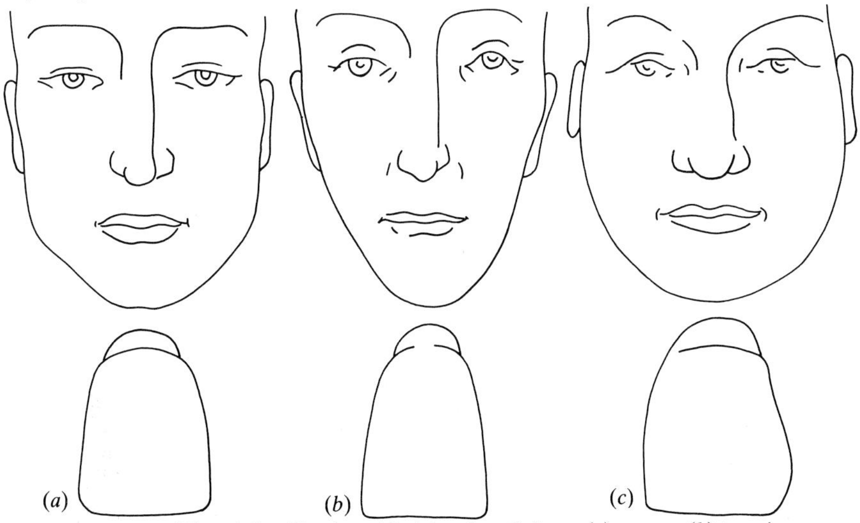

Figure 7.3 Leon Williams' classification of facial and tooth form: (*a*) square; (*b*) tapering; (*c*) ovoid

and through the angle of the jaw. If these lines are almost parallel the type is square; if they converge towards the chin the type is tapering; and if they diverge at the chin, ovoid (Figure 7.3). Having determined the general type to which the patient belongs it only remains to select teeth which are suitable in length, width and colour, for that individual.

Size

Length and width are the only two dimensions which need to be considered at this stage, the thickness being a variable of less aesthetic importance. This statement must not be taken to mean that the thickness of the anterior teeth is unimportant, for it has a considerable bearing on phonetics, but it can be easily varied by the technician without alteration to the form, length or width.

Length

The length of the upper six anterior teeth is normally such that the necks of the teeth will overlap the anterior ridge by 2–3 mm cervically, and the incisal edges of the centrals will show below the relaxed lip. The amount of the central incisors visible below the lip is about 3 mm in a young person and less than half that amount in an elderly patient (Figure 7.4). This is not a hard and fast rule, however, and wide variations will frequently be found necessary because the amount of tooth which an individual shows varies, depending on the following factors.

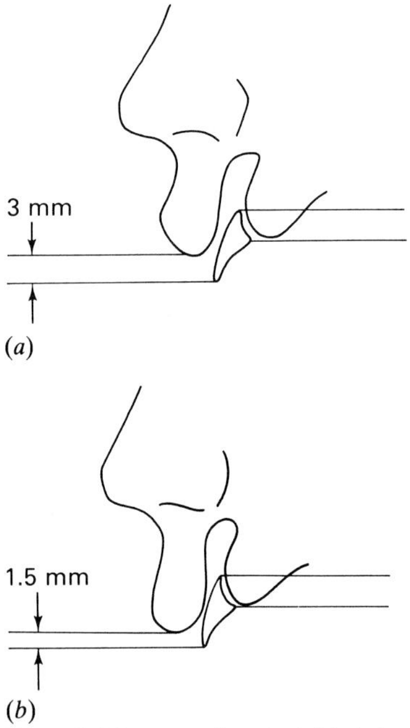

Figure 7.4 Amount of tooth visible below the upper lip in: (*a*) young patient; (*b*) an elderly patient

Length of the upper lip

Some people have long lips which almost completely cover their natural teeth, while others have short, curved lips which, even in the relaxed position, expose sometimes more than half the length of the teeth.

Mobility of the upper lip

This also is a variable factor. Some individuals expose all the upper anterior teeth and a considerable amount of gum when they smile while others show very little tooth and merely stretch the lips laterally.

Vertical height of occlusion

Reduction in the vertical height will cause the lips to bunch up and cover the teeth, while an increase will cause an excessive amount of the teeth to show.

Vertical overlap

A deep vertical overlap results in the exposure of a much greater length of tooth than an edge-to-edge incisal relationship.

Width

Probably the most satisfactory way of selecting teeth of a suitable width for a given case is to choose a set which is wide enough to allow the canines to be mounted on the canine eminence when set up. When using this method, it must be remembered that in very narrow V-shaped mouths, the natural teeth were, in all probability, crowded, and wider

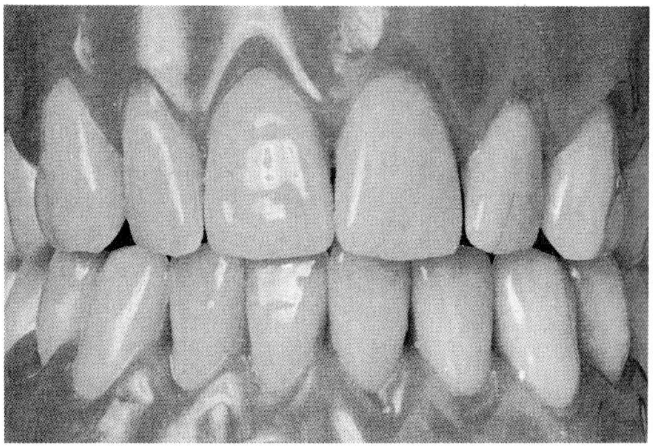

Figure 7.5 Mild irregularity of the maxillary incisors in a V-shaped mouth

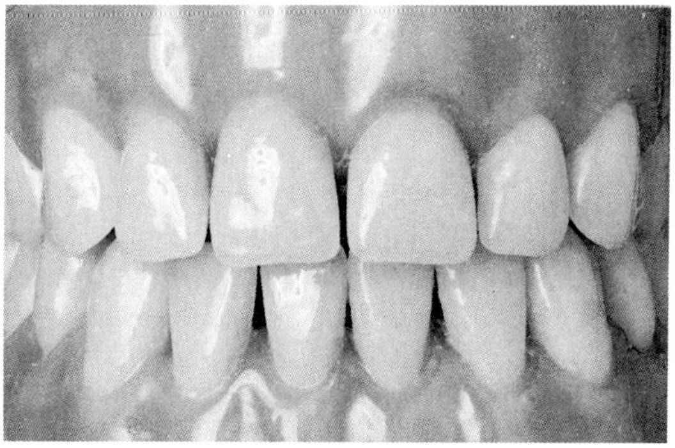

Figure 7.6 Teeth slightly spaced in a broad mouth

teeth should be selected than will reach without irregularity from one canine eminence to the other; overlapping of the centrals and laterals will enable the canines of the wider set to be placed in their correct positions (Figure 7.5).

Similarly, to satisfy the above method, broad teeth would be required in broad mouths, but narrower teeth can be used if they are slightly spaced or if a diastema is placed between the central incisors (Figure 7.6). Natural anterior teeth vary greatly in size, but as a rule they are much larger than is generally realized and one of the commonest prosthetic errors is to use teeth which are too small, thus making them appear obviously false.

The width of most natural maxillary central incisors is over 8.5 mm and any tooth less than 8 mm is rare. The combined width of the maxillary six anterior teeth is normally 46 mm or more and anything less than 45 mm is very unusual.

Harmony

Having considered the length and breadth of the teeth, the final selection with regard to size should be made according to the general characteristics of the patient's features, bearing in mind that harmony of the various dimensions should be the aim. The relationship between the length and breadth of the face and that of the selected teeth should be studied, and for this purpose the face-length is taken from the supra-orbital ridge line to the inferior border of the chin, and the breadth as the distance between the lateral aspects of the zygomatic processes. If the length and breadth of the face appear about equal, then the dimensions of the teeth should follow a similar pattern; the face which appears long in relation to its breadth would indicate teeth of those proportions, irrespective of their shape.

Colour

Natural teeth vary as much in colour as they do in size and shape, and the selection of a suitable shade for any edentulous person is a matter of individual judgment. There are, however, a few generalizations which help in making a decision. Fortunately colour is not critical for the edentulous patient provided that it is compatible with the general colouring of the skin, hair and eyes. Harmony can be obtained over quite a wide range of colour. This statement will be obvious if it is remembered that the natural teeth remain almost constant in colour, merely darkening very slightly with age, but remain in harmony with hair which may first be black, then grey, then white. The colour of the skin may change from a ruddy complexion in health to pallor in sickness, the same teeth remaining in harmony with both conditions.

The following facts are true of nearly all natural teeth, exceptions being very rare:

1 The neck of the tooth has a more pronounced colour than the incisal edge.
2. The incisal edge, if unworn, is more translucent than the body of the tooth and is usually of a bluish shade because it is composed entirely of enamel.
3. Maxillary central incisors are the lightest teeth in the mouth; maxillary laterals and mandibular incisors are slightly darker; canines are darker still.
4. This variation in shade is appreciated by the manufacturers, most of whom make the desired grading in each set of six anteriors, and the prosthetist selects only the shade of the centrals.
5. Posterior teeth are usually uniform in colour and very slightly lighter than the canines.
6. Teeth darken slightly with age.
7. More natural and pleasing effects can be obtained by using teeth of different shades from different sets of six anterior teeth.

The three dominant tooth colours of yellow, grey and opal are each found in a wide variety of shades and intensity. Many attempts have been made to correlate tooth colour with the skin, hair and eyes, but only vague generalities may be stated:

1. Yellow is dominant with fair hair, blue eyes and a fresh complexion.
2. Grey sometimes tinged with blue is dominant with dark hair, brown eyes and dark complexion.
3. Opal is dominant with a clear, pale complexion, irrespective of the colour of the hair and eyes.
4. A person of powerful build and with large teeth usually has teeth of a dark shade and a rather pronounced colour.
5. Small, pearly-white teeth are so rare that they always look false.

The following suggestions may be useful:

1. Always moisten the shade guide because, when in the mouth, the teeth are always moist and this

has an effect on the reflection and refraction of light and hence the colour.

2. Always place the teeth under consideration in the shade of the upper lip in the position they are to occupy; they will appear darker in this position than in the hand.
3. When in doubt, select a tooth which is obviously too dark and view it in position, then try one which is obviously too light, gradually merging these two extremes until a pleasing shade is found.
4. The assistance of the patient, and any friend or relation who may be available, may be useful but only let them see the tooth in the shadow of the upper lip, otherwise too light a colour will invariably be chosen.
5. Attempt to look at the face as a whole rather than focus entirely on the teeth and, whenever possible, select teeth under natural light or colour-corrected artificial light.
6. Remember that the lighter the shade the more artificial the tooth looks; many female patients insist on lighter teeth than the dentist thinks desirable but, unless the selection is glaringly wrong, the dentist should consider giving way to the patient, as after all, it is she who will have to wear the denture.

Posterior tooth form

Early artificial dentures were carved from solid blocks of ivory (Figure 7.7) and their fit, occlusion and appearance were all extremely poor, but with the discovery of vulcanite in 1839, followed soon after by the use of porcelain teeth, the modern conception of artificial teeth began. Dentists found, before the end of the nineteenth century, that natural tooth forms with their interlocking cusps caused instability of the dentures, and investigations were begun on how this difficulty could be overcome. Research into this problem followed two quite distinct lines:

1. To alter the shape of the posterior teeth so that cusps could be eliminated without sacrificing efficiency.
2. To retain natural tooth forms and to prevent their causing instability; this was attempted by designing articulators which copied the mandibular movements of the individual patient (see Chapter 9).

A large number of tooth forms have been designed and marketed over the years but, for practical purposes, the selection of posterior teeth may be made as follows.

For plane-line (hinge) articulators

Inverted cusp teeth

The lack of projecting cusps reduces the lateral drag on the dentures when functioning. When setting teeth to functionally generated paths or preformed templates, inverted cusp teeth should be used, otherwise the occlusal plane will not conform

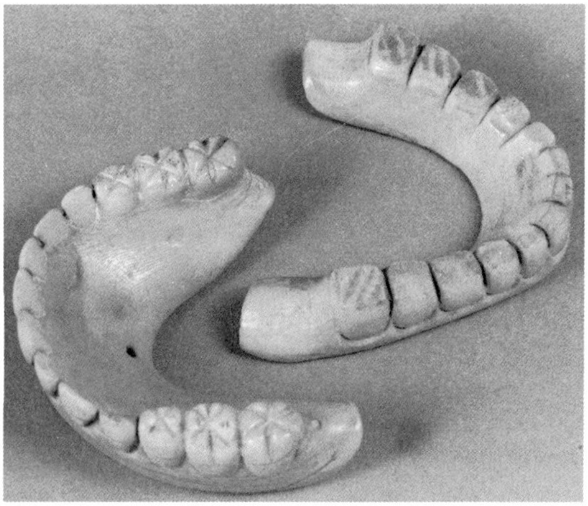

Figure 7.7 Dentures carved from ivory

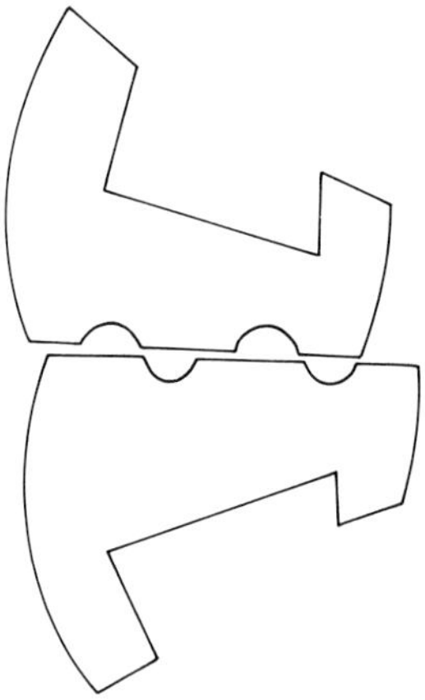

(*a*)

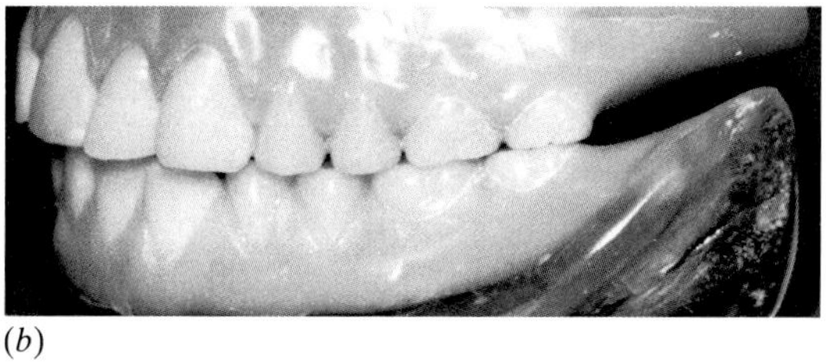

(*b*)

Figure 7.8 (*a*) Inverted cusp teeth, illustrated in section. The design of the occlusal surface takes the form of an intaglio. (*b*) Lateral view of complete dentures on which inverted cusp teeth were used. These teeth are also called zero-cusp or monoplane sufficiently closely to the curves of the occlusal rim or template. Inverted cusp teeth may also be used whenever poor resistance to lateral movement of the dentures is anticipated.

Shallow cusp teeth

These teeth are commonly used when setting up dentures on plane-line articulators, and provided the cusps are not too high, they produce tolerable results. Many patients will adapt themselves to the limitation of lateral mandibular movement imposed by any cuspal interference, and there is no doubt that the presence of cusps does facilitate the trituration of food.

One disadvantage of cusps on teeth is that as alveolar resorption progresses the vertical dimension reduces and the interlocking of the cusps causes the lower denture to be displaced forwards and the upper backwards, causing damage to the underlying tissues. The use of flat inverted cusp teeth (Figure 7.8) prevents or reduces this trauma.

For adjustable or moving-condyle articulators

Ideally the cusp angle and height of the cusps of all the posterior teeth should be accurately related to the paths of the mandible when functioning. Practically this is not possible, but certain teeth are available for which the manufacturers publish the cusp angle, e.g. 2O° posteriors, and teeth of this type can be satisfactorily employed with most adjustable or moving-condyle articulators. This is discussed further in Chapter 9.

Chapter 8

Setting teeth on the articulator

It is not intended that this chapter should be an authoritative description of laboratory techniques, but in order to understand the necessity and value of oral records, the clinician must know how they are used by the technician. Further, it is impossible for the clinician to criticize intelligently and fairly a technician's work, or alter such work, without some knowledge of the technique of setting teeth.

The parts of a denture

A denture (Figure 8.1) consists essentially of two parts which, though united, serve different functions:

1. The base, which may best be described by enumerating its functions:
   (a) To provide the retention and stability of the denture.
   (b) To carry and support the teeth.

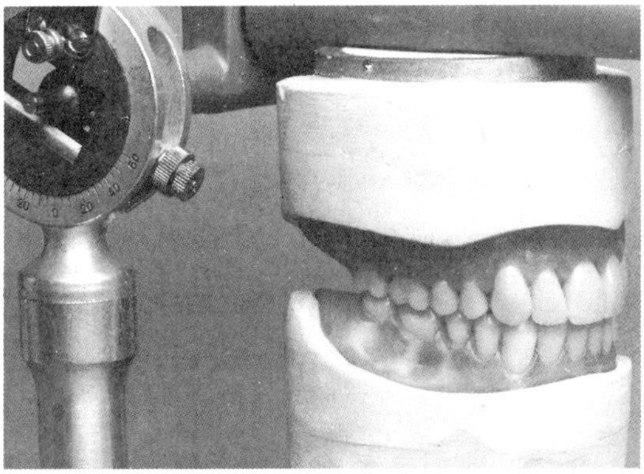

Figure 8.1 The denture bases and the teeth

   (c) To represent the gums and mucosa.
   (d) To assist the teeth in supporting the cheeks and lips.
2. The teeth, whose functions are:
   (a) To provide a comfortable and atraumatic occlusion.
   (b) To assist in preparing food for deglutition.
   (c) To impart a pleasing and natural appearance.
   (d) To assist in speech.

In every case the artificial teeth are first mounted in wax on a base-plate which may be either temporary or permanent (see Chapter 6). The process of arranging the teeth is usually termed setting-up, that of moulding and carving the wax supporting them as waxing-up.

The position of the teeth

Before the artificial teeth can be arranged to form dentures the placing of each tooth, and the reasons why it is so placed, must be understood, because if each tooth is not positioned and angled correctly, the dentures will be functionally inefficient and aesthetically poor.

The casts, in their correct retruded jaw relationship, are mounted on a hinged piece of apparatus called an articulator (see Figures 6.4 and 6.5). This is to enable the technician to set the teeth in correct relationship to each other. An articulator may be of the simple hinge type, producing 'plane-line' occlusion, or it may imitate to some extent the mandibular movements and so produce 'anatomical' occlusion.

The teeth must be set in very definite positions, only variable within rather small limits, and these

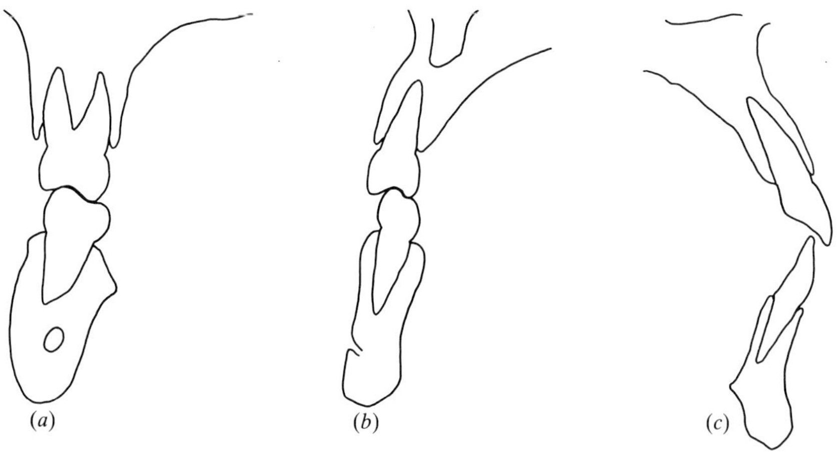

Figure 8.2 Illustrating the relationship of the natural teeth to their supporting bone in the: (*a*) molar region; (*b*) premolar region; (*c*) incisor region

will be described in relation to: the casts; the occlusal plane; the vertical axis; and the other teeth.

The following description of the arrangement of the teeth is the normal intercuspal occlusion unless otherwise stated, but this must frequently be modified for individual cases. This is particularly true of the upper anterior teeth where irregularities are frequently introduced for aesthetic reasons, and these alterations must be made at the chairside by the dentist or detailed instructions of what is required given by the dentist to the technician.

The relationship of the teeth to the casts

When the natural teeth are present in the mouth their crowns are situated over the centres of the alveolar ridges. In the mandible the alveolar ridge supporting the molar teeth forms a buttress of bone on the lingual aspect of the so-called basal bone or body of the mandible. The ridge supporting the premolars is immediately above the body of the mandible and the ridge supporting the lower incisors and the canines is slightly labial to the main body of the mandible. The maxillary alveolar process is situated on the external, inferior surface of the maxilla (Figure 8.2).

In the horizontal plane, the position of the teeth and the alveolar ridges which support them is determined by the interaction of the forces of the muscles surrounding them. Lingually this force is provided by the tongue, and buccally and labially by the cheeks and lips; thus the teeth may be regarded as lying in a zone of neutral muscular force (Figure 8.3), and if the development and function of the tongue, cheeks and lips are normal the teeth form two catenary curved arches which, when occluded, interdigitate perfectly with one another. When the natural teeth are lost, the alveolar ridges, being no

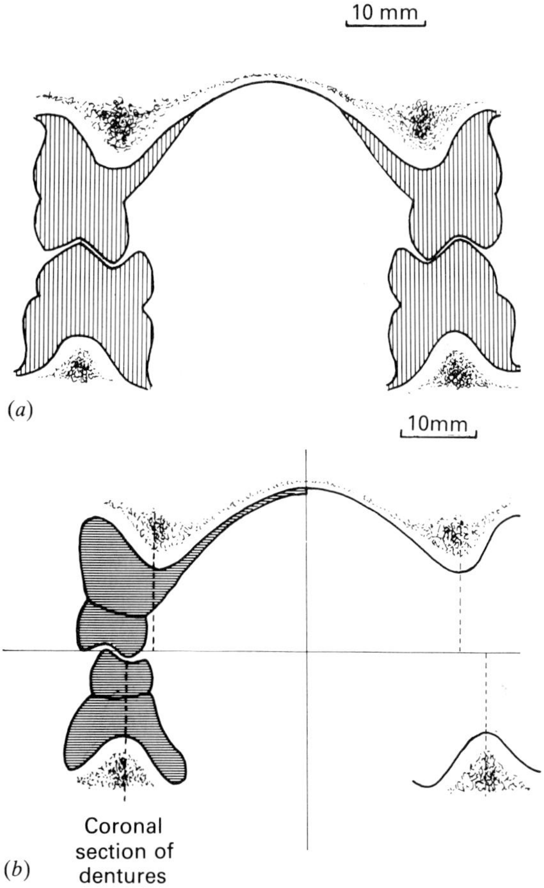

Figure 8.3 (*a*) Outline of natural teeth and supporting tissue (hatched) lost after teeth are extracted. This represents the denture space. (*b*) Position and outline form of dentures. The teeth and bases maintain the balance of tongue and cheek muscular forces

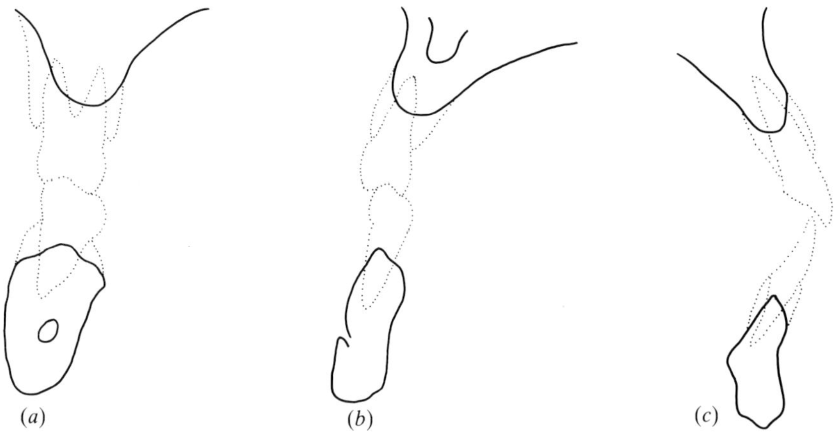

Figure 8.4 Illustrating the form of the residual alveolar ridge after the natural teeth have been extracted. Dotted line indicates tissue which is lost. (*a*) Molar region; (*b*) premolar region; (*c*) incisor region

longer required to support them, resorb. In the mandible this bone loss occurs from both buccal and lingual sides in a downwards direction, while in the incisor region it occurs more from the labial side. The edentulous residual alveolar ridge, by which the dentures will be supported, appears to be situated slightly more buccally than was the dentate alveolar ridge in the molar regions and slightly more lingually in the incisor region because of the normal lingual inclination of the molar crowns and the labial inclination of the incisor crowns of the natural teeth. In the maxilla the loss is entirely from the buccal and labial surfaces and thus the residual ridge lies slightly more palatally all round (Figure 8.4).

The problem now arises: where to set the teeth in relation to the residual alveolar ridges. In view of the fact that dentures only rest on the tissues and are held in place by comparatively weak forces, it would obviously be desirable from a mechanical point of view to set the teeth right over the centres of the ridges so that the forces applied to the teeth when occluding and chewing were directed straight through the ridges, thus tending to seat the dentures firmly on them. If this is done, although stability when chewing is enhanced, several undesirable features develop. From Figure 8.5 it can be seen that when the upper teeth are set over the centre of the upper ridge, the lower teeth require to be set slightly inside the lower ridge. The tongue space when compared with that which existed when the natural teeth were present is considerably reduced and the teeth now no longer occupy the neutral zone, but are cramping the tongue.

The tongue is a very potent factor in the control of dentures and in the majority of patients, if it is allowed its normal space, it will soon learn to control the dentures against tip and tilt by applying a compensating force to them in the correct place. If, however, the tongue is cramped, the patient will be uncomfortable and movements of the tongue will tend to unseat the dentures. Another undesirable feature which develops if the teeth are set over the alveolar ridges relates to the appearance. Because the natural upper and lower front teeth are positioned outside the basal maxilla and mandible they support the lips and cheeks and give them a natural fullness. When the natural teeth are lost and the ridges resorb, the cheeks and lips fall in to produce an aged and unpleasant appearance. If, however, the artificial teeth are placed as nearly as possible in the positions occupied by the natural teeth, support is once again provided for the lips and cheeks and the patient's appearance restored. It can

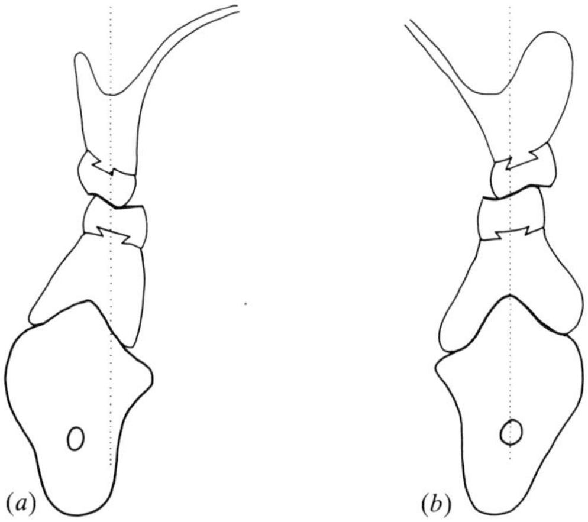

Figure 8.5 Showing the incorrect (*a*) and correct (*b*) relationships of the artificial cheek teeth to the ridges

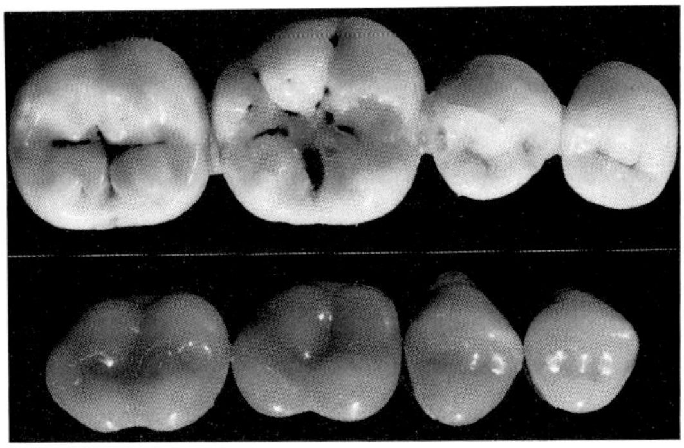

Figure 8.6 Comparison between natural and artificial posterior teeth

be seen therefore that the correct position to set artificial teeth bears less relationship to the ridges than to the positions occupied by the natural teeth. This is not absolutely true in every case, however, and when setting artificial teeth one may wish to achieve a compromise of setting the teeth as near the ridges as possible without cramping the tongue or spoiling the appearance.

Artificial posterior teeth are considerably narrower than natural teeth (Figure 8.6) and this allows some latitude in positioning them in the horizontal plane, that is, in the buccolingual direction. It is also a fact that the forces retaining the lower denture in place are very much less than those retaining the upper, due to the smaller surface area of the lower and therefore, from a mechanical point of view, it is desirable to reduce the tipping forces on the lower denture by setting the posterior teeth over the centre of the residual alveolar ridge. In view of the fact that the natural molars, and to a lesser extent, the premolars inclined lingually and that the artificial teeth are narrower than the natural teeth, they can usually be set right over the lower ridge without encroaching on the space occupied by the cheeks or tongue. This is the only rule which applies to setting up so far as the relationship of the teeth to the ridge is concerned. If the lower teeth are set in this position in occlusion with the upper posterior teeth then the latter will lie lateral to the upper ridge (see Figure 8.5), the amount depending on the degree of maxillary resorption which has occurred. This varies between individual patients.

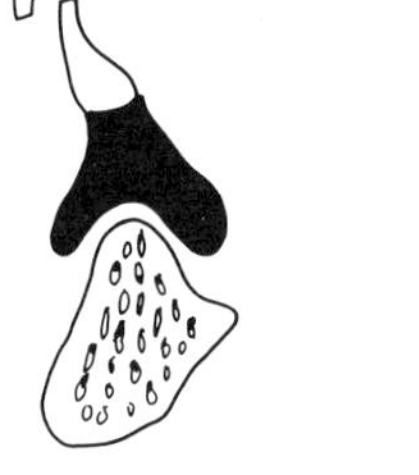

Figure 8.7 The anterior teeth of complete dentures are always set in front of the residual alveolar ridges

The anterior teeth, both upper and lower, are always set in front of the ridge, the amount depending on the degree of resorption which has occurred (Figure 8.7). As a general rule, the cervical part of the artificial tooth is set in the pre-extraction position of its natural predecessor but the angulation of the crown may be altered according to the clinical circumstances, such as activity of the lip muscles and aesthetics. The position of the labial surfaces of the anterior teeth is determined in the patient's mouth when the jaw relations are being recorded. This information is available from the record blocks when setting the teeth.

The orientation of the teeth

When setting the teeth they are placed one by one, not only in their correct positions in space, but also with the correct angulation of their long axes and unless each tooth is correctly positioned and orientated the final arrangement of teeth will result in the trial denture being functionally useless and aesthetically displeasing.

The important thing, therefore, when beginning to set teeth, is to learn perfectly the position and angulation of each individual tooth, so that you know exactly where you are going to place each tooth. In order to describe the position and orientation of individual teeth, two imaginary references are employed: the horizontal and vertical planes.

When recording the jaw relations in the patient's mouth, the occlusal surface of the upper record block is trimmed parallel to the naso-auricular line, which is a line joining the lower border of the ala of the nose to the external auditory meatus, and positioned at a height so that the incisal edges of the patient's future artificial central incisors and the mesiopalatal cusps of the upper first molars will just touch it. This is the occlusal plane (Figures 6.12 and 8.8).

When the casts are mounted on the articulator by means of the record blocks, the occlusal plane of the blocks is lined up parallel with the laboratory bench which is taken to be the horizontal. Thus with this method, the occlusal plane and horizontal plane are one and the same. The occlusal or incisal edges of each tooth are set to the occlusal plane.

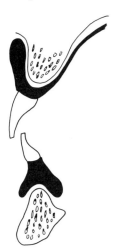

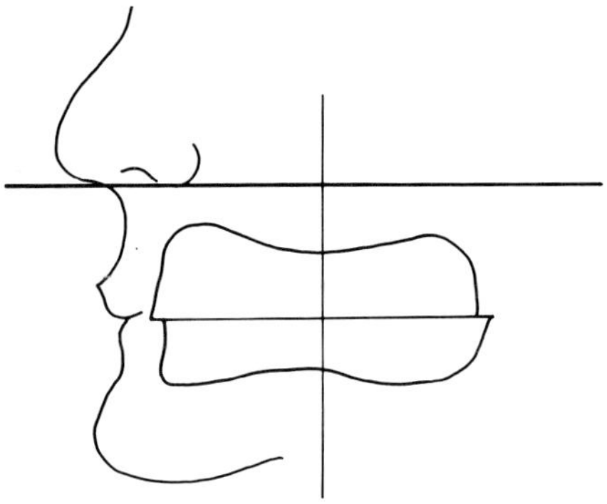

Figure 8.8 Occlusal rims of record blocks parallel to naso-auricular line. The vertical axis is at right angles to the line

The vertical plane or axis can be imagined as a plumb-line, hanging and passing straight through the casts when the articulator is standing on the bench (Figure 8.9). Three points of reference now exist to which each tooth can be referred as it is set: the alveolar ridge, the occlusal plane (the horizontal) and the vertical plane or axis.

The position of the upper teeth (Figures 8.10, 8.11 and 8.12)

Central incisor

Its long axis inclines slightly towards the vertical axis when viewed from the front, and slopes labially about 15° when viewed from the side. The incisal edge is in contact with the occlusal plane.

Lateral incisor

Its long axis slopes rather more towards the midline of the mouth when viewed from the front, and is inclined labially about 20° when viewed from the side. The incisal edge is about 1 mm short of the occlusal plane.

Canine

Its long axis is parallel to the vertical axis when viewed from both front and side. The bulbous cervical half of the tooth provides its prominence. Its cusp is in contact with the horizontal plane.

First premolar

Its long axis is parallel to the vertical axis when viewed from the front or the side. Its palatal cusp is about 1 mm short of, and its buccal cusp in contact with, the occlusal plane.

Second premolar

Its long axis is parallel with the vertical axis when viewed from the front or the side. Both buccal and palatal cusps are in contact with the occlusal plane.

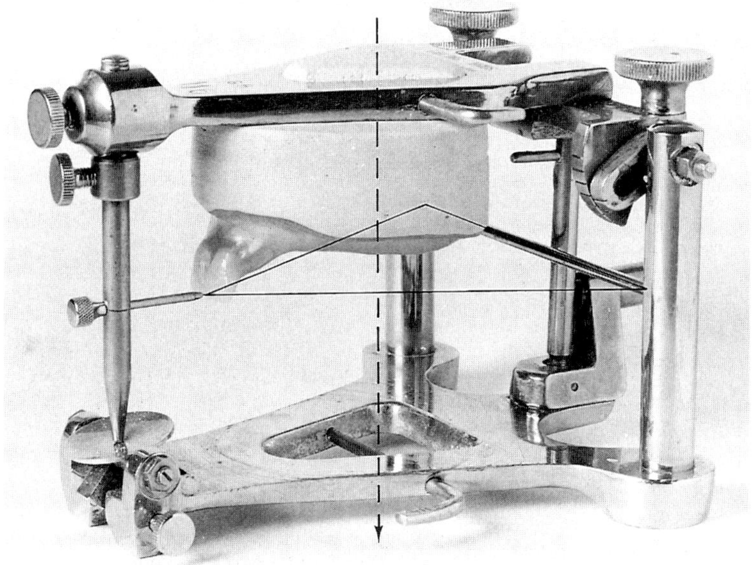

Figure 8.9 The horizontal is represented by the triangular plane joining the incisal pin (the mesio-incisal point) and the sighting bar between the condylar pillars. The dotted line at right angles to this represents the vertical axis

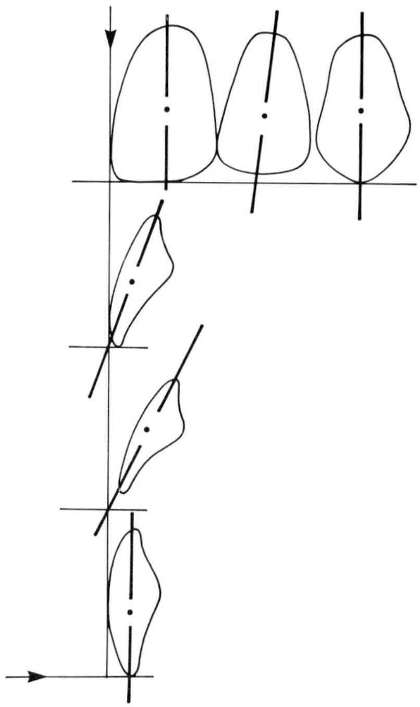

Figure 8.10 The relation of the upper anterior teeth to the horizontal plane and the vertical axis

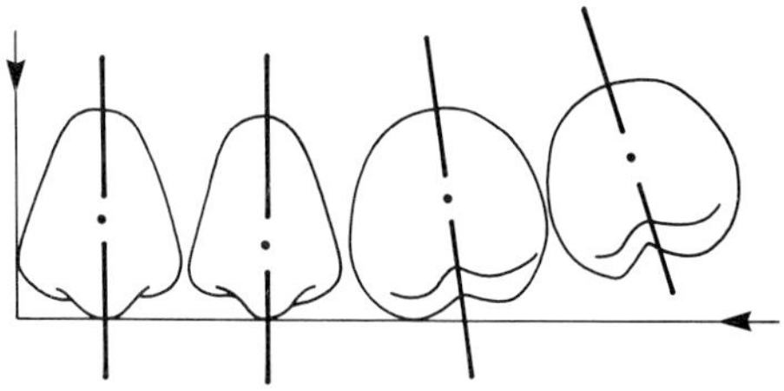

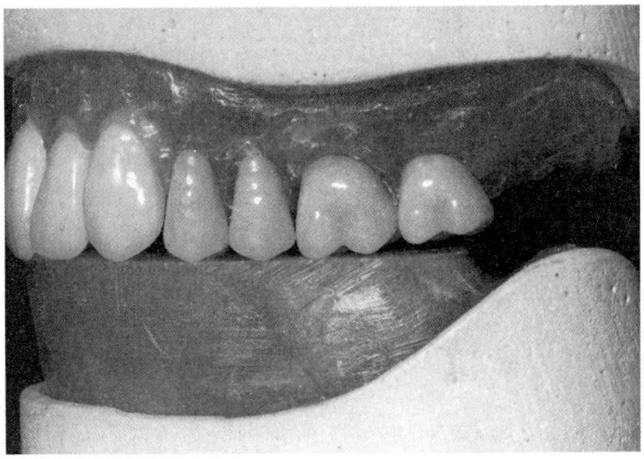

Figure 8.11 The relation of the upper posterior teeth to the horizontal plane and the vertical axis. Lateral view

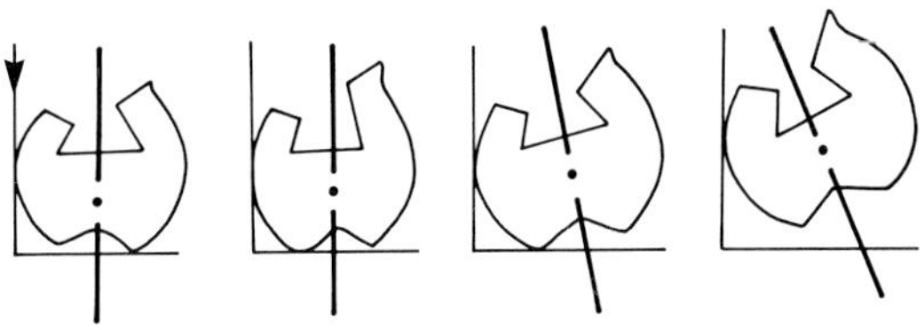

Figure 8.12 The relation of the upper posterior teeth to the horizontal plane and the vertical axis. Anterior view

First molar

Its long axis slopes buccally when viewed from the front, and distally when viewed from the side. Only its mesiopalatal cusp is in contact with the occlusal plane.

Second molar

Its long axis slopes buccally more steeply than the first molar when viewed from the front, and distally more steeply than the first molar when viewed from the side. All four cusps are clear of the occlusal plane, but the mesiopalatal cusp is nearest to it.

The position of the lower teeth

Central incisor

Its long axis inclines slightly towards the vertical axis when viewed from the front, and slopes labially when viewed from the side. The incisal edge is about 2 mm above the occlusal plane although the amount depends on the overjet.

Lateral incisor

Its long axis also inclines to the vertical axis when viewed from the front, and slopes labially when viewed from the side but not so steeply as the central incisor. The incisal edge is about 2 mm above the occlusal plane.

Canine

Its long axis leans very slightly towards the midline when viewed from the front, and very slightly lingually when viewed from the side. Its cusp is slightly more than 2 mm above the occlusal plane.

First premolar

Its long axis is parallel to the vertical plane when viewed from the front and from the side. Its lingual cusp is below the horizontal plane and its buccal cusp about 2 mm above it as it contacts the mesial marginal ridge of the upper first premolar.

Second premolar

Its long axis is also parallel to the vertical plane when viewed from the front and from the side. Both cusps are about 2 mm above the occlusal plane, the buccal cusp contacting the fossa between the two upper premolars.

First molar

Its long axis leans lingually when viewed from the front, and mesially when viewed from the side. All the cusps are at a higher level above the occlusal plane than those of the second premolar, the buccal and distal cusps being higher than the mesial and lingual. The mesiobuccal cusp occludes in the fossa between upper second premolar and first molar.

Second molar

The lingual and mesial inclination of the long axis of this tooth is more pronounced than in the case of the first molar. All the cusps are at a higher level above the occlusal plane than those of the first molar, the distal and buccal cusps more so than the mesial and lingual. The mesiobuccal cusp contacts the fossa between the two upper molars.

Compensating curves

From the foregoing descriptions of the orientation of the teeth it will be seen that they are arranged so that the posterior teeth, when considered as a whole unit, form two curves, an anteroposterior and a lateral curve.

Anteroposterior curve

Compensating curves are the artificial curves introduced into dentures in order to facilitate the production of balanced articulation: they are the artificial counterparts of the curves of Spee and Monson which are found in the natural dentition.

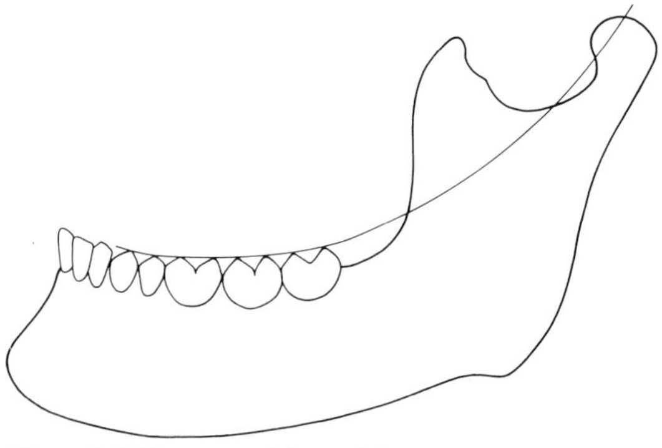

Figure 8.13 The curve of Spee of the natural dentition

The anteroposterior curve follows an imaginary line touching the buccal cusps of all the lower teeth from the lower canine backwards, and approximates to the arc of a circle. A continuation of this curve backwards in the natural dentition (curve of Spee), will nearly always pass through the head of the condyle (Figure 8.13).

The arrangement of the posterior teeth in this anteroposterior curved manner may best be appreciated by reference to Figure 8.14. If the path followed by the condyles is horizontal, then the teeth could be set to conform to a horizontal plane. When the mandible moves forwards the teeth will remain in contact.

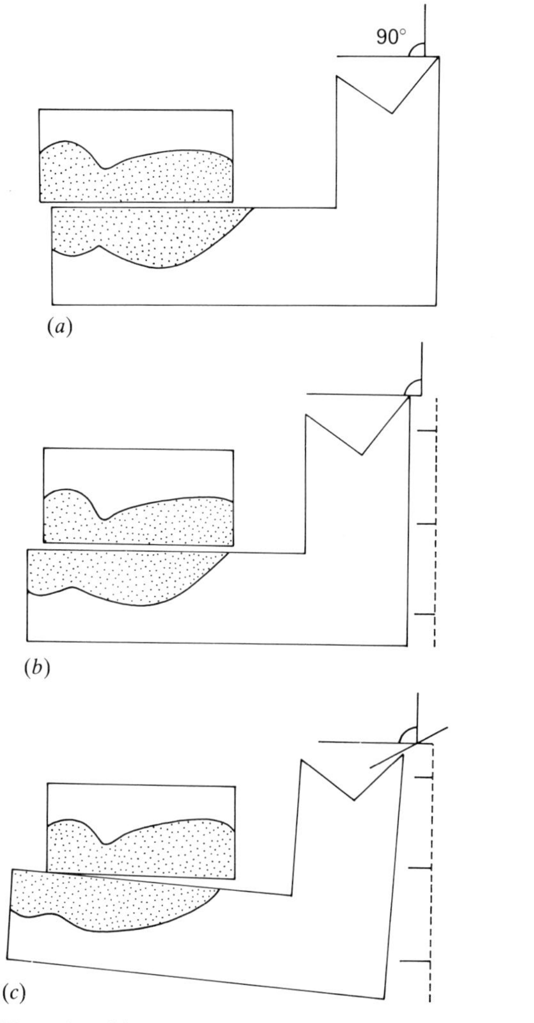

Figure 8.14 (*a*) Retruded contact position. (*b*) Protrusion with a condylar path parallel to the occlusal plane: contact maintained. (*c*) protrusion with a condylar path sloped at an angle to the occlusal plane: contact lost posteriorly

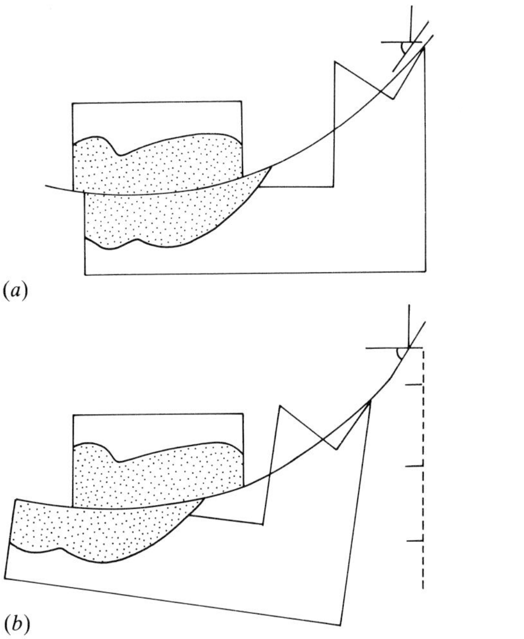

(*a*)

(*b*)

Figure 8.15 (*a*) Retruded contact position with an occlusal surface which is an arc of the circle of which the condylar path is also an arc. (*b*) In protrusion, contact is maintained

If the path travelled by the condyles is at an angle from the horizontal plane (as it always is to some extent), then as soon as the mandible moves forwards the condyles commence to descend, and the posterior teeth will lose contact if they have been set to conform to a horizontal plane.

If the posterior teeth, instead of being set on a horizontal plane, are set to an anteroposterior curve then as the mandible moves forwards and the condyles travel downwards all the teeth can remain in contact (Figure 8.15).

The lateral curves

In the natural dentition there are two lateral curves, one involving the molar teeth (the curve of Monson), and the other involving the teeth anterior to the second premolars. The second premolars are not involved in any curve as they lie on a horizontal plane.

The posterior curve has its concavity facing upwards and increases in steepness from before backwards, the occlusal surfaces of the upper molars facing outwards and downwards. The anterior curve is a reverse of the posterior curve just described (Figure 8.16).

When the mandible is moved laterally the rotating condyle on the working side (i.e. the side towards which the mandible is moved) remains in the glenoid fossa and moves very slightly outwards and backwards (Bennett movement). The orbiting condyle on the other side (balancing or non-working side) travels downwards and forwards.

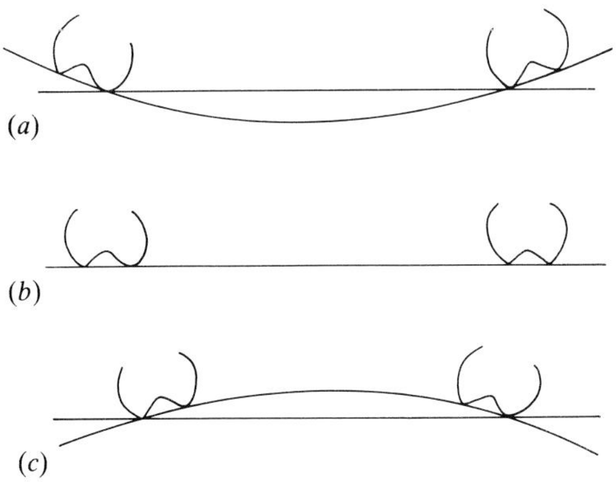

(*a*)

(*b*)

(*c*)

Figure 8.16 Lateral compensating curves greatly exaggerated. (*a*) Molar curve; (*b*) second premolar; (*c*) first premolar curve

If the teeth are set on a horizontal plane, those on the non-working side will lose contact, due to the downward movement of the condyle on that side. If, however, the teeth are set to conform to a curve, the steepness of which relates to the steepness of the condylar path, then the teeth will remain in contact during the lateral and downward movements (Figure 8.17).

Position of the teeth relative to one another

The teeth of one jaw occlude with those of the other. Occlusion means 'the act of closing or the state of being closed' and relates to the position of the teeth when in contact.

Three types of occlusal reationship exist:

1. Retruded
2. Protrusive
3. Lateral.

These are dependent on the position of the mandible relative to the maxilla. When setting teeth on a plane-line articulator the technician is only interested in the relationship of the teeth in retruded contact position, which is given below.

1. The six upper front teeth overlap the six lower front teeth by about 2 mm. This overlap is in both a horizontal and a vertical plane. In the vertical plane it is known as the *overlap* and in the horizontal plane as the *overjet* (see Figure 2.48).
2. The buccal cusps of the upper premolars and molars overlap those of the lower; the palatal cusps of the upper posterior teeth and the buccal

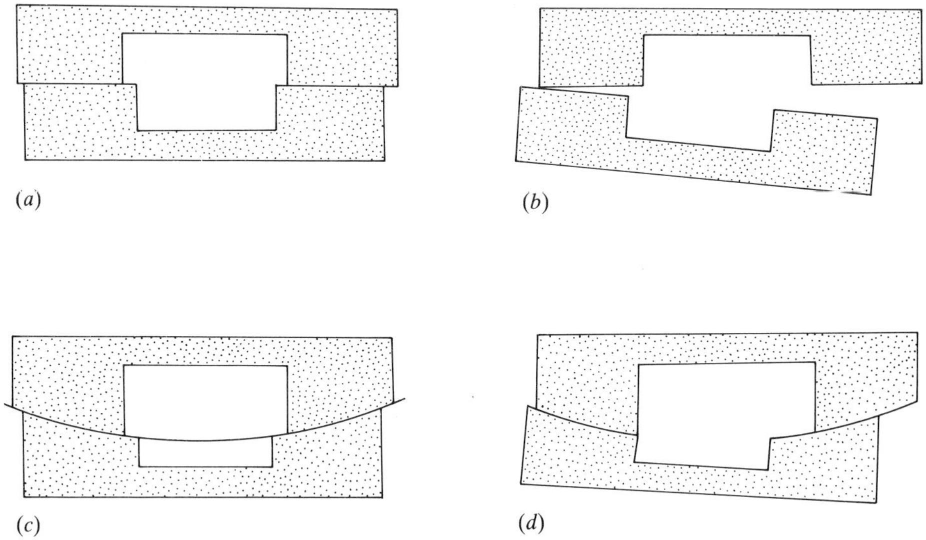

Figure 8.17 A diagrammatic representation of form of the occlusal surface in the molar region and its relation to lateral mandibular movement. (*a*) Retruded contact position with a horizontal occlusal plane (seen from front). (*b*) Lateral movement of the mandible to the right, the left side losing contact. (*c*) Retruded contact position with an occlusal surface forming an arc of a circle concentric to that followed by the mandible. (*d*) Lateral movement of the mandible to the right; contact maintained on both sides

cusps of the lower posteriors interdigitate with the opposing teeth and are known as the supporting or holding cusps as they support or hold the mandible in the intercuspal position (Figure 8.18).

3. Every tooth except the two lower central incisors and the two upper last molars occludes with two teeth in the opposing jaw; this may best be appreciated by reference to Figure 8.18.
4. The labial surfaces of the six anterior teeth present a curve when viewed from the occlusal surface, the shape of this curve depending on the shape of the underlying alveolar ridge, the width of the sulcus and the outline of the occlusal rim as it was carved at the chairside.
5. The posterior teeth should be set in such a way that their buccal surfaces make contact with a straight-edge laid from the labial surface of the canine, backwards (Figure 8.19).

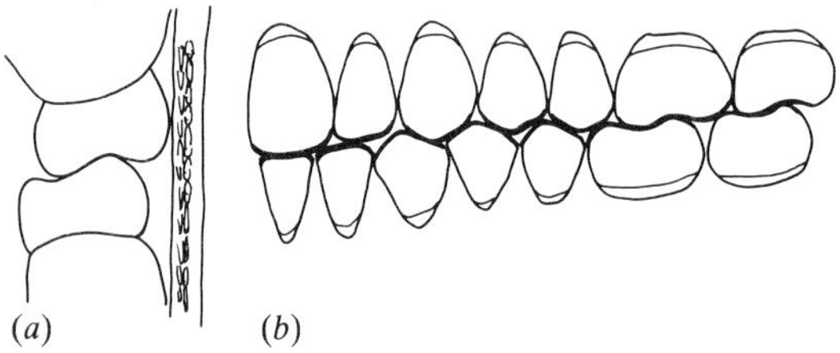

Figure 8.18 The occlusal relationship of the teeth. (*a*) Anterior view; (*b*) lateral view

Articulation is a term which is constantly being used in relation to both natural and artificial teeth and is apt to be confused with the term occlusion. Occlusion is a static state used when opposing teeth are in contact without movement. Articulation is a dynamic state used when opposing teeth are in contact during movements of the mandible.

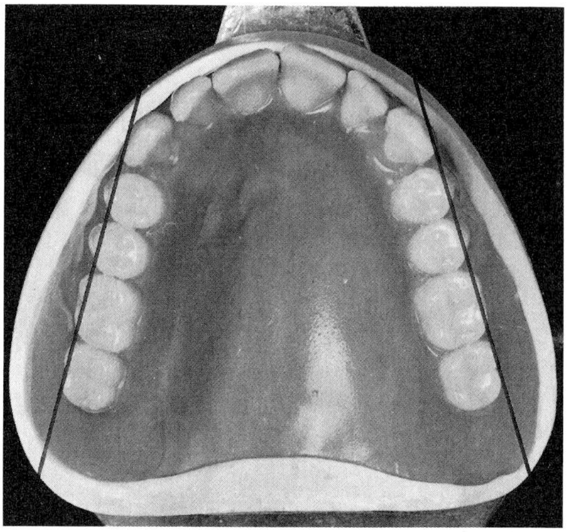

Figure 8.19 Posterior teeth are set with buccal surfaces contacting a straight-edge

Materials from which teeth are made

Both anterior and posterior teeth may be made from either porcelain or acrylic resin. Each of these materials has advantages and disadvantages.

Porcelain is hard and resists abrasion and wear. The appearance of teeth made from it is reasonably natural but somewhat opaque and false unless the very best quality teeth, which are expensive, are used.

Porcelain teeth cannot readily be altered or modified by the addition of stains and characterization lines. The bonding of porcelain teeth to the denture base is purely mechanical, the posterior teeth being held by the acrylic flowing into the diatoric holes in the teeth, the anterior teeth by their pins. The different coefficients of expansion of acrylic and porcelain result in the acrylic base being stressed in the regions of the teeth, but in practice this is of little significance. Porcelain teeth can chip in use particularly if the material has been overheated by grinding on a carborundum stone which may be carried out to modify their shape or occlusal form. They also fracture easily on impact if dropped.

Acrylic has a poor abrasion resistance and wears rapidly but the appearance of the teeth made from it is very natural, except in the cheaper grades. Acrylic teeth can be stained and modified with ease in the laboratory. The bonding of this material to the denture base is by a chemical union and no stresses occur in the region of the teeth. The density of acrylic is about half that of porcelain and so the denture is much lighter in weight.

So far as anterior teeth are concerned, either material may be used with safety and satisfaction. The choice between acrylic and porcelain for posterior teeth, however, is not so simple. Porcelain teeth being hard tend to jar on occlusion and transmit the full masticatory load to the ridge. They do not readily wear into a smooth even articulation to accommodate tiny occlusal faults when the dentures are fitted, or changes of articulation due to bone resorption throughout the life of the dentures, although polished facets do develop on them slowly. Porcelain teeth maintain the vertical occlusal dimension and are hard and sharp enough to produce efficient mastication.

Acrylic teeth produce a cushioning effect when chewing somewhat akin to that provided by the periodontal membrane in natural teeth. They wear to accommodate changes in occlusion, but unfortunately they usually wear so rapidly that they allow the vertical dimension to close and the mandible to posture forwards. They do produce less efficient mastication.

The wear of acrylic posterior teeth, resulting in loss of vertical dimension and eventually uneven occlusion, is a serious fault and for this reason alone such teeth should not as a general rule be used, although there is a wide range of abrasion resistance in different manufactured teeth. In patients presenting with narrow painful ridges, or in the older patient when the biting power is small, or where the mucosa need protecting as in any patient with a problem connected with the supporting tissues, a case may be made for them.

The claim that the wear of acrylic teeth is supposed to allow the occlusion to adjust itself to the gradual closure of the vertical dimension which occurs throughout the life of the denture, due to ridge resorption, is not usually substantiated in practice. At any rate, dentures should never be worn for so long that closure of the vertical dimension and habitual protruded posture, due to ridge resorption and tooth wear, is allowed to occur, for in these cases the denture bases will be so poor a fit that they will cause tissue damage. As a general rule most dentures require replacing within five to ten years with yearly review and modification during this time.

Waxing the trial dentures

When the teeth have been mounted in their correct positions and in proper occlusion, more wax is added to the base and the whole made to conform to certain definite requirements. The periphery of the upper denture must fill out the sulcus of the master cast with the posterior palatal border thinned down almost to a knife edge. The buccal and labial surfaces must be shaped to allow for comfortable and free movement of the buccinator and orbicularis oris muscles.

The lower denture must be similarly finished on the buccal and labial surfaces and periphery, but the lingual surface should be inclined inwards, from above downwards, affording no undercut areas in which the tongue might lodge and unseat the denture.

In both dentures the wax distal to the second molar must be made thin to allow the tongue as much room as possible at the back of the dentures and also to avoid any contact between the heels of the dentures.

As a general rule the distance from the distal surface of the second molars to the posterior edge of the denture should be at least 10 mm. If it is less, either the teeth have been placed too far back or the denture base is underextended.

Gum-fitted anterior teeth

In some patients the maxilla is overdeveloped in the incisor region, and if a wax flange is placed over this region it pushes the upper lip out, making the

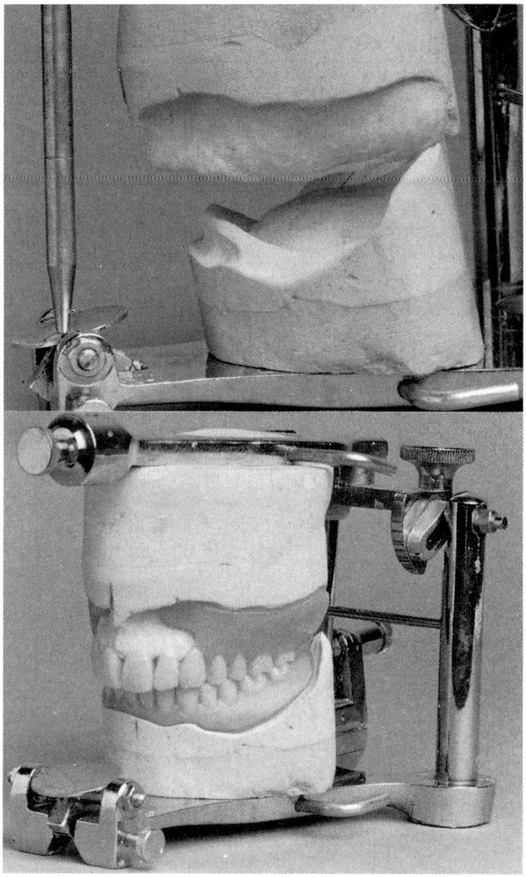

Figure 8.20 The upper six anterior teeth are fitted to the gum. Often known as an open-faced denture. Note the extensions of the denture base in the labial sulcus in the form of 'wings' or Tuerkheim retainers

patient appear to have a swollen lip. In these cases the six upper anterior teeth may be fitted directly on to the alveolar ridge without any labial flange (Figure 8.20). These dentures are known as 'open-faced'.

Indications for this type of denture are rare but they may be necessary where the labial cortical plate is bulbous. This may be developmental or pathological (e.g. Paget's disease of bone) in origin and it may be exaggerated by minimum bony resorption or expansion of the labial plate during extraction.

Retention of this type of denture is unsatisfactory owing to the peripheral seal being ineffective, and the loss of the stabilizing effect of the labial flange. Sometimes two extensions, known as 'wings' or Tuerkheim retainers, are added in an attempt to overcome these deficiencies (Figure 8.20).

In these cases it is better to avoid gum-fitting the teeth because of the poor retention and because of the diminished support and subsequent tissue damage. Either a very thin labial flange may be used or surgical reduction of cortical bone considered.

Setting teeth for abnormal jaw relationships

When the casts have been mounted on the articulator it may be found in a number of cases that they present deviations from the normal relationship and thus present problems in setting the teeth.

Superior protrusion

The lower ridge is narrower than the upper and the prominent maxilla is often associated with a receding chin (Figure 8.21).

The upper posterior teeth may need to be set more palatally than usual in order that they may occlude with the lower teeth. The lower teeth should never be set outside the ridge (Figure 8.22). Setting

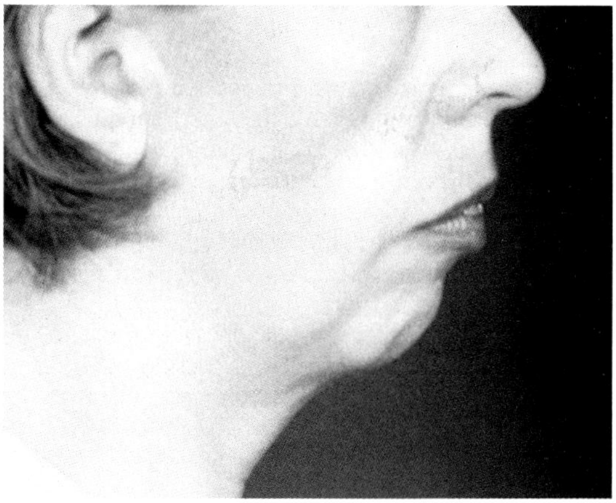

Figure 8.21 Angle class II division 1 malocclusion showing a typical profile

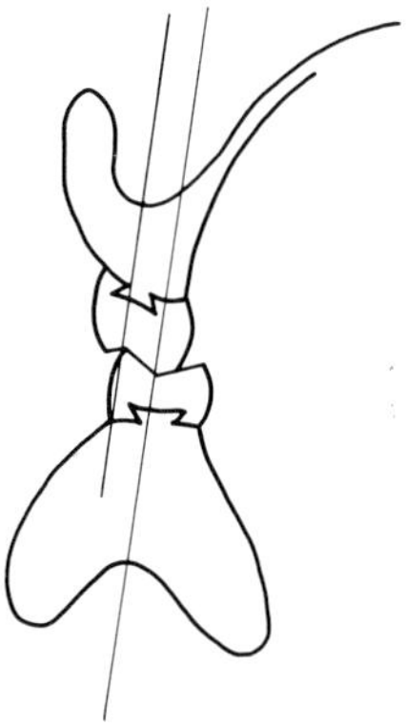

Figure 8.22 Upper posterior teeth set slightly inside the ridge in a case of superior protrusion

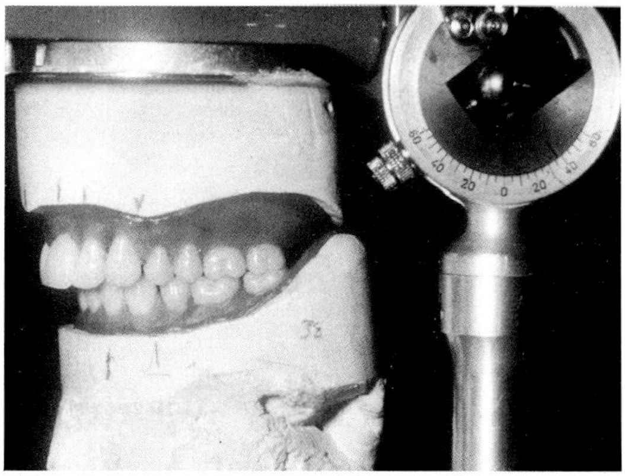

Figure 8.23 Superior protrusion with a large horizontal overjet

the upper teeth in this position does not produce marked instability, although it reduces the tongue space, but as the tongue is used to being cramped by the narrowness of the lower ridge this will not be serious. Setting the lower teeth outside the ridge, however, will lead to instability.

Cases of superior protrusion always present a large horizontal overjet and no attempt should be made to reduce this by leaning the upper incisors backwards or the lowers forwards (Figure 8.23). Such angulation of the teeth will, in the case of the upper, give the patient a rabbity appearance and in the case of the lower tend to unstabilize the denture by placing the lower teeth in the way of the lower lip (Figure 8.24).

A large overjet always exists in the natural dentition of individuals with a superior protrusion and they are rarely capable of approximating their upper and lower incisors; for this reason it is neither necessary nor desirable to attempt to make that possible with the artificial teeth.

It is permissible, however, to set the upper incisors at a higher level than the natural predecessors if that is deemed necessary for the improvement of appearance. This has the effect of maintaining an adequate overjet but reducing the vertical overlap.

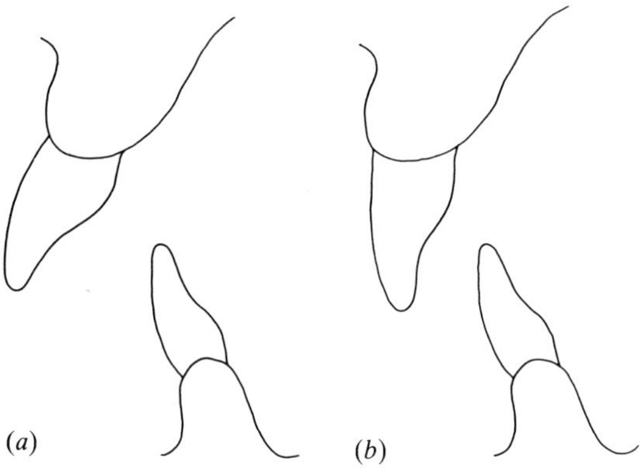

Figure 8.24 (*a*) Correct, (*b*) incorrect setting of the anterior teeth for a case of superior protrusion

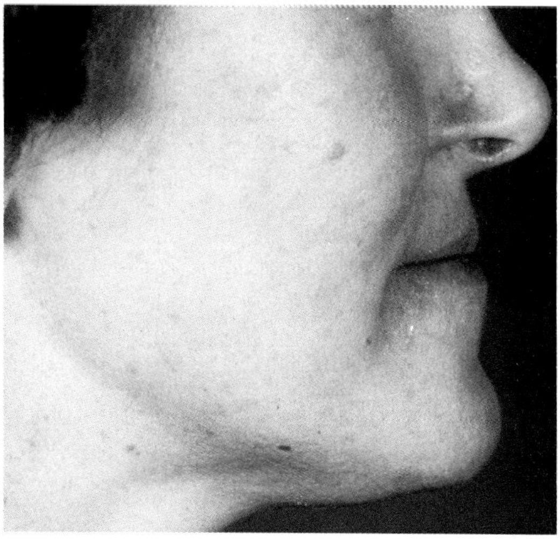

Figure 8.25 Inferior protrusion. Typical profile with prominent chin and obtuse mandibular angle

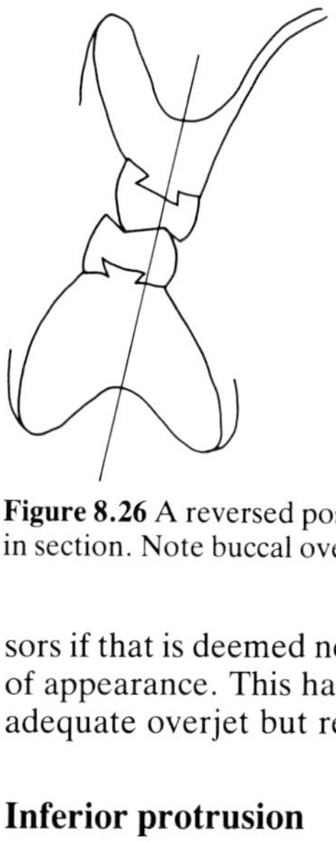

Figure 8.26 A reversed posterior tooth relationship shown in section. Note buccal overjet of lower molar

Inferior protrusion

The lower ridge is broader than the upper and usually associated with a prominent chin (Figure 8.25). When setting the posterior teeth it is often difficult to occlude them in a normal relationship because of the discrepancy between the ridges, particularly in the molar region. In extreme cases it may be necessary to reverse the tooth relationship (Figure 8.26). This means that instead of the buccal cusps of the lower molars fitting into the fossae of the upper molars, the reverse occurs. Sometimes the crossing of the occlusion has to be applied to all the posterior teeth, but more commonly it is only the molars which are affected. Occasionally the width of the lower ridge is so great in relation to the upper

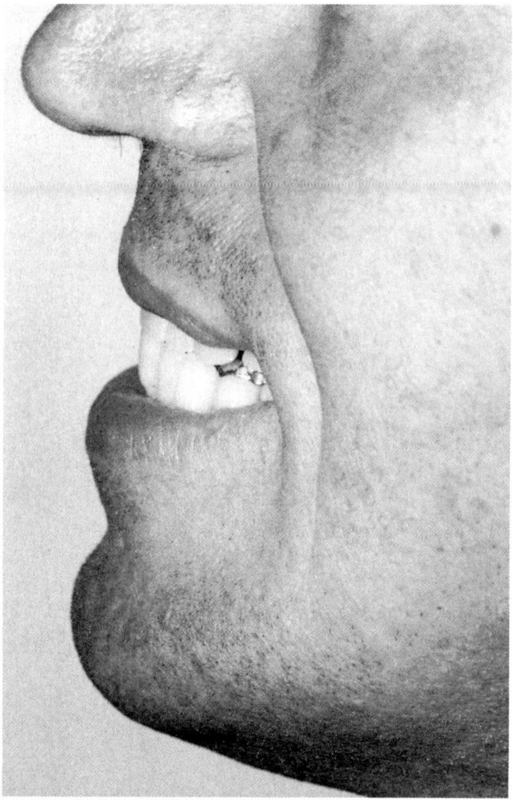

Figure 8.27 Marked case of inferior protrusion. The anterior teeth have been set edge to edge and the maxillary labial flange made sufficiently wide to reposition the upper lip

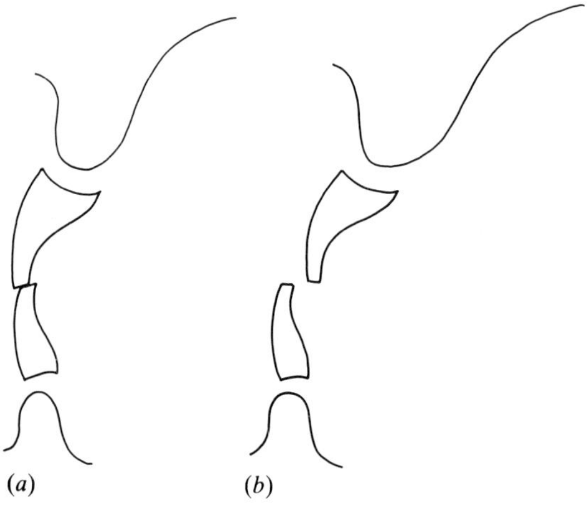

(*a*) (*b*)

Figure 8.28 (*a*) The method of setting the anterior teeth so that they occlude edge to edge in a moderate case of inferior protrusion. (*b*) The method of setting the anterior teeth in a gross case of inferior protrusion

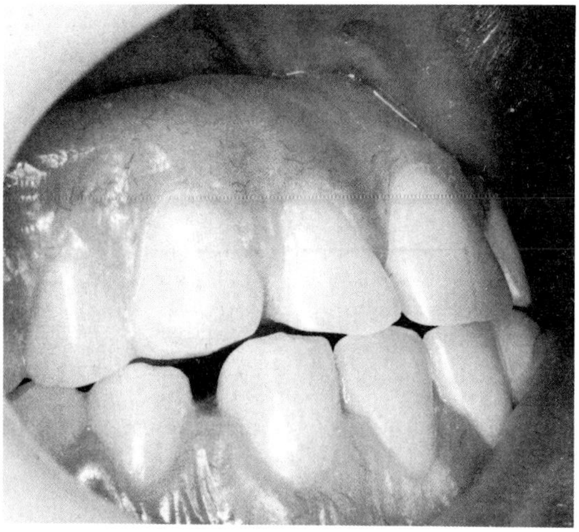

Figure 8.29 Edge-to-edge incisor relationship in an Angle class III malocclusion. Lower incisors in this edentulous patient have been retro-inclined and the upper labial flange is wide

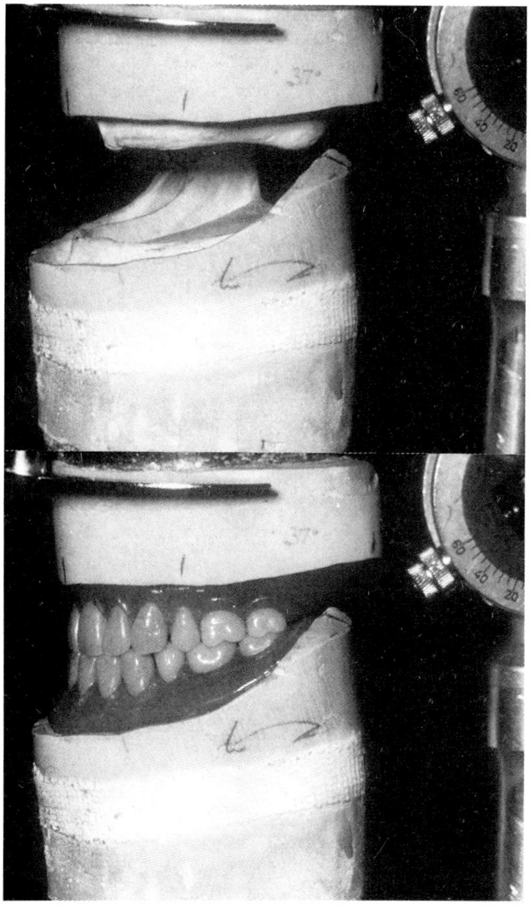

Figure 8.30 Inferior protrusion showing cast relationship in the retruded contact position and method of setting the teeth of the complete dentures

that the second molars cannot be made to occlude at all. In such cases they are best left off the denture and as mastication is mainly performed in the premolar and first molar region their loss is not serious.

In cases presenting marked inferior protrusion it is frequently necessary to set the upper teeth far outside the ridge and it is then important that the buccal flange is sufficiently wide that the polished surface has the correct shape (Figure 8.27). If the retention of the denture is satisfactory the only trouble likely to result from setting teeth over the buccal sulcus is a midline fracture of the denture due to its continual flexion, particularly if the occlusion is not balanced, and a metal palate may be incorporated.

The anterior teeth are best set edge to edge or, in extreme cases, with a negative overjet (Figure 8.28). An edge-to-edge relationship, although it may appear difficult to accomplish, is almost always possible by retro-inclining the lower incisors and setting the upper incisors more labially, especially at the incisal edge. A wide labial flange will produce a satisfactory polished surface (Figure 8.29).

The incisal edge of each anterior tooth should be ground to a chisel-like shape to produce an efficient occlusion (Figures 8.28 and 8.30).

In all cases of inferior protrusion, a negative overjet of anterior teeth and a reverse relationship of posterior teeth should be avoided wherever possible as these produce inefficient occlusions from the point of view of patient comfort and mastication.

Setting teeth for patients who have satisfactory old dentures

It is important when making replacement dentures for patients who already possess a satisfactory set not to reduce the tongue space. If the tongue is cramped with new dentures they will never be successful. If the tongue has more space than in the old denture it is all right. One method of ensuring that the new dentures do not cramp the tongue is to measure the space provided by the old ones and copy it (Figure 8.31). Another method is to copy the existing dentures and make replica dentures which are then used as a recipe for new replacement dentures. This technique is described in Chapter 16.

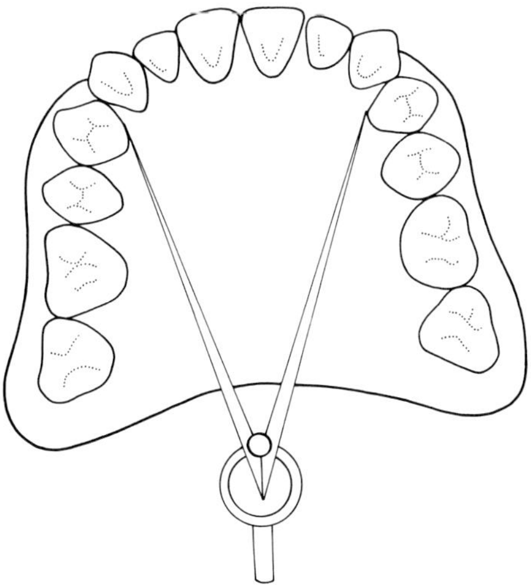

Figure 8.31 A method of measuring the tongue space on the old dentures

The posterior border of the upper denture

In many cases it will be found that the posterior border of an existing upper denture finishes far forward on to the hard palate and one must decide, when making a new denture, whether to place it in its correct location on the soft palate, or copy its old position. Although it is obviously desirable to place the posterior border correctly and so increase the retention of the denture, many patients who have been used to the back edge of their denture finishing on the hard palate may resent it being placed further back. It must be remembered that a patient who has been wearing a denture for years has become adept at holding it in position, subconsciously, with his tongue. The best way to discover a patient's reaction to the position of the posterior border is to carry the base-plate of the record block on to the soft palate and sense the reaction, always remembering that the base-plate is slightly thicker and less well-fitting than a denture. If there is any protest or retching, finish the new denture to the same line as the old.

Chapter 9

Adjustable articulators and occlusion

The term 'anatomical articulation' is sometimes used to denote an arrangement of the artificial teeth whereby the patient with complete dentures can make normal closed mandibular movements with comfort and efficiency. This result is obtained by setting the teeth in balanced occlusion, i.e. with as many teeth as possible in occlusion in any lateral or protrusive jaw position (Figures 9.1, 9.2, and 9.3). The teeth must also be set to give balanced articulation, i.e. with the teeth arranged so that they maintain an even sliding contact between one position of balanced occlusion and the next, and during masticatory movements, without causing any cuspal interference.

Shortcomings of plane-line articulators

Provided the records have been taken correctly, dentures can be constructed on a plane-line articulator which will occlude in retruded contact position, but the articulation is often unsatisfactory for the following reasons.

Tilting of the dentures

Pressure applied to only one or two teeth when the upper and lower teeth come into contact in eccentric positions may cause tilting of the dentures (Figure 9.4).

Cuspal interference

Any attempt at lateral or protrusive movement, with the teeth in occlusion, will either prove impossible or the dentures will be dragged bodily in the direction of the mandibular movement with consequent damage to the underlying tissues. This will tend to occur even with low-cusp or zero-cusp teeth. The damage is often of a chronic or insidious nature so that the patient is not aware of anything being amiss.

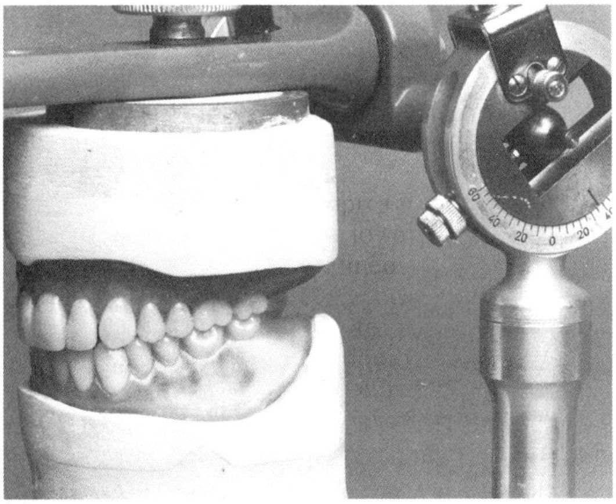

(*a*)

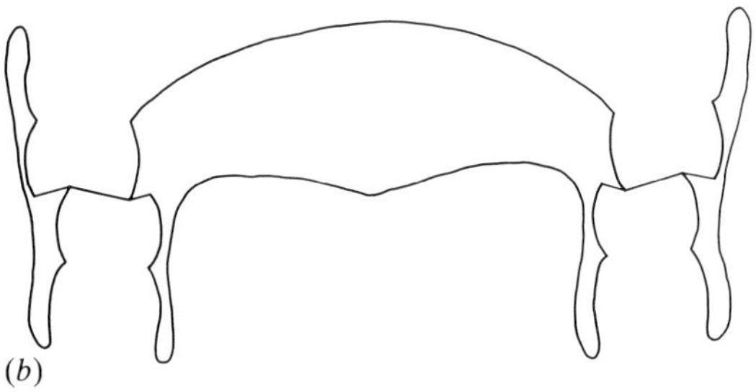

(*b*)

Figure 9.1 Anatomical articulation. (*a*) Illustrating the occlusion of the teeth with the mandible in the retruded contact position. (*b*) Cross-sectional diagram of (*a*)

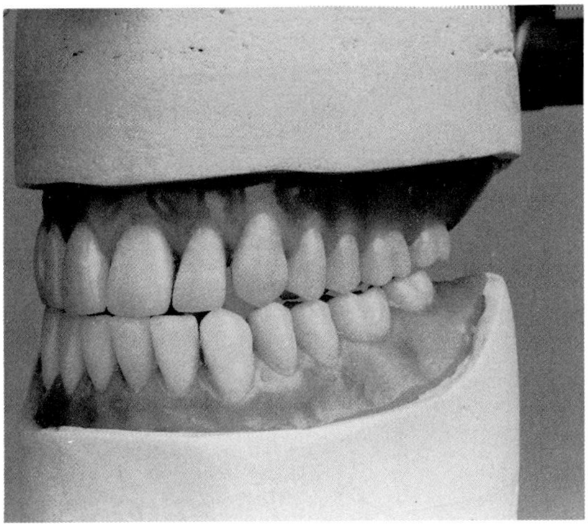

Figure 9.2 Illustrating the occlusion of the teeth with the mandible protruded

Reduced efficiency

As a result of these faults, patients wearing dentures set on a plane-line articulator learn to avoid lateral and protrusive movements and to chew with a hinge-like or chopping action, ensuring that their teeth always occlude in the intercuspal position. This hinge movement will only produce a crushing of the food because cutting and grinding requires some lateral movement. A good example of grinding is that of a pestle and mortar where one surface is moved over another, while in cutting with a knife-edge less pressure is required. From this explanation it can be readily understood why the efficiency of the occlusion is relatively poor.

Pain

In either lateral or protrusive positions only one or two teeth are in contact, and since these teeth will sustain the entire occlusal load, the tissues under them sometimes become painful (Figure 9.5). It should be realized that teeth are in contact many times in the course of the day other than during eating and it is at these times, the so-called empty mouth movements, that the dentures display their most inefficient and damaging features.

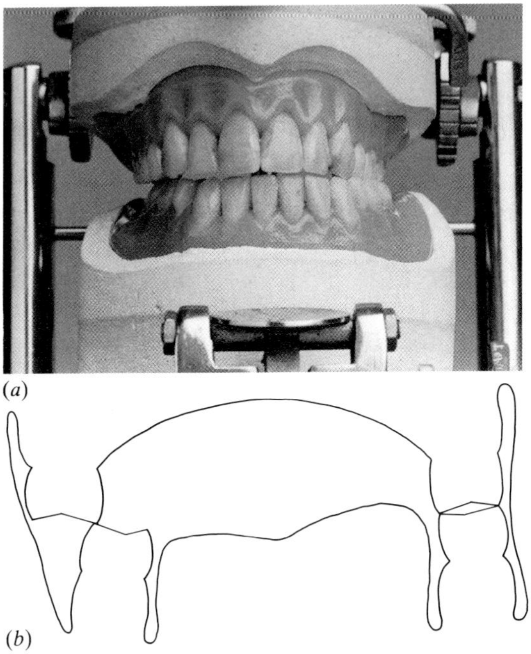

Figure 9.3 Illustrating the occlusion of complete dentures with the mandible in a lateral position. (*a*) Dentures in left working contact and right non-working (balancing) contact. (*b*) Cross-sectional diagram to show how balance is maintained in lateral occlusion

Advantages of adjustable articulators

Balanced occlusion

In any closed mandibular position, retruded or eccentric, the maximum number of teeth is in contact and therefore the occlusal load is distributed over the supporting tissues.

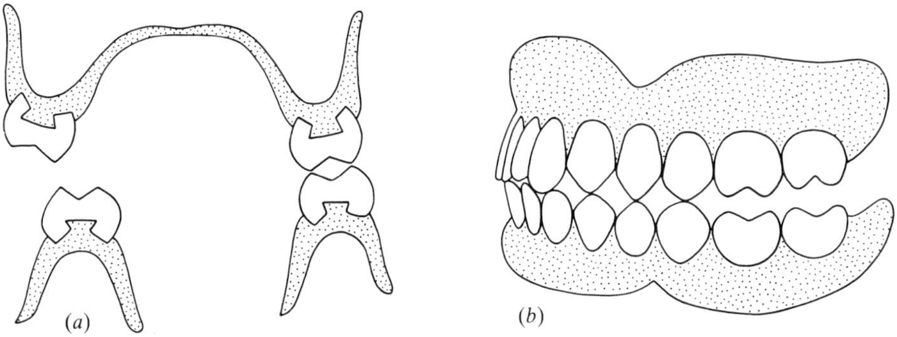

Figure 9.4 The unilateral and haphazard occlusion that occurs in dentures set on a plane-line articulator. (*a*) Lateral occlusion; (*b*) protrusive occlusion

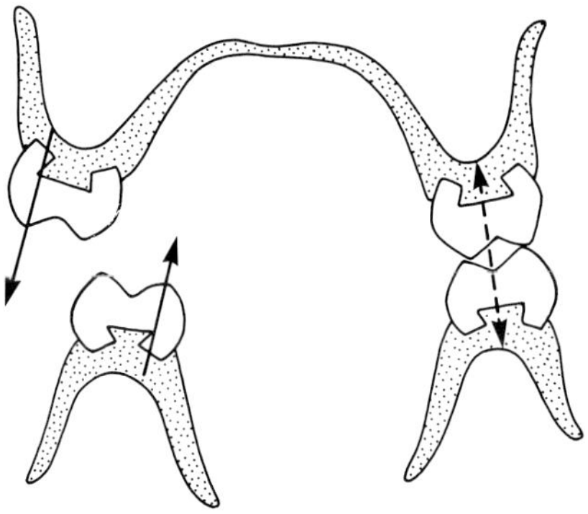

Figure 9.5 Tilting forces acting on dentures that have been set with an unbalanced occlusion

Stability

Since the maximum number of teeth is always in contact, tilting of the dentures is less likely to occur, and as cuspal interference has been eliminated, there will be little tendency for the dentures to be dragged across the mucosa.

Reduced trauma

Since there will be no tilting of the dentures and the occlusal pressure will be distributed as evenly as possible, the minimum amount of damage will occur in the supporting tissues and, provided the hygiene of the patient is good, the health of the oral tissues will be maintained.

Functional movements

Most patients will become accustomed to dentures which have been set on an adjustable articulator far more readily than a plane-line articulator because the former allows for normal mandibular movements, while the latter requires an entirely new pattern of muscle-controlled movement to be learnt.

Efficiency

Grinding and cutting of foodstuffs are possible because lateral and protrusive movements can be made while still maintaining balanced articulation. It has been suggested that the introduction of food on one side of the mouth will prevent the teeth of the opposite side from maintaining balance and that therefore balanced articulation is of no advantage. While this statement is obviously true for a large, hard morsel of food, it is not correct for the majority of foodstuffs which require much less pressure before the opposing cusps have penetrated it and have come into contact with each other. Maximum pressure is only exerted when the mandible encounters maximum resistance at the beginning of the return from a lateral or protrusive position to intercuspal occlusion, and at this stage the cusps have penetrated the food to some extent and are nearly in contact. From this it follows that very little tilting would be required before the teeth on the opposite side made contact and restored balance. This slight tilting is even further reduced by the fact that the soft tissues on the working side are under pressure and therefore are slightly compressed. Even if the statement 'enter food, exit balance' were correct, an articulation built correctly on an adjustable articulator would still be worth while, because any position of occlusion will re-seat such a denture but only in retruded contact position will this be possible with a plane-line articulator.

Saving time

When complete dentures have been made with balanced articulation there remain only minor occlusal corrections to be done and thus a considerable amount of clinical time is saved.

Balanced articulation

By balanced articulation is meant an arrangement of the teeth so that in any jaw relationship as many teeth as possible are in occlusion, and when changing from one position to another they move with a smooth, sliding motion, free from cuspal interference and maintaining even contact.

In order that the teeth can be arranged so that they fulfil these requirements, four factors are needed:

1. An articulator which can be adjusted to copy the movements and reproduce the relationships of the jaws of the patient for whom the dentures are being made.
2. A means whereby these movements and relationships can be measured and transferred to the articulator.
3. An understanding of the factors which influence the arrangement of the anterior and posterior teeth to produce balance.
4. Posterior teeth with cusp angles which will permit them to be set in balanced articulation.

These four points will now be described in greater detail.

Adjustable articulators

There are many articulators, sometimes called moving-condyle articulators, which are designed to reproduce mandibular movements, but the majority of them are, for the sake of simplicity, arranged to give only the average of such movements. For example, the condylar mechanism may work on a

35° angle while the incisal guidance table is set at 10° The more the patient differs from the average the less valuable do these non-adjustable types become, and therefore only the type of articulator which is adjustable to individual movements will be considered. The influence of the Bennett movement or lateral side-shift on occlusal balance of complete dentures is small and, from a clinical point of view, can usually be ignored.

Recording jaw relationships

The anatomical relationships and the controlling factors in mandibular movement, which are peculiar to the individual patient, and which must be accurately transferred to the articulator before it can be used to set teeth in balanced occlusion, can best be appreciated from a study of Figure 9.6. This represents a schematic sagittal section of a patient with record blocks in place in retruded contact position, and a transverse section showing the maxilla and condyles. From it the following list of relationships, which are fixed for individual patients but vary from patient to patient, can be drawn up:

1. The relationship of the maxilla A to the heads of the condyles B in retruded contact position is a fixed, unalterable factor peculiar to each patient.
2. Once the vertical jaw relation has been determined, the relationship of the mandible C to the maxilla and to the heads of the condyles in retruded contact position, is a fixed, unalterable factor peculiar to each patient.
3. The slope of the condylar path PQ is a fixed factor peculiar to each patient and therefore the angle QPH, which it makes with the horizontal plane, will be constant; note that the condylar path on one side may be different from the other.

In addition, the surfaces of the record blocks are parallel to the naso-auricular (ala–tragus) line GH and if all these factors are known and can be transferred to an articulator, it will be possible, within the limits of these factors, to reproduce the patient's masticatory mechanism.

Methods of measuring the patient's fixed factors

All the measurements are obtained through the agency of record blocks which have been trimmed parallel to the naso-auricular line and to the correct vertical height, as described in Chapter 6. The blocks should be notched to receive wax occlusal wafers.

Relating the mandible in retruded contact position (RCP) to the maxilla

This entails securing the normal RCP relationship as for plane-line articulators.

Recording the condylar angle

The condylar path is the curved path taken by the head of the condyle when moving down the articular eminence and up into the glenoid fossa, and for practical purposes this is considered to be a straight line. The angle which this makes with the horizontal plane is known as the condylar angle (or condylar guidance angle).

1. Place the upper record block in the mouth. Prepare a softened wax wafer as for normal record taking and place it on the lower block.
2. Place the lower record block in the mouth and request the patient to move his jaw forwards and close the blocks together. Chill the wafer in the mouth, remove the united blocks from the

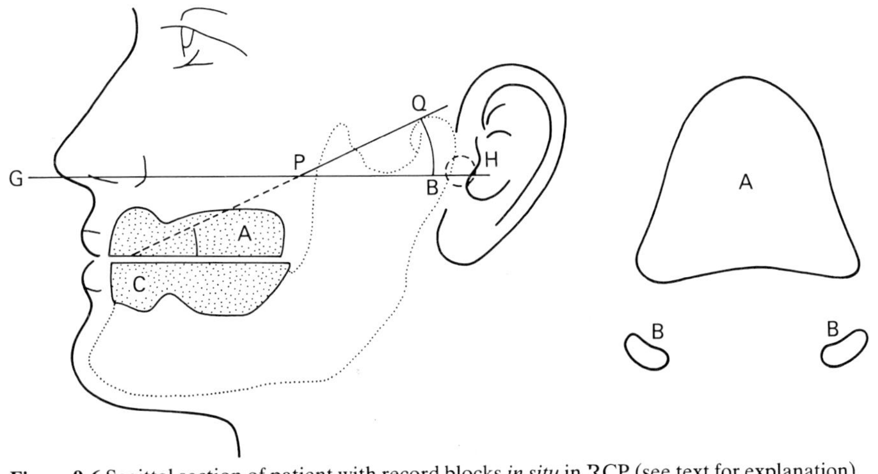

Figure 9.6 Sagittal section of patient with record blocks *in situ* in RCP (see text for explanation)

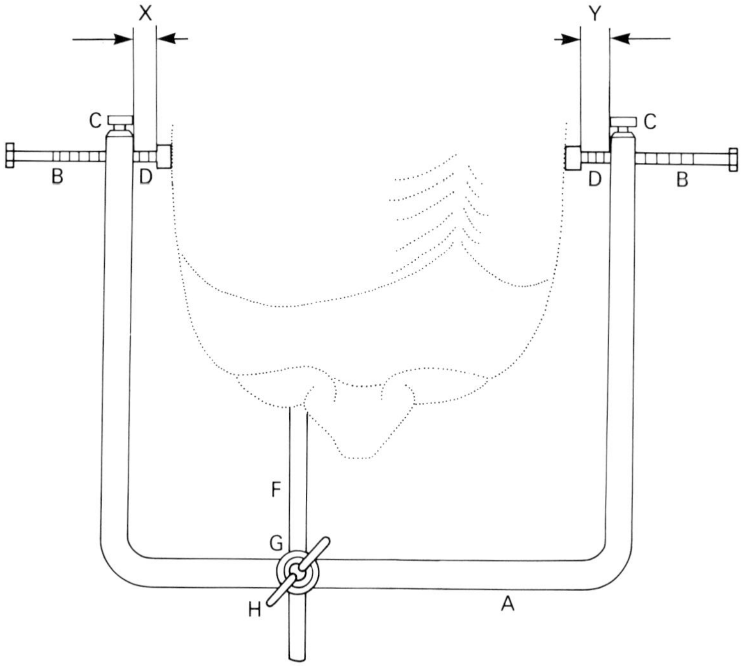

Figure 9.7 The facebow in position as seen from above. See text for explanation

mouth, and separate the wax wafer from the blocks. Use a second wafer to repeat the same protrusive movement which brings both condyles forwards. The patient should protrude at least 7 mm to record the condylar movement sufficient to adjust the articulator satisfactorily.

Recording the relation of the maxilla to the glenoid fossae

For this a piece of apparatus called a facebow or transfer bow is used (Figure 9.7). It consists of a metal bow A carrying in channels at its extremities two graduated rods B which slide inwards and outwards for adjustment. The rods may be fixed by tightening the finger screws C. The rods bear at their inner ends two cups D; a flat metal fork is attached eccentrically to a rod F which is united to the centre region of the bow through the agency of a universal joint, G. This joint can slide along and rotate around the bow and may be fixed when required by tightening the finger screw, H. The construction of the facebow endows it with considerable versatility for adjustment.

It is used as follows:

1. The position of the middle of each glenoid fossa is marked on the patient's face. These positions may be arrived at by placing a straight edge from the outer canthus of the eye to the apex of the tragus of the ear, and marking a cross with a wax pencil or felt pen on this edge 1 cm in front of the anterior border of the tragus (Figure 9.8). It is easier to measure the distance between two fixed points than between two moving ones, so the measurements are taken from the maxilla to the glenoid fossae rather than from the mandible to the heads of the condyles. While taking these measurements the actual positions of the heads of the condyles can be entirely ignored. It should be appreciated that there is an element of approximation in locating the hinge axis by surface markings on the face. For this reason this type of facebow is sometimes known as an arbitrary facebow.
2. Adapt a wax wafer to the upper record block and, by warming the fork, fix it to the wafer, taking care that the rod F is placed on the right side of the centre line. Place the upper record block, carrying the fork, into the patient's mouth (Figure 9.9) and then insert the lower block and ask him to close. The position of the lower jaw in relation to the upper is of no importance; it is merely being used to hold the upper block in place. Alternatively, an assistant may place a finger against the palate of the upper block in which case the lower block is not necessary.
3. Loosen all the finger screws on the facebow and slip the universal joint on to the rod F which is projecting from the mouth. Adjust the cups D so that they are in contact with the crosses on the

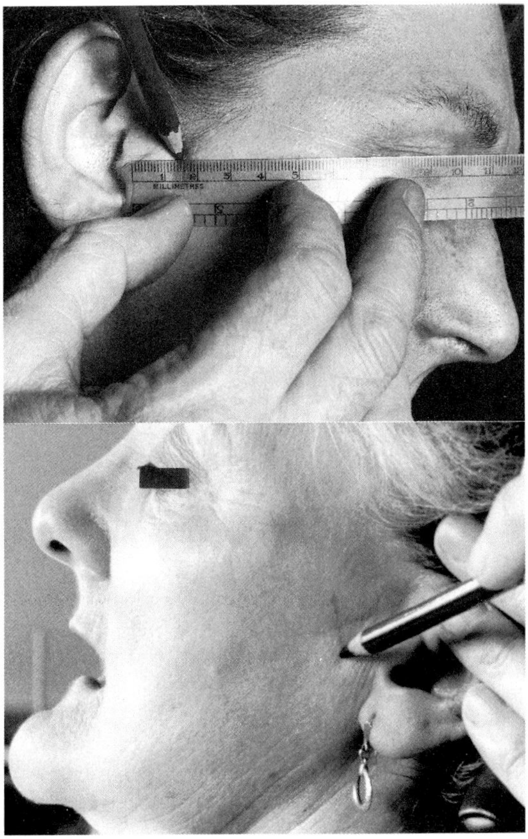

Figure 9.8 Determining the position of the glenoid fossae

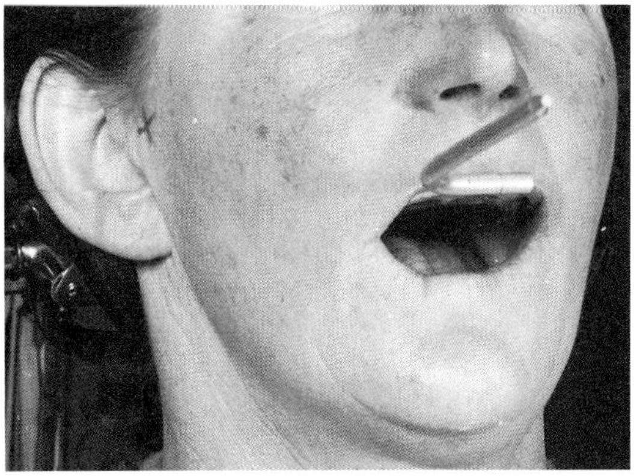

Figure 9.9 Facebow fork attached to upper record block in position. Note stem exits from mouth on right side but parallel to the median sagittal plane of the face

skin locating the glenoid fossae. Ensure that the facebow is central in relation to the head by making certain that an equal number of graduations appear on both the rods B. When the facebow is correctly adjusted, tighten the finger screw. Run the orbital rod against the lowest point of the left bony orbit to locate the anterior mark of the Frankfort plane and tighten its finger screw. The facebow will then appear as in Figure 9.10. With this type of facebow the condylar rods are difficult to locate on the surface marks on the face and the marks are also liable to be approximate. For these reasons some clinicians prefer the ear-piece bow where the cups fit into each external auditory meatus.

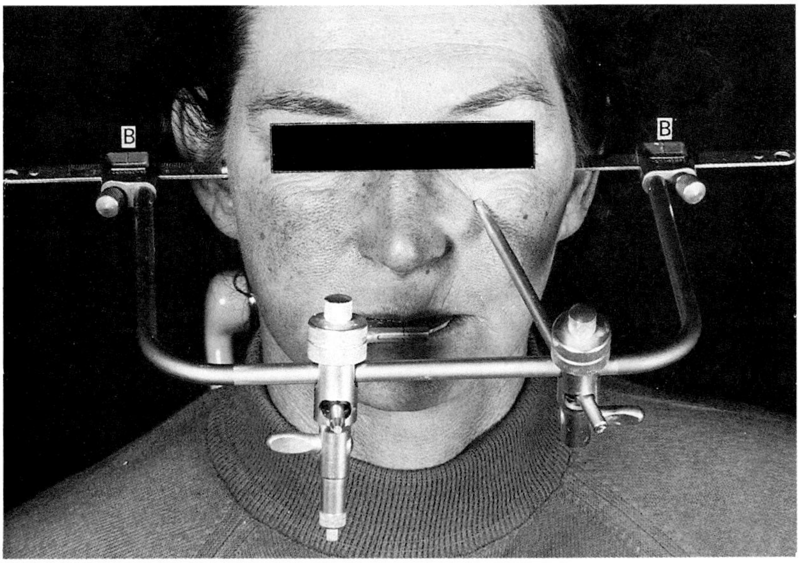

Figure 9.10 The facebow in position. Note that the readings on the condylar rods B are the same on both sides

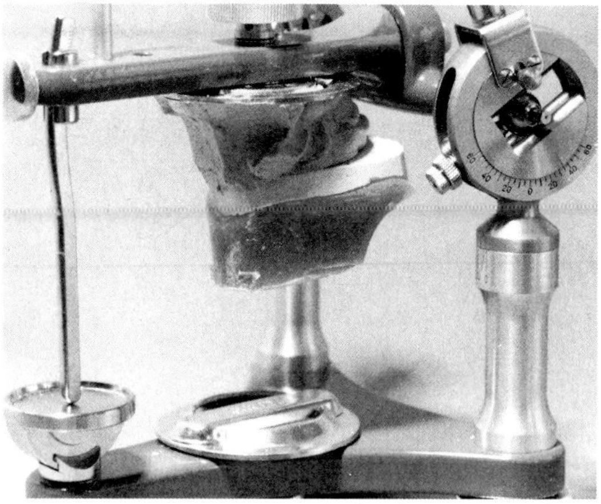

Figure 9.11 The upper cast attached to the upper member of the articulator by means of the facebow

4. Loosen the finger screws C and remove the facebow with the fork, orbital rod and upper record block attached. Remove the record block, leaving the wax wafer attached to the fork. The duplication in the wafer of the V-shaped grooves in the occlusal rim will enable it to be replaced in its correct position when required.

Mounting the casts on the articulator

1. Attach the facebow to the articulator, making certain that it is correctly centred. The graduation marks should be equal on both sides, though they may not be the same measurement as they were on the patient as the intercondylar distance is a fixed factor on most articulators, but is variable from one patient to another.
2. Place the upper record block together with the upper cast in place on the wax template of the facebow fork. Raise or lower the front of the facebow until the orbital pointer touches the undersurface of the orbital plane flag. Support the facebow in this position, check that the incisal post graduation mark is at zero and, by means of plaster, attach the upper cast to the upper member of the articulator which must also be parallel to the base (Figure 9.11).
3. The relationship of the lower cast to the upper is obtained by means of the record blocks and the wax wafer recording retruded contact position. The lower cast is attached to the base of the articulator with plaster.

The upper cast has now been fixed to the articulator in the same relationship to the hinge axis of the articulator as the patient's maxilla bears to his glenoid fossae (Figure 9.12). Further, the lower cast is fixed to the articulator in the same relationship to the upper cast as the patient's mandible bears to his maxilla in retruded contact position, and thus both casts are related to one another and to the hinge axis of the articulator in a similar manner to the way in which the patient's maxilla and mandible are related to one another and to his intercondylar axis. The whole is related to the Frankfort plane which is taken as the horizontal.

For all practical purposes the arbitrary or ear-piece facebow is adequate but if greater

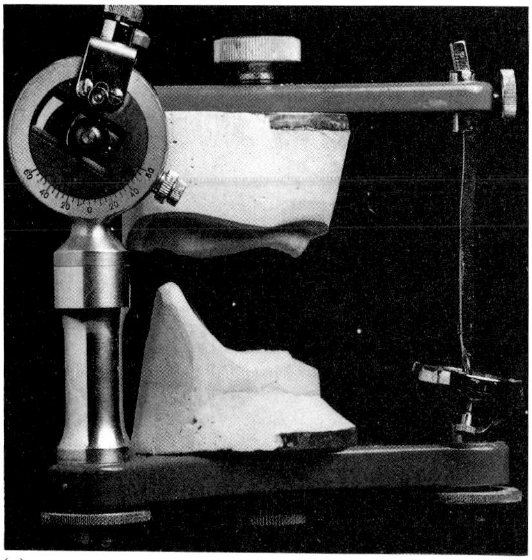

(*a*)

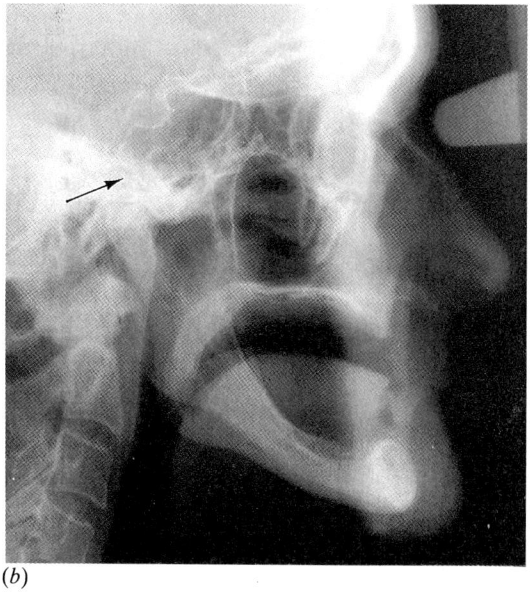

(*b*)

Figure 9.12 Mounted casts (*a*) and lateral skull radiograph (*b*) of same patient. Both casts are related to one another in the retruded contact position and to the hinge axis in a similar manner to the way the patient's jaws are related to one another and to his intercondylar axis (arrow indicates head of right condyle on radiograph) precision is thought desirable a kinematic facebow may be used. With this, the bow is attached to a clutch on the mandibular alveolar ridge and as the mandible opens and closes on the terminal arc the actual hinge axis can be accurately located on the face.

Adjusting the condylar angle

1. Loosen the condylar elements and replace the retruded contact position wafer, which is between the record blocks, with one of the protrusive wafers.
2. Move the upper arm of the articulator and the adjustable condylar path until this wafer is accurately seated between the record blocks. Lock the adjustments on each side and note the condylar angle readings.
3. Repeat the operation using the other protrusive wafer.
4. It is often found that the first reading is slightly different from the second and, if so, set the condylar angle at the average of the two.

Factors influencing balance

For clarity of description in the section that follows, the mandible is described as moving from the retruded position to eccentric positions of occlusion with the occlusal surfaces of the teeth in contact. During mastication, of course, the reverse action actually occurs, the teeth occluding in an eccentric position and the lower teeth then moving in contact with the upper teeth back into the retruded position. However, provided the records have been taken correctly, the articulator adjusted properly and the teeth set in balance, it makes no difference which way the mandible moves. Before the factors influencing the position of the teeth can be formulated, and before the articulator can be given the final adjustment which will enable it to be used for setting the teeth, the factors influencing the movements of the mandible with the teeth in contact must be understood. Given a motive force derived from the muscles, two factors influence these movements: the condylar paths, and the inclination of the contacting surfaces of the teeth

During protrusion with the teeth in contact there must be a vertical drop equal to the depth of the vertical overlap of the incisors or to the depth of the posterior cuspal inclines, and this drop must be obtained during a forward movement equal to the horizontal overjet (Figure 9.13). With natural dentitions under consideration, the depth of the anterior overlap is greater than the posterior cusp height with the result that when the incisors are in edge-to-edge contact the posterior teeth are out of occlusion. This apparently unbalanced situation is satisfactory with natural teeth supported by periodontium in bone, and indeed it is considered advantageous for disclusion or separation of posterior teeth to occur at the beginning of eccentric mandibular movement, but it is a very unsatisfactory arrangement for an artificial occlusion. Tipping and rocking of the denture is almost certain and the strains so imposed are apt to cause pain, excessive alveolar resorption and instability of both dentures, particularly during empty mouth movements.

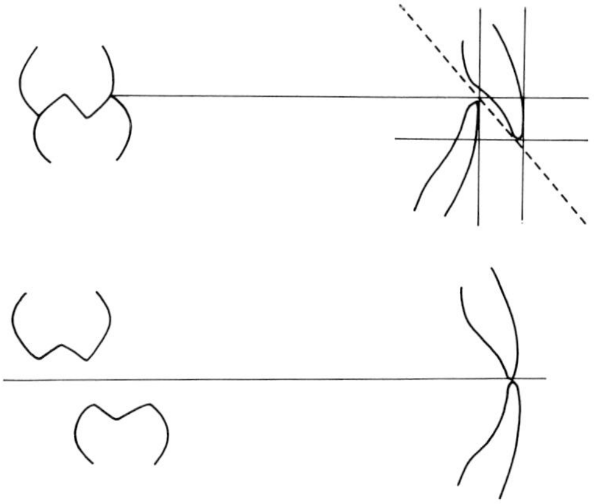

Figure 9.13 Deep vertical overlap leading to loss of contact of the posterior teeth when the mandible is protruded

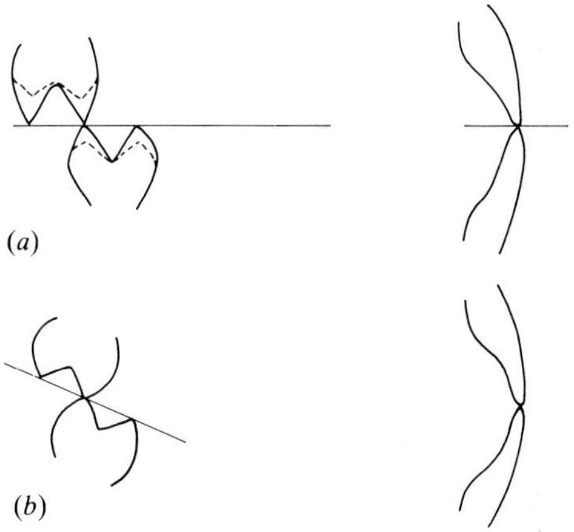

(*a*)

(*b*)

Figure 9.14 Correction of the fault illustrated in Figure 9.13 by: (*a*) Increasing the height of the cusps; (*b*) increasing the steepness of the compensating curve

This lack of balance can be corrected in dentures by increasing the steepness of the compensating curve, by using posterior teeth with steeper cusps, or by a combination of both of these (Figure 9.14). Only within narrow limits will these expedients prove satisfactory and beyond these limits the stresses introduced will cause instability and pain.

Since the condylar control of the patient is a fixed factor which cannot be altered by the dentist or

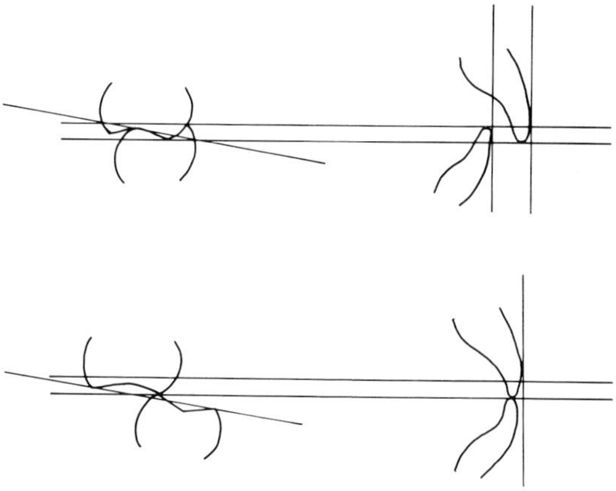

Figure 9.15 A reduction in the amount of vertical overlap allows the use of shallower cusps and a less extreme compensating curve

technician, and the setting of the anterior teeth is capable of wide variation, it is obvious that the latter must be modified from the original when complete dentures have to be constructed. This modification usually takes the form of a reduction in the amount of overlap, thus reducing the amount of vertical opening necessary to bring the incisors edge to edge; this in turn allows shallower cusped teeth to be used and a less extreme compensating curve (Figure 9.15). It will be clear from a study of the diagrams that a steepening of the anteroposterior compensating curve will decrease the cusp angle, and vice versa. A general rule in complete dentures is the flatter the alveolar ridge (i.e. the less it can resist lateral pressure), the less should be the anterior overlap and the shallower the cusps.

The same lack of balance of natural teeth is found during lateral movements of the mandible. The rotating condyle on one side remains virtually stationary, although it may shift sideways, and therefore the posterior teeth on that side remain in contact, with the lower cusps moving down the cusp inclines of the upper. On the opposite side the head of the orbiting condyle moves downwards and forwards, thus tending to move the teeth on that side out of contact. In dentures the same conditions apply as for protrusion, i.e. that lack of contact in lateral movement produces unsatisfactory dentures and that balance restored by very steep cusps, or a very steep compensating curve, will produce unstable dentures.

The mandibular path

In a protrusive movement with the teeth in contact the path of the mandible is directed at the back by the movements of the condyles down their respective paths, and in the front by the movement of the lower teeth against the inclines of the upper teeth.

In lateral movement the mandibular path is directed by the path of the orbiting condyle and the inclines of the teeth on the side towards which the mandible moves. To fix the movements of the mandible to certain well-defined channels, both the condylar angles and the slope of the tooth inclines must be known. We already know, and have transferred to the articulator, the slope of the condylar path but we do not know the cusp angles suitable for the individual patient. Fortunately, however, we can fix these cusp angles within the limits set by the effect of the condylar paths, and make the mandible follow our dictates.

The movement of the frame of the articulator is governed at three points, i.e. posteriorly by the two condyle guidances and anteriorly by the incisal post which rests on the incisal guidance table. While each of these can be varied on the articulator, the condylar angles are determined by the patient and only the incisal angle is decided by the dentist or technician. Varying the angle of the incisal table will alter the angle which the path of the contacting surfaces of the anterior teeth makes with the horizontal, i.e. the incisal guidance angle. The way in which one chooses the angle of the incisal guidance table is explained later in the chapter.

It is obvious that there is no incisal guidance table present in the mouth and when the dentures are inserted it is only the condyles and the teeth which govern lateral and protrusive movements when the teeth are in contact. The incisal guidance table is in fact merely a convenient substitute for the teeth as each tooth is set on the articulator.

Figures 9.16 and 9.17 illustrate the effect on the protrusive path of the mandible when the incisal guidance is altered while the condylar guidance remains the same. For any given setting of the condylar angles and incisal table the protrusive path followed by the mandible can be determined as follows. A line is drawn at right angles to the condylar path from the centre of the condyle, and another at right angles to the incisal guidance table from the point of the incisal post. The point where these lines meet is the rotation centre for the path of the mandible on that side. It must be understood that the rotation centre is constantly changing as the mandible travels its path but, as the mandible moves, any given point on it moves with it and maintains the same relationship to each successive rotational centre. It may thus be stated that, for a given condylar angle, the steeper the angle of the incisal guidance, the steeper the path of the mandible, and vice versa. The effect of variations of steepness of the mandibular path, on setting the teeth in balanced occlusion for protrusive movements, is best shown diagrammatically, and Figures

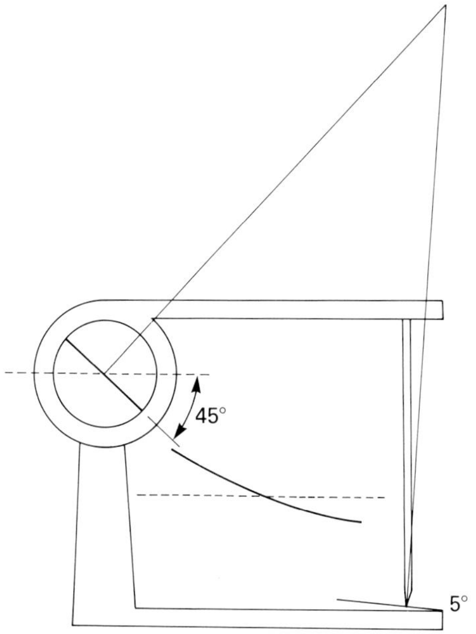

(*a*)

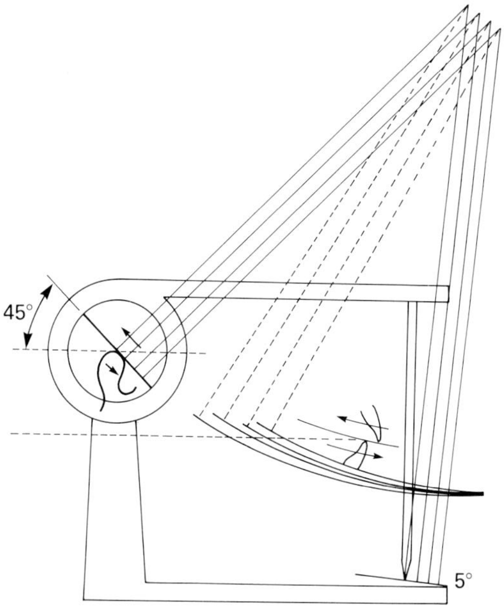

(*b*)

Figure 9.16 (*a*) The thick black curved line represents the path of the mandible in protrusion with a condylar angle of 45° and an incisal angle of 5°. (A 45° condylar angle is seldom encountered in practice, but it simplifies the illustration). (*b*) See text

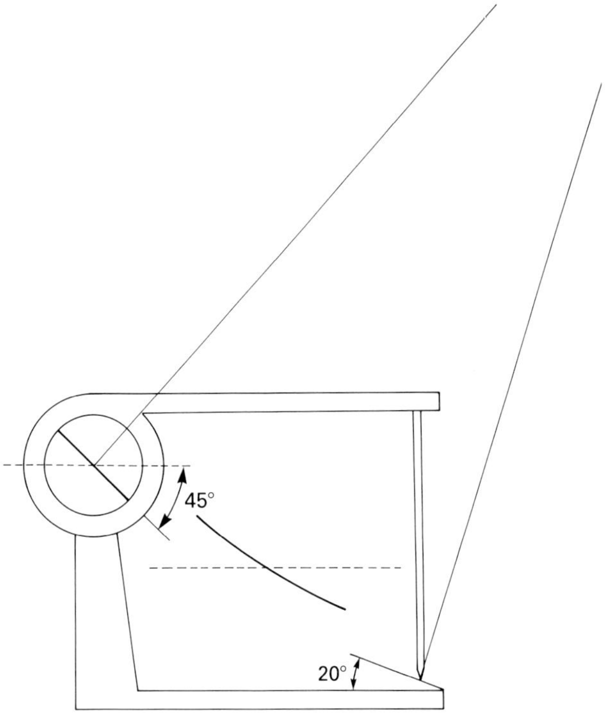

Figure 9.17 The thick black line represents the path of the mandible in protrusion with a condylar angle of 45° and an incisal angle of 20°

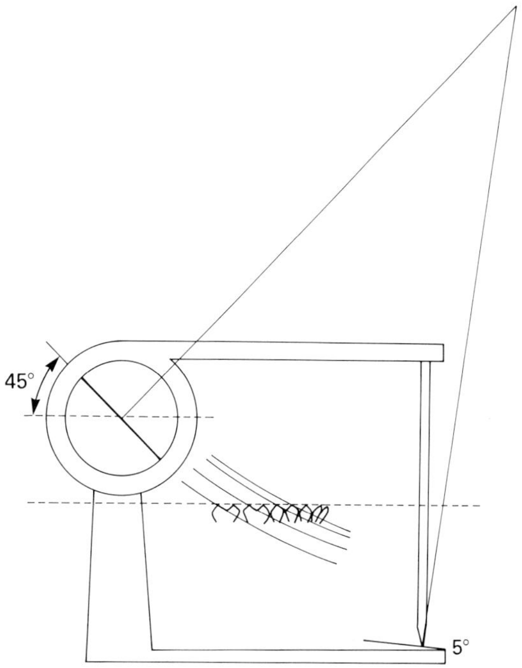

Figure 9.18 Illustrating the steepness of the cusps necessary when the teeth are set to a horizontal occlusal plane

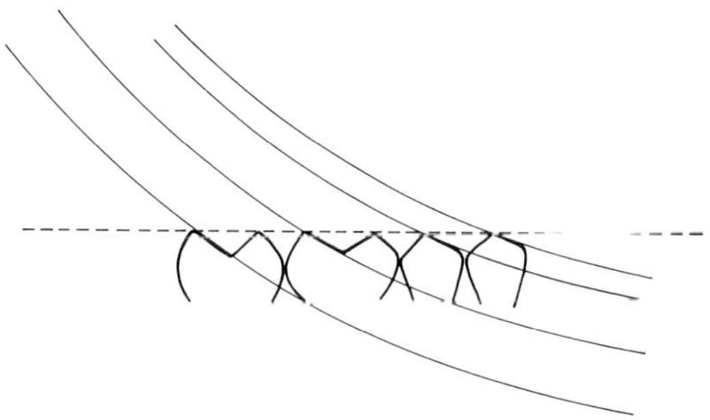

Figure 9.19 Enlargement of teeth in Figure 9.18 to show parallelism of cusp angles with the mandibular path

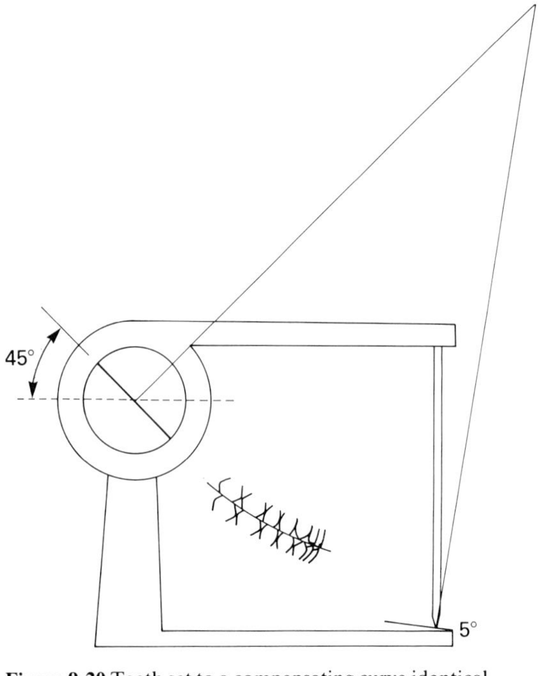

Figure 9.20 Teeth set to a compensating curve identical with the mandibular path. Zero cusp or monoplane teeth

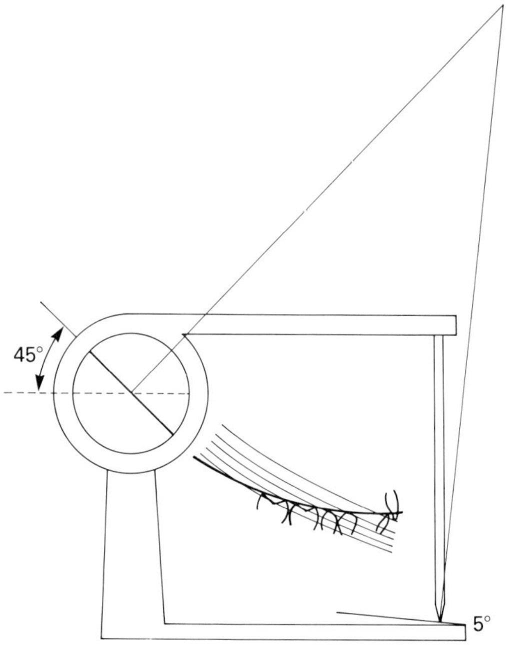

Figure 9.21 Teeth set to a reasonable compensating curve requiring cusps of average height

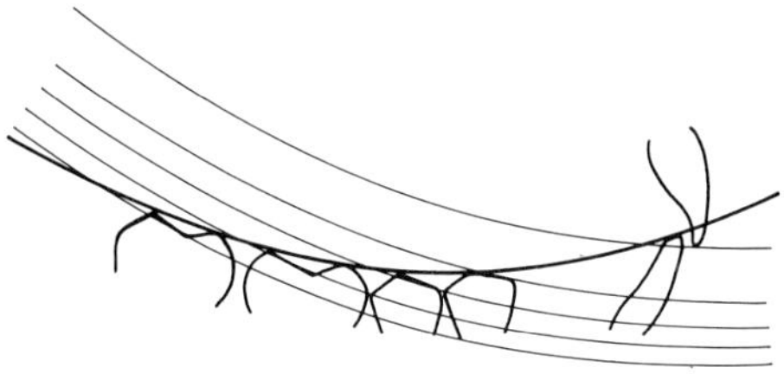

Figure 9.22 Enlargement of teeth in Figure 9.21 to show how the parallelism of the cusp angles to the mandibular path is obtained by tilting the long axes of the teeth

9.18–9.22 depict the variation in the cuspal angles of the teeth when they are set to:

1. A horizontal occlusal plane (Figures 9.18 and 9.19).
2. A compensating curve identical with the mandibular path (Figure 9.20).
3. A reasonable compensating curve; the articulator shown has a condylar guidance of 45° and an incisal guidance of 5° (Figures 9.21 and 9.22).

It will be observed that, to maintain balanced articulation, the cuspal angles must be such that they are parallel to the path followed by the mandible. Thus, if the teeth are set to a horizontal occlusal plane, these cusp angles must be steep and the cusps high, becoming progressively so towards the back. The introduction of a compensating curve allows these angles and heights to be reduced. It will also be noticed that the overlap and overjet of the front teeth must be related to the mandibular path, so that

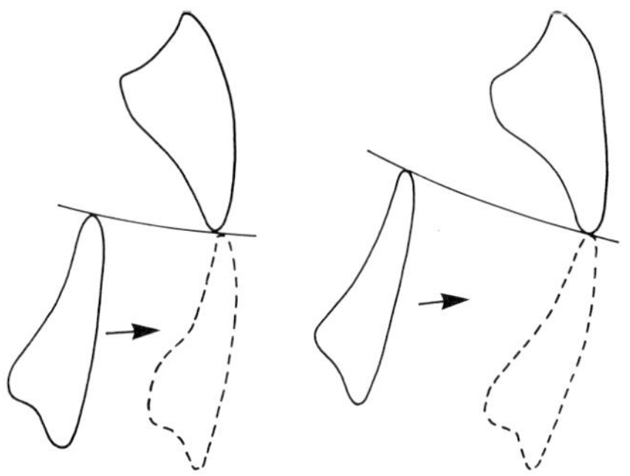

Figure 9.23 Illustrating how the overlap and overjet are related to the mandibular path

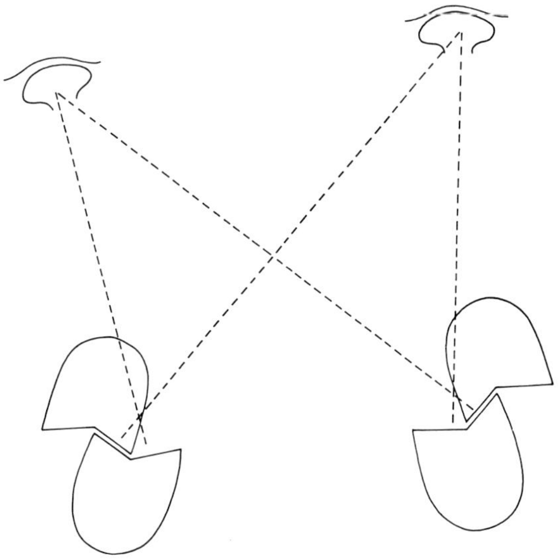

Figure 9.24 Diagram to illustrate how each condyle becomes a rotational centre depending on which side the person is chewing

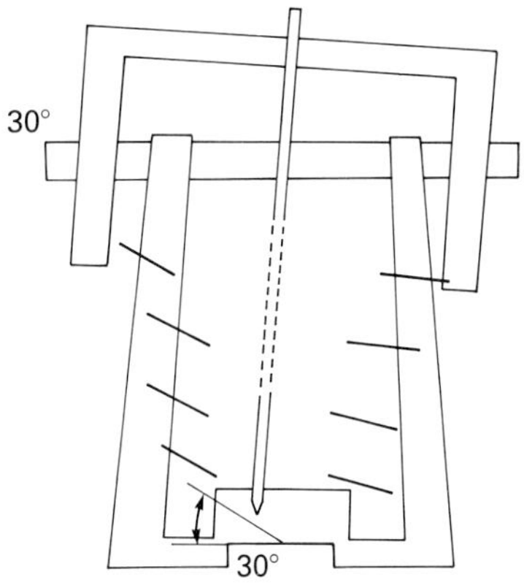

Figure 9.25 Diagrammatic representation of the paths of the posterior teeth during a lateral mandibular movement with a condylar and incisal guidance both of 30°. The paths represent in ascending order those of the first premolar, second premolar, first molar and second molar teeth. The left side in the diagram is the balancing side and the right the working side, because on the articulator it is the upper member which moves

as the mandible moves forwards, the incisal edges of the lower front teeth meet and slide upon the incisal edges of the upper front teeth (Figure 9.23). This may be summed up by saying that within the limits set by the path of the mandible the greater the vertical overlap, the greater must be the horizontal overjet, and vice versa.

The rotational centres for the lateral movements are more difficult to show diagrammatically because they alter according to the part of the mandible being considered. Thus in the molar region the condylar guidance is the stronger influence and the incisal guidance the weaker, while in the first premolar region these conditions are reversed. Thus Figure 9.24 shows diagrammatically how each condyle becomes a rotational centre when it is on the working side and Figure 9.25 shows the effect of an identical condylar and incisal guidance, i.e. both set to 30°, which gives an even lift to the moving frame of the articulator along the whole length of the balancing side. The side towards which the mandible moves is termed the working side, and the side from which it moves, the balancing or non-working side. On the working side the condylar guidance is nil, because that condyle does not move (except for the Bennett movement or side shift which is not allowed for in many articulators). Thus the only upward movement of the working side is controlled by the incisal guidance, which decreases in influence from before backwards.

Figure 9.26 shows the effect on the mandibular path in the regions of the various teeth, with a condylar guidance of 30° and an incisal guidance of 5°. The angles of the path given are rough approximations, but they enable a picture to be formed of the influence on lateral mandibular movements of the condylar and incisal guidance, and show clearly how an alteration of the incisal guidance alters the mandibular path.

Thus if a composite diagram is drawn showing the paths followed in both right and left lateral movements, of a case with both condylar guidances of 30° and the incisal guidance 5°, then AB is the path followed when the left side is the balancing side and CB the path when it is the working side (Figure 9.26).

Thus in order that the teeth shall maintain contact during lateral mandibular movements, they must be

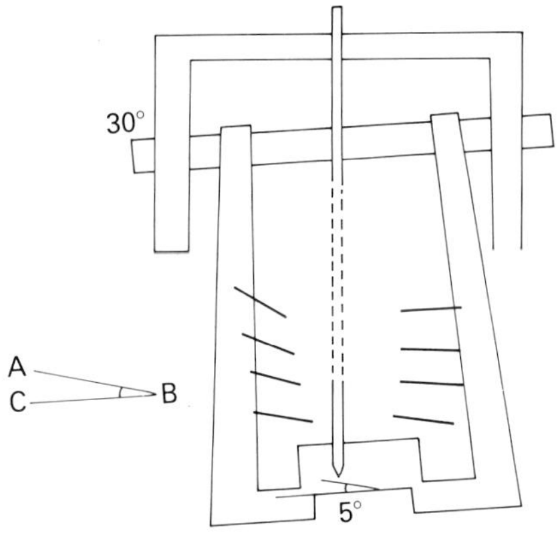

Figure 9.26 Diagrammatic representation of the paths of the posterior teeth during a lateral mandibular movement with a condylar guidance of 30° and an incisal guidance of 5°. AB represents the path followed by the second premolar when the left side, in the diagram, is acting as the balancing side, and CB represents the path followed by this tooth when the left side is acting as the working side

set as shown in Figure 9.27*a* while Figure 9.27*b* shows how they maintain cusp contact on the balancing side, and Figure 9.27*c* when in working occlusion. The palatal inclines of the maxillary teeth, and the buccal inclines of the mandibular teeth, must be parallel to the path AB, and the buccal inclines of the maxillary teeth, and the lingual inclines of the mandibular teeth, must be parallel to the line CB.

Figure 9.28 shows how cuspal interference will occur if teeth are set to a horizontal occlusal plane, and how the introduction of the lateral compensating curve corrects this.

Figure 9.29 shows how cusp locking can also occur in a protrusive movement if the anteroposterior cuspal angles are not in harmony with the protrusive path of the mandible.

Setting the incisal guidance table

From the foregoing it will be realized that the angle of the incisal guidance table will markedly affect the cusp angles, cusp heights, the vertical overlap and the horizontal overjet. A method of setting the table for any given patient is indicated below.

Set the upper and lower six front teeth to the required overlap and overjet as determined by aesthetics and function, and then alter the incisal guidance table so that in protrusion, and right and left lateral movements, the incisal edges of the upper and lower teeth just slide upon one another. Remember, however, that the steeper the slope of the table, the higher and steeper will need to be the cusps of the premolar and molar teeth, and even

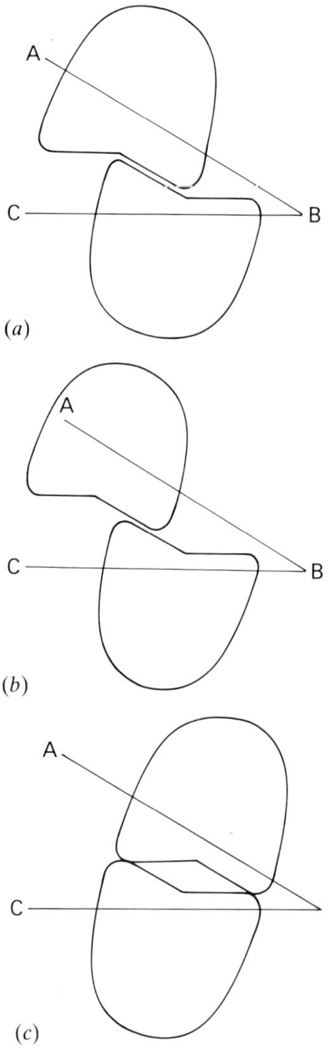

Figure 9.27 (*a*), (*b*), (*c*) Setting of teeth (see text)

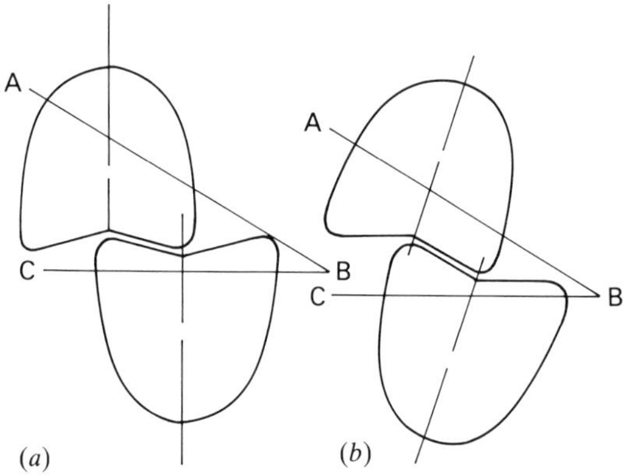

Figure 9.28 (*a*) Teeth set with long axes vertical. Cuspal inclines not parallel to planes of movement. (*b*) Long axes of teeth inclined to lateral compensating curve. Cuspal inclines are now parallel to planes of movement

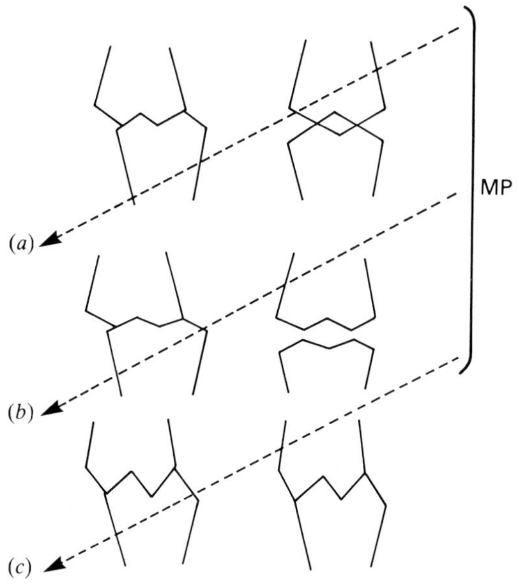

Figure 9.29 Diagrammatic representation of cusp locking and loss of cuspal contact. MP = mandibular path. (*a*) The cuspal inclines are parallel to the mandibular path and therefore tooth contact can be maintained during mandibular movement. (*b*) The cuspal inclines are of a lesser angle to the horizontal than the mandibular path, thus tooth contact will be lost during mandibular movement. (*c*) The cuspal inclines are of a greater angle to the horizontal than the mandibular path: thus cusp locking occurs if mandibular movement is attempted

with balanced articulation on the articulator high steep cusps are liable to cause instability of the dentures in the mouth because of limitations in the accuracy of simulating the patient in the laboratory. Therefore, when setting the teeth, make the vertical overlap as small as possible. This is particularly true when the mandible is atrophic and almost without any alveolar ridge. In such a case the posterior teeth must be virtually cuspless if functional stability is to be attained.

Teeth for balanced articulation

Many varieties of teeth have been manufactured over the years for use with complete dentures, and in some the occlusal design is arranged to facilitate occlusal balance; in a few instances the cusp angle, i.e. the angle between the slope of the cusp and the horizontal plane through the tip of the cusp, is stated.

Cusped teeth

Posterior teeth with cusps should generally be used in preference to cuspless or zero-cusp ones for two reasons:

1. Greater efficiency: a convex surface makes point contact with a flat or convex surface and this point contact, moving under pressure, results in a cutting action. The cusps also produce a grinding action when moving through the intercuspal spaces which help to hold the food in position while it is being ground. Provided that the cusps and sulci are correctly shaped, there is ample clearance for the ground and cut particles to escape from the occlusal surfaces. Flat, cuspless teeth, while able to crush and grind food, cannot possibly cut vegetable or animal fibres, which must therefore be reduced to a length suitable for swallowing before being placed in the mouth.
2. Balance: with cusped teeth a balanced articulation can be built on the articulator and then modified by grinding any areas of occlusal contact where pressure is slightly excessive. With cuspless teeth it is very difficult to obtain balance and the most satisfactory way of doing so is to use a technique employing plaster and pumice record blocks which will shortly be described.

Inverted cusp teeth

There are several types of teeth which are described as having 'inverted cusps'. These are in effect flat-surfaced or zero-cusp teeth with hollows ground into the occlusal surface. The claim is made for these teeth that food fibres are cut between the edges of the hollows, while the flat surfaces allow lateral movements without cuspal interference. With most teeth of this type the first claim is quite inaccurate as the hollows are not provided with escape grooves for the food, and soon become filled up and clogged. The second claim is correct in that they will avoid cuspal interference but, on the other hand, it is difficult to grind these flat surfaces to produce balanced articulation, especially if they are made of porcelain.

Plaster and pumice record blocks

The techniques which have been described so far have all left the degree of curvature of the compensating curves to the discretion of the technician. The object of this technique is to obtain the individual curves of a given patient. Briefly, this is attained by inserting record blocks with abrasive rims and allowing the patient to grind them together until they are in balanced articulation. This is a type of functionally generated path technique and is very suitable for patients with marked translatory movements of the mandible.

Bases

Stability of the record blocks is essential for accuracy since there will be a considerable lateral and protrusive drag, owing to friction, during the process of grinding. Ideally the bases should be made of heat-cured acrylic resin.

Occlusal rims

These are made of a mixture of plaster and an abrasive, such as coarse carborundum, pumice or sand. The buccolingual width should be approximately 1 cm which is necessary to define the lateral and anteroposterior curves, and for strength.

It is essential when employing this technique that the jaw relationship is first recorded with wax blocks which are then mounted on a simple articulator. The blocks with abrasive rims are then constructed with the vertical height opened a few millimetres to allow for the closure which will result from the grinding.

One method of constructing the rims is to make them of composition to within 5 mm of the estimated correct height, to groove the composition for retention and then build up the plaster–pumice for a further 4–5 mm (Figure 9.30).

Developing the occlusal curves

The patient is instructed to grind the blocks together with both lateral and protrusive movements but only to use the minimum pressure necessary to keep the blocks in contact. The necessity for using very light pressure must be emphasized since the high proportion of abrasive needed for rapid cutting weakens the plaster which will crack or crumble if anything approaching full gnathic pressure is used.

Denture adhesive may be used to assist stability of the blocks, or the dentist may support the blocks with his fingers to prevent any movements of the bases in the preliminary stages of grinding. The patient should be instructed not to swallow the debris. The record blocks are removed from time to time for cleaning and inspection and to allow the patient to rinse his mouth and also to rest.

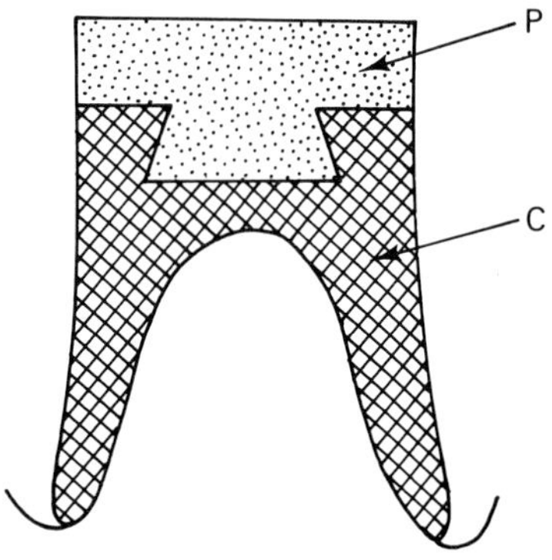

Figure 9.30 Details of the construction of a plaster–pumice occlusal rim: P, plaster–pumice; C, impression compound

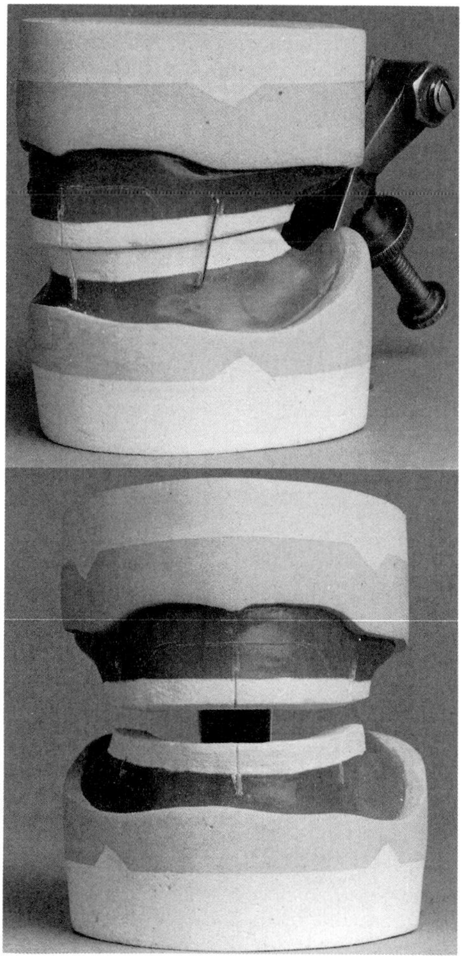

(*a*)

(*b*)

Figure 9.31 Plaster–pumice blocks after having been ground in the mouth. (*a*) The blocks are sealed in retruded contact position in the mouth by wire staples. (*b*) shows the definite curves produced by this technique

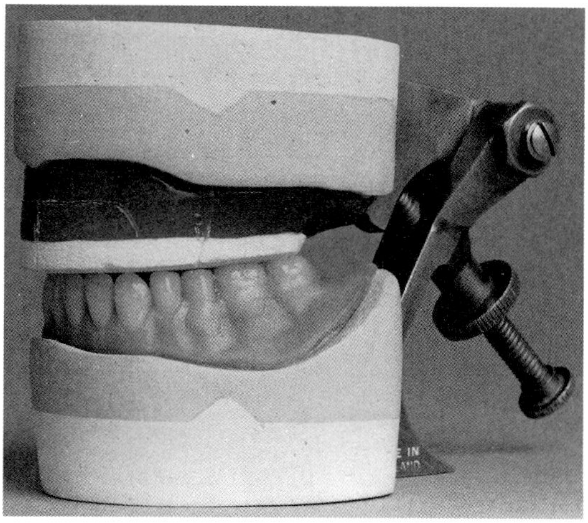

Figure 9.32 Lower teeth set to upper block

The grinding is continued until the correct vertical height is obtained, usually within a few minutes. The occlusal surfaces of the rims now show correct balancing curves for the patient (Figure 9.31). The curves are reproduced in the denture by mounting the casts on a plane-line articulator and setting the lower zero-cusp teeth to occlude with the upper block and then the upper teeth to occlude with the lower ones (Figure 9.32).

It should be appreciated that there are numerous balancing curves suitable for every patient and that curves obtained by this grinding technique under different conditions are not interchangeable. The form of curve will vary with the height of the occlusal surfaces and also with the original shape of the plaster–pumice blocks, whether flat or curved. It is usually best to make the surface of the rims conform to a segment of a 100 mm radius sphere, i.e. similar to the architecture of natural teeth. This average curve is then modified by the patient.

Plaster–pumice rims tend to be rather messy and a good alternative is modelling wax mixed with a little carding wax to render it displaceable. The rims are covered with tin foil to prevent them sticking together while the patient squeezes them into his own individual occlusal curves.

Chapter 10

Phonetics

Mechanism of speech

The voice is principally produced in the larynx, while the tongue, by constantly changing its shape and position of contact with the lips, teeth, alveolar processes and hard and soft palates, gives the sound form and influences its qualities. The oral cavity, nasal cavities and the sinuses act as resonant chambers, and the muscles of the abdomen and thorax control the volume, and rate of flow, of the air stream passing into the speech mechanism.

The soft palate in conjunction with the pharynx controls the direction of the air stream after it passes from the larynx. In all the vowel, and most consonant sounds, the air stream is confined entirely to the oral cavity, but a few nasal sounds do occur, e.g. M, N and NG, in which the air is expelled entirely through the nose. The former are produced by raising the soft palate into close contact with the pharynx, thus sealing off the nose and forcing the air to proceed through the mouth.

With the nasal sounds the soft palate is pressed downwards and forwards and, for the NG sound, the dorsum of the tongue humped up to meet it, thus sealing off the oral cavity and forcing the air stream to proceed through the nose. For M and N it is the closure of the lips and the contact between the tip of the tongue and the alveolar ridge that prevents oral egress of air. The vowel sounds are formed by a continuous air flow, the alteration in size of the mouth and the change in shape and size of the lip opening giving the various sounds their characteristic form.

The consonant sounds are produced by the air stream being obstructed in its passage through the mouth by the formation of complete or partial seals or stops. These are produced by the tongue pressing against the teeth or palate, or by closing of the lips. The sudden breaking of the seal brought about by the withdrawal of the tongue, or the opening of the lips, produces the sound. In many sounds there is a build up of air pressure behind the stop which when the seal is released produces an explosive effect. Examples of these are: the lip closure of the P and B sounds; the tongue and anterior hard palate contact in T and D sounds.

In some cases the seal or stop is not complete, but the channel through which the air stream must pass is made extremely narrow: an example of this is the production of an S, Z or C soft sound, in which the tongue separates itself from the anterior aspect of the hard palate by about 1 mm, forming a thin slit-like channel through which the air stream hisses.

Speech, therefore, is largely a matter of the control of the size and shape of the mouth, which is chiefly governed by the position of the tongue and its contact with the teeth, alveolar processes and palate.

Fortunately for the prosthetist, the tongue possesses remarkable qualities of adaptability, and rapidly becomes accustomed to changes occurring in the mouth. After the extraction of teeth, or the insertion of a denture, some difference may be noticed in the quality of the speech, but improvement quickly follows as the tongue adjusts itself to the new conditions. In extreme cases, such as the edentulous state or when poorly designed complete dentures are worn, the previous tone and quality are not always re-established. The tongue's adaptability is illustrated by the number of individuals wearing dentures, designed with little regard to their effect on phonation*, who exhibit no obviously apparent speech defects, the reason being that in the construction of those dentures the general principles of setting teeth were followed, coupled with due

* The correct word is not phonation but articulation; in the science of phonetics, phonation refers to the action of the vocal and ventricular folds.

regard to the aesthetic requirements and the attainment of the correct vertical dimension. This has produced the occlusal plane at a level corresponding to that of the natural dentition, the anterior teeth in approximately the same position anteroposteriorly as the natural teeth, and the new dental arch conforming to that of the previous arch, thereby allowing the correct tongue space. Thus the dentures replacing the lost tissues have conformed closely to the state which existed naturally, the main difference being the increase in bulk, a factor for which the tongue must compensate. However, some knowledge of phonetics in relation to dentures is necessary, in order to correct the speech defects that may occur in denture wearers, and also to act as a guide for the more accurate design of complete dentures.

Factors in denture design affecting speech

The vowel sounds

These sounds are produced by a continuous air stream passing through the oral cavity which is in the form of a single chamber. All vowel sounds involve the tongue having a convex configuration. The position of the hump of the tongue in relation to the hard and soft palates determines the quality of the sound. The tip of the tongue, in all the vowel sounds, lies on the floor of the mouth either in contact with or close to the lingual surfaces of the lower anterior teeth and gums. The application of this in denture construction is that the lower anterior teeth should be set so that they do not impede the tongue positioning for these sounds; i.e. they should not be set lingual to the alveolar ridge. The upper denture base must be kept thin, and the posterior border should merge into the soft tissue in order to avoid irritating the dorsum of the tongue, which might occur if this surface of the denture were allowed to remain thick and square-edged.

The consonant sounds

For convenience, these sounds may be classified thus:

1. Bilabials: formed mainly by the lips (e.g. B, P, M).
2. Labiodentals: formed by the lips and teeth (e.g. F, V).
3. Dentals: formed by the tongue and teeth (e.g. Th). Note that Th in thick, and Th in then, are different sounds.
4. Linguopalatals: formed by the tongue and palate.
   (a) Tongue and anterior portion of the hard palate (e.g. D, T, C (soft), S, Z, R). In phonetics, these are known as alveolar sounds.
   (b) Tongue and portion of the hard palate posterior to that of (a) (e.g. J, CH, SH).
   (c) Tongue and soft palate (e.g. C (hard), K, G, NG); these are velar sounds.
5. Nasal (e.g. M, N, NG, also belonging to the other groups).

Unless careful consideration is given to the following aspects of denture construction, speech defects will occur, varying from the almost indiscernible to the unpleasantly obvious.

Denture thickness and peripheral outline

The prosthetist's aim is to produce dentures which are mechanically functional, aesthetically pleasing and permit normal speech. The most satisfactory attainment of the first two requirements may cause slight defects in the patient's speech but this should not be allowed to happen and some compromise will often be required satisfactorily to equate these three aims. One of the reasons for loss of tone and incorrect articulation of speech is the decrease of air volume and loss of tongue space in the oral cavity resulting from unduly thick denture bases. The periphery of the denture must not be over-extended so as to encroach upon the movable tissues, since the depth of the sulci will vary with the movements of the tongue, lips and cheeks during the production of speech sounds. Any interference with the freedom of these movements may result in indistinct speech, especially if the function of the lips is in any way hindered.

Most important is the thickness of the denture base covering the centre of the palate, for here no loss of natural tissue has occurred, and the base reduces the amount of tongue space and the oral air volume.

The production of the palatolingual group of sounds involves contact between the tongue, and either the palate, the alveolar process, or the teeth. With the consonants T and D, the tongue makes firm contact with the anterior part of the hard palate, and is suddenly drawn downwards, producing an explosive sound; any thickening of the denture base in this region may cause incorrect formation of these sounds. When producing the S, C (soft), Z, R and L consonant sounds, contact occurs between the tongue and the most anterior part of the hard palate, including the lingual surfaces of the upper and lower incisors to a slight degree. In the case of the S, C (soft) and Z sounds, a slit-like channel is formed between the tongue and palate through which the air hisses. If artificial rugae are too pronounced, or the denture base too thick in this area, the air channel will be obstructed and a noticeable lisp may occur as a result.

To produce the Ch and J sounds the tongue is pressed against a larger area of the hard palate, and in addition makes contact with the upper alveolar process, bringing about the explosive effect by rapidly breaking the seal thus formed. The Sh sound is similar in formation, but the air is allowed to escape between the tongue and palate without any explosive effect, and if the palate is too thick in the region of the rugae, it may impair the production of these consonants.

Vertical dimension

The formation of the bilabials, P, B and M requires that the lips make contact to check the air stream. With P and B, the lips part quite forcibly so that the resultant sound is produced with an explosive effect, whereas in the M sound lip contact is passive. For this reason M can be used as an aid in obtaining the correct vertical height since a strained appearance during lip contact, or the inability to make contact, indicates that the record blocks are occluding prematurely. With the C (soft), S and Z sounds the teeth come very close together, and more especially so in the case of Ch and J; if the vertical dimension is excessive, the dentures will actually make contact as these consonants are formed, and the patient will most likely complain of the teeth clicking together.

Occlusal plane

The labiodentals, F and V, are produced by the air stream being forced through a narrow gap between the lower lip and the incisal edges of the upper anterior teeth. If the occlusal plane is set too high the correct positioning of the lower lip may be difficult. If, on the other hand, the plane is too low, the lip will overlap the labial surfaces of the upper teeth to a greater extent than is required for normal phonation and the sound might be affected.

Anteroposterior position of the incisors

In setting the upper anterior teeth, consideration of their labiopalatal position is necessary for the correct formation of the labiodentals F and V. If they are placed too far palatally the contact of the lower lip with the incisal and labial surfaces may be difficult, as the lip will tend to pass outside the teeth; the appearance usually prevents the dentist from setting these teeth forward of their natural position. If the anterior teeth are placed too far back some effect may be noticed on the quality of the linguopalatals S, C (soft) and Z, resulting in a lisp due to the tongue making contact with the teeth prematurely. The tongue will more readily accommodate itself to anteroposterior errors in the setting of the teeth than to vertical errors.

Postdam area

Errors of construction in this region involve the vowels U and O and the palatolingual consonants K, NG, G and C (hard). In the latter group the air blast is checked by the base of the tongue being raised upwards and backwards to make contact with the soft palate. A denture which has a thick base in the postdam area, or a posterior edge finished square instead of chamfered, will probably irritate the dorsum of the tongue, impeding speech and possibly producing a feeling of nausea. Indirectly, the postdam seal influences articulation of speech, for if it is inadequate the denture may become unseated during the formation of those sounds that have an explosive effect, requiring the sudden repositioning of the tongue to control and stabilize the denture; this applies particularly to singers. Speech is usually of poor quality in those individuals whose upper denture has become so loose that it is held in position mainly by means of tongue pressure against the palate. Careful observation will show that the denture, in such cases, rises and falls with tongue movements during speech.

Before passing to the next factor it should be mentioned that the consonants M, N, NG, belong to the nasal group in which the air stream is allowed to escape into the nasal cavity through a channel formed by the incomplete approximation of the soft palate and pharynx.

Width of dental arch

If the teeth are set to an arch which is too narrow the tongue will be cramped, thus affecting the size and shape of the air channel; this results in faulty articulation of consonants such as T, D, S, N, K and C, where the lateral margins of the tongue make contact with the palatal surfaces of the upper posterior teeth. Every endeavour should be made, consistent with general principles of denture design, to place the lingual and palatal surfaces of the artificial teeth in the position previously occupied by the natural dentition.

Relationship of the upper and lower anterior teeth

The chief concern is that of the S sound which requires near contact of the upper and lower incisors so that the air stream is allowed to escape through a slight opening between the teeth. In abnormal protrusive and retrusive jaw relationships, some difficulty may be experienced in the formation of this sound, and it will probably necessitate adjustment of the upper and lower anterior teeth anteroposteriorly so that approximation can be brought about successfully. The consonants Ch, J and Z require a similar air channel in their formation.

Summary

To summarize, it will be seen that speech requirements call for dentures having a correct vertical dimension, an accurate periphery and a dental arch formation permitting natural tongue space, so that adequate freedom for movement is ensured. The setting of the anterior teeth should be such that they follow that of the natural teeth, thus fixing the occlusal plane at thc correct level and preventing the placing of the artificial teeth inside or outside the pre-extraction position, which would require the tongue to adapt itself to new circumstances. Finally, denture bases should be made suitably thin, but consistent with the other factors of denture construction, so that contact by the tongue takes place in as near a natural and normal manner as is possible.

Chapter 11

Trying the dentures in the mouth

Having set the teeth on the articulator according to the information obtained at the record stage, it is necessary to try the waxed dentures in the patient's mouth before finishing them, so that they may be checked and the occlusion verified. Once the dentures have been processed in acrylic it is laborious and difficult, and sometimes impossible, to effect any alteration, whereas in the wax stage changes can easily be made. Since so many points require checking, it is sound practice to get into the habit of working to a definite plan during the trial stage, and the following order is suggested.

1. The lower denture by itself
   - (a) Peripheral outline
     - (iii) Buccal and labial
     - (ii) Lingual
     - (iii) Posterior extension
     - (iv) Underextension
   - (b) Stability to occlusal stresses
   - (c) Tongue space
   - (d) Height of the occlusal plane
2. The upper denture by itself.
   - (a) Peripheral outline
     - (i) Buccal and labial
     - (ii) Posterior border
   - (b) Stability to occlusal stresses
   - (c) Retention.
3. Both dentures together
   - (a) Position of occlusion
     - (i) Horizontal relationship (retruded contact position)
     - (ii) Vertical dimension (occlusal face height)
   - (b) Evenness of occlusal contact
   - (c) Balanced occlusion
   - (d) Appearance
     - (i) Centre line
     - (ii) Anterior plane
     - (iii) Shape of the teeth
     - (iv) Size of the teeth
     - (v) Shade and blend of the teeth
     - (vi) Profile and lip form
     - (vii) Amount of tooth visible
     - (viii) Regularity of the teeth
   - (e) Approval of appearance by the patient.

Before carrying out these checks, remove the dentures from the articulator and place them in a bowl of cold water. It is important that the waxed dentures should be frequently placed in cold water as wax softens appreciably at mouth temperature and, if left in the mouth too long, the teeth may be displaced and the bases may distort. The method of carrying out these checks is as follows.

Trying the lower denture by itself

Place the denture in the mouth and seat it on the ridge.

Peripheral outline

The entire periphery should be checked to ensure that it is not over-, or under-extended.

The buccal and labial periphery

Hold the denture in place with light pressure on the occlusal surfaces of the teeth and move the cheek on one side upwards and inwards, thus simulating the action it makes when chewing. Now relax the pressure on the teeth and observe if the denture rises from the ridge. If it does, trim the periphery where it is seen to be over-extended until little or no movement occurs. Pay particular attention to the buccal frena and ensure that they have adequate

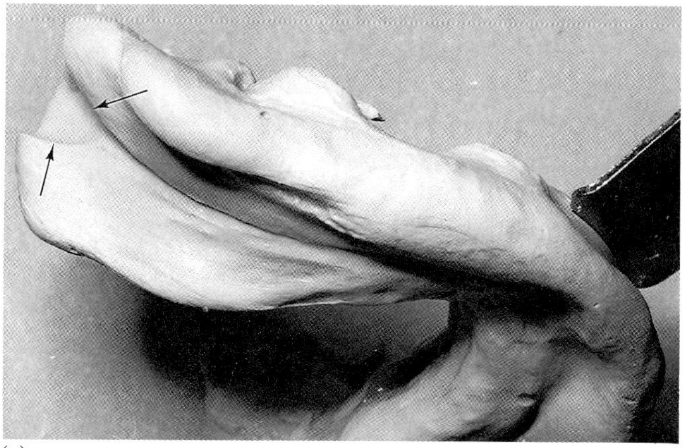

(*a*)

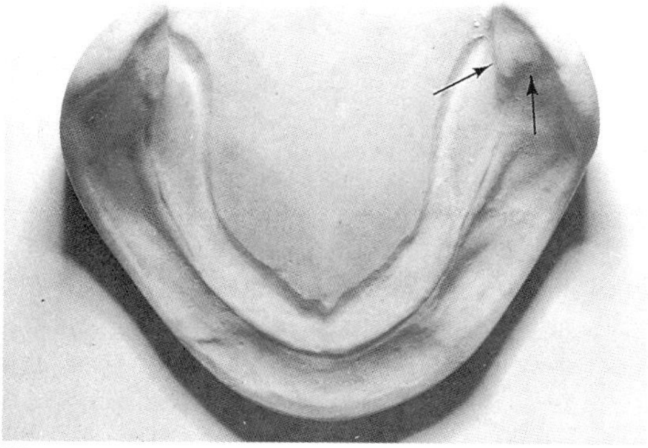

(*b*)

Figure 11.1 (*a*) The posterior edge of the lower denture should cross the retromolar pad (arrowed). (*b*) On the cast of another case the retromolar area is well defined in the form of a pear-shaped pad (arrowed)

clearance. Repeat for the opposite side and for the lip. Note the bulk and shape of the buccal aspect of the denture. It should take the form of a gentle convexity in the molar region but concave in the premolar region (see Chapter 2). Such a contour will aid the muscular control of the denture as the cheek will tend to fit against the surface and hold the denture down.

The lingual periphery

Hold the denture in place with light pressure and ask the patient to protrude his tongue sufficiently to moisten his lips; if the denture lifts at the back, it is over-extended in the region of the lingual pouch. Next, ask the patient to put the tip of his tongue up to the back of his palate; if the denture lifts in the front, it is over-extended anteriorly, probably in the region of the lingual frenum. Such over-extension must be relieved, but care should be taken to avoid over-trimming, which occurs very easily owing to the difficulty of seeing the functional depth of the lingual sulcus when the denture is in place. Final adjustments are more easily and more accurately made after the finished denture has been worn for a few days, when areas of slight inflammation will indicate the precise location of over-extension.

Posterior extension

Ensure that the heels of the lower denture are extended as high up the ascending ramus of the mandible as is practicable; the purpose of this is to buttress the denture against the backward pressure of the lower lip (Figure 11.1).

Under-extension

Though of less common occurrence than over-extension, it is equally important that the periphery should not be under-extended since dentures must cover the greatest possible area if maximum retention and support are to be obtained. If the denture is found to be under-extended in any part of the periphery as shown by the presence of a gap between it and the functional position of the surrounding mucosa, replace the denture on the cast and check whether the base has been carried to the full extent of the impression at this point. If it has, it implies an inaccuracy in the impression which must be retaken before proceeding further. An alternative is to proceed to the finish stage and then rebase the denture to rectify the peripheral error.

Stability under occlusal load

This test is used to determine if occlusal stresses will be transmitted unfavourably. Apply pressure with the ball of the finger in the premolar and molar regions of each side alternately; this pressure must be directed at right angles to the occlusal surface. If pressure on one side causes the denture to tilt and rise from the ridge on the other side, it indicates that the teeth on the side on which pressure is applied are set too far outside the ridge. It may also indicate lack of adaptation of the base on the side being loaded or under-extended flanges on the side which rises.

Tongue space

Natural teeth occupy a position in the mouth where the inward pressure of the cheeks and lips is equalled by the outward pressure of the tongue, and it is into this zone of neutral pressure that the artificial teeth must be placed. The tongue, being more mobile than the cheeks, will cause greater instability of the lower denture if the teeth are set on the lingual side of the neutral zone than if they are set on the buccal side. If the tongue is cramped by the denture, lateral pressure will be exerted, producing instability when the tongue moves. You can test for lack of tongue space as follows: Ask the patient to relax the tongue, making sure that the denture is seated on the ridge, and then request him to raise the tongue. If the tongue is cramped, the denture will begin to rise immediately the tongue moves. This immediate reaction of the denture tends to differentiate the movement caused by a cramped tongue from the movement caused by lingual flange over-extension; movement due to the latter cause does not occur until the tongue has risen some distance.

The causes of lack of tongue space are:

1. Posterior teeth set inside the ridge.
2. Molar teeth which are too broad buccolingually. Such teeth should be replaced by smaller ones or their width reduced by grinding the lingual aspect (if the teeth are porcelain take care not to damage the retentive diatoric hole; if they are acrylic they should be polished before being finally set).
3. Molar teeth leaning inwards. This will not always cause cramping of the tongue, but should never be allowed to occur as it interferes with the free vertical movements of the tongue.
4. Setting the upper teeth over the ridge almost invariably leads to the occluding lower teeth lying too far lingually.

Height of the occlusal plane

To obtain maximum stability of a lower denture, the occlusal plane of the lower teeth should be very slightly below the bulk of the tongue, so that the tongue performs the majority of its movements above the denture and thus tends to keep the denture down (see Figure 2.41).

The denture must therefore be examined to see if the tongue, when relaxed, lies above or below the occlusal plane. Ask the patient to relax and place the tip of the tongue comfortably and without strain behind the lower front teeth, which is the normal relaxed position of the tongue, and then open his mouth without moving his tongue. If the height of the occlusal plane is correct, the tongue will be seen to lie on top of the lingual cusps.

If the lower denture still tends to rise unduly after the lingual periphery has been checked, and as much lateral space as possible for the tongue has been allowed, it may be necessary to reset the teeth completely, lowering the occlusal plane. This may be especially necessary in those patients who have a low tongue position (see Chapter 2).

The height of the occlusal plane is also of importance for the following reason: the greater the height of the lower denture, the longer will be the lower front teeth and the greater the surface exposed to the unfavourable pressure of the lower lip.

This concludes the examination of the lower denture alone, and it should be removed from the mouth and placed in a bowl of cold water.

Trying the upper denture by itself

Place the upper denture in the mouth and examine in the following manner.

Peripheral outline

1. The buccal and labial periphery is checked as for the lower denture.
2. The position of the posterior border is verified to check that the posterior edge is situated on the soft palate and that the postdam area on the cast has been placed correctly (see Figure 2.7).

Stability

Stability under occlusal load may be carried out as for the lower denture, but is intended to check the closeness of adaptation of the base against the mucosa and the future support of the denture in those cases where the mucosa is unevenly displaceable.

Retention

Retention is checked by seating the denture with a finger on the vault of the palate and then attempting to remove the denture at right angles to the occlusal plane. Load is then applied upwards and outwards in one canine region to check the retentive force in the contralateral corner of the denture, i.e. in the region of the tuberosity vestibular space and pterygomaxillary notch. Then check the other side in the same way.

Both dentures together

Remove the upper denture from the mouth, replace on its cast to confirm the fit, and chill in cold water for a few seconds. Then place both dentures in the mouth. If it is found necessary to improve the retention of the dentures when using a shellac type of base-plate, adhesive powder may be sprinkled on their fitting surfaces.

Position of occlusion

Horizontal relation (retruded contact position)

Hold the lower denture in position on the ridge and ask the patient to relax, then to 'close on your back teeth' gently and maintain them in occlusion while the examination is carried out. If the registration is accurate, the teeth will interdigitate in the mouth in exactly the same manner as they do on the articulator, but if the registration is wrong, the teeth will not interdigitate correctly and may even occlude cusp to cusp on one or both sides. The clinician must make quite certain that the occlusion he sees in the mouth is not due to movement of the dentures on the ridges, tilting of either denture or dropping of the upper denture. This is best tested by asking the patient to keep the teeth together and then trying to separate the posterior teeth by means of a thin spatula or Le Cron blade; this test should be carried out on each side of the mouth alternately. The teeth should be brought into occlusion several times, using any of the registration aids, in order to make certain that the position of occlusion is correct or, if it is incorrect, to ascertain the type of error, i.e. whether the mandible can be retruded from the previously recorded jaw relationship, whether a lateral deviation has occurred, or whether there is a premature contact on one side before the other.

Observation of the upper and lower centre lines in relation to each other, with the dentures on the articulator and then in the mouth, will indicate a lateral deviation, if present. When the lower centre line is seen to be to one side of the upper centre line, with the dentures in the mouth, in contrast to the coincidence of these lines when viewed on the articulator, it is possible that the original registration was incorrect and that a lateral position has been recorded; this may be checked by the occlusion of the posterior teeth. If the original position was incorrect, the lower cusps will be slightly farther back on one side indicating a greater retrusion of the condyle on that side. Should the lower cusps be slightly forward on one side, it indicates that the original recording of the occlusion was correct and the patient is now giving a lateral position (Figure 11.2). Major errors in the position of occlusion are easily detected, but minor errors may pass unnoticed; therefore it is extremely important to watch for any slight movement of the dentures on their respective ridges from the time the teeth first make contact until they reach the position of complete interdigitation, the reason being that the cusp inclines of the teeth guide the dentures into occlusion and will move the dentures in relation to the ridges when only a slight error of jaw relationship exists from that which was obtained when taking the records. Care is needed when holding the lower denture in place on the ridge to avoid pushing it backwards. When errors of occlusion are noted at this trial stage they must be corrected by re-recording the position of occlusion as follows.

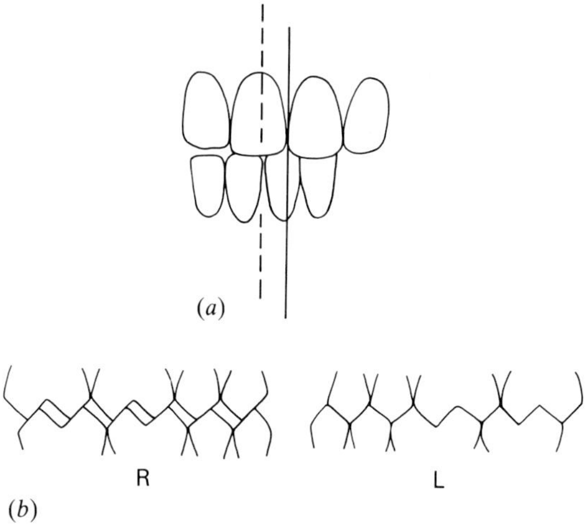

Figure 11.2 Incorrect recording of the occlusion (lateral mandibular swing) as it appears at the trial stage: (*a*) A right swing seen from the front. Note lack of continuity of upper and lower centre lines. (*b*) A right swing seen from the side. Posterior teeth on left side appear to interdigitate but have shifted medially, those on right do not interdigitate

The dentures are seated on the casts on the articulator and the posterior teeth removed from one of the dentures and replaced by wax which should be trimmed to occlude with the posterior teeth of the other denture without altering the vertical dimension as set on the articulator (Figure 11.3). In this way considerable time may be saved in trimming the blocks in the mouth, as then only minor adjustments are necessary to produce evenness of occlusal contact. The position of occlusion is recorded by adding a little softened base-plate wax to the chilled blocks, placing the dentures in the mouth and asking the patient 'to close on the back teeth', thus impressing the cusps of the opposing teeth into the wax without effecting any alteration in the vertical height (Figure 11.4). Care must be taken to see that the new position of occlusion gives the necessary correction. Points which may help in this

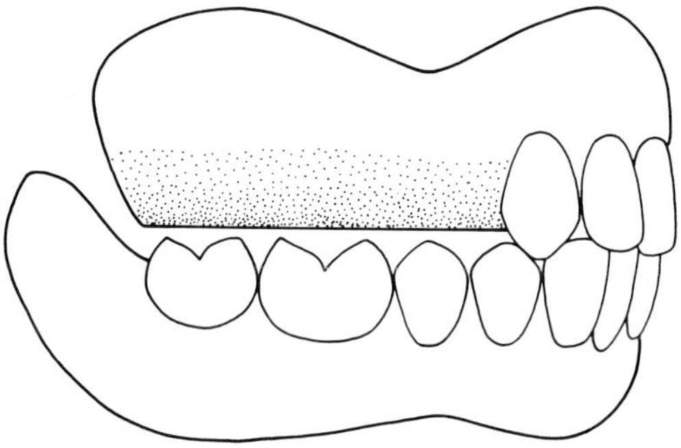

Figure 11.3 Re-recording retruded contact position (RCP). Posterior teeth replaced by wax

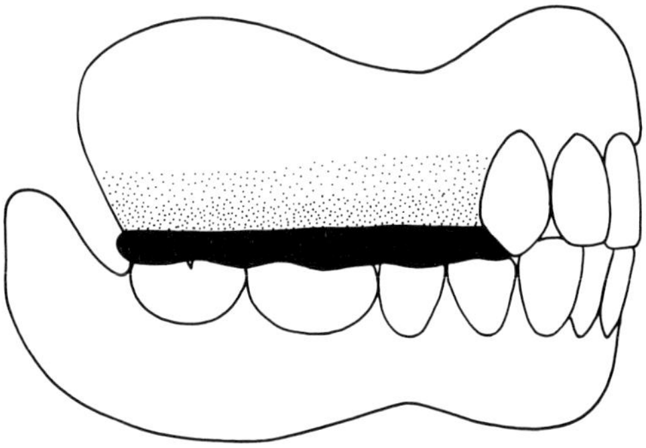

Figure 11.4 Re-recording RCP. Uniformly softened wax is added and the patient induced to the correct position

are observations of overlap, overjet, and the relation of the centre lines. When correcting a lateral deviation care must be taken to see that the lower anterior teeth do not impinge on the upper teeth, as this may cause the mandible to be guided into another incorrect position, or the dentures to tilt. If any contact of the anterior teeth occurs the offending lower teeth should be removed and the position retaken.

The advantage of removing posterior teeth from the upper trial denture is that in the re-recording the softened wax on the occlusal surface of the blocks is not interfered with by the operator's index fingers which are being used to control the lower denture; the disadvantage is that the orientation of the occlusal plane, as determined by the upper posterior teeth, is temporarily lost. Removal of lower posterior teeth, on the other hand, means that the softened wax replacing the teeth is almost bound to be displaced or disturbed by the controlling index fingers. It is better, therefore, to remove the upper teeth rather than the lower when rectifying an occlusal error.

Check the vertical height

Ask the patient to relax with the lips closed. Watch the point of the chin and then ask the patient to close the teeth together; the chin should move upwards a small but definite amount (see Chapter 6). If it is impossible to obtain this movement in spite of repeated attempts, it can be assumed that the vertical height is too great and, if this is excessive, there will also be a strained appearance when the lips are brought into contact with each other. It should be remembered that patients who are mouth breathers relax with their lips parted, and frequently have a large freeway space. An over-closed vertical height will be associated with a large freeway space, and when the teeth are in occlusion the lips will be seen to be pressed too firmly together with some loss of the vermilion border.

In order to correct the vertical height the posterior teeth are removed from one of the dentures and replaced by wax blocks. The articulator should be closed or opened approximately the amount assessed to establish a suitable freeway space, and the blocks then trimmed to occlude with the opposing teeth at the new vertical height. Final adjustments for evenness of occlusal contact, and for the production of the correct freeway space, are carried out in the mouth. Once these are satisfactory, the record blocks should be chilled in cold water, and a little registration paste added to their occlusal surfaces to record the impressions of the opposing teeth when registering the retruded contact position. The chilled blocks resist the occlusal load during this stage and prevent over-closure.

With cases set on an adjustable articulator the articulator may be closed or opened 1 or 2 mm without taking a further occlusal registration, provided the facebow record is correct, the reason being that the articulator reproduces the patient's individual jaw and hinge-axis relationship, and that a closure or opening of this amount on the articulator will not produce any translatory movement in the patient. Such changes of vertical dimension occurring in the patient may be considered as a hinge movement, although the danger of doing this on the articulator without reference to the patient is that the facebow transfer was not absolutely accurate.

Evenness of occlusal contact

Provided the horizontal and vertical relationships are correct, the evenness of the occlusion is next checked.

As the teeth close, they should occlude evenly and with equally distributed pressure all round. It frequently occurs that the teeth on one side of the mouth occlude slightly before those on the other, or the molars before the premolars. This may be due to:

1. Pressure on the blocks being heavier on one side than the other when the records were taken.

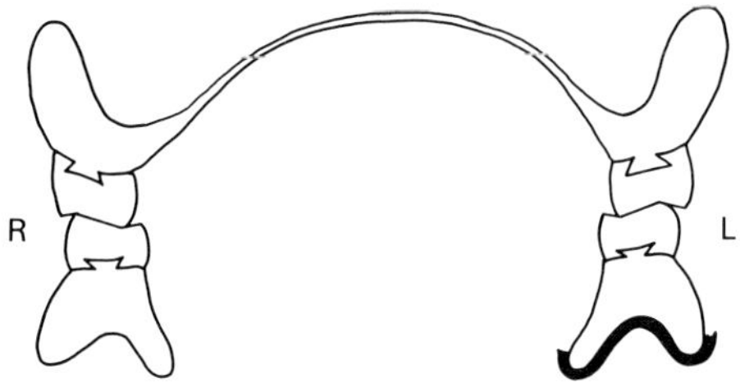

Figure 11.5 Section through a complete upper and lower denture at the trial stage. Inspection in the mouth would reveal apparently even contact between the molar teeth on both sides. What has actually occurred, however, is that heavy pressure on the right side has caused the lower denture to lift from the ridge on the left side until the teeth make contact. The use of mylar strips to check occlusal pressures will help to reveal such an error

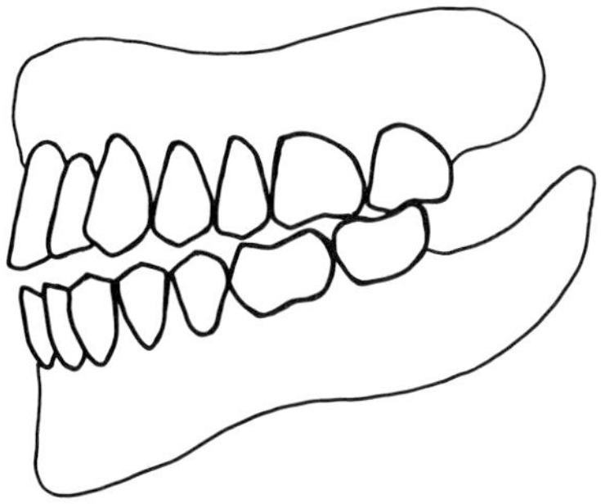

Figure 11.6 Incisor relationship error due to the molars occluding too early

2. A slight error when sealing the casts and blocks together or when mounting them on the articulator.
3. Warpage of the base-plates.

Such errors may escape notice at the trial stage as the waxed dentures readily tilt because the fit of the base-plates is less than that of finished dentures, thus allowing the teeth to be in occlusion when in fact they should not be in contact on the side on which the dentures have tilted (Figure 11.5). Such irregularity of pressure may only be slight, but if it escapes notice at the trial stage, the teeth in the finished dentures will be held apart in the area of heavy pressure and may require excessive grinding to correct the error. It may be so gross as to necessitate remaking one of the dentures. Teeth out of contact in the incisor and premolar region, due to the molars occluding too early, is frequently due to this cause (Figure 11.6).

To test for evenness of occlusal pressure, place two pieces of thin mylar tape between the teeth in the molar region, one on each side. Request the patient to close and then endeavour to remove the tapes simultaneously, holding one with each hand, by pulling them out between the closed teeth. Any difference in the force required to remove the strips will be readily appreciated, and if this force is interpreted in terms of occlusal pressure, an assessment may be made of whether or not it is even. Repeat the test in the premolar regions.

Before doing this, the patient should be asked, as the dentures close together, 'which side meets first?' Normal sensations of touch enable patients to respond accurately to such a question, although the method is less reliable if the contact of the record block base against the mucosa is not perfect.

Remember at all times to hold the dentures in place with the index fingers until final contact (Figure 11.7).

To test whether the front of the denture is rising slightly from the ridges when the back teeth are occluding, insert the point of a wax knife between the upper and lower incisor teeth and attempt to push the upper denture upwards and the lower denture downwards. Any appreciable movement may be interpreted as excessive contact in the molar region.

If the unevenness of contact is very slight, soften the wax supporting the teeth of one of the dentures on the offending side. Replace the dentures in the mouth and, holding the lower firmly in place, request the patient to close. The teeth on the side of heavy pressure will sink slightly into the softened

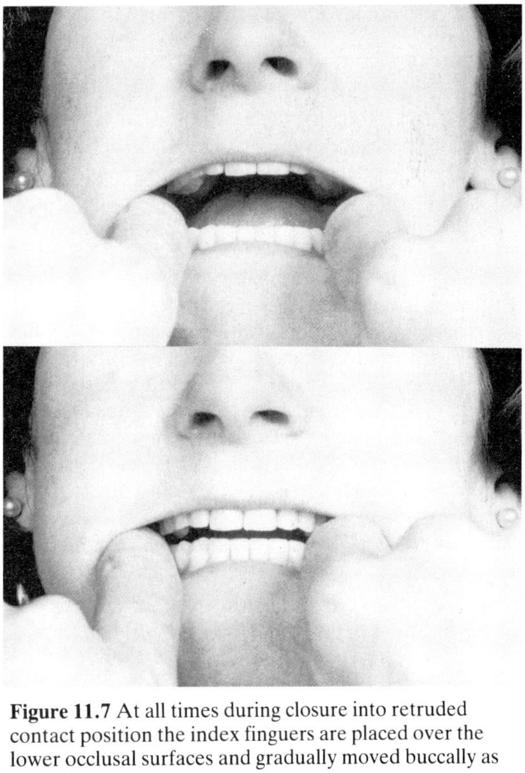

Figure 11.7 At all times during closure into retruded contact position the index finguers are placed over the lower occlusal surfaces and gradually moved buccally as the patient closes

wax until the occlusion of the teeth on the opposite side arrests them, thus evening the occlusal pressure. If the unevenness is more than very slight, this technique is not advisable as the initial contact on one side will either compress the supporting mucosa on that side or cause deviations of the mandible as the first tooth contact acts as a pivot. Complete retaking of the retruded contact position (RCP) record with built-up wax blocks is the only solution.

In cases in which difficulty is experienced with the position and evenness of occlusion it frequently simplifies the problem if the upper denture is finished in acrylic first and then the waxed lower denture is re-tried against this denture. Small alterations in the occlusion can easily be made to the waxed lower denture before it is finished, and with the closely fitting, well-retained upper denture in place patients seem to find it simpler to produce a correct position of occlusion. If this method is used, the technician must remount the acrylic upper denture on the articulator in occlusion with the wax lower denture as the purpose of the re-trial is to confirm or refute the accuracy of the articulator mounting.

Balanced occlusion and articulation

The first check is for retruded contact position which, if found to be incorrect, necessitates the removal of the upper posterior teeth and the recording of the correct position on the wax blocks replacing them. The lower cast is then removed from the articulator and reset according to the new position, thus keeping the upper cast in the same position as it was mounted by means of the facebow. When the retruded contact position is found to be correct, the testing of the waxed dentures continues in the following way.

Make sure the teeth have been correctly balanced on the articulator in lateral and protrusive positions. In the mouth check for evenness of occlusal pressure in the retruded contact position with mylar tape and then test for occlusal balance with gentle lateral and protrusive movements. With the teeth in a working position of occlusion, insert a thin blade between the teeth on the balancing side and attempt to separate them; if they do separate, it shows that the occlusion of the teeth on that side is apparent and not real and is resulting from the displacement of the denture bases from the alveolar ridges. This error may be due either to an incorrect facebow transfer or to an incorrect condylar path registration. When the error is considerable, these registrations should be taken again, the casts remounted on the articulator and the teeth reset; but if the error is only slight, it may be corrected by perfecting the occlusal surfaces of the teeth when the dentures are finished. Minor errors of cuspal interference are best left until the dentures have been finished and fitted.

Appearance

This aspect of the trial stage is a matter more for individual judgement, and sometimes the patient's ideas, than for set rules. However, certain factors need to be checked as routine.

Centre line.

Stand in front of the patient, some distance away; a wrong centre line will be obvious, but if in doubt any of the aids described in Chapter 6 may be applied. Minor errors may be corrected by adjusting the maxillary anterior teeth at the chairside but if the error is more than 1 mm the whole case may have to be reset.

Anterior plane.

This may be observed from the same position and any tendency for this plane to slope markedly up or down should be noted and corrected (Figure 11.8).

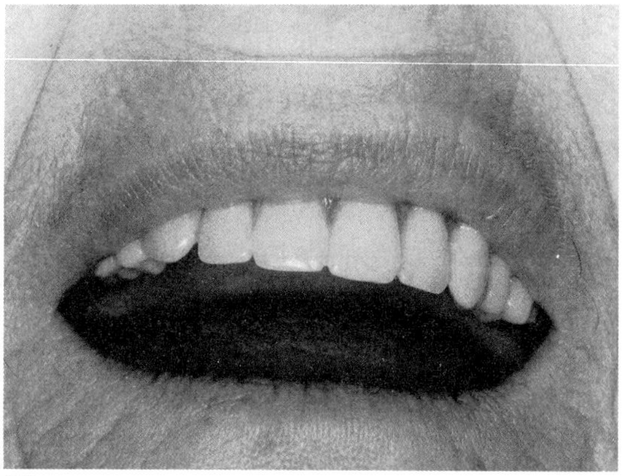

(*b*)

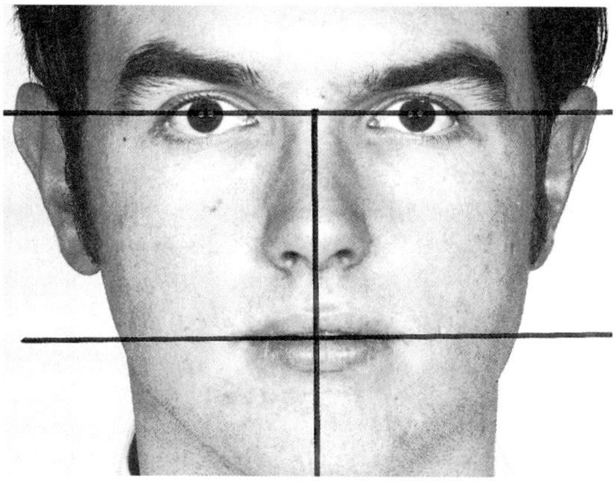

(*a*)

Figure 11.8 (*a*) The plane of the anterior teeth is sloped and it should also be noted the width of the teeth is too small. (*b*) On the face of another person the interpupillary line is not at right angles to the median sagittal plane and is an unreliable data line to orientate the occlusal plane

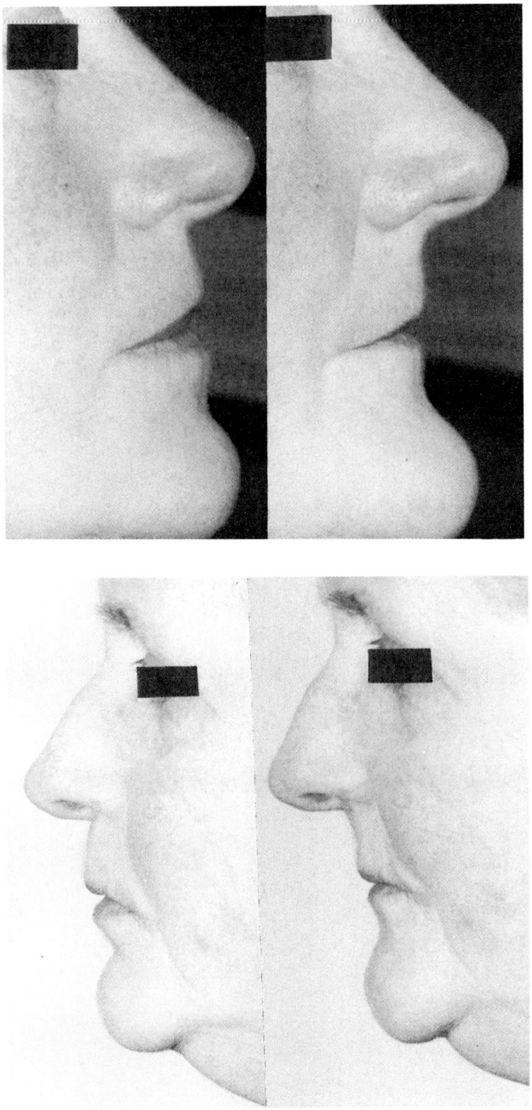

Figure 11.9 Restored and unrestored profiles of edentulous patients. Note the change in the line angle between the lateral aspect of the lip and the side of the face. Some patients comment that their nose is becoming bigger and these photographs show why

It is important to ask the patient to smile and if one side of the face rises more than the other it is good practice to set the anterior plane to run slightly up towards the elevated side. This has the effect of making the smile less crooked and harmonizes the lip–tooth relationship. Thought should also be given to the smile curve, i.e. the incisal edges of the maxillary incisors lying parallel to the smiling lower lip, as in most faces this produces a pleasing appearance.

Shape of the teeth.

Ensure that the selected teeth conform with the patient's facial type (see Chapter 7), but remember that the shape is influenced by the wax around them and this will require checking and altering before consulting the patient's views.

Size of the teeth.

Individual judgement must be relied on here together with the patient's opinion. Slight irregularities in tooth setting, such as a mesially rotated lateral, will affect the apparent size of a tooth as will another tooth adjacent to it, e.g. a maxillary canine will look larger against a small first premolar. Such effects are often very subtle and may lead to disappointment unless these fundamental aspects of aesthetics are understood.

Shade and blend of the teeth.

The shade is affected by the colour and density of the surrounding wax which is an entirely different environment than the acrylic in the finished denture.

Profile and lip form

Observe the patient's profile and note if the lips are either excessively distended or unduly sunken (Figure 11.9). In the first case, remove some wax from the labial flange and try the dentures again. If

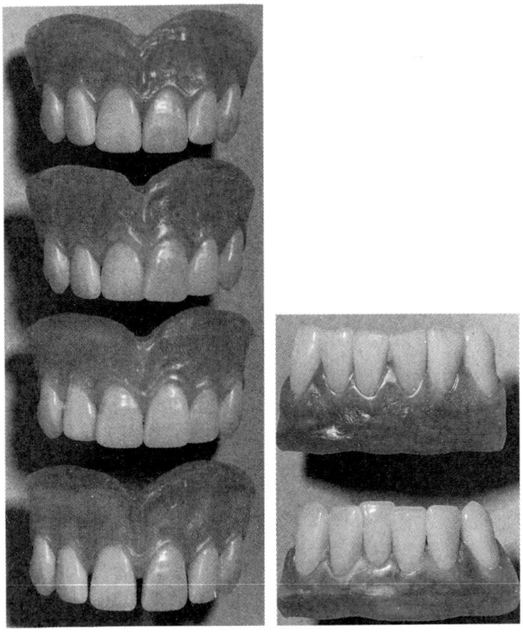

Figure 11.10 Some common types of irregularity used in anterior tooth arrangements

this produces insufficient improvement, examine the denture to see if the teeth should be set farther in, or if smaller teeth can be used. If the lips are sunken and inverted consider the need to set the anterior teeth further forward.

Amount of tooth visible.

Ask the patient to say the days of the week 'Sunday, Monday .... ', and note how much tooth shows. In this connection remember that a smiling person usually only shows the upper teeth; if much of the lower incisors are visible, or only these teeth show, examine the amount of overlap and, if excessive, reduce it by altering the lower teeth. If this does not effect an improvement, the position of the occlusal plane may require to be altered.

Regularity of the teeth.

Few natural dentitions exhibit perfection, and to set teeth absolutely regularly in the incisor region, especially in persons of middle or advanced age, tends to emphasize that the teeth are artificial. Therefore a little irregularity is usually desirable. Some common types of irregular tooth arrangements are illustrated in Figure 11.10. If the patient already has dentures and likes the appearance it is best to copy the tooth setting since it is always inadvisable to alter a patient's appearance radically, without his or her consent.

Approval of appearance by the patient

It is always wise for the dentist to obtain the patient's approval of the appearance of the trial dentures before they are returned to the laboratory for finishing, as this allows for any necessary adjustments. Some patients are quite prepared to leave the question of appearance to the dentist, while others are extremely fussy over the smallest detail. When dealing with the former, the dentist should still insist that they consider the matter of their appearance, otherwise when the dentures are finished the patient may react unfavourably. In the case of the fussy patient, much time and trouble must be spent on getting the shade, shape and setting of the teeth just as the patient wishes, but it is very important to obtain final approval before finishing the dentures. In this connection the dentist often needs to use his restraining influence to avoid extremely bad errors of aesthetics and much waste of time.

It should be remembered that other people will see more of a patient's dentures than the patient will, and if the dentures are not aesthetically pleasing in the opinion of his relations and friends he will usually become dissatisfied. It is, therefore, advisable to ask the patient to bring a relation or candid friend with him at the trial denture stage and the approval or criticism of this second individual should be sought as well as that of the patient himself.

Chapter 12

Delivering finished dentures

Examination of the dentures

Before fitting the dentures they should be inspected to ensure that they have been correctly finished by the technician, the following points being most important.

1. The fitting or contact surface must show no irregularities that are not present in the mouth. The commonest defects arise from cuts and scratches on the cast, or air bubbles present just below the cast surface which break under the pressures of flasking and packing acrylic. These faults result in excrescences or blebs on the fitting surface which should have been removed by the technician, although they should not occur at all.
2. The entire periphery should be only lightly polished otherwise there is a danger of destroying the peripheral seal. The posterior edge of the upper denture should be thinned down almost to a knife-edge.
3. The edges of any relief area should be rounded and not left square and sharp.

Place the dentures, which have previously been stored in cold water, in the mouth and examine them as at the trial stage. Test the retention of the upper by attempting to withdraw the denture at right angles to the occlusal plane and then, by placing a finger behind the incisor teeth, push in an outward and upward direction. If the postdam of the denture has been correctly placed, considerable force should be needed to break the peripheral seal. Note that the retention will increase after the patient has worn the dentures for a few days, due to the adaptation of the soft tissues to the denture.

Checking the occlusion

If the laboratory work has been done carefully, the occlusion should be almost perfect. Slight unevenness often occurs, however, due to processing errors, and so the occlusion should be checked with articulating paper or marking tape; these are impregnated with different colours of dye. There is a wide range of papers and tapes produced in various dimensions, but the thinner ones (approx 0.05 mm) give the most reliable results as they interfere least with the occlusion. Place a piece between the teeth and induce the patient to close in retruded contact position. Remove the dentures from the mouth and examine them. The occlusal surfaces will exhibit areas of coloration where the cusps and fossae of the opposing teeth have been in contact. These marks should be evenly spread over the occlusal surface, but particularly the holding or supporting cusps i.e. upper palatal, lower buccal. Areas of hard or uneven pressure will show up as darker and broader spots; areas of low pressure, or no contact, as very lightly coloured spots, or not coloured at all. To equalize the contact the fossae opposite the holding cusps are lightly ground with a carborundum stone. The denture is then wiped to remove the dye and a further test with marking paper made, and so on until there is simultaneous and even contact all round the dental arch in retruded contact position. This may be further tested with strips of mylar tape between each occluding tooth.

The use of occlusal wax

Articulating paper has a number of disadvantages:

1. It will colour a tooth even if it only rubs against it and thus areas which are not in occlusion are frequently marked.

2. The paper is stretched across the cusps so that the hollows or fossae between the cusps fail to be marked.
3. It is difficult to place paper or tape between the occlusal surfaces on both sides while at the same time ensuring that the dentures do not shift and thus give erroneous marks.

A more satisfactory way of adjusting the occlusion is by using wax. Two strips of casting or occlusal indicator wax 6 mm wide are laid one on either side of the upper denture on the occlusal surfaces of the posterior teeth. The dentures are then inserted in the mouth and the patient induced into retruded contact position. The dentures are removed from the mouth, and the wax peeled off. If these are then viewed by transmitted light, those areas where the occlusion is heavy will be seen as thinned, completely transparent wax or even as holes right through the wax. Replacement of the wax on the denture enables the exact areas of the teeth to be marked through the wax with a graphite pencil and then modified by grinding.

Another advantage of wax is that, by fitting the upper and lower dentures into their correct positions in one wax wafer, the actual position of occlusion on the opposite side of the dentures as it exists in the mouth may be observed, and gross errors readily seen.

It requires to be emphasized that the even adjustment of the occlusion is most important to the success of dentures, as faults in the occlusion are a very common cause of problems. This should not be overlooked if a patient returns complaining of pain or looseness because frequently the periphery of a denture is blamed for what is in reality a fault of occlusion. Uneven occlusion will also increase the patient's difficulties when attempting to eat because the new dentures will feel uneven and uncomfortable when in contact.

Remounting

To achieve perfection of occlusion a check record should be taken, the dentures remounted on the articulator and the occlusion refined as described in Chapter 13. It is then that attention will be paid to eccentric positions of occlusion and refinement completed in working, balancing and protrusive contacts. This procedure of remounting, however, is best delayed until the next visit of the patient as this gives a few days for the dentures to settle and the mucosa time to adapt to the denture fitting surfaces.

Dentures finished with an occlusal error

If the occlusion is discovered to be incorrect at the finished stage, as will occasionally occur in spite of the greatest care being taken at the trial stage, it may be due to a slightly more retruded position of the mandible, i.e. the dentures have been made to a position slightly forward of the retruded contact position (RCP). If this is not more than 1 mm it may be corrected by means of a check record (see Chapter 13). When the error is greater it will require the removal of all the posterior teeth from the lower denture.

Gently flame the posterior teeth of the lower denture, playing the flame actually on to the porcelain and not the acrylic base; conduction of the heat through the porcelain softens the acrylic without burning it, and the teeth may be prised off the denture with a wax-knife. Acrylic teeth, of course, may be ground away with a carborundum stone. Wax blocks are then built to replace the teeth, trimmed to the correct height by trial, and the RCP retaken. The dentures are then remounted on the articulator and new lower teeth set. If the overjet resulting from the new record is abnormal, the lower anterior teeth must also be removed from the denture and reset.

When the error is severe the denture needs to be comletely remade although in some cases a master impression may be taken in the denture with zinc oxide–eugenol (ZOE), thus avoiding the need for conventional impressions.

Improving the appearance

When the upper and lower incisors erupt, the incisal edges present three small tubercles. As the teeth come into use for incising, these tubercles are gradually worn away by the grinding of the lower teeth against the upper. This attrition results in the formation of even incisal edges which as age advances become irregular, due to uneven wear, sometimes assuming a chisel-like form when viewed from the side.

Many acrylic and porcelain teeth present a regular, even edge and if no attempt is made to simulate the wear of natural teeth they appear obviously false. A little grinding of the incisal edges of the teeth with a carborundum stone makes a remarkable difference and enhances the natural appearance of the dentures (Figure 12.1). The older the patient the greater will be the effects of attrition and the observation of people who possess their own teeth will disclose much about the wear of the incisal edge.

Examination of the labial surface of a natural incisor will disclose that two vertical grooves separate three ridges; canines usually have one ridge separating two depressions. The rest of the surface, although smooth, is not regularly contoured and is built up from a large number of facets.

All these irregularities result in the incident rays of light which strike the tooth surface being

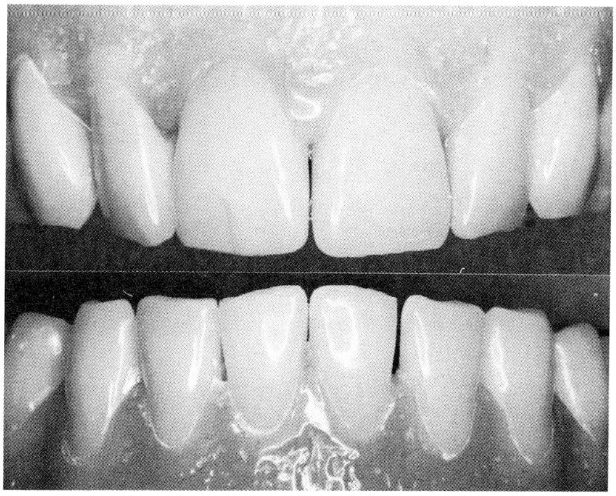

Figure 12.1 Appearance of incisors of these complete dentures is improved by simulating the normal wear of teeth

scattered as they are reflected, and only one or two of the more prominent ridges reflect light evenly as high spots. If artificial teeth are to appear natural, therefore, they must scatter the incident rays, and the breaking up of the surface of the tooth by judicious grinding, followed by gentle polishing, can considerably enhance the appearance.

Instructions to the patient

Many patients will have had experience with complete dentures and may thus not require an explanation of the points about to be considered, but those patients having dentures fitted for the first time will need, and benefit by, information concerning the following.

Wearing dentures at night

Dentures occupy space in the mouth and at the beginning the patient will be extremely conscious of their presence. In order to reduce this period of discomfort to a minimum, the dentures should be worn at night, thus allowing the tongue, cheeks and lips to become accustomed to the bulk during the hours of sleep. Once the patient has become used to the dentures it is no longer necessary for them to be worn at night, but the final decision should be left to the individual who may have personal reasons for wishing to continue the practice. From the point of view of the health of the tissues, it is preferable to remove the dentures at night, although in some cases there appears to be no clinical difference between the mouths of patients who wear their dentures continuously and those who remove them at night.

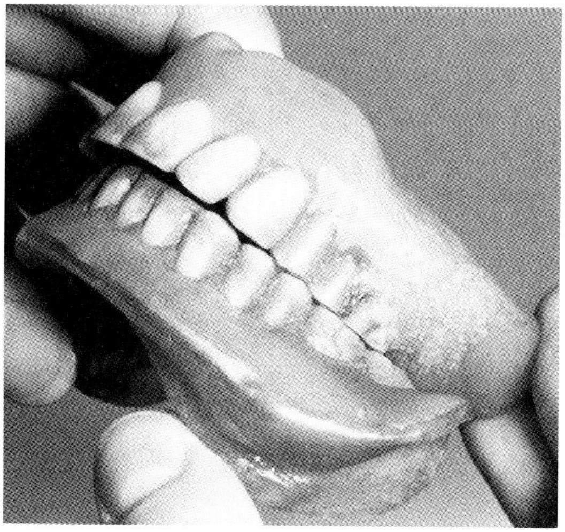

Figure 12.2 Complete dentures coated with plaque and calculus caused by patient neglect

Cleaning

Whenever possible dentures should be removed after every meal and food debris washed away, particular attention being given to the deep parts of the fitting surface so that no food remnants remain to stagnate and irritate the tissues (Figure 12.2). At least once a day the dentures should be thoroughly cleaned with a brush and liquid detergent, or any recognized brand of denture cleaner. If not worn at night, they should be placed in water. In the case of acrylic bases and teeth, strong solutions containing sodium hypochlorite must be avoided as they are liable to bleach the surface of a denture. The patient should be warned against using harsh abrasive materials and hard bristle brushes, since both will wear away the surface detail of the teeth and denture base. It is important to mention that very hot water may cause warpage.

As a precaution against chipping teeth, or fracturing a denture, the hand basin should be half-filled with water during the cleaning operation to act as a cushion if the denture slips from the fingers.

Eating

All complete denture patients have to pass through a period of learning before they can eat with comfort since mandibular movements are generally much more restricted, and the tongue has to control the lower denture as well as the food. The following suggestions to patients are useful during the period of learning to eat:

1. The food should be cut into small pieces and only a little placed in the mouth at a time.

2. Commence by chewing in the premolar region on one or both sides.
3. Soft and non-sticky foods are easier to eat than the more fibrous types.
4. Chewing with the posterior teeth should be mastered before any attempt is made to bite with the incisors.

Talking

People who have been edentulous for a considerable period will have adapted themselves to the prevailing conditions, and will have corrected some of the speech defects arising from the loss of the teeth. With the insertion of dentures, the conditions are suddenly changed. The tongue is affected by the reduction of space, and may be cramped temporarily by the bulk of the lingual flange of the lower denture. This may lead to difficulty in forming some of the speech sounds until the tongue has had sufficient time to adapt. Patients who are likely to experience speech difficulties should be advised to read aloud, and practise any word which causes trouble. A few hours spent in this manner will enable most patients to speak naturally and with complete ease. Occasional sips of water during this speaking programme are often helpful.

Easing the dentures

With the delivery of correctly constructed dentures, and instructions to the patient, the dentist's part in the rehabilitation is almost complete. Except for refinements of the occlusion, it is now the patient's perseverance and ability to learn to use the dentures that decide the final success of the case. The patient should be asked to attend for examination two or three days after the insertion of the dentures so that the dentist may carry out any necessary adjustments. Soreness may occur in that time due to the fact that the peripheries of the impressions rarely reproduce all the functional movements, and when the dentures are first worn there is probably slight over-extension somewhere. The flange of the denture may be too deep and press into the tissues of the sulcus, forming first an inflammation which later breaks down into an ulcer, the depth and extent of which depends on the degree of damage by the denture. In the first day or two the dentures settle on the compressible mucosa with possible slight changes in the evenness of occlusion. The over-extended flange must be trimmed and the occlusion modified with carborundum stones. A further visit may be necessary for final corrections as it is never wise to remove too much of the periphery at one time, since over-easing may lead to loss of peripheral seal. Other causes of soreness, and complaints made by patients, are discussed in Chapter 13.

If, after being worn for a short time, the dentures hurt, they should not be removed by the patient immediately unless the pain is severe, since perseverance will often overcome slight soreness. If the dentures have to be left out because of pain, they should nevertheless be worn for a few hours immediately before visiting the dentist because, unless this is done, there probably will be no sign in the mouth to indicate where the denture is over-extended.

Pressure-indicating paste

It is essential to locate exactly which part of the denture base is over-extended or causing excess pressure. Sometimes this is obvious but frequently the area cannot be seen. In these instances a mark is made on the mucosa which will transfer itself to the

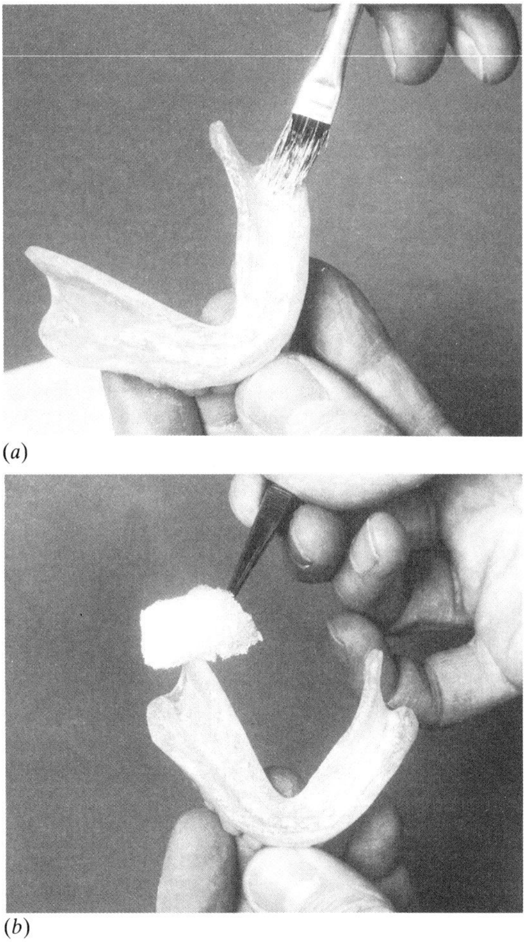

(*a*)

(*b*)

Figure 12.3 Pressure-indicating paste is applied to the denture with (*a*) a stiff brush or (*b*) a piece of polyurethane sponge

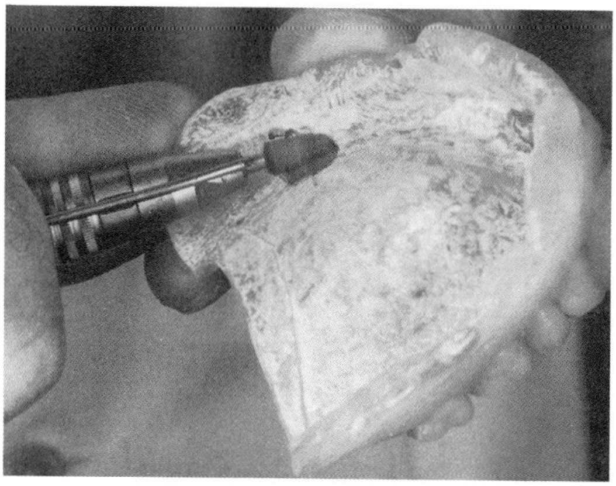

Figure 12.4 An area of wipe-off is eased with a carborundum stone or metal bur

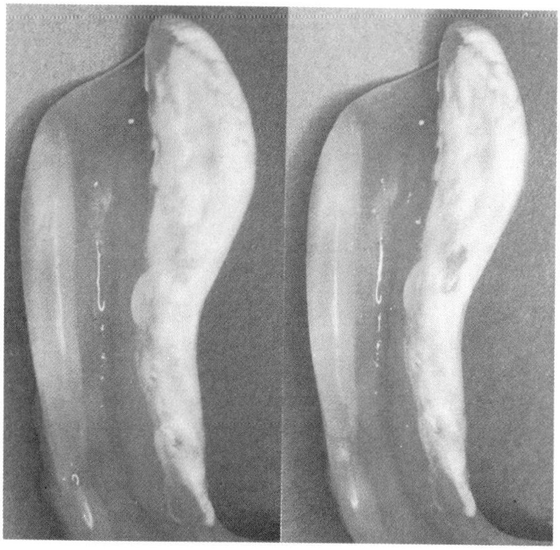

Figure 12.5 Indicator wax may be used instead of paste to locate areas of pressure seen here on the anterior part of the left mylohyoid ridge

denture. The tissues are dried and a mark made with a wet indelible pencil. The denture is inserted and pressed into place. When it is removed the gentian violet will have transferred itself to the denture base.

A better method, and one which can be employed when fitting the denture, is to coat the whole or part of the periphery and fitting surface with a pressure-indicating paste. This is applied to the dried denture either with a stiff brush or dabbed on with a piece of polyurethane sponge (Figure 12.3). The denture is then inserted and pressed firmly into position taking care not to rub off any paste on the lips or tongue. Do not allow the patient to occlude unless the occlusion is perfect.

The denture is removed and if over-extension or pressure exists it will be readily visible as an area of acrylic uncovered by the paste (Figure 12.4 and 12.5). This area of the denture is trimmed with a stone or bur, the debris removed, paste again applied and the denture reinserted. This procedure is continued until there is no obvious 'wipe-off' area and thus no pressure. Polish any trimmed areas and return the denture to the patient.

In cases of gross over-extension resulting in severe ulceration, the patient should be instructed to leave the denture out for 24 h in order to allow the swelling to subside, otherwise the denture will require to be over-trimmed and this will reduce its accuracy.

When adjusting the periphery or fitting surface it should always be remembered that soreness and ulceration are frequently caused by faults in the occlusion, or cuspal interference, that apply excessive pressure to small areas of mucosa under the denture bases. It is therefore sound practice always to check the occlusion before easing a denture.

Chapter 13

Check records for complete dentures

Reasons for errors

The efficiency and comfort that a patient experiences when using complete dentures depends to a large extent on the harmony of the occlusion.

A suitable impression technique, carefully carried out, will result in dentures that are stable provided there is no over-extension and the polished surfaces are correctly shaped. With care the correct retruded jaw position may be obtained and, if an adjustable articulator is used with a facebow and occlusal records, a satisfactory balanced articulation will be produced. These procedures should result in comfortable and efficient dentures with accurate occlusion and articulation. Unfortunately, however, occlusal faults occur during the construction that are undetectable when the dentures are examined in the mouth; these faults may be clearly seen when the dentures are mounted on an articulator after check records have been taken. Such dentures may cause pain and discomfort to the patient and result in reduced efficiency and damage to the supporting tissues unless the faults of occlusion are rectified. The errors which occur are due to one or a combination of the following:

Incorrect registration of retruded contact position (RCP)

This is probably the most common cause of error in the occlusion of finished dentures. During registration considerable care is taken to obtain a correct vertical dimension and the physiological fully retruded position of the mandible, but often, when brought together, the record blocks exert uneven pressure on their respective supporting alveolar ridges, and this condition passes unnoticed. The uneven pressure may be due to premature contact of the blocks on one side of the mouth, in the second molar region of both sides, or in the incisor region. This causes uneven compression of the mucosa and often displaces the blocks from the ridges in areas away from the region of premature contact. When the casts are placed in the record blocks obviously no such compression or displacement occurs and therefore the occlusion as registered on the articulator differs from that registered in the mouth. Thus an error in occlusion has been established which possibly may be passed over at the trial stage due to the poor fit of the trial denture bases allowing movement to take place. On finishing the denture the teeth are found to occlude only in the area where the premature contact of the occlusal rims occurred, the remainder of the teeth being slightly out of contact. The degree of separation will be related to the degree of premature contact occurring between the rims. This will vary from the almost indiscernible to a larger fault where a knife blade may be inserted between the non-occluding teeth.

Another fault causing errors in the occlusion of the finished dentures results from slight movement of record blocks on the ridges during registration due to their imperfect fit and inadequate retention. The retruded contact position of the finished dentures will be slightly inaccurate for this reason and the dentures will tend to move on the ridges as the cuspal inclines of the teeth guide the dentures into their slightly inaccurate position of occlusion when the mandible assumes its correct retruded relationship with the maxilla. This continual denture movement during tooth contact causes soreness of the ridge, particularly the lower since this denture is not only the more unstable of the two but also covers about half the mucosal territory of the upper.

Finally, an error of occlusion may result from the manner in which the casts and record blocks are mounted on the articulator. The casts may not be seated accurately in the blocks, or the articulator may not be handled with due care when the casts are being attached with plaster.

All these errors can usually be lessened by using an accurately fitting acrylic base in preference to a shellac base which invariably warps slightly. The errors cause discrepancies in the occlusion of the teeth and will probably pass unnoticed at the trial stage, and often at the finished denture stage, and are observed only when carrying out an RCP check record.

Irregularities in setting the teeth.

When setting up teeth the technician is unlikely to produce a perfectly even contact in retruded, protruded and lateral occlusions. Some teeth will be in good occlusion while others will be slightly out of occlusion, thus producing areas of heavy pressure. When setting and testing the occlusion for eccentric contacts the teeth, held in wax which exhibits a certain amount of resiliency, permit tooth movement to occur when heavy occlusal contacts are encountered. This cannot happen when the teeth are held firmly in the final denture base material and results in premature tooth contacts in the occlusion and articulation of the finished dentures.

During the setting of teeth it is possible for them to move slightly due to the contraction of wax on cooling, thus causing irregularities in the occlusion of the finished dentures.

These possibilities point to the need for a final adjustment of occlusion once the dentures are finished.

Tooth movement when flasking and packing.

Movement of the teeth may occur at the time of boiling out the wax trial base after the dentures have been flasked and if such teeth are not correctly repositioned they will cause occlusal irregularities. When packing acrylic dough, teeth may be driven into the investing plaster, particularly when packing follows soon after flasking and the plaster has a low crushing strength. The possibility of such an error occurring is increased when the polymethyl methacrylate is used in a slightly advanced stage of dough, and when the posterior teeth have been ground to fit close to the ridge. Rapid closure of the flask in the bench press will add to the hazard. Injection moulding techniques for packing acrylic are an obvious improvement.

Incomplete flask closure

Such an occurrence not only causes an increase of vertical dimension because of the alteration in tooth/cast relationship but also results in derangement of the occlusion which usually necessitates the total remake of the denture.

Remounting dentures with check records

It can be appreciated that even with care on the part of the dentist and technician errors may occur which influence the final occlusion and articulation of finished dentures (Figure 13.1). In some instances, these errors may be corrected by careful use of

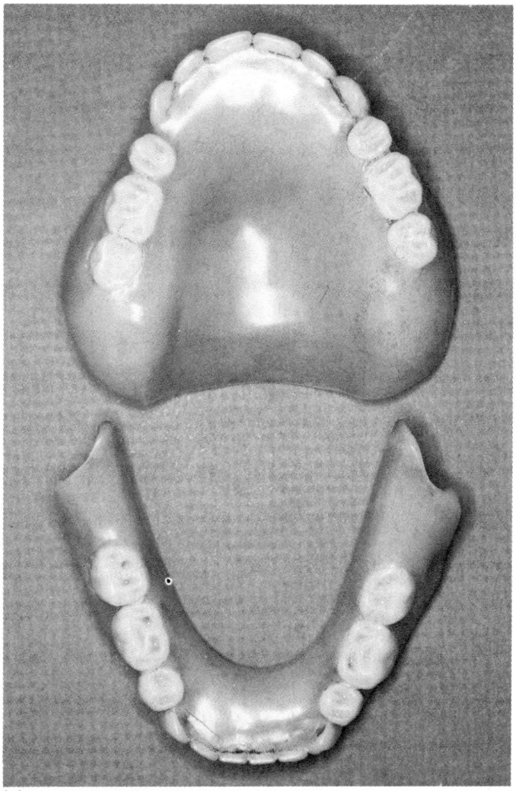

(*a*)

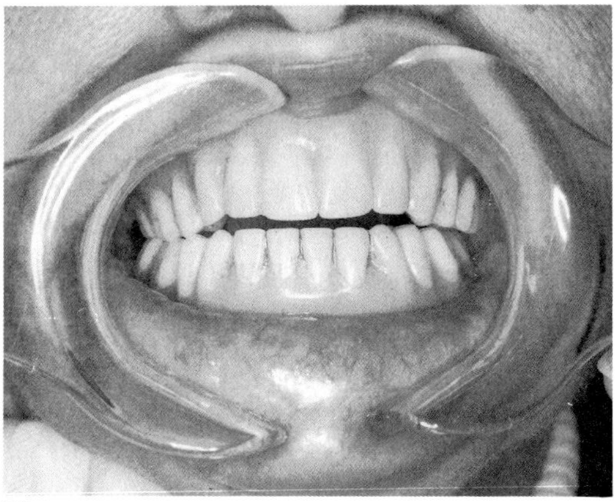

(*b*)

Figure 13.1 (*a*)The finished dentures. (*b*) In the mouth, as the patient closes into the retruded contact position (RCP) the occlusal error is seen marking paper or tape at the chairside, but such correction is often proved false when check records are taken for confirmation. It is far more satisfactory, and often less time-consuming clinically, to register the retruded contact position of the finished dentures with a check record, mount the finished dentures on an adjustable articulator and then refine the occlusion either at the chairside or in the laboratory.

Method of remounting dentures

Facebow mounting

If the dentures were made on an adjustable articulator it is likely that the original maxillary cast, or holding cast, is still located to the upper member of the articulator in its correct relationship to the mandibular hinge-axis as determined by a facebow.

If this cast has been destroyed, or if the dentures were made on an articulator without the aid of a facebow, then the first stage in remounting dentures to refine the occlusion is to locate the maxillary denture in an accurate position on an adjustable articulator with a facebow transfer. The details of this technique have already been covered in Chapter 9 and only an outline will be given here.

Wrap soft impression compound on the warmed prongs of a facebow fork. Lay the upper denture into it so that the midline of the fork coincides with the mesio-incisal point of the denture and the stem, lying parallel to the occlusal plane, projects on the right side of the denture (Figure 13.2). Chill the compound. Insert the denture. An assistant holds the denture and fork while the facebow is located in position over the hinge-axis and correctly centred so that the readings are the same on both sides (Figure 13.3). Tighten the thumb screw and locate the orbital plane indicator rod. Remove the whole facebow and assemble on the articulator.

Lay the upper denture in the facebow fork, block out any undercuts in the fitting surface with tissue paper and mount the denture to the upper member of the articulator with quick-setting plaster (Figure 13.4). This is a clinical procedure and should be

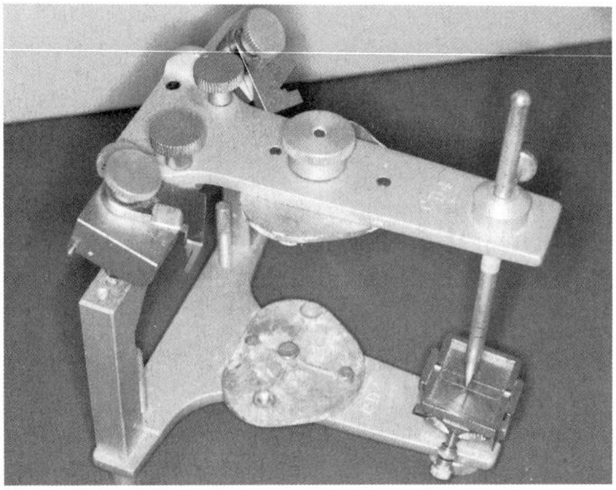

(*a*)

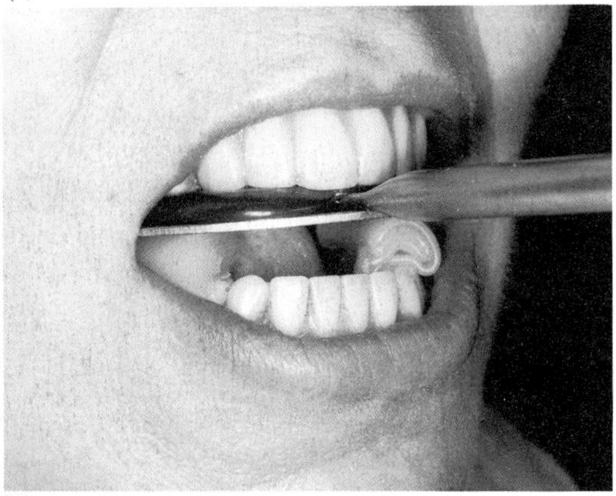

(*b*)

Figure 13.2 (*a*) A Whipmix (semi-adjustable) articulator is being used to remount the dentures. (*b*) Facebow fork located on the upper denture (the lower denture is in the mouth only to hold the fork in position: note roll of wax to act as a prop)

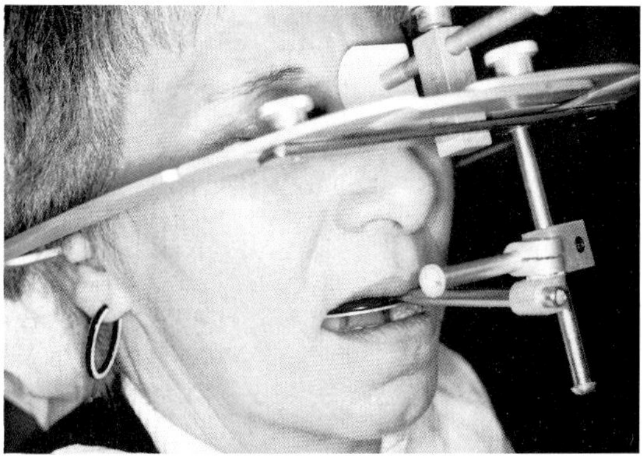

Figure 13.3 The facebow located on the head and fixed to stem of facebow fork

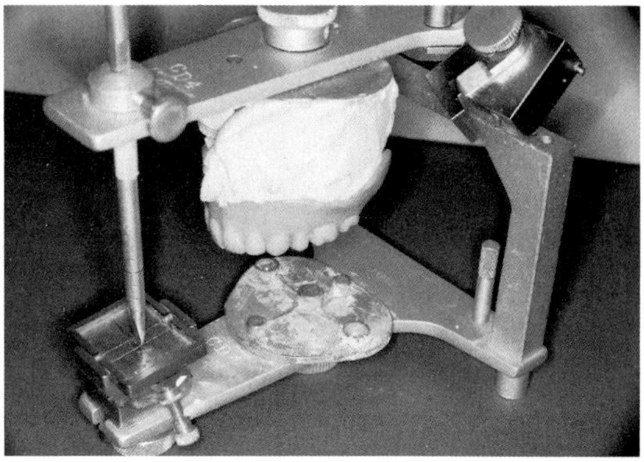

Figure 13.4 Maxillary denture fixed to upper member of the articulator

carried out at the chairside. When the plaster has set, dismantle the facebow and remove the upper denture. The next stage is to locate the lower denture to the upper by means of a check record. Note that some clinicians dispense with the orbital pointer and mount the upper denture so that its occlusal surface orientates at 10° to the horizontal, i.e. the bench surface. This figure of 10° is the average angle of the occlusal surface of natural teeth to the Frankfort plane.

Check record

A D-shaped piece of base-plate wax is cut to cover the maxillary teeth without projecting beyond the buccal cusps. Two small tags are left to cover the labial surface of each canine. Soften the wax that covers the teeth as uniformly as possible and seat both dentures. Induce the patient into the retruded position but stop the closure just prior to tooth contact and thus avoid any mandibular or denture deviation that might be caused by faulty tooth contact. The separation between the teeth should be about 0.5 mm, but at no point should the wax be penetrated. This is often called a 'pre-centric' check record (Figure 13.5). It is very important that the lower denture is held firmly against the lower ridge as any last-moment shift which might not be noticed will invalidate the accuracy. This apparently simple procedure is one of the most difficult in prosthetic dentistry.

The thin wax record chills against the opposing teeth fairly quickly so that the patient can open in a few seconds. Place a dab of registration paste on the surface of the wax record in the molar and premolar regions and close again into the retruded position. A quick-setting paste should be used otherwise the patient's mandible may elevate on one side or deviate during a long setting period and introduce errors. The paste not only makes the record more accurate but also makes it more rigid.

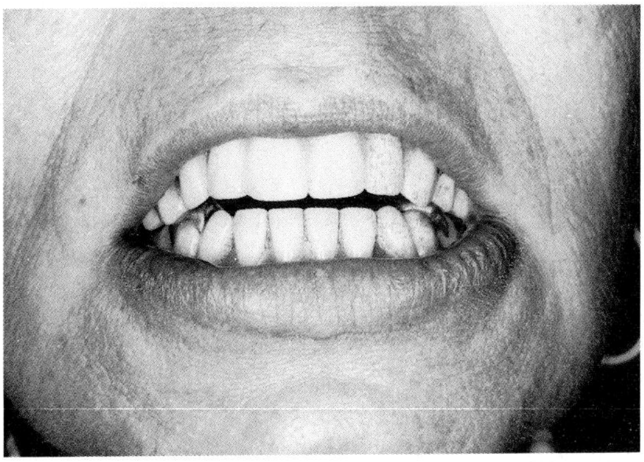

Figure 13.5 RCP check record with teeth slightly out of contact (the 'pre-centric' record)

Both dentures are removed and laid in cold water to chill the wax record before mounting on the articulator.

Mounting the lower denture (Figure 13.6)

Without separating the dentures, locate the upper on its cast and locate the previously prepared lower holding cast in the lower denture. Do not press the dentures together with excessive force as this may distort the wax record. Mount the lower cast to the lower member of the articulator with quick-setting plaster.

Second check record

There may be errors in the wax check record that cannot be recognized by the clinician. This is important when one remembers that the reason for remounting dentures is to correct errors in the occlusion. If one then remounts in a faulty position the errors are compounded and the situation can only worsen.

Remove the wax record. Allow the articulator to close on the incisal post when a small space will be seen between the occlusal surfaces of the dentures.

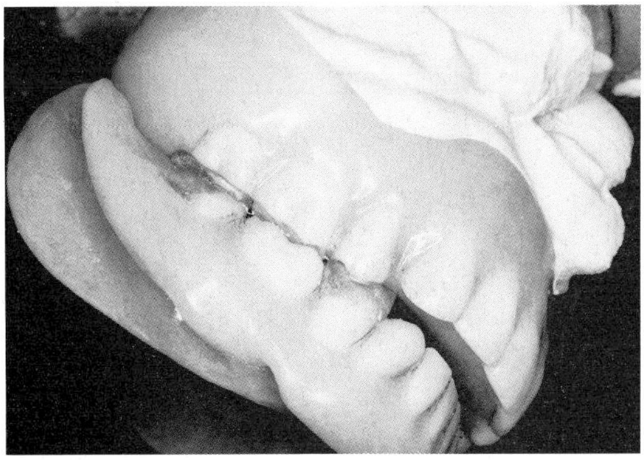

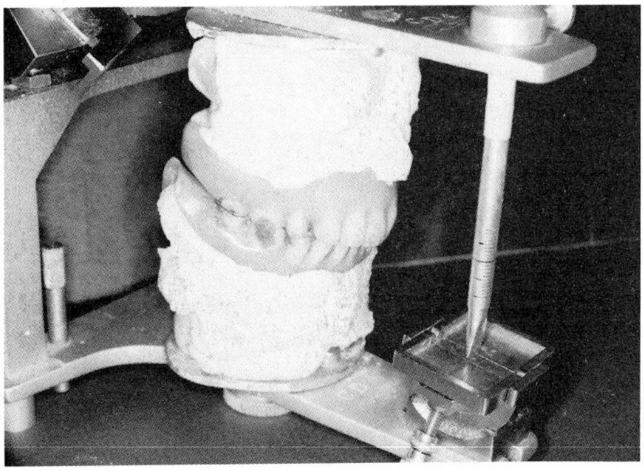

Figure 13.6 The mandibular denture located into the RCP check record and fixed to the lower member of the articulator

Make another wax check record similar to the first and record the retruded jaw position on the patient. The vertical distance between the occlusal surfaces of the dentures will probably be different but this is irrelevant as long as the patient is in the retruded position i.e. the terminal hinge-axis. Chill the wax record and separate the dentures.

Verifying the two records

Free the movement of the condylar spheres in the condylar tracks of the articulator. Lay the second check record in position and bring the upper member of the articulator into the record and, as it does so, watch for any movement, forwards or backwards, of either of the spheres in its track. If both records are identical there will be no alteration in position of the spheres in the tracks thus indicating that the dentures are mounted correctly in the retruded position. If there is alteration of position of one or both spheres this indicates a movement of one or both condyle heads of the mandible of the patient during the check records and means that the mandible was not in the retruded position. The procedure is then to make another check record, dismount the lower denture and remount it to the lower member of the articulator. In other words, go through the same procedure until such time as two records are obtained that are coincident. There are occasions when this can be very tedious and time-consuming, but proceeding beyond this stage without knowing that the dentures are correctly mounted on the articulator in the retruded position is totally pointless. This cannot be emphasized too often.

Lateral or protrusive records (Figure 13.7)

A strip of softened wax of double thickness is placed on the occlusal surface of the upper denture, the denture placed in the mouth and the mandible moved to the right lateral position and closed almost to tooth contact. A second wax wafer records the left lateral position. If the patient experiences difficulty in making lateral movements then a protrusive record should be taken with the mandible protruded approximately 7 mm. These records are used to set the sagittal condylar paths of the articulator. The lateral guidance or Bennett angles on the condylar pillars are set by the formula

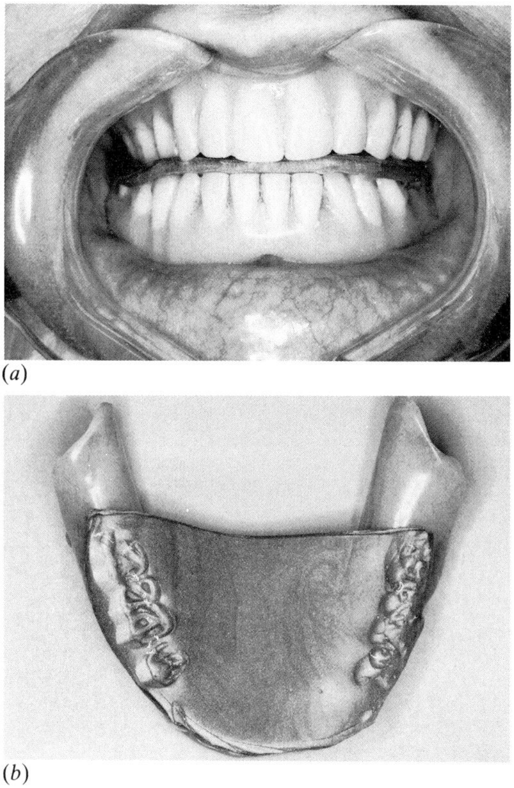

(*a*)

(*b*)

Figure 13.7 Right lateral check record being made in the mouth (*a*) and shown laid on the lower denture (*b*) for photographic purposes

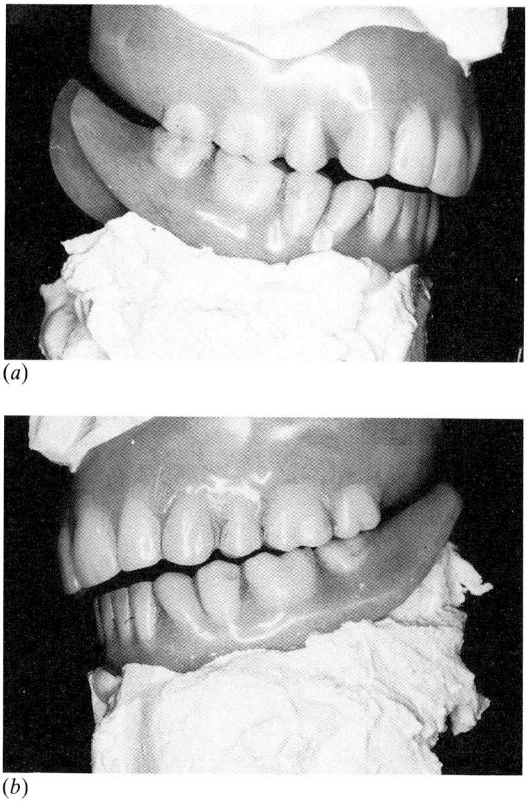

(*a*)

(*b*)

Figure 13.8 As the articulator is hinged together the occlusal errors in retruded contact position (RCP) are seen

L = (H/8) + 12, where H is the angle of the condylar path as related to the horizontal plane as viewed in the sagittal plane. Setting the lateral guidance angle allows the Bennett or side shift to take place during lateral movements of most adjustable articulators.

Correcting the occlusion

The incisal post is removed and the articulator hinged until the teeth contact. The occlusion is studied for points of premature contact or change in the maxillo-mandibular relationship (Figure 13.8). In order to produce a satisfactory result it is important to carry out the occlusal correction systematically to ensure that:

1. The vertical dimension is maintained.
2. An even distribution of contact is obtained in the retruded jaw position.
3. An even distribution of contact is maintained in lateral and protrusive positions.

The vertical dimension is controlled by the lower buccal cusps and the upper palatal cusps, which are the holding or supporting cusps, and their opposing fossae. It is essential therefore that these zones receive careful consideration when establishing retruded, lateral and protruded occlusions.

Adjusting RCP

Place thin marking paper on the occlusal surface of the lower teeth and tap the articulator with sufficient pressure to record the first contact areas (Figure 13.9). Observe the prominent cusp or cusps and decide whether the cusp or its opposing fossa and marginal ridges should be ground by checking this cusp in its working position and then its non-working position. If the cusp makes premature contact in both retruded and lateral positions then the cusp, and not the fossa, should be ground to produce even occlusion (Figure 13.10). However, when a cusp producing premature contact in the retruded position does not cause premature contact when in working and non-working positions, then the fossa and marginal ridges are ground to accommodate the cusp (Figure 13.11). This principle is followed until an even RCP is obtained on both sides (Figure 13.12).

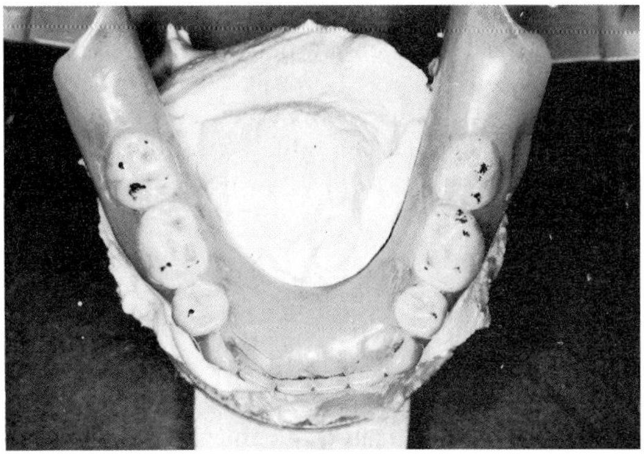

Figure 13.9 Contact areas on mandibular teeth shown after tapping into RCP on marking paper

In all modifications of teeth with carborundum stones or burs it is important to maintain the shapes of cusps and fossae. This means that grinding is done on the sides of cusps rather than the tips which has the effect of changing the angle but not the height. Large round stones or burs usually destroy tooth shape and should not be used. Small wheel or inverted-cone stones or, in the case of acrylic teeth, small round burs are effective in developing point contacts and tracks of cusps against grooves, fissures and fossae.

Adjusting lateral contacts

To enhance the retention and stability of the dentures and to reduce the stress applied to the alveolar ridges as the mandible moves laterally, it is most important to provide a free sliding lateral articulation all round the dental arch.

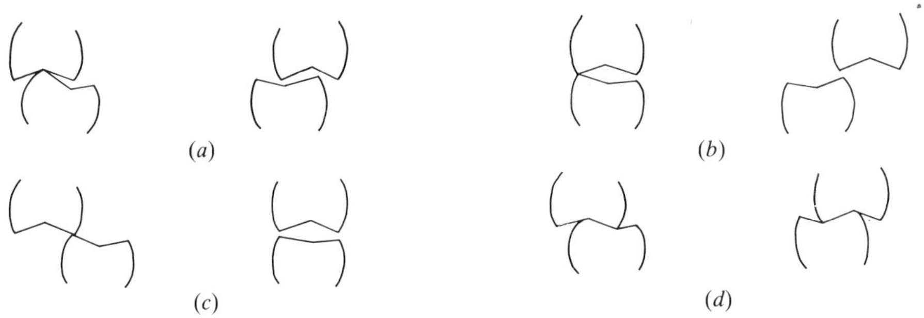

Figure 13.10 (*a*) The lower right buccal cusp occludes prematurely in RCP. (*b*) When tested as a working-side, contact it is found to be in premature occlusion, and also (*c*) when tested as a balancing-side contact. Therefore the lower buccal cusp is ground to produce even contact in RCP as in (*d*)

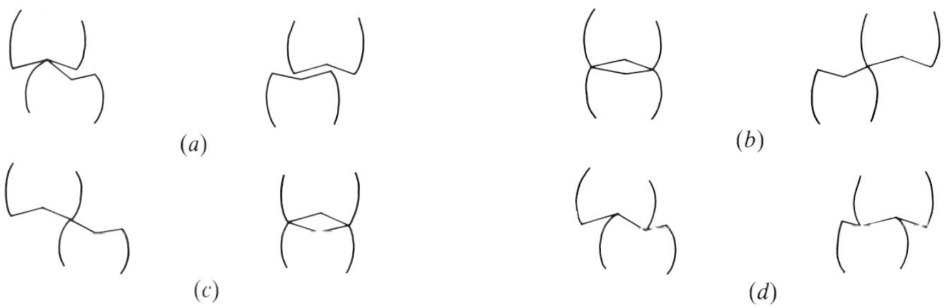

Figure 13.11 (*a*) The lower right buccal cusp occludes prematurely in RCP. (*b*) When tested as a working-side contact, occlusion of the teeth on the balancing side occurs. (*c*) If the lower right buccal cusp is checked in its balancing-side contact it would be observed that the working side (left) also shows tooth contact. Therefore the fossa of the upper right tooth should be deepend to produce even contact in RCP as in (*d*). (Note: The checking and grinding is carried out in stages and it may be necessary to grind fossa and cusp in order to produce the desired balance in retruded and eccentric occlusions)

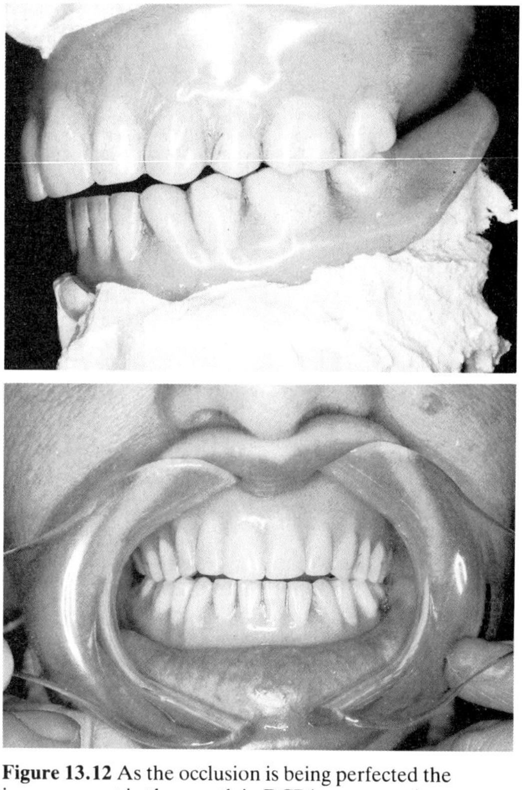

Figure 13.12 As the occlusion is being perfected the improvement in the mouth in RCP is apparent (compare with Figure 13.1). More correction is needed to improve the premolar occlusion

Red marking paper is placed between the occlusal surfaces of the teeth and the dentures moved with firm pressure from RCP into right lateral occlusion. If the upper and lower buccal cusps make premature contact and the non-working side is out of occlusion then the upper buccal cusp is ground (Figure 13.13) as the lower buccal cusp is required to maintain vertical dimension and even pressure in RCP (Figures 13.14 and 13.15).

When the lower lingual and upper palatal cusps occlude prematurely in this lateral position the lower lingual cusp is ground to produce contact of both sides of the denture (Figure 13.16). as the upper palatal cusp is required for the maintenance of vertical dimension in RCP. The grinding of the *b*uccal *u*pper and *l*ingual *l*ower cusps to produce balance in working movements is often referred to as grinding to the BULL rule. Remember the aim is not to reduce the cusp tip but to re-shape the slopes of the cusps, i.e. faults are corrected by grinding lingual-facing slopes of buccal upper cusps and buccal-facing slopes of lower lingual cusps.

Should the non-working or balancing side exhibit premature contact between the lower buccal cusp and the upper palatal cusp, it will be necessary to grind the buccal-facing slopes of the palatal upper cusps and the lingual-facing slopes of the lower buccal cusps. This might involve some shortening of these cusps and as these are responsible for maintaining the vertical dimension (i.e. the supporting cusps), it is necessary to check and adjust the occlusion in retruded contact position.

When the procedure has been completed for the right working position it is then repeated on the left, so that in both working excursions the contact is slightly firmer than on the balancing side. This is an arrangement more suitable in the mouth as the firmer contact takes into account the mucosal compression that occurs on the working side.

Adjusting protrusive contacts

As we are dealing with an artificial dentition, and are not concerned with the possible over-eruption of teeth as may occur with a natural dentition, most of the grinding for correction of premature contacts of incisal edges of anterior teeth, when in protrusive occlusion, can be carried out at the expense of the

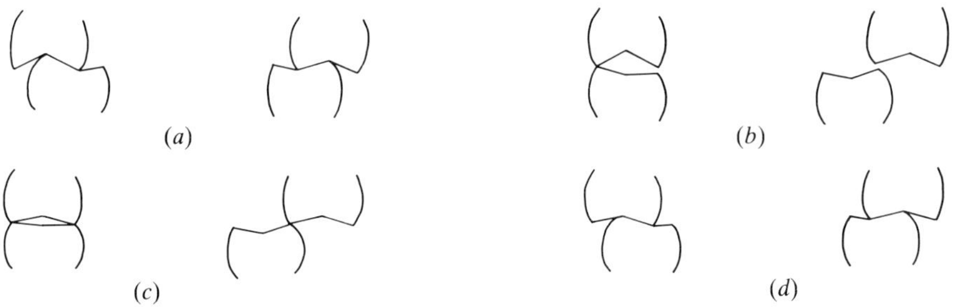

Figure 13.13 (*a*) RCP. (*b*) The upper right buccal cusp is seen to be in premature contact when the right side is acting as the working side. (*c*) The upper buccal cusp is reduced to bring the teeth on the balancing side into contact. This does not alter the evenness of RCP (as in (*a*) and (*d*)

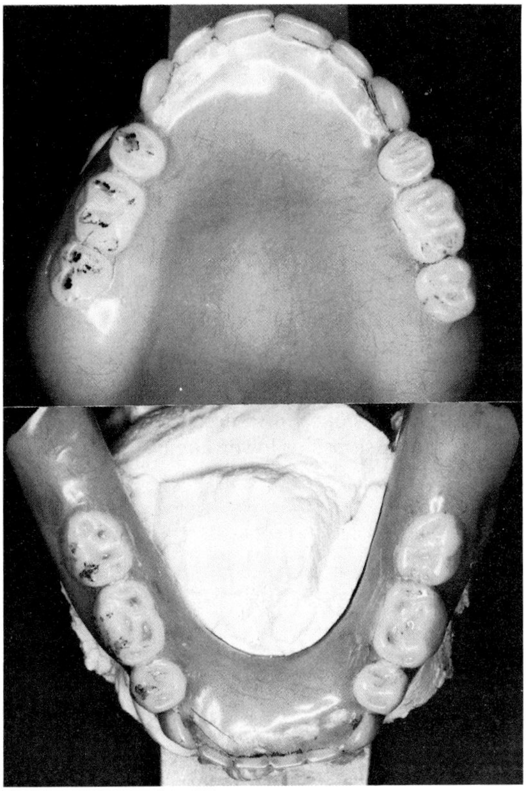

Figure 13.14 Right working movement. Marks on upper and lower teeth

lower incisors (Figure 13.17). A limited amount of grinding, however, of the upper anterior teeth to simulate attrition, related to the patient's age, can enhance the appearance of the dentures.

Place a piece of marking paper across the incisors and slide the dentures into edge-to-edge contact. Use a wheel carborundum to grind the lingual aspects of the upper incisors and the buccal aspects of the lower incisors (Figure 13.18). Removal of tooth substance, as indicated by the marking paper or tape, should not reduce the length of the teeth if grinding is carried out in this way. If the cusp angles of the posterior teeth are too small, of course, it may be found impossible to achieve protrusive balance without reducing the length of the incisors. This may not be acceptable from an aesthetic point of view and the only solution then is to remove the posterior teeth and reset teeth with the correct cusp angle.

If, on protrusion, there is lack of contact of the incisors, and the error is not too great, balance may be restored by inserting marking paper on both sides and sliding forward. Contact marks will be found on the posterior teeth. Grind the marks on the distolingual slopes of the upper buccal cusps and the mesiobuccal slopes of the lower lingual cusps and, in addition, any marks on the ridges crossing the fissures of the upper premolars or lower molars.

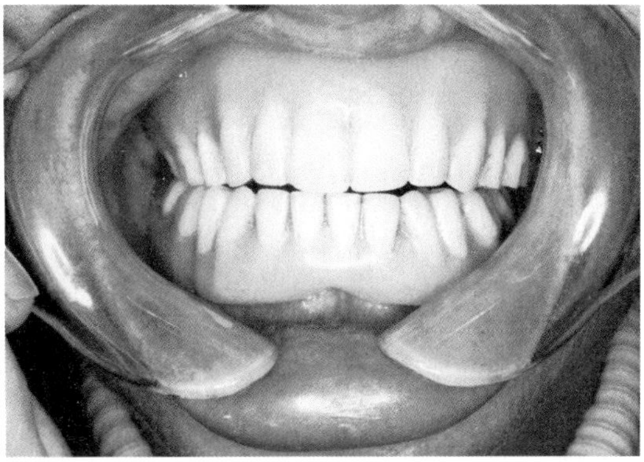

Figure 13.15 Right working movement in the mouth after modification of contacts shown in Figure 13.14

Perfecting articulation with grinding paste

The main correction of occlusal irregularities is made with small abrasive stones in a hand-piece but final occlusal freedom can be gained by placing a

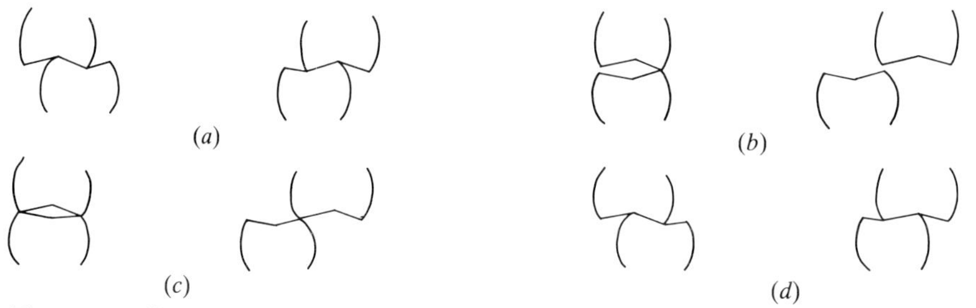

Figure 13.16 (*b*) The lingual cusp of the lower right tooth occludes prematurely when the right side becomes the working side. In order to produce contact on the balancing side the lingual cusp must be reduced (*c*) and not the upper palatal cusp which is required to maintain even contact as in (*a*) and (*d*)

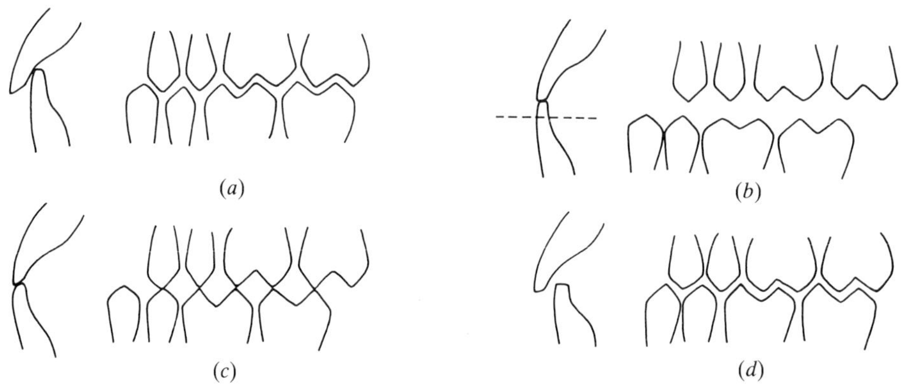

Figure 13.17 If in protrusion the incisors meet edge to edge (*b*) with the posterior teeth out of occlusion, the lower incisors may be ground to restore posterior contact (*c*). This will reduce the vertical overlap but cause no change in the even contact of the posterior teeth in RCP (this should not be done when dealing with natural dentitions as further eruption of the lower anteriors may occur to restore contact with the upper incisors). Some reduction of the incisal edge of the upper incisors together with an increase in its palatolabial slope will also help, but excessive grinding should be avoided as the appearance may be spoiled

paste of no. 150 silicon carbide powder on the lower denture and working the posterior teeth through lateral and protrusive excursions. The amount of adjustment made with grinding paste must be small as this will reduce all occluding surfaces and if excessive will result in loss of vertical dimension. A paste of powder mixed with petroleum jelly or toothpaste is used to smooth the previously ground tooth surfaces and produce a perfectly even occlusion. Grinding paste may be used in the mouth when the dentures are returned to the patient if it is considered desirable, but if carried out a warning must be given to the patient not to swallow while the paste is in the mouth.

Reduction of sharp edges of ground teeth

On the completion of all occlusal correction sharp edges occurring buccally and lingually must be rounded and polished to prevent tongue and cheek irritation (Figure 13.19).

Dentures constructed on a plane-line articulator

The same check record technique should be used with dentures made on a plane-line articulator and, although it is not possible in every case to produce a completely free occlusion in the anterior region, reasonable results may be obtained for a very large majority of patients. The depth of overlap, however, in a few cases restricts the free movement and can only be eliminated by mutilation of the appearance. Nevertheless, if a low incisal guidance angle is used when the teeth are being set up, and compensating curves are introduced, there should be no difficulty in establishing a reasonably free articulation.

Even where the depth of vertical overlap restricts lateral movements it is possible to provide a reduction of cuspal interference and the technique of remounting with an RCP check record has the considerable advantage of permitting correction of minor errors in retruded contact position and the

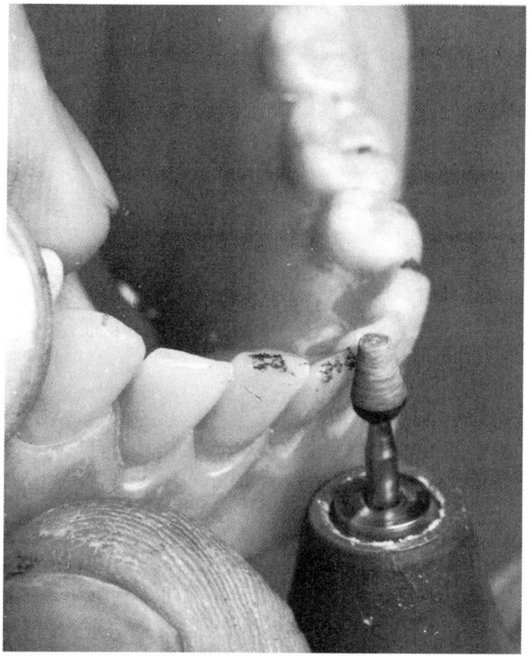

Figure 13.18 Using a rotary carborundum stone to grind the labial aspects of the lower incisors

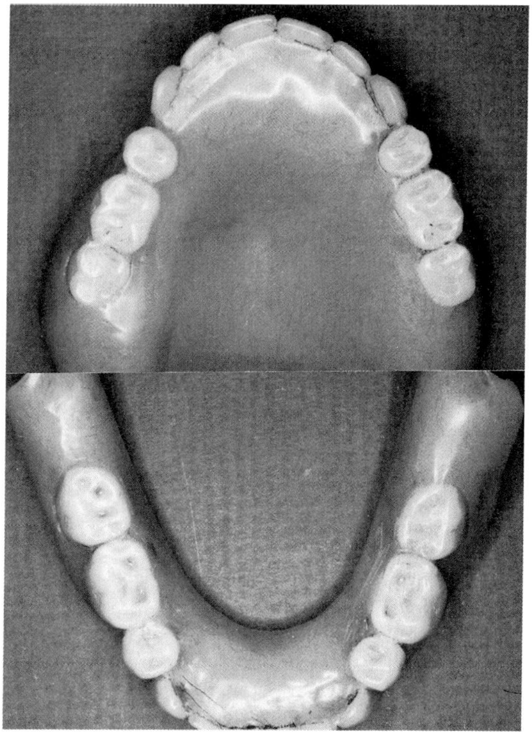

Figure 13.19 The occlusion in RCP and eccentric positions has been perfected and the surfaces of the teeth smoothed and polished prior to returning to the mouth

establishment of even pressure in retruded and, to a certain extent, eccentric occlusions, and for this reason should be carried out for all cases mounted on plane line articulators. Increased comfort of the patient and improved clenching and masticatory ability follow the check record adjustments.

Complete denture opposed by a partial denture

Frequently a condition arises in which a complete upper denture opposes a partial lower denture and natural teeth, or occasionally a complete lower denture opposes a partial upper denture and natural teeth. These cases can be approached in a similar way by check records. The variations to be borne in mind are the necessity of obtaining an impression of the lower partial denture *in situ* and the limited grinding of any natural teeth. When pouring the impression the denture must be retained in it and care is taken that the denture does not shift. Certain parts of the partial denture, such as clasps or connectors, may require blocking out with soft wax before pouring in dental stone otherwise the denture may be locked into the cast. If it is necessary to grind the represented natural teeth on the cast a note of the areas ground must be made so that a similar adjustment can be carried out to the natural teeth when the dentures are returned to the patient.

Chapter 14

Complaints

It is impossible to discuss every complaint which may be made by a patient but the following are the most common and will give a comprehensive outline of how the dentist may diagnose their causes and how they should be treated.

Most complaints will fall under one of the following headings, although frequently a patient will have more than one complaint:

1 Pain and discomfort.
2 Appearance.
3 Inability to eat.
4 Lack of retention and instability.
5 Clicking of teeth.
6 Nausea.
7 Inability to tolerate dentures.
8 Altered speech.
9 Biting the cheek and tongue.
10 Food under the denture.
11 Inability to keep denture clean.

Pain

Over-extension of the periphery

This is by far the most common cause of pain with new dentures. It is due to incorrect moulding of the impression or incorrect outlining of the denture on the cast and is visible in the mouth as an area of hyperaemia or an ulcer, depending upon how continuously the denture has been worn, or how gross is the over-extension.

Treatment: apply pressure-indicating paste to the periphery and insert the denture. On removal an area of wipe-off will be seen. An alternative method is to dry the mucosa, touch the inflamed area with methylene blue or an indelible pencil and insert the denture. Remove the denture and ease the periphery with a small carborundum stone or a bur. Except in cases of severe ulceration this will give immediate relief, but remember that the area is slightly oedematous and therefore only the minimum material should be removed from the denture. Where there is an ulcer, additional relief is gained by applying tincture of benzoin compound to the dried mucosa. Polish the abraded periphery before dismissing the patient.

If the denture is an old one, the over-extension may be due to alveolar resorption and the slow, chronic irritation may have caused a local hyperplasia. Cut back the denture periphery and line the fitting surface with tissue conditioner or black gutta percha.

When the hyperplasia has reduced, or been removed surgically, construct new dentures.

Poor fit

This is easily detected by the poor retention, rocking, tilting and inability to seat the denture accurately in any position. The movement of the denture rubbing the mucosa causes pain, and patches of redness are sometimes visible.

Treatment: new dentures, but the old ones can be worn in the meantime with a lining of tissue conditioner.

Insufficient relief

This may occur over a prominent bony area, such as the buccal canine region where the bone has been expanded at the time of extraction. The denture moves over the hard area causing pain. The painful area is red and possibly ulcerated.

Treatment: apply pressure indicating paste to demarcate the area and ease the contact surface with a carborundum stone.

Occlusal faults

This may be any one of the following faults, or a combination of them.

Wrong anteroposterior relationship

When the teeth occlude the mandible will not be fully retruded. Attempts to retrude it will drag the dentures against the mucosa as they are locked together by the interdigitation of the teeth. This is often difficult to diagnose but can be seen by watching closely while the patient slowly approximates the teeth and increases the occlusal load. At some stage in this movement the lower denture will be seen to shift. This is often associated with a complaint of looseness.

Treatment: if only slight it can be cured by a check record, remounting and grinding of the dentures; if gross, place occlusal pivots to reposition the lower denture (see Chapter 16).

Uneven pressure

This may be the result of faulty setting of the teeth and, if so, is usually very slight. More commonly it is the result of tilting of the record blocks, undetected at the trial stage. Pain is due to trauma caused by the one-sided pressure and is then confined to the crest of the alveolar ridge on that side; sometimes small hyperkeratinized areas are to be seen, as in an excessive vertical dimension. Pain may also be due to tilting of either denture, more usually the lower, and is then situated near the buccal periphery on the side of excesssive pressure and near the lingual periphery on the opposite side. Diagnosis can be made by trying to insert a thin blade between the posterior teeth, first on one side, and then on the other, with the teeth in firm contact. Lesser degrees of error can be detected by inserting a thin mylar strip on either side between the occlusal surfaces of the posterior teeth while the patient closes just sufficiently to hold them in place. The strip on the side of the heavy pressure will be immovable while that on the opposite side will be easily withdrawn.

Treatment: if the error is small the areas of heavy contact are detected by marking paper and the fault corrected by grinding or, better still, by remounting with a check record and adjusting the occlusion on the articulator. If the error is large, temporary improvement can be effected by adding cold-cure acrylic to the side of lighter pressure. When symptoms have abated either replace the posterior teeth or remake the dentures.

Excessive vertical dimension

This is due to an error at the registration stage and is almost always due to increasing the vertical height beyond normal limits. Pain is associated with the crest of the lower ridge, as distinct from the lateral surfaces, and small white patches may be seen in the painful area. Easing the denture over these white patches gives immediate relief from pain, but within a few days the patient usually returns with the same complaint in a different site. In nearly all cases of excessive height the patient also complains that the teeth jar, clatter, are 'in the way' or 'too high' when eating, and sometimes when talking.

Treatment: if the occlusal plane of the upper is judged to be correct make a new lower denture to a decreased vertical dimension; otherwise, new upper and lower dentures.

Insufficient vertical dimension

Pain from this cause is not normally associated with new dentures. It is almost always the result of loss of vertical height through alveolar resorption. The pain is often indefinite in locality and may be associated with temporomandibular joint dysfunction and its symptoms of facial or joint pain.

Treatment is aimed at restoring the vertical height and stabilizing the occlusion by occlusal pivots, followed by new dentures.

Cuspal interference

A dragging action will be exerted on both upper and lower dentures during all lateral and protrusive movements with the teeth in contact if cusped posterior teeth are used:

1. With a plane-line articulator.
2. With a moving-condyle articulator if care has not been taken to obtain balanced articulation.

The same effect may result from an excessive vertical overlap or an incorrect incisal guidance angle (Figure 14.1).

This dragging will cause pain with well-fitting dentures and also instability with those having poor retention. The pain is usually widely distributed and often only experienced when attempting to eat, although 'empty mouth' grinding movements exacerbate the problem. Sore areas may be found on the labial or buccal surfaces of the alveolar ridges, and on the lingual surfaces of the lower ridge. The patient often removes the dentures after a few hours because of the discomfort. This condition can easily be detected by asking the patient to grind the teeth, when shifting of the dentures can be seen. Another simple method of diagnosing this fault is to hold the upper denture in place between the finger and thumb above the canine teeth and ask the patient to grind the teeth. The dragging can easily be felt.

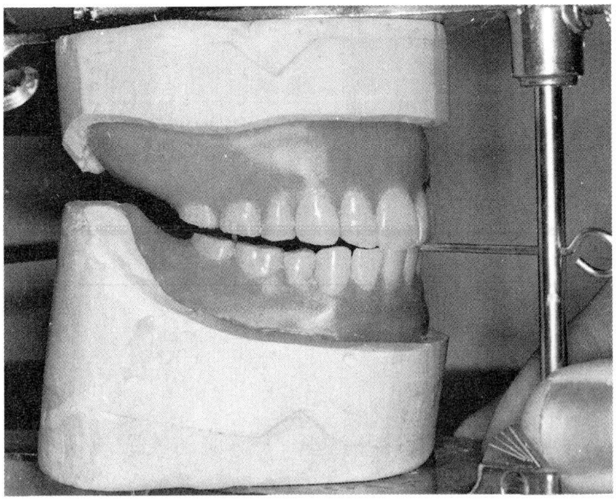

Figure 14.1 Complete dentures with a marked fault in protrusive occlusion giving rise to pain in the lower anterior ridge and looseness of the upper denture

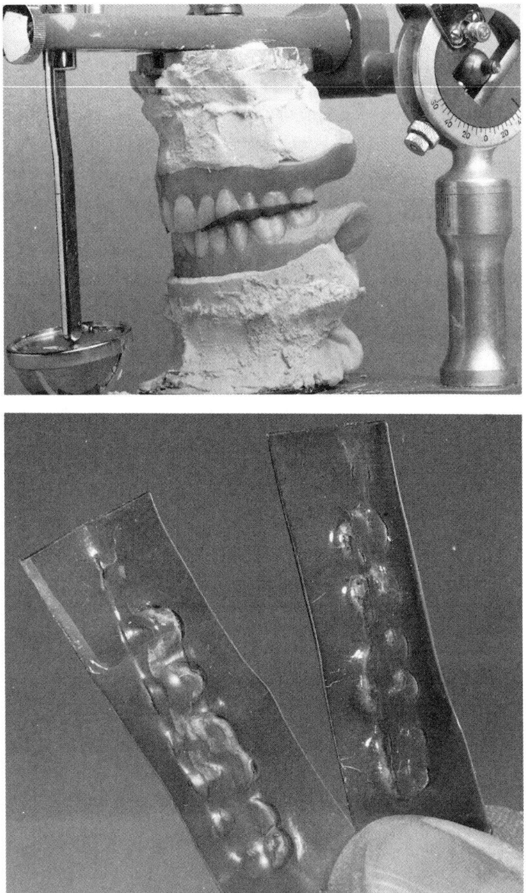

Figure 14.2 If a diagnosis of cuspal interference is made the dentures may be remounted with 'pre-centric' check records and the occlusal fault corrected or at least markedly improved

Treatment: if the cuspal interference is slight, or confined to only one or two teeth, it can be corrected by the careful use of marking paper and grinding. The taking of a check record and adjusting the occlusal surfaces on the articulator is the most accurate method of correcting this error (Figure 14.2). If the interference is gross, new dentures with balanced occlusion will be required.

Teeth off the ridge

Pain from this cause is confined chiefly to the upper buccal sulci and maxillary tuberosities. It is usually the result of setting the upper teeth too far buccally in an attempt to overcome marked discrepancies between the size of the upper arch and that of the lower, combined with lack of peripheral seal and incorrectly shaped polished surfaces. During mastication the upper denture tilts, digging the periphery of the denture into the mucosa on the working side, and pulling it down over the tuberosity, or other undercut area, on the opposite side. The actual tilting can be seen if the patient bites on a wooden spatula placed on the posterior teeth, first on one side and then the other.

Treatment: some relief may be obtained by removing all four last molars and reducing the bulk of base acrylic over the tuberosity. This gives more space for the tongue to control the upper denture. New dentures, with the above faults corrected, are the most effective treatment.

Retained root or unerupted tooth

Pain may be caused by direct pressure on an area which is already tender and will be felt very soon after inserting new dentures. It may also be caused by a well-fitting denture preventing draining from an undetected sinus. Well-fitting, functional dentures appear in some cases to stimulate the eruption of unerupted teeth. The painful area will usually be localized and often close inspection will reveal the cause. Diagnosis should be confirmed by radiograph (Figure 14.3).

Treatment: extraction of the root or tooth followed by relining of that part of the denture. If for some reason extraction is contraindicated, then relief may be given by easing the denture over the area.

Narrow resorbed ridge

This is more usually associated with the lower, and caused by the denture pressing the mucosa against the sharp ridge of bone during mastication. The pain is worst on the side habitually used for eating, but it may be widespread with an associated burning sensation. It is most severe during, and immediately following, a meal, and is increased by perseverance on the part of the patient.

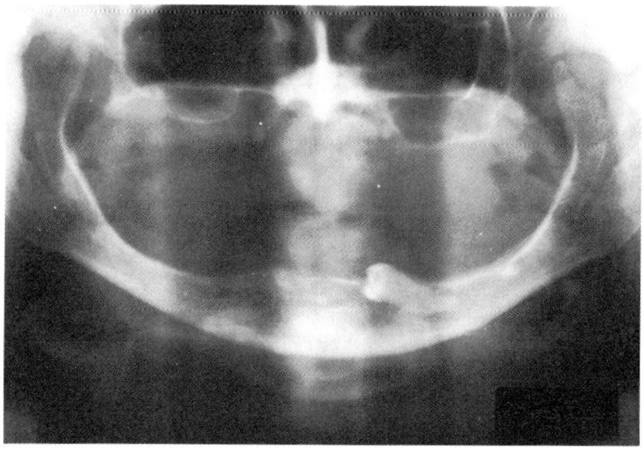

Figure 14.3 Panoramic radiograph shows position of unerupted lower premolar and possibly two apices which would require additional intra-oral radiographs

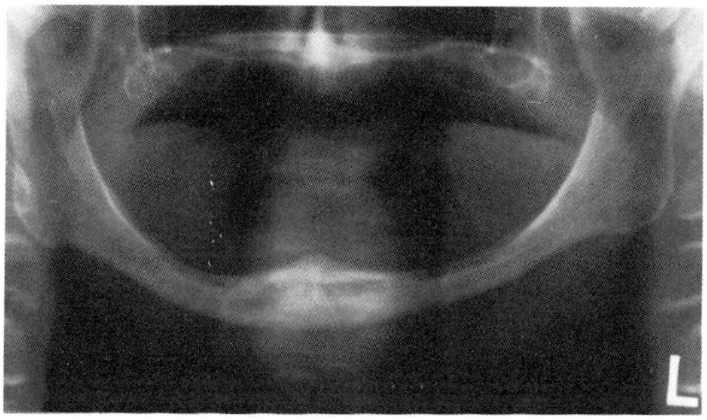

Figure 14.4 Radiograph showing dehiscence of mandibular canal

Treatment: in the lower, alveolectomy followed by relining the denture may be considered but relief over the bony irregularities is often the best treatment. In the upper, relief over the crest of the alveolus is usually sufficient since the palate can resist the masticatory loads.

Mental foramen

Under normal conditions the mental foramen is situated on the buccal surface of the mandible below the lower alveolar ridge and is thus outside the denture-bearing area. If, however, gross resorption of the alveolar and basal bone has taken place, the foramen may come to lie on the crest of the ridge and so be subject to pressure from the denture (Figure 14.4). When a new denture is constructed to these altered conditions, adequate relief should be given for the mental nerve. The pain may be localized to the immediate vicinity of the mental foramen, or it may be referred, and is then felt as a pain in the side of the face or in the lips and chin. It can usually be diagnosed by locating the mental foramen by radiograph.

Treatment: relieve the denture so that the nerve cannot be subjected to pressure.

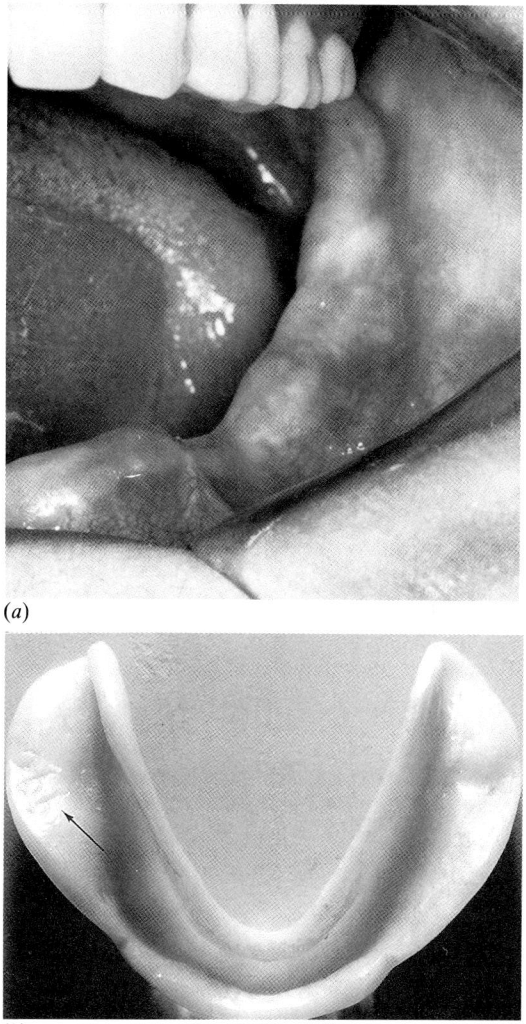

(*a*)

(*b*)

Figure 14.5 (*a*) Rough irregular surface of alveolar ridge on left mandibular area. (*b*) The patient's symptoms of discomfort were increased by the rough surface of the denture (arrowed) made by an identification number

Irregular resorption (Figure 14.5)

Sometimes, because of alveolar resorption, an area is found which is rough, with a number of sharp spicules of bone, and if the mucosa covering it is thin, pain will be caused by pressure on it. This is very similar to the pain associated with narrow resorbed ridges except that it is localized. The uneven alveolus can be detected by gentle palpation and confirmed by radiograph.

Treatment: surgical smoothing of the affected area followed by relining the denture. Treatment by surgery in such cases is often disappointing as the area remains tender for a long time and so simply relieving the denture may be a better treatment.

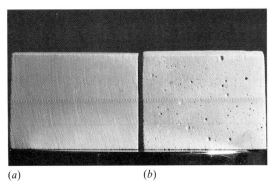

(*a*) (*b*)

Figure 14.6 Photographs of specimens of dental stone poured (*a*) under vacuum and (*b*) without vacuum to show the marked difference in surface

Rough contact or fitting surface

If a denture has been processed on a cast with a porous surface small pimples or blebs will be found on the contact surface where the acrylic has been forced into the small air bubbles of the cast (Figure 14.6). Normally these pimples are removed by the technician, but if they are overlooked the patient will complain of pain under pressure and a local area of inflammation can be seen.

Treatment: remove the roughness from the denture and polish lightly. Always inspect a denture when it is dry, under a good light and magnification, to detect surface roughness or blebs.

Swallowing and sore throat

These two complaints are listed together as they are different ways of describing pain arising from the over-extension of a denture. The cause in the upper is extension on to the soft palate with trauma in the postdam region or excessive pressure in the hamular notches, while in the lower it is over-extension distally in the lingual pouch. The pain ceases if the denture is left out, and starts again soon after its reinsertion.

Treatment: the patient will usually know which denture is at fault and examination of the regions described will show a slight redness or ulceration. Reduction of the over-extension produces relief, although the symptoms may persist for some time.

Undercuts

Sometimes the dentist will make use of an undercut area which, in his judgement, is unlikely to cause pain, and although the new denture was inserted with comfort, the patient returns with the complaint that inserting and removing the denture is becoming increasingly painful. The maximum bulge of the alveolus in this area is found to be red and painful, and in some cases ulcerated.

Treatment: it may be possible to insert this side of the denture first, quite painlessly, and then the opposite side, removing it in reverse order. If this manoeuvring is not successful the fitting surface must be cut away until the denture can be inserted comfortably but the periphery must not be reduced in height. Often the flange will be too thin to allow acrylic to be removed from the fitting surface and if this is so the flange must be thickened by the addition of more material. Should this easing ruin the retention, as is likely to be the case if much has to be cut away, an alveolectomy will be necessary followed by a new buccal or labial flange.

Summary

It might be helpful to list the causes of pain or discomfort following the fitting of dentures.

1. Localized painful areas *with* ulceration:
   Blebs and surface irregularities.
   Periphery too sharp.
   Postdam too deep.
   Edges of relief areas.
   Lack of relief.
   Occlusal error.
   Excess periphery.
   Tissue displacement by impression:
     pterygomaxillary notch
     frenum
     pear-shaped pad.
2. Localized painful areas *without* ulceration:
   Upper displaceable ridge.
   Rough bony alveolar ridge.
   Dental remnant.
   Mental foramen.
   Mylohyoid ridge.
   Buccal prominence of tuberosity.
   Lack of relief, e.g. incisive papilla.
   Occlusal error.
   Excessive vertical dimension.
   Peripheral over-extension.
   Denture into undercuts.
   Cramped tongue space.
   Mucosal displacement.

Appearance

In spite of the greatest care on the part of the dentist to obtain the patient's full approval of the appearance at the trial stage, there will always be some patients who are dissatisfied with their appearance when wearing the finished dentures. The patient should not be condemned too severely for this inconsistency, as it is difficult to form a considered opinion on all details of facial appearance when sitting in a dental chair, in strange surroundings, with trial dentures in the mouth, and being asked to criticize the work of a professional person. The number of patients who are dissatisfied with their appearance with the final dentures can be much reduced if the dentist insists on a relation or candid friend being present at the trial stage, although it has to be stressed that the appearance cannot be fully assessed until four to six weeks after insertion of the finished dentures. This is because of the adaptation of the lip and facial muscles to the underlying teeth and denture bases. This is the basis of the problem of judging the appearance at the trial stage.

The following examples of complaints about appearance are by no means comprehensive but will be found to cover the main points.

Facial appearance

Patients may complain that the nose and chin are more prominent or are approximating. This is due, in the case of old dentures the patient is wearing, to continuing alveolar resorption and the spatial change of position of the dentures in relation to the skull as a whole. If this complaint is voiced after delivery of the new dentures it means a failure to restore the occlusal face height correctly. The same causes operate in complaints of the lips and cheeks falling in, although this is more likely to be due to the teeth of new dentures being set too far lingually and to insufficient width of the buccal and labial flanges (Figure 14.7).

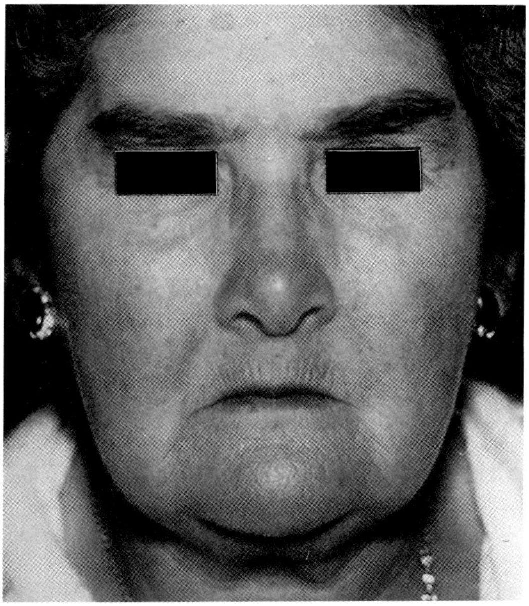

Figure 14.7 Patient wearing new complete dentures which failed to restore lips and cheeks to the correct form. (Note vertical folds on upper lip caused by very early loss of maxillary teeth and subsequent dentures of incorrect design.)

Dissatisfaction with teeth

Colour

This complaint is almost invariably that the teeth are too dark or too yellow, but before changing them it must be explained to the patient that natural teeth darken with age and that very light-shaded teeth look more artificial than darker ones.

Treatment: comply if possible with the patient's request for lighter teeth, usually by a compromise between the shade chosen by the operator and that chosen by the patient. If the dentist feels that a patient is insisting on such an unreasonably light shade that the dentures will look absurd, it may be best to delay treatment or refer the patient to a colleague.

Shape

Few people are sufficiently observant to be able to describe the shape of their lost teeth and are likely to say vaguely, when referring to their dentures, that 'they don't look right'. Shape is closely bound up with size, and a different make of tooth of the same basic shape and size may well look more natural. Artificial teeth usually look larger than natural teeth of identical size, probably because their mesial and distal surfaces are not so rounded, and so the eye is able to focus on their width more accurately.

Treatment: remove the teeth complained of and replace them with others mounted in wax until by a process of trial and error, mutually suitable ones are obtained.

Position

The complaint may be that the teeth are too far back in the mouth, or too far forward. If the setting is left entirely to the technician without any instructions he may place them as nearly over the alveolar ridge as he can, but if the patient has been edentulous for some time the labial resorption of the upper alveolus makes this the wrong position for the anterior teeth. A fear is sometimes expressed that moving the teeth anterior to the ridge into the position the natural teeth occupied will affect the stability of the denture, but this is not so. Stability will be jeopardized much more by encroaching on the tongue than by setting the teeth in the neutral zone where the pressures of tongue and lip are equalized.

Treatment: the patient may complain that the incisal edges are too low and, therefore, that too much tooth is showing. Adaptation of the lip will often satisfy the patient but the fault may be in placing the occlusal plane in an inferior position. If the dentures are finished in acrylic the anterior teeth may be removed and replaced at a higher level but this is usually unsatisfactory as it spoils the acrylic matrix and ruins the protrusive tooth contacts.

Often the best solution in such cases is to remake the dentures but great care must be taken to get the periphery of the master impression right, to select the position of the occlusal plane and to pay strict attention to tooth position at the trial stage.

General dissatisfaction

One of the most difficult cases to deal with is that of the patient, fitted with new dentures, who returns a few days later with the vague remark that he 'does not like them'. He can specify no particular complaint and it will be found on questioning that comfort, retention, stability and efficiency are not at fault; so the conclusion, which is invariably right, is that it is a question of appearance. It may be due to diffidence on the part of the patient unwilling to make a specific complaint that would appear to criticize the dentist's skill. If the dentist is fortunate enough to have the right type of sympathetic surgery assistant, he is well advised to leave it to her to find out what is really in the patient's mind, although it may take some time. Sometimes the patient will bring a photograph to illustrate what he used to look like and what he was expecting the dentist to reproduce. These photographs are little help as they were invariably taken many years previously, often 30 or more. If the complaint can be pinned down to one particular point it can usually be remedied, at least partially, but if it is a longing for lost youth it will take much tact to satisfy the patient that the colour of the hair, the complexion and the tone of the muscles have all altered, and that the teeth alone cannot produce the desired effect. These patients are often at the climacteric; impatience or harshness will only antagonize them but with tact, kindness and genuine sympathy they can almost always be brought to see the matter in its true proportions, and thereafter may be among the dentist's most grateful patients.

Inability to eat

This complaint is mainly confined to patients who are wearing complete dentures for the first time, and are impatient at the time spent in acquiring new habits of eating. Careful attention by the operator to the psychological approach to denture wearing, as described in Chapter 3, will eliminate this complaint except in rare cases, and these must be persuaded to persevere, so that they will either learn anew how to eat or will define some specific complaint which can then be remedied.

Difficulty may be encountered with certain fibrous foods and this is likely to be due to low-cusp or zero-cusp posterior teeth, lack of interdigitation of posterior teeth, the use of acrylic teeth in a patient used to porcelain, unbalanced occlusion, or a locked occlusion arising from setting teeth on a plane-line articulator. These faults may also cause the dentures to dislodge during eating, a further complication being a restricted tongue space which may occur if the upper teeth are set directly over the ridge, if the lower posterior teeth overhang the tongue or if the posterior teeth, particularly the lowers, are too broad.

An over-extended periphery may cause a denture to dislodge. It is quite possible for a denture to be slightly over-extended and yet to be stable during speech and swallowing. This is because movements during eating are more extensive than those employed when moulding the periphery of the impression. The commonest place for this to occur is in the region of the posterior lingual pouch. It is frequently difficult in these cases to locate the exact area of over-extension, since the tissue contact with it is too intermittent to cause pain or ulceration. Intelligent observation by the patient of the exact movement which causes the instability will eventually enable the operator to locate the over-extension.

The posterior natural teeth are often lost some time before the anterior ones, with the result that a habit is formed of eating on the anterior teeth. When complete dentures are being worn for the first time, it is only natural that the patient should try to continue his previous eating habits with bad results. Most experienced complete denture patients have such good, though unconscious, control that they can bite an apple or eat corn off the cob with little difficulty, but this automatic skill is only acquired with time and patience. Biting, the function of the anterior teeth as opposed to chewing, the function of the posterior teeth, is an action the new denture patient should not attempt, although when he has mastered this he has learnt denture control.

Lack of retention and instability

When opening the mouth

Patients more often complain that the lower denture lifts than that the upper one drops. If this lifting only occurs when the mouth is widely opened it may be explained by what is commonly known as a low tongue position (Figure 14.8). When a dentate person opens the mouth wide the tongue remains back in the mouth to protect the oropharyngeal isthmus while in an experienced denture wearer the tongue falls forward to stabilize the lower denture. If the low tongue position persists in edentulousness then the denture is likely to rise on wide mouth opening. Explanation of this will help the patient to counteract the problem. Other causes are given below.

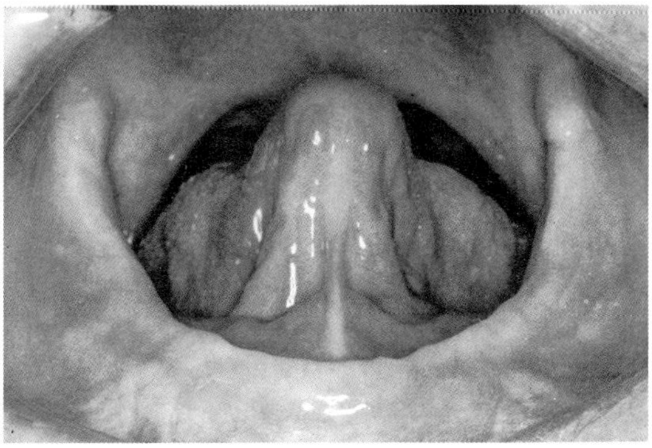

Figure 14.8 The low tongue position when the mouth is opened (sometimes called the defensive tongue)

Over-extension

This has already been discussed under the heading of pain, the difference in these cases being that the over-extension is so slight that the tissues do not make constant contact with it, and consequently soreness does not arise. The treatment is identical.

Tight lips (Figure 14.9)

These can be a most difficult problem when in conjunction with a flat, atrophic lower. The inward pressure from the lips will seat the upper denture more firmly in position but will push the lower denture backwards and up the ascending ramus.

Treatment: remake with the lower anterior teeth set more lingually, with a labial concavity on the denture, and with the maximum extension in the region of the retromolar pads. Denture space techniques are useful (see Chapter 16) and surgical vestibuloplasty must be considered.

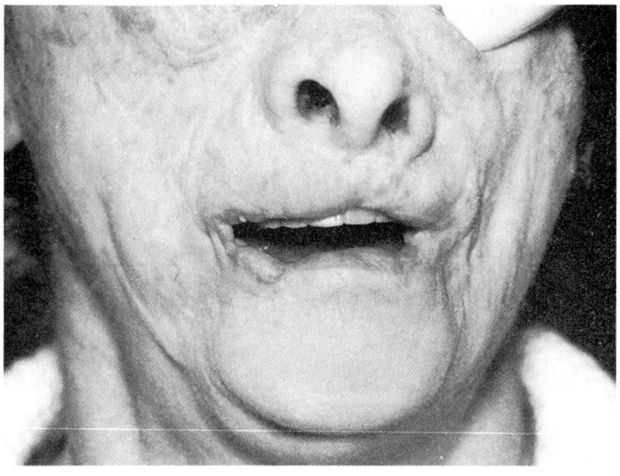

Figure 14.9 An edentulous patient with lupus vulgaris presenting great difficulty with tight lips and atrophic alveolar ridges

Tongue space

If the lower posterior teeth are tilted or set lingually they produce an undercut area into which the wide middle-third of the tongue will press. Movements of the tongue then lift the denture.

Treatment: reduce the width of the lower posterior teeth by grinding off the lingual cusps. This effectively alters the downward facing lingual surface to an upward facing one more favourable to tongue control.

Under-extension and lack of peripheral seal

This fault is by no means uncommon, and its effect on the retention of the denture is most marked. Maximum retention cannot be obtained without covering the greatest possible denture-bearing area. Some clinicians produce this fault by placing excessive tension on the soft tissues during the peripheral moulding of the impression, through their desire to avoid over-extension. Where this cause is suspected of being the fault, it can be checked by adding tracing stick round the periphery, moulding it carefully and noting the result. A conventional reline can then be undertaken (see Chapter 15).

Lack of saliva

There is no specific treatment for this condition but palliative treatment such as artificial saliva will help the patient (see Chapter 16).

When coughing or sneezing

Occasionally a new denture wearer will complain that his upper denture falls and his lower denture lifts, whenever he coughs or sneezes violently.

Treatment: it must be explained to the patient that when coughing or sneezing the soft palate rises suddenly and there is a moment when the pressure of air in the mouth is considerable so that the peripheral seal of the upper denture is broken and it is liable to fall; the unusual muscular movement causes the lower denture to lift. There is no way of preventing these movements of the dentures, but covering the mouth with a hand or handkerchief is an obvious suggestion.

Clicking of teeth

Patients are often less disturbed by contact of teeth than relatives who are irritated by the noise. The main causes are:

1. Excessive vertical height causes the dentures to contact during speech, particularly the sibilant sounds, as the mandible moves vertically through the speaking space.

2. Movement of the lower denture from whatever cause is very liable to lead to clicking of the teeth, particularly the molars if the distal part of the denture rises.
3. Cuspal interference or lack of balanced occlusion is a likely cause of faulty tooth contacts. Particular attention should be paid to the retruded contact position as faults here are often missed in the examination of the occlusion.
4. Excessive incisal guidance angle usually infers that the horizontal overjet is inadequate in relation to the vertical overlap. This means that during speech, in which there is often a pronounced horizontal movement of the mandible as well as vertical, the incisors contact each other and cause clicking.
5. Porcelain teeth by nature of the material create more impact noise than acrylic, a problem increased if the patient has been used to acrylic for many years.

Nausea

Although this subject has been mentioned from the point of view of impression taking, there are some essential differences when considering nausea in relation to wearing a complete upper denture. The cause of the sickness is the same in both cases, light or intermittent contact on the soft palate or back of the tongue, and the patient's complaint is almost invariably 'that the upper denture goes too far back and makes me feel sick'. The causes are given below.

Denture slightly over-extended

Movements of the soft palate cause intermittent contact with the denture and this may be diagnosed by observing the relation of the posterior border to the vibrating line.

Treatment: remove the excess and readapt the postdam if necessary.

Denture under-extended

If the posterior border of the upper denture does not extend beyond the hard palate it cannot compress the soft tissues sufficiently to maintain close contact under all normal conditions, and this will often cause nausea because of the intermittent contact and tickling effect at the back of the palate. A posterior edge which lies too far forward is detected by the dorsum of the tongue and is a common cause of nausea.

Thick posterior border

This is a very common cause of nausea resulting from the dorsum of the tongue being irritated by the thick edge. The edge of the upper denture should be thin, and slightly embedded in the compressed mucosa, so that the tongue is unable to detect any definite junction between denture and palatal mucosa.

Protrusive imbalance

If the occlusion is not balanced in protrusive imbalance there is a heavy contact on the incisors and no contact between the molars. This produces movement of the back of the upper denture which causes saliva to collect at the posterior border and a tickling effect, leading to nausea.

Inability to tolerate dentures

Patients sometimes complain that new dentures are not comfortable but can give no specific cause for complaint. These cases are difficult to diagnose since they are not accompanied by pain, and retention appears to be satisfactory, but as the patient has nearly always previously worn dentures a careful comparison of the new with the old will generally give a clue to the cause (Figure 14.10).

Cramped tongue space

This is the most common reason for this complaint, the teeth on the new upper denture having been set on the crest of the alveolar ridge which has resorbed considerably since the older denture was made. Since the resorption is greatest on the buccal and labial aspects of the upper ridge, the teeth are now mounted nearer to the midline, so decreasing the tongue space.

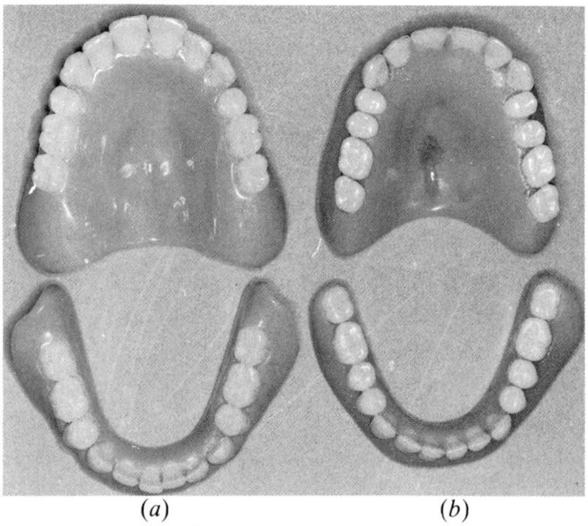

(*a*) (*b*)

Figure 14.10 Dentures for the same patient.
(*a*) Replacement dentures with adequate tongue space and teeth in the pre-extraction position. (*b*) Existing dentures which the patient could not tolerate (note cramped tongue space)

Altered vertical height

The vertical height of new dentures may have been increased only a few millimetres but it may be sufficient for a sensitive patient to notice a difference, particularly if the original dentures were made with a very small freeway space.

Altered occlusal plane

As in the case of an altered vertical height, the position of the occlusal plane is unlikely to have been changed by more than a few millimetres, but even a slight alteration will require some adjustment of muscular movement and control, particularly the tongue.

Unemployed ridge

This type of ridge was discussed in Chapter 5 and is a common cause of discomfort and inability to wear a new complete lower denture because the latter applies pressure on tissue not previously loaded.

Changes in shape

Very often when new dentures are made with marked changes in form and dimension of the periphery or polished surface as compared with the patient's existing dentures there is difficulty in tolerating the change, particularly in older patients.

Treatment: unless any of the above-mentioned factors are gross the patient should be encouraged to persevere for several weeks, by which time, in most cases, the discomfort or intolerance will have disappeared; if not, then nothing remains but to modify the dentures or remake them if the cause of the problem has been diagnosed.

Altered speech

Reference should be made to Chapter 10. When complete dentures are first worn there is always some temporary alteration in speech owing to the thickness of the denture covering the palate, necessitating slightly altered positions of the tongue. Commonly this is only a temporary inconvenience, most rapidly overcome by the patient reading aloud; when there is an altered position of the upper incisors, a change in their palatal shape, any reduction of tongue space, or alteration in occlusal level, adaptation may be very difficult even with perseverance.

Treatment: the dentures must be remade paying particular attention to the principles laid down in Chapter 10 and to the correct restoration of the denture space, defined as the space in the edentulous mouth formerly occupied by the teeth and supporting tissues which have since been lost.

Biting the cheek and tongue

Cheek biting

Insufficient overjet

The normal occlusal relationship of the posterior teeth is with the buccal cusps of the upper teeth outside those of the lower teeth; this arrangement, along with the correct peripheral width on the dentures, normally prevents the cheeks getting caught between the teeth. If for any reason this arrangement has been altered, or if a patient has very lax cheeks, cheek biting may occur.

Treatment: increase the buccal overjet and make sure the peripheral form is adequate in width and height; in some cases it may be necessary to remove the last molar teeth or grind the buccal surfaces of the teeth.

Reduced vertical height

If the vertical occlusal dimension of the dentures is reduced, the resultant bunching of the cheeks allows them to be trapped between the occlusal surfaces of the teeth as they occlude. This may also occur if the occlusal plane of either denture is incorrectly positioned. It should be remembered that when the natural teeth are lost there is no record of the occlusal position of either the upper or lower teeth and the selection of the occlusal plane in complete dentures is entirely empiric.

Treatment: restore the vertical dimension or change the occlusal plane.

Biting the tongue

This is almost invariably due to a decrease in the tongue space occurring when fitting new dentures for patients already wearing dentures, but it may also be due to changes in occlusal level as mentioned above.

Food under the denture

This complaint is usually made by patients wearing dentures for the first time and who have not yet learnt how best to control the food. Undoubtedly a perfect peripheral seal will prevent the ingress of food beneath the denture, but perfection is not always attained and, owing to alveolar resorption, never maintained. Scraping a groove on the cast, along and near the entire periphery of the denture, is sometimes carried out, but this food-line, as it is termed, causes inflammation and ulceration and should not be undertaken.

Treatment: this usually consists of covering the maximum possible area and obtaining an adequate peripheral seal; thereafter, only perseverance by the patient can bring about any improvement.

Inability to keep denture clean

This complaint may be caused by:

1. Inadequate laboratory work by the technician, especially failure to polish all round each tooth before setting in wax. Careless waxing and flasking are common faults. It is not possible to polish acrylic in the interdental space, or the col between teeth, if the original wax was rough or incorrectly designed.
2. Loss of original polish by patient's use of hard household abrasives.
3. Failure of patient to clean the dentures regularly or efficiently. Many denture patients also wear spectacles but often the dentures are cleaned in the bathroom under poor light when the spectacles are not worn. Cleaning is therefore not always done properly.
4. Incorrect use of denture cleansers. These cleansers may be listed:
   (a) Oxygenating cleansers containing alkaline percarbonates or peroxides.
   (b) Hypochlorite solutions containing dilute sodium hypochlorite.
   (c) Mineral acid, usually dilute hydrochloric acid.
   (d) Powders and pastes containing mild abrasives, precipitated chalk or hydrated alumina.
   (c) Liquid detergent.

Summary

At the conclusion of this chapter it is worth stressing the eight most common causes of problems with complete dentures:

1. Incorrect anteroposterior relationship of the mandible to the maxilla.
2. Premature contacts in retruded contact position.
3. Lack of occlusal balance in eccentric mandibular positions.
4. Vertical dimension excessive and therefore inadequate freeway space and interference with speaking space.
5. Cramped tongue space and teeth set too far lingually.
6. Inadequate periphery leading to poor retention and failure to restore lips and cheeks to the pre-extraction form.
7. Underextended denture bases.
8. Failure to recognize design of existing dentures.

Chapter 15

Relining, rebasing, resilient bases and repairs

The term 'relining' is used to denote the production of a new fitting surface in an existing denture; rebasing is the replacement of most of the base material. It should be noted that the terms are often used interchangeably and it is only a matter of degree between relining and rebasing a denture.

Reasons for relining and rebasing

Owing to the fact that alveolar resorption is a continuous process, though varying in degree, the comfort, efficiency, stability, retention and appearance of dentures are all liable to become impaired with the passage of time. The reasons for relining and rebasing are listed below.

To improve retention and stability

Loss of fit will make the maintenance of the peripheral seal impossible and will greatly impair the retentive effects of adhesion and cohesion. It may also permit a rocking or tilting of the denture during function and, in extreme cases in the lower, a lateral movement.

To improve the appearance

One effect of alveolar resorption in the mandible is that the lower denture sinks below the original occlusal level and thus the patient has to close beyond the original vertical dimension in order to occlude the teeth. This overclosure is frequently noticed by the patient as a protrusion of the mandible and an undue approximation of the nose and chin, giving an appearance of age. Resorption of the upper alveolar ridge will also have a marked effect on appearance because, although the hard palate does not materially alter, the upper denture slides upwards and backwards on the curve of the palate to lie under the upper lip.

To restore the vertical dimension

Relining and rebasing are clinical techniques sufficiently versatile to have little effect on the vertical dimension or to increase it to any desired amount.

To restore the occlusion

Resorptive changes in the edentulous jaws produce large changes in the position of the mandible in relation to the maxilla and hence changes in the occlusion of dentures. This is combined with wear and abrasion of the occlusal surfaces.

Relining and rebasing can reposition the dentures to correct the maxillo-mandibular relationship, but occlusal pivots (see Chapter 16) are usually necessary to rectify the occlusal surface wear prior to more permanent restoration in the laboratory.

To alleviate pain

If a denture has been worn with comfort and then becomes painful, it may be due to the fact that the supporting tissues have altered allowing the dentures to tilt, rock or move, and thus transmit undue pressure to one area. Relining will alleviate pain arising from this cause but adjustment of the occlusion will also be necessary.

Impression materials

Those in general use for the purposes of relining and rebasing are:

1. Zinc oxide–eugenol paste.
2. Elastomers.
3. Tissue conditioners.
4. Composition and tracing stick.
5. Black gutta percha.
6. Cold cure acrylic.

Alginate is not suitable as an impression material because it is dimensionally unreliable in thin section.

Clinical techniques

The periphery of the existing denture should be carefully examined for its relationship to the functional position of the sulci. If the denture border was positioned accurately when the denture was originally constructed, it may now appear slightly over-extended in height due to alveolar resorption. The denture flange is trimmed until the periphery is a fraction short of the functional position of the sulci. Parts of the base which fit into undercut areas are relieved so that the impression within the denture can be readily removed from the stone cast without fear of fracturing the ridge. A further point to consider is whether or not any substantial increase of the vertical dimension is desired, as this influences the type and quantity of material used for the impression.

When improved retention is the only consideration, a very thin layer of zinc oxide–eugenol paste (Figure 15.1) is spread evenly over the entire fitting and peripheral surface of the denture, which is then seated in position in the mouth and the teeth brought into occlusion; a slight pressure is maintained and the periphery trimmed by suitable lip and cheek movements to record their functional positions. The tongue presses against the anterior teeth to define the lingual periphery.

Where the vertical dimension has to be re-established in addition to the fit, the layer of impression material used must be of greater thickness. Zinc oxide–eugenol paste is not suitable as the sole material in cases which require a restoration of 3–4 mm. The lower denture is first lined with composition and an impression taken with the teeth in occlusion. The thickness of composition used should be such that it almost restores the desired vertical dimension. The periphery may be adjusted with tracing stick. The composition is then dried, and the final impression to the correct height taken with a wash of zinc oxide paste.

If the vertical dimension is being increased beyond 3–4 mm, and both dentures are being rebased, the question arises which denture should accommodate the greater part of this opening. The lower ridge, in the majority of cases, will have resorbed more than the upper, and the hard palate scarcely at all. As a general guide, the incisal level of

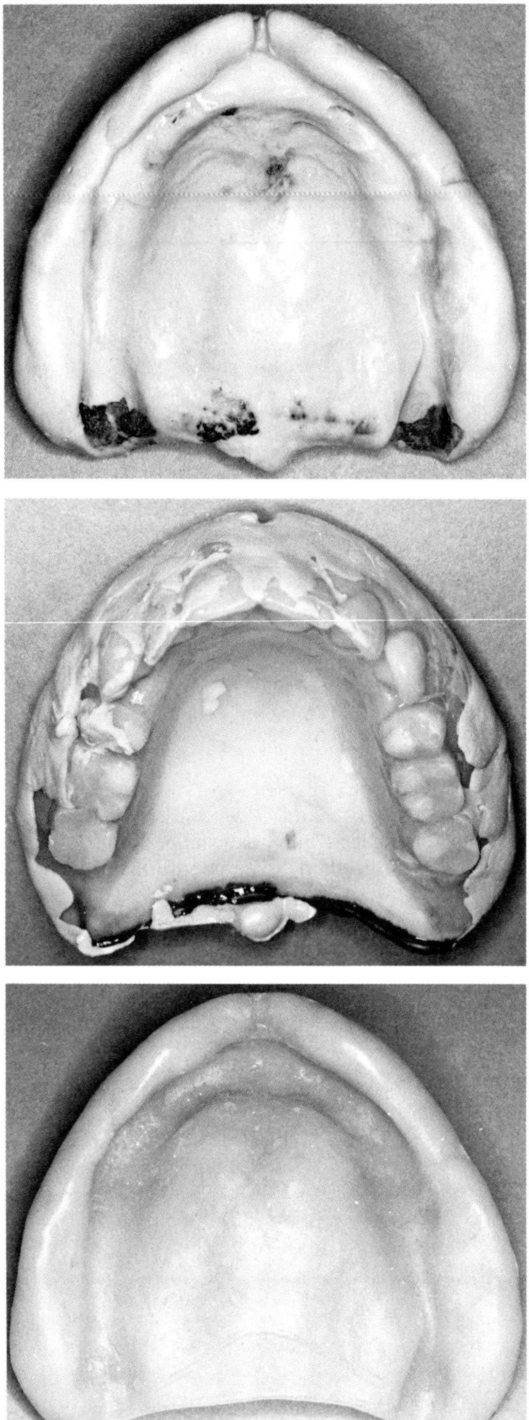

Figure 15.1 Rebasing a maxillary denture. Before applying the zinc oxide–eugenol (ZOE) paste the postdam area is perfected with tracing stick. Note how the impression paste sweeps round the periphery on to the polished surface. The finished denture is an exact reproduction of the impression

the upper anterior teeth should be studied in relation to the lip line, and the upper impression taken first, with sufficient thickness of material to bring the upper incisors into the desired position.

Although there is no apparent resorption of the hard palate, it will frequently be found that the incisors, which originally showed to the extent of 1–2 mm below the lip, have completely disappeared when the lip is at rest. This effect is caused by upper alveolar resorption allowing the denture to tilt and rise anteriorly, together with alterations of muscular tone and age changes of the upper lip.

The rebasing is completed by lining the lower denture with impression material of sufficient thickness e.g. one of the elastomers or tissue conditioners to complete the increase in vertical dimension.

Alternatively the whole impression may be carried out with composition alone. Whenever composition is being used, it is an advantage to grind away about 2 mm from the fitting surface of the lower denture, except in cases of flat lower ridges, in order to allow for a greater thickness of material. It will be found that if there is only a wafer of composition it is very difficult to keep it in a soft, workable condition when inserting it into the mouth as it cools too rapidly; the greater thickness overcomes this difficulty.

Black gutta percha, unlike composition, possesses the ability to flow slightly after it has been softened, and can be used in either thin or thick sections. It is an excellent space-filling material and, in this sense, is more versatile than tissue conditioner. A strip is cut from the sheet of gutta percha, placed in boiling water for a few minutes, dried and laid on the dry fitting surface of the denture and then inserted in the mouth. As the patient occludes, the gutta percha flows until the denture is seated. Peripheral movements are reproduced by gutta percha and the patient may wear the denture for some days to allow adaptation before the gutta percha is replaced with acrylic.

Should the upper denture need a thick layer of impression material to adjust the occlusal plane in relation to the lip line, or to eliminate excessive rock across the torus, the seating of the denture can be more accurately effected if an impression of the anterior and posterior ridges is obtained first in composition, gutta percha or cold-cure acrylic. The stops so formed will prevent loss of vertical height when the teeth are brought into occlusion during the zinc oxide–eugenol impression stage or temporarily relining with tissue conditioner.

Improved retention and stability are obtained, when relining a denture, if the periphery is carefully adapted to the functional level of the sulci with tracing compound. In an upper denture this includes the postdam region.

Cold-cure acrylic has been suggested as a material for relining dentures since it avoids any laboratory technique and the inconvenience caused to the patient by being temporarily deprived of his dentures. The procedure involves lining the cleansed, dried denture with a thin layer of acrylic dough and placing it in position in the mouth, the mucosa having previously been protected with a smear of petrolatum or vegetable oil. The dough is allowed to polymerize in the mouth for a few minutes. The denture is then removed before the peak exothermic reaction, and polymerization completed in a warm water bath. The denture borders must be trimmed and polished.

A serious disadvantage to the use of this material is the fact that acrylic dough often causes considerable irritation of the mucosa by monomer but the rigid cold curing resins for direct use in the mouth, consisting of polyethyl methacrylate polymer and butyl methacrylate monomer, are clinically acceptable as temporary relining materials.

Resiliant bases (Figure 15.2)

When other causes have been eliminated and pain under a lower denture is considered to be due to the type of alveolar bony ridge and a mucosa which cannot withstand the transmitted pressure of clenching and denture-base movement, some relief of the symptoms may be obtained by lining the denture with a resilient material. The clinical procedure calls for an accurate impression in the existing denture with no tissue displacement, the remainder of the technique being carried out in the laboratory. Tissue conditioners are particularly useful as impression materials in such cases as they allow the mucosa to recover from the trauma of the denture for a week or two. When the denture is comfortable, and the mucosa is normal, the tissue conditioner is replaced by the resilient lining.

At the present time a large number of proprietary resilient linings are available and many of these produce a comfortable denture. The life of most is limited to a year or two and then they require renewal, but if the patient is comfortable then frequent renewal is well worthwhile.

The two groups of materials are acrylics and silicones.

1. Heat-cure acrylics are copolymers of ethyl or butyl methacrylate with the addition of plasticizers.
2. Cold-cure acrylics, essentially the same, but activated by a peroxide-amine system.
3. Some acrylics are produced in the form of a soft pliable sheet which is laid on the clean, dried denture. These are sold over the pharmacy counter and some patients cause oral damage by adding sheet upon sheet which increases the

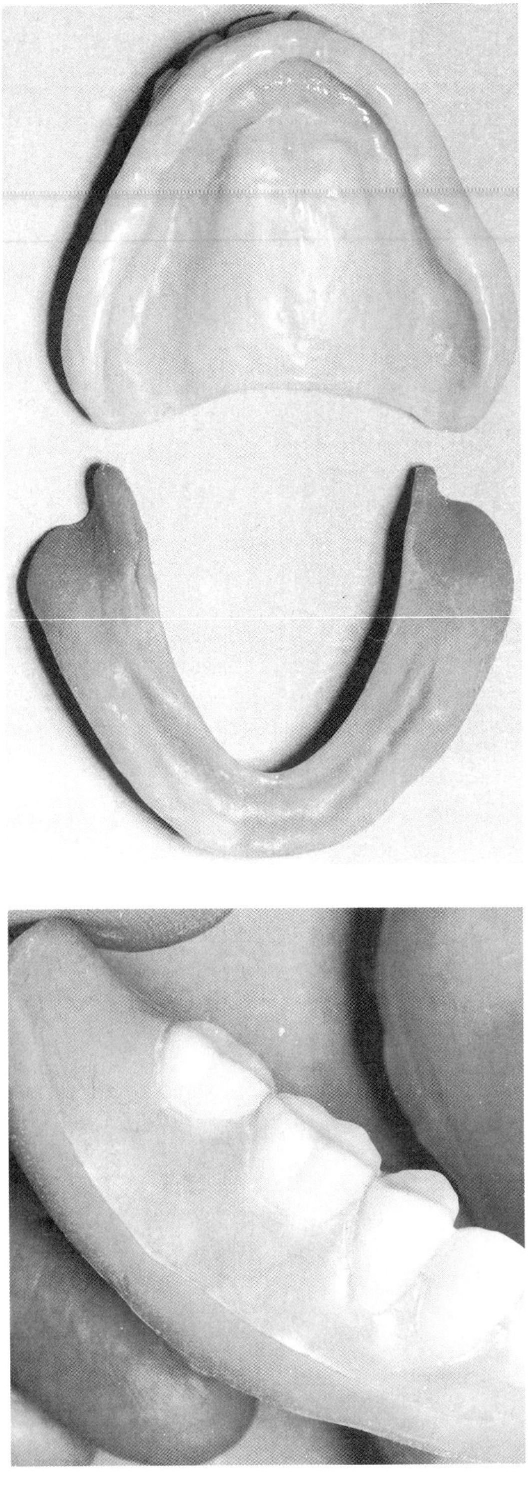

Figure 15.2 Soft resilient lining (heat-cure silicone). Note thickness of lining. Thin linings are useless to relieve pressure pain

vertical dimension and, in turn, alveolar resorption, occasionally quite severe.

4. Heat-cure silicones, in some cases with a methacrylate group to increase bonding with the acrylic denture base.
5. Cold-cure silicones which are essentially the same as silicone impression materials.

If the resilient lining is thick and is attached to a lower acrylic denture, the latter may fracture as a result of flexion. In these cases a cast metal strengthener may be incorporated on the lingual side of the denture.

Repairs

There is a tendency to regard denture repairs as a nuisance, without any necessity to find out the cause of the breakage, with the result that many dentures are mended only to break again shortly afterwards, when they should be either relined or replaced. No denture which breaks in the mouth should be repaired without the cause of the breakage being ascertained.

A number of dentures which are brought by patients as having cracked in the mouth have in fact been dropped. The crack, started by the accident, passes unobserved and the stresses of mastication complete the fracture. These cases are difficult to diagnose as patients will rarely, either through forgetfulness or untruthfulness, admit that they have ever dropped the denture.

Breakage of a denture in the mouth almost invariably starts with a small crack spreading across the denture, rather as though it were being torn instead of broken. Often the first thing to be noticed by the patient is the sensation of a hair on the denture and a very close inspection is often required to see the small crack at this stage.

Fracture of the denture base

Poor fit

This is a very wide term and can more readily be described under separate headings.

Alveolar resorption

This will be found to be the cause of breakage in dentures which have been worn for some considerable time, or which were made shortly after the extraction of the teeth. The alveolar resorption causes the denture to be unevenly supported and is a common cause of fracture.

Warpage

Dimensional change of acrylic is a cause of further fracture of a denture which has already been repaired.

Relief areas

Failure to relieve the cast in prominent bony areas, like a torus palati, may lead to excessive flexure of a denture. On the other hand, excessive relief may make the denture palate so thin that its weakness causes fracture.

Inaccurate impression

If the impression or cast on which the denture was constructed was not accurate, considerable stresses will be induced in the denture base during mastication owing to the unevenness of its support, and eventually the base may fracture. The length of time before this happens depends on the stresses induced and also on the physical properties and thickness of the material used.

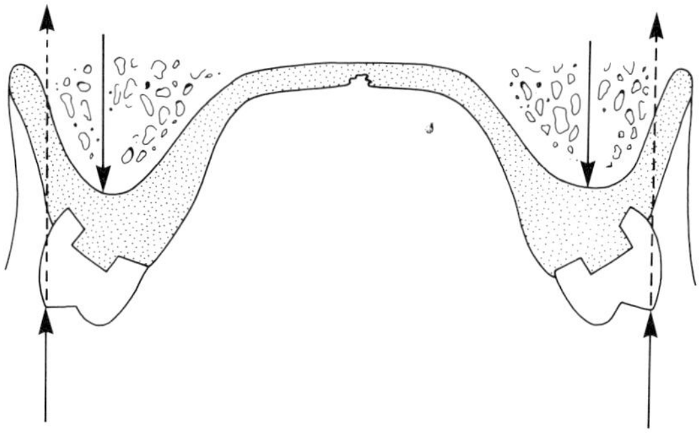

Figure 15.3 Illustrating a cause of midline fracture. The long partially broken arrows represent the forces of mastication applied outside the ridge, which is itself acting as a fulcrum. This would not be the case if the peripheral form was correctly designed (see text)

Position of teeth

It is often assumed that if the upper teeth are set outside the ridge the force of mastication is also applied outside the ridge, the ridge itself becoming a fulcrum point, thus causing a large component force to be transmitted to the midline of the denture; the result is a midline fracture (Figure 15.3).

However, this is an unsound argument provided the periphery is sufficiently wide to ensure a retentive force on the contralateral side as this shifts the fulcrum around which the denture tilts and the load is more evenly distributed. A balanced occlusion is also very important as a factor resisting midline fracture.

Various denture base materials with greater impact and fatigue strength are available, including vinyl copolymers and rubber-acrylic graft copolymers. Another method is to incorporate carbon fibres into the acrylic as this enhances mechanical properties but, at the same time spoils the appearance. Inserting so-called strengtheners, such as wire or mesh, into acrylic has the opposite effect and usually leads to areas of weakness.

In cases of repeated fracture another satisfactory treatment is to provide a cobalt–chromium palate carried up the lingual surfaces of the anterior teeth (see Figure 2.21). This prevents the initial fracture which invariably occurs between the upper incisor teeth, particularly if the teeth are spaced or if there is a labial frenal notch. If a conventional metal palate is used, the acrylic uniting the front teeth still cracks.

Breakage of teeth

Cuspal interference

Where this is confined to one tooth, or in cases where the force is heavier on one tooth than elsewhere, it will frequently cause the tooth to split. An anterior tooth may be broken off if there is excessive overlap with insufficient overjet. In dentures worn for some time the upper anterior teeth are often chipped along the incisal edges. This is due to the progressive alveolar resorption, the shift forwards of the lower denture, the backward shift of the upper denture and the resultant traumatic contact of incisal edges.

Faulty tooth

This is almost entirely confined to porcelain teeth and is very rare when one considers the number of these teeth in use. An undetected flaw in the porcelain usually results in the tooth breaking across the line of the pins and excessive grinding of either the occlusal or ridge surface of a porcelain posterior tooth to facilitate setting will weaken it and cause its fracture in use.

Chapter 16

Techniques for overcoming difficulties encountered in complete dentures

From the facts obtained during the examination and history, the prosthetist should be in a position to anticipate difficulties and by selecting suitable materials and techniques be able to overcome them. There follows a list of problems which may cause varying degrees of difficulty, with suggested methods for obtaining a satisfactory result. Many of the points are discussed elsewhere in the book but are presented here for convenience.

Occlusal pivots

Introduction

After complete dentures have been worn for a number of years and alveolar resorption has continued, changes occur in the occlusion so that load tends to concentrate towards the front of the mouth as the mandible rotates around the condylar axis to compensate for the resorption. This is a most unstable situation and, if new dentures are made without previously correcting it, the occlusal instability produces problems often to the point where the patient rejects the new dentures or, at least, has constant difficulty and mucosal discomfort. The patient who presents with a bag of dentures, none of which has been comfortable, comes into this category.

Action

Occlusal pivots (Figure 16.1) transfer the occlusal load to a transverse axis across the middle of the

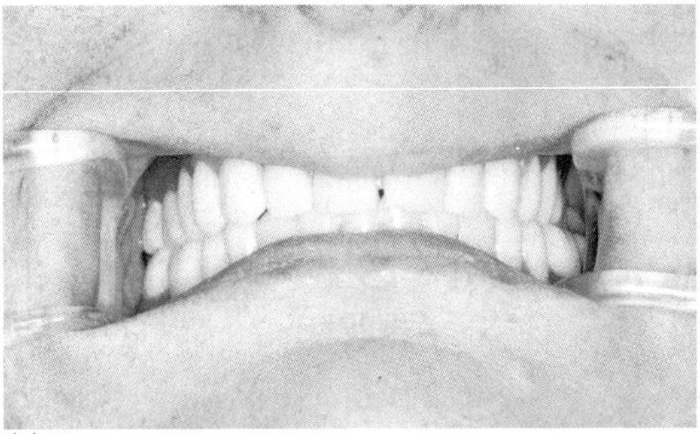

(*a*)

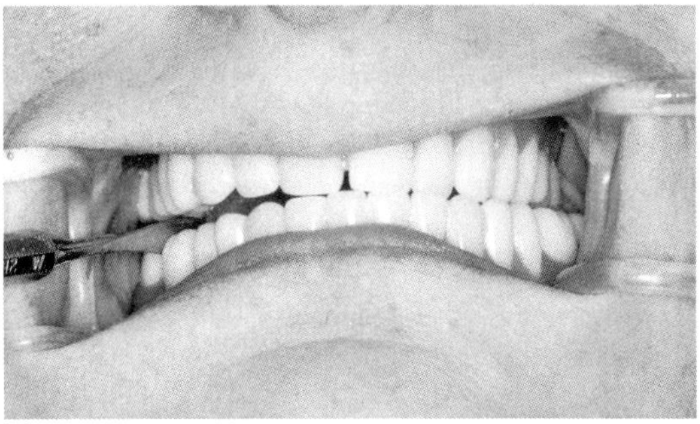

(*b*)

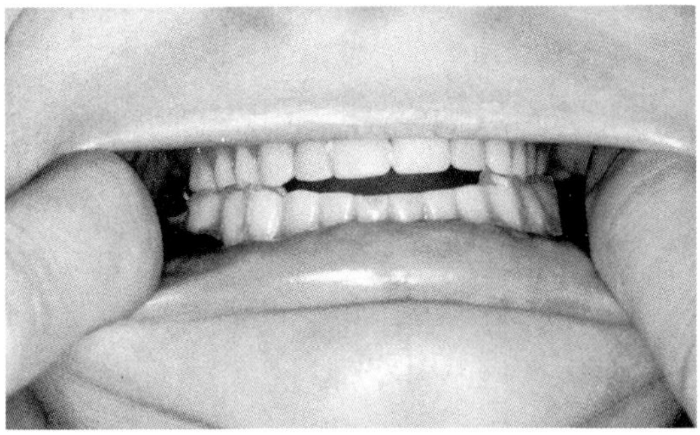

Figure 16.1 Occlusal pivots. (*a*) The dentures which the patient has worn for many years appear to be in good occlusion but (*b*) separation with an instrument is easy. In such cases, (*c*) the occlusion can be temporarily restored with pivots

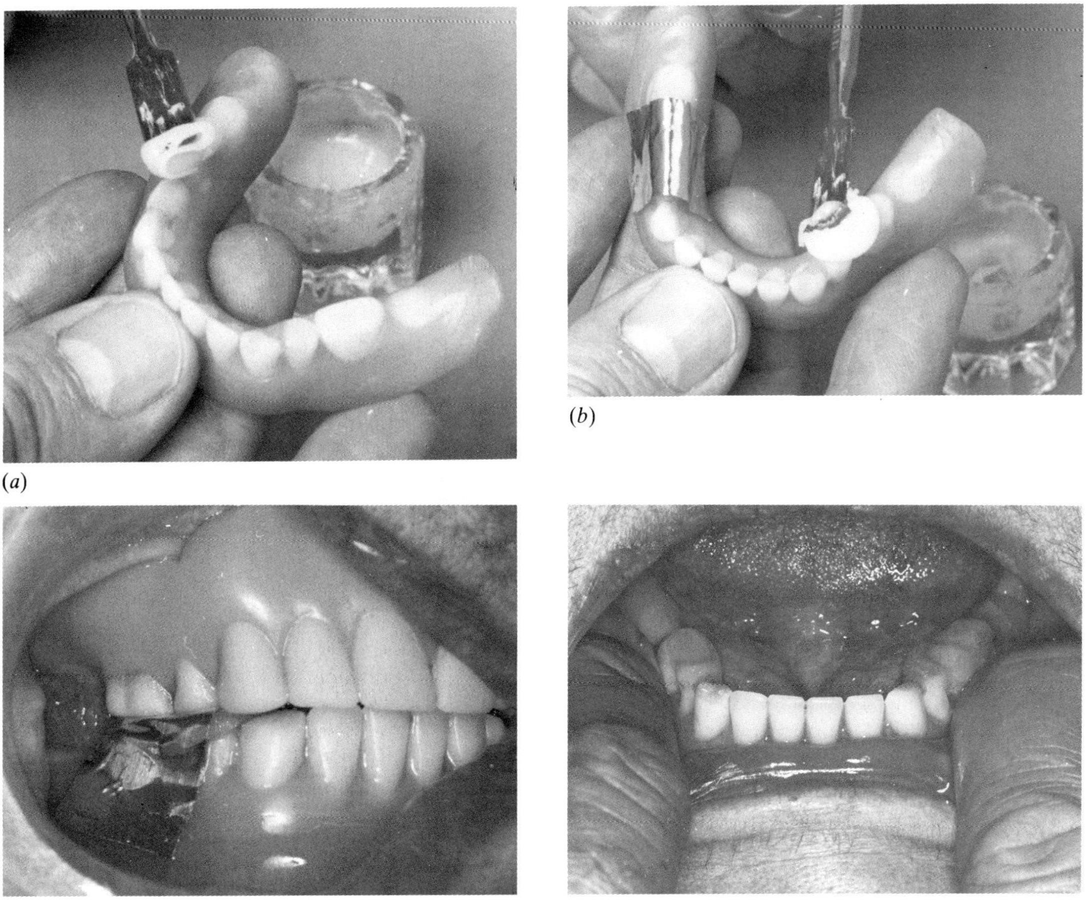

(*a*) (*b*) (*c*) (*d*)

Figure 16.2 Occlusal pivot technique. (*a*) Last molars removed and cold-cure acrylic applied to posterior teeth. (*b*) Protect with thin metal foil. (*c*) Induce patient into a retruded position. (*d*) Pivots stabilize the mandibular position prior to replacement dentures

denture and cause the mandible to take up a more posterior position; this has the effect of spreading loads more evenly over the supporting mucosa. Because pivots are temporary, modifications can be made until the patient is more comfortable. New dentures can then be made.

Technique

The cusps of the upper posterior teeth and canines are reduced with a stone to create a flat occlusal table (Figure 16.2). Broad lower posterior teeth should be narrowed to increase the tongue space. Remove all four second molars to provide lingual shelves so that the patient will have better control of the dentures. Reduce the occlusal surface of the lower posterior teeth if the vertical dimension is too great. If the incisal guidance angle is excessive, reduce the length of the lower incisors.

A square of tin foil is cut to cover the teeth of each lower posterior quadrant. The foil is removed and laid aside. A mix of clear, cold-cure acrylic is adapted to the occlusal surfaces of the second premolars and first molars on each side of the lower denture. The prepared foil hood is laid on the acrylic, both dentures inserted and the patient induced into a retruded position. Care is taken that the patient closes gently on the foil while the dentures are held in place by the operator's index fingers. The lower denture is removed and placed in hot water to hasten the polymerization of the cold-cure resin and returned to the mouth before polymerization is complete, at which time the patient is asked to close more firmly on the foil. The denture is again returned to hot water until polymerization is complete, the foil peeled off, and the excess resin removed by cutting stones. The denture is returned to the mouth when there should be a simultaneous contact on both sides but, if not, the newly polymerized resin can easily be adjusted. The pivots are then polished.

Follow-up treatment

In spite of the relatively small occlusal surface of the pivots, many patients remark on the improved comfort and masticatory efficiency. In some cases, where the habitually protruded or lateral mandibular positions have developed over many years, a number of modifications to the pivots will be required until the mandibular position is stable.

Tissue conditioner

Because of occlusal faults or changes and continuing alveolar resorption the mucosa under complete dentures is liable to be injured by traumatic loads. The health of the tissue may also deteriorate if the hygiene is neglected.

Under these conditions the mucosa should be rehabilitated before further corrective prosthetic treatment is undertaken. Tissue conditioners, consisting of ethyl alcohol, aromatic esters and small particle acrylic polymer, can be used for this purpose (Figure 16.3).

Technique

The dentures are dried, a mix of tissue conditioner added to the fitting surfaces and both dentures inserted into the mouth; the patient occludes lightly and the tissue conditioner is adapted around the lingual and buccal peripheries of the dentures and left in the mouth for a few minutes. The excess tissue conditioner is trimmed off with curved scissors or a scalpel blade. The patient is instructed not to distort the material with a brush but to clean the denture only under running water.

At the recall visit a few days later modifications or additions may be necessary to the tissue conditioner. This may have to be done over a few visits until the mucosal health is improved. Between visits the patient should be instructed in careful oral hygiene. Brushing the mucosa with a soft badger hair toothbrush is very useful but this should be done lightly for the first few days otherwise the mucosa may be damaged.

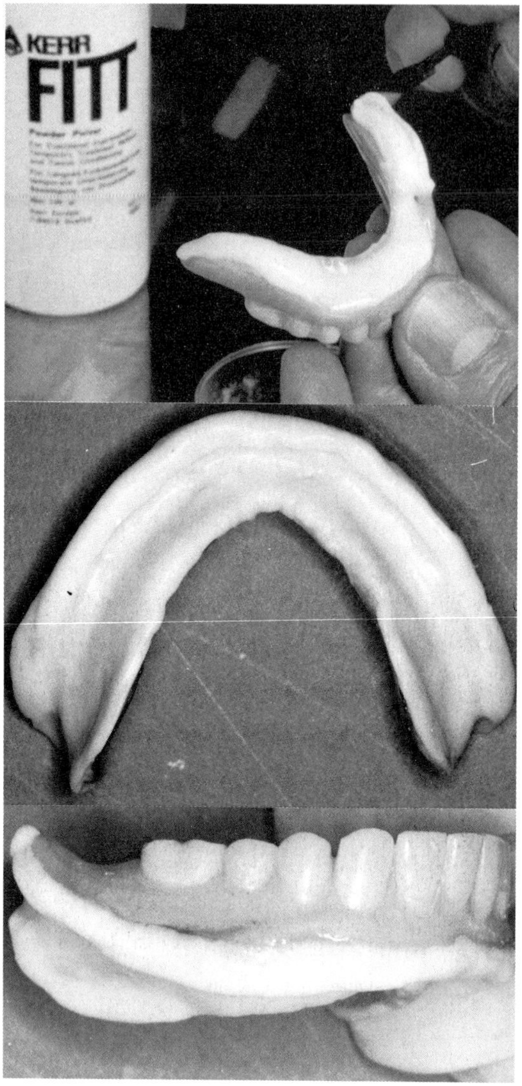

Figure 16.3 Tissue conditioner on complete lower dentures

Replica dentures

A technique in use for many years, and which has gained increasing popularity recently because of the advent of reliable duplicating methods and pouring acrylics, is that of copying a patient's existing denture to produce a replica. An impression is taken with the replica in the mouth and the new denture made to the same shape and size of the replica which is then discarded.

It is a technique particularly suitable for older patients who have had the same dentures for many years. These dentures may have obvious faults and discrepancies according to the dentist, but to the patient they are perfectly comfortable and acceptable. The patient consults the dentist because the dentures feel a little slack or because the teeth are becoming worn away. In other respects there are no complaints. If the dentist decides it would not be prudent to make any alteration to these dentures then the replica technique has much to commend it.

At an arranged appointment the patient's dentures are embedded in a flask and an alginate, agar or silicone impression made of the whole of each denture. The dentures are removed and returned to the patient who is then dismissed. The impressions are poured in cold-cure acrylic to produce the replicas.

At the second appointment impressions are taken in each replica, the usual material being zinc oxide–eugenol paste but other impression materials may be used. The periphery may be altered by adding tracing stick compound. The replicas are usually in occlusion during this procedure and so a closed-mouth impression technique is used. If the occlusion is very disrupted modifications can be made on the replicas (Figure 16.4).

The replicas are poured in the laboratory and mounted on the articulator with or without a facebow according to choice. Buccal and lingual registers are poured to ensure exact copying of the polished surfaces and tooth position. The replicas are removed, discarded and replaced by wax, and the teeth set in position. These wax dentures may then be checked in the mouth or they may be flasked and finished in acrylic, the choice depending on circumstances.

There are many variations of the replica technique but the essential aims are the same. The advantages for older patients, and particularly those who are handicapped or housebound, are the easy transition from old dentures to new, the repetition of familiar polished surfaces, the relatively unaltered occlusal form and less clinical time.

The disadvantages of the technique are that design faults are repeated, facial form is seldom fully restored, inefficiencies of existing dentures are not eliminated and special impression techniques cannot be used.

The advantages in most cases, however, outweigh the disadvantages.

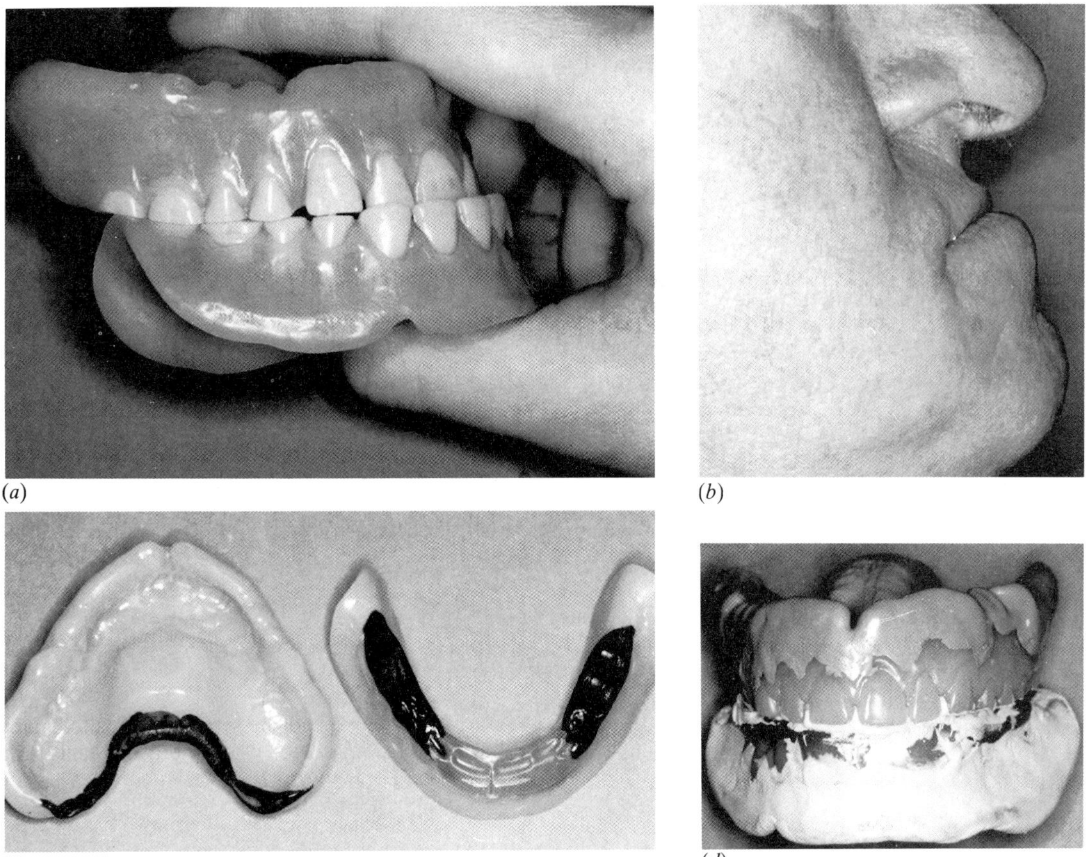

Figure 16.4 Replica dentures. (*a*) After some years the acrylic teeth have been abraded and the mandible postures forwards with loss of occlusal face height. (*b*) The prognathic appearance. (*c*) On the replica dentures a postdam is placed and a correct jaw relation record made. (*d*) Closed-mouth impressions: upper polysulphide, lower zinc oxide–eugenol paste

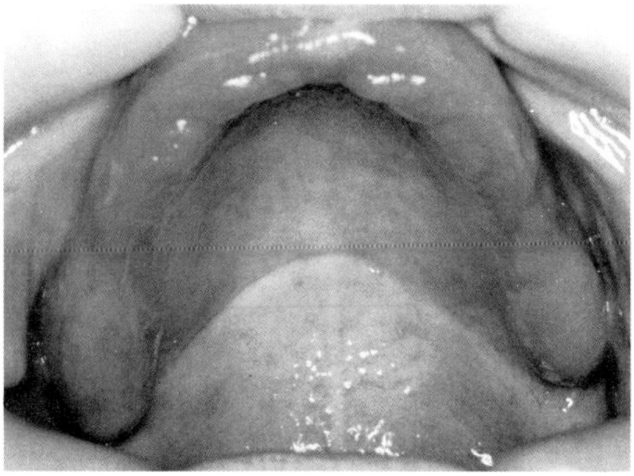

Figure 16.5 Denture-induced stomatitis

Denture-induced stomatitis

This is sometimes termed denture sore mouth but it is usually symptomless and so denture stomatitis is a more appropriate term. It is an expression of oral candidiasis as the yeast-like fungus *Candida albicans* is usually implicated.

In a typical patient the maxillary denture-bearing area appears inflamed and oedematous and the oral hygiene is poor (Figure 16.5). The denture is usually worn night and day and there is often an associated angular cheilitis of the lips. The patient is often unaware of any problem although the stomatitis is of a chronic nature.

Treatment

The dentures are thoroughly cleaned and polished. An ultrasonic cleansing bath with a detergent solution is useful. Instructions in strict oral hygiene and a fungicide are prescribed, e.g.

Nystatin ointment	(100 000 units/g)
Amphotericin B	(50 mg 6-hourly)
Miconazole	(250 mg 6-hourly)

Nystatin ointment is smeared on the dried fitting surface of the denture which is removed after meals, scrubbed with detergent and fungicide reapplied. The denture is best worn at night during this treatment as this also helps the angular cheilitis. The carbohydrate intake should be reduced.

This regimen may be continued for about a week after which the dentures are removed at night and immersed in hypochlorite solution. At this stage any

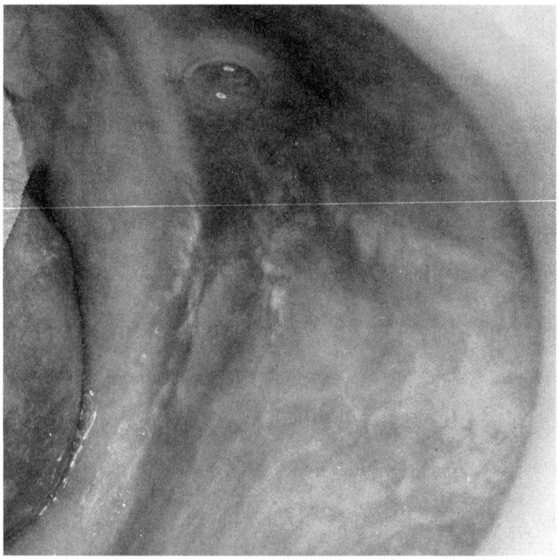

(*a*)

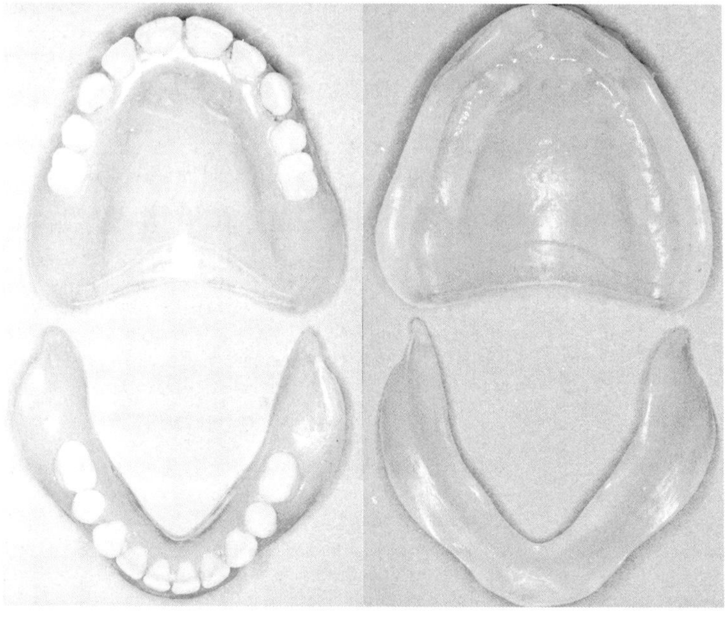

(*b*)

Figure 16.6 (*a*) Lichen planus in the lower left buccal sulcus of an edentulous patient. Trauma from dentures must be avoided. (*b*) Note the shape of the lower denture, the polished periphery and the long lingual shelf to allow tongue control. The lower cast was metal-foiled to ensure a smooth surface and the occlusion carefully equilibrated obvious faults in the dentures are rectified and steps taken to replace the dentures as soon as the stomatitis has cleared. The mucosal oedema is reduced by tissue conditioner combined with brushing by the patient with a soft badger toothbrush.

The folds at the corners of the mouth are reduced by the replacement dentures partly by ensuring an increase in vertical dimension but mostly by restoring the lips and cheeks to their pre-extraction form. In persistent cases there is advantage in burnishing 0.06 mm metal foil over the master cast to produce an atraumatic acrylic fitting surface, or to make the denture with a swaged stainless steel or yellow gold base which produces a non-porous surface with good thermal conductivity, factors favourable to prevention.

It should be realized that denture-induced stomatitis, which can take the form of pin-point hyperaemia, diffuse hyperaemia or granular enlargement, can be difficult to treat and continuing supervision of patients is essential.

Other mucosal problems are shown in Figures 16.6 and 16.7.

Allergy

An allergic or hypersensitive state is one of specifically altered reaction to a particular substance. It may be induced by continuous or frequently repeated exposure to an allergenic substance.

Signs are often singularly lacking in patients complaining of allergy and too much reliance cannot be placed on symptoms only, the latter ranging from general intolerance to dentures to areas of irritation or discomfort. Burning mouth is a common symptom but it is important to differentiate between a primary irritant and a truly allergic reaction.

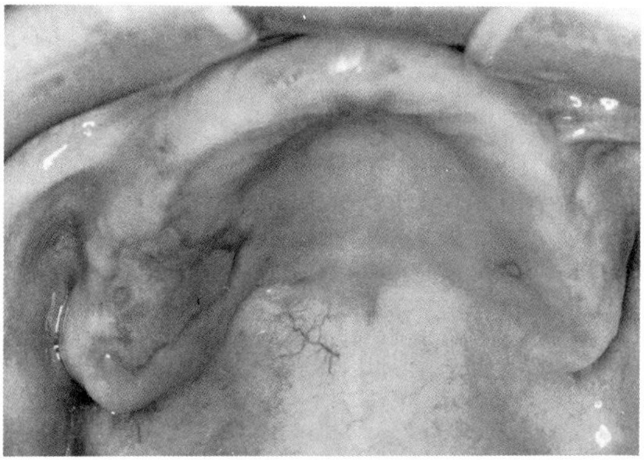

Figure 16.7 Benign mucous membrane pemphigoid. As the mucosa is easily traumatized the denture fitting surface should be as smooth as possible (see Figure 16.6). Stability and occlusal balance are essential to reduce movement

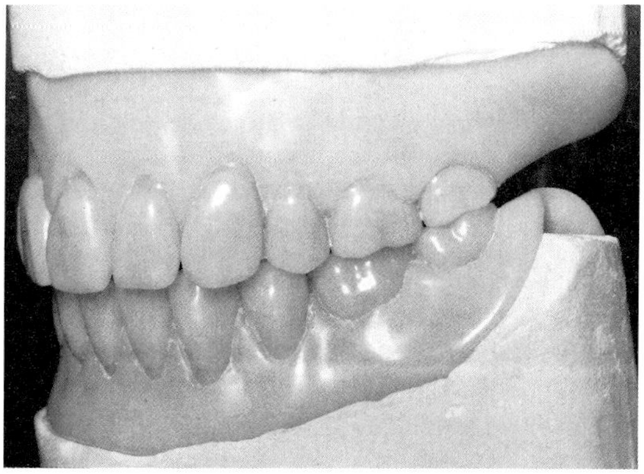

Figure 16.8 The use of nylon 12 as denture base material and porcelain teeth in a case of acrylic hypersensitivity. Note the difficulty of finishing this material around the gingival margins

In spite of the undoubted qualities and excellent properties of standard heat-cured polymethyl methacrylate as a denture base material, there is occasionally a need for a different polymer either because of limitations in the mechanical properties of acrylic or because of the possibility of a hypersensitivity (allergy) to one or other of its components.

The type of situation in which either nylon or high molecular weight acrylic might be used as a denture base material is where there is a suspected hypersensitivity or allergy to a particular constituent (Figure 16.8). Such cases can be investigated by a contact hypersensitivity test in which small stainless steel chambers contain the potential allergen in a vehicle of petroleum jelly or distilled water. These chambers are adhered to the skin on the patient's back with Stanpore (similar to micropore) and the site identified with an indelible pencil or similar mark. The allergens are made up according to international laboratory concentrations and comprise a wide range of different materials depending on the nature of the patient's history and complaint. The skin site is examined after 48 h and again at 96 h for any obvious reaction. In some cases there is a delayed reaction which may occur some time after the 96 h period. In the event of a positive reaction it may be assumed that the particular allergen should be omitted from a denture. This usually means turning to an entirely different material, e.g. polycarbonate, vulcanite, nylon or high molecular weight acrylic.

Hypersensitivity can be confusing and fraught with pitfalls for the clinically unwary and very often signs and symptoms can easily be explained without having to make a diagnosis of allergy.

Burning mouth

Some patients complain of a burning or tingling sensation when wearing complete dentures. The symptoms are often so severe that the dentures cannot be tolerated for more than a few hours. The feeling may be restricted to parts of the mouth, e.g. anterior tongue or palate, or it may be widespread including the lips.

It is a complex problem and the following list is helpful in deciding on the aetiology:

Deficiency: vitamin B12, folate, iron
Infections: staphylococcal, candidiasis
Psychogenic: cancerophobia, depression, hypochondria, climacteric
Idiopathic: erythema migrans
Prosthetic: occlusal faults, bony irregularity, denture trauma.

The possible prosthetic causes will be discussed further. Movement of the denture bases tends to exacerbate the symptoms of burning and so the occlusion should be balanced in all positions and, for the same reason, attention paid to the form and shape of the polished surfaces. It is usually said that dentures of high quality will reduce the symptoms considerably. Sometimes the burning is restricted to the anterior third of the tongue. This is often assumed to be a cancerophobic feeling about oral cancer but, in most cases, it is due to a restricted tongue space in the denture either because the upper anterior teeth are set back on the ridge and so the tongue continually taps them, or because the lower posterior teeth are set so far lingually that they irritate the sides of the tongue.

Burning may also be due to a spiky or rough lower alveolar ridge which can be tested by finger palpation and confirmed by radiograph, but a less commonly observed cause of burning, and one which is often missed by clinicians, is a rough cortical border in the upper jaw which is difficult to detect by finger palpation or by radiograph. Examination of a dried skull, however, shows how this can easily occur as the labial cancellous bone resorbs to leave the sharp palatal cortex (Figure 16.9). Pressure of the mucosa on this sharp bone has an itching, irritant effect which tends to build up in the form of burning. Another cause of this complaint is pressure on the various foramina in the mouth, particularly the incisive foramen beneath the incisive papilla which is often distorted by the impression or by the denture. Burning mouth is often confused with allergy and hypersenstivity to various dental materials and many patients with burning mouth become convinced that this is the root cause of the problem. This is seldom the case. Allergy is discussed elsewhere in this chapter.

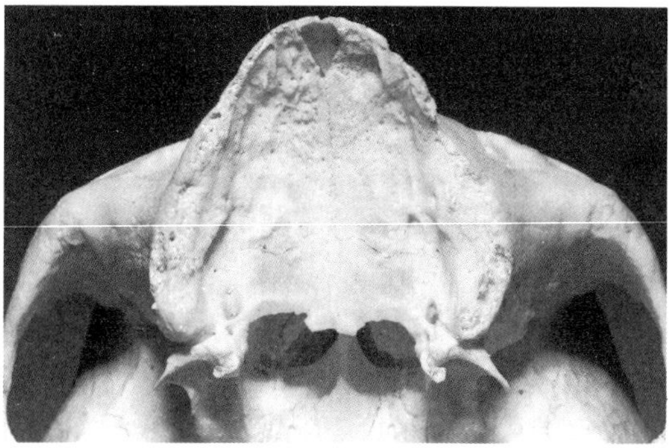

Figure 16.9 Resorption of residual alveolar maxillary bone results in a sharp palatal cortical ridge

Dry mouth

Dry mouth or xerostomia is characterized by a reduction in salivary flow, although it has to be said that some patients complain of a dry mouth when in fact the amount of saliva is normal.

The effect of reduced saliva in complete denture patients is twofold: liability to trauma and reduction in retention.

Saliva is a lubricant and in its absence the mucosa is more vulnerable to trauma from denture movement. Impressions should be recorded in one of the elastomeric materials or zinc oxide–eugenol paste and poured in a vacuum mixed stone to eliminate porosity. The surfaces of the casts should ideally be covered with thin metal foil (0.06 mm) to produce a smooth denture surface. Movement of the dentures is reduced by ensuring the occlusion is balanced in all mandibular positions and the polished surfaces designed to be in harmony with the dry lips and cheeks.

Retention depends partly on the surface forces of adhesion and cohesion; in the absence of saliva these forces are reduced. However, the main retentive force is derived from the peripheral seal and this is only marginally affected by lack of saliva if the periphery of the denture is correctly designed with the emphasis on width rather than height. Retention problems experienced in the presence of dry mouth are more related to the tense unyielding mucosa found in such patients, rather than the absence or reduction of saliva.

Nevertheless, a dry mouth is unpleasant for a complete denture patient and particularly if it has developed in a short time such as occurs after irradiation in the treatment of neoplasms. The following list of palliative treatments is useful to help these patients:

1. 50% solution of glycerine in water flavoured with lemon juice before meals.
2. Sucking a sour (tart) sugar-free candy or chewing sugar-free gum.

3. Drinking alkaline water (Vichy).
4. Increase the intake of fresh fruit and vegetables, with a decrease of carbohydrate. Nicotinamide is occasionally prescribed.
5. Application of bland creams e.g. almond oil, lanolin or cocoa butter to lips and mucosa.
6. Pilocarpine to stimulate gland secretion.
7. Gum tragacanth mixed with glycerine or paraffin oil applied to dentures.
8. Silicone spray or cream.
9. Various synthetic salivas containing polyethylene oxide or hydroxypropyl methylcellulose (Hypromellose) or sodium carboxymethylcellulose (Glandosane).

Retching

Retching or gagging may be a problem when impressions are being recorded or when dentures are inserted. Some patients start to retch weeks or months after dentures have been satisfactorily fitted. The range or degree of severity is very wide and the following list describes different types of patients:

Very severe: these patients seldom seek dental treatment
Severe: they tend to retch at the beginning of examination
Difficult: retching takes place in spite of the most careful clinical technique
Problem: these patients can wear dentures for only a few minutes
Occasional: they manage with dentures but certain movements, e.g. grinding the teeth, cause retching.

There are a number of methods of dealing with the problem. It is important to give the patient a feeling of confidence and, probably more important, a feeling of confidence on the part of the dentist. It is likely that in the past the patient has had some unfortunate dental experience, or very badly designed dentures, that has made him retch and it is natural that he is apprehensive.

The palate may be sprayed with surface anaesthetic or ethyl chloride prior to recording the impression. Other methods include local analgesia to anaesthetize the palate combined with refrigerant spray of the posterior third of the tongue which is often implicated as much as the palate in the retching reflex. Hypnotherapy is also used, as are various types of behaviour therapy. Barbiturates may be used to depress the central nervous system, antihistamines to lower the feeling of sickness, or parasympathetic depressants to reduce the salivary flow which increases at the outset of retching.

It is usually wise to have the patient's head upright and to record the lower preliminary impression first; an impression material with minimum flow such as impressions compound is recommended. Either silicone or heavy-bodied polysulphide is suitable for master impressions.

One method of conditioning the patient is to make an acrylic base-plate which he wears as much as possible over a few weeks. Teeth and denture matrix are then added after the patient is sufficiently confident. It is important that the base-plate is retentive as any detectable looseness will undermine progress.

The retching reflex can be gradually extinguished by having the patient press on the palate with a toothbrush without making himself retch. Over a few weeks the brush is laid further and further back on the palate until it can touch the soft palate without causing distress. This is a very useful technique as it goes to the core of the problem, i.e. the patient has to come to terms with his excitable reflex which he himself has to learn to control. As soon as the patient can demonstrate his success to the dentist, impressions are recorded and the dentures made.

Dentures that cause retching usually have obvious faults. Lack of retention, under-extended bases, restricted tongue space and marked occlusal faults are common. Less common is the heavy incisal contact on protrusion which causes minor movements of the postdam region of the upper denture. This milks glandular secretions under the denture and as this mucus collects it irritates the mucosa and causes a feeling of retching. If the patient removes the denture and washes it the feeling of retching disappears and such a history is diagnostic.

Whenever dentures are made for a patient with a history of retching it is important to see him the day after the dentures are delivered, and frequently thereafter, to maintain the progress and to avoid any relapse. In this sense, treatment can be very time-consuming.

Metal denture bases

Stainless steel (Figure 16.10)

Stainless steel was introduced as a denture base material around 1921. Swaging was carried out by means of a hydraulic press and was prolonged and laborious. Nowadays hydraulic high energy forming is used with oil under compression.

Because of its high ductility it is easily formed to give an accurate reproduction of the surface of a die. Strain hardening during the forming process raises the proportional limit to develop sufficient strength in the finished denture base. With its high resistance to corrosion it does not tarnish in the mouth, and since a high gloss finish is easily obtained, this further increases resistance to tarnish.

Modern casting methods have tended to supersede swaging techniques and, since the advent of

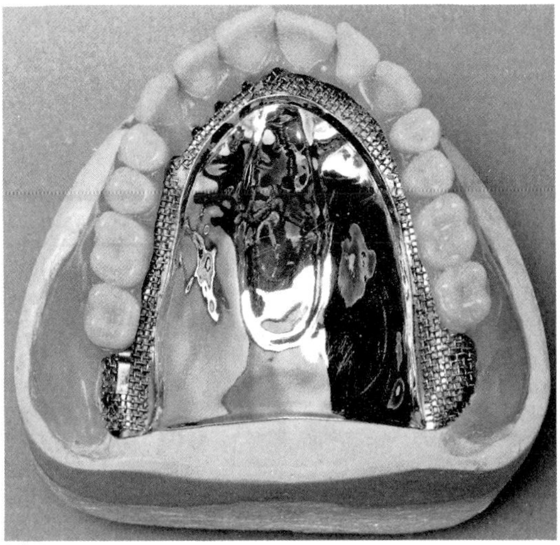

(*a*)

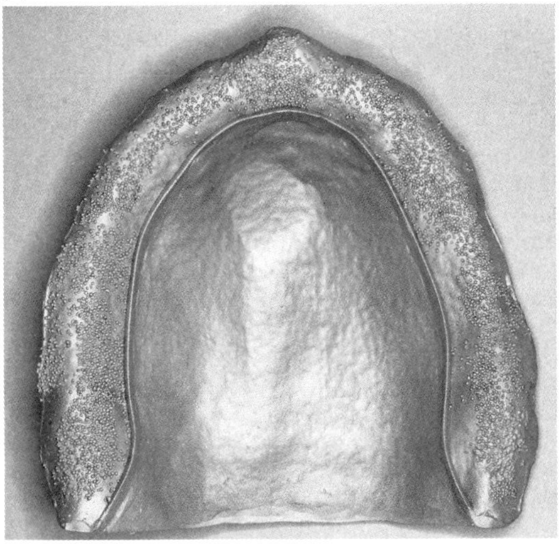

(*b*)

Figure 16.10 (*a*) Stainless steel base for complete upper denture. Tooth position should always be determined first to ensure correct location of palatal stop, (*b*) (cast cobalt–chromium base shown for comparison)

cobalt–chromium alloys, the vast majority of metal bases are now cast. However, in certain clinical situations, a place still exists for the stainles steel base in dentistry. The smooth fitting surface can be an advantage in some cases; the fact that stainless steel is the thinnest denture base possible is good for patient tolerance; and in those cases where opposing teeth leave little space to accommodate a denture base, a thin stainless steel base is of great use.

Cast alloys

Cast cobalt–chromium or yellow gold alloy may be used as alternatives to acrylic to form bases of complete dentures. Metal has several good features:

1. Greater impact, flexural and fatigue strengths.
2. Because of these superior physical qualities alloys can be used in thin section and so the palate feels less bulky to the patient.
3. High thermal conductivity enables normal sensations of heat and cold to be appreciated.
4. A metallic surface is easier to keep clean and less liable to plaque deposit.
5. The presence of a metallic palate in an upper denture, or a metal base in a lower denture, eliminates much of the dimensional change taking place during and after polymerization of acrylic. This is especially beneficial in complete lower dentures because of their horseshoe-shape and their medial distortion after de-flasking.

V-shaped palate

Retention by adhesion is diminished because the palate, having sloping sides, offers only a small area which is horizontal to a vertical displacing force. Acrylic denture bases tend to warp during curing and the imperfect fit at the sharp angle of the palate further reduces the surface forces.

Satisfactory results will depend on the excellence of the peripheral seal obtained in the impression technique, because the main retentive factor in these cases is atmospheric pressure. In the midline there is often a fissure and the acrylic must fill this, especially in the postdam region, to maintain seal.

Flat palate with shallow ridges

The denture may easily be displaced during mastication through lack of ridge offering no lateral

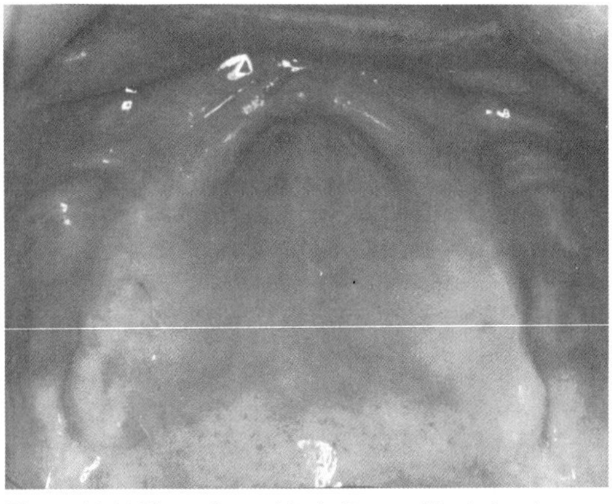

Figure 16.11 Flat palate with shallow residual alveolar ridge. The incisive papilla is anterior to the ridge. Note the absence of definable tuberosities and the generalized hyperaemia

resistance; the shallow sulci adversely influence peripheral seal (Figure 16.11).

An impression technique which ensures adequate peripheral width is essential so that seal is maintained between the cheeks, lip and the buccal surface of the denture. The denture periphery should not be polished. Balanced occlusion with a low cusp tooth is advisable.

Undercut ridges

Retention may be reduced as the denture will have to be trimmed so that it may pass over the bulbous ridge, thus causing loss of peripheral seal.

Treatment: (a) The most satisfactory result is obtained when an alveolectomy is carried out, as the operator is then able to construct a denture having the maximum peripheral seal. (b) When a denture is trimmed, or the undercuts blocked out on the cast, some reduction in peripheral seal may result unless care is taken to maintain seal against the cheek i.e. on the buccal side of the denture border.

Spiky lower ridge

The patient with a ridge of this type frequently complains of pain during mastication and clenching as the pressure on the denture compresses the soft tissue between the fitting surface and the spiky process forming the crest of the alveolar ridge (Figure 16.12).

Treatment: (a) surgery to reduce the sharp alveolar crest; (b) relieve the ridge area of the cast with an adequate thickness of tin foil; (c) an unemployed ridge impression technique; (d) a resilient lining, but this may not succeed as the silicone rubber drags the mucosa across the spiky ridge.

Reducing the vertical dimension in such cases may be advantageous as this reduces the force applied during mastication.

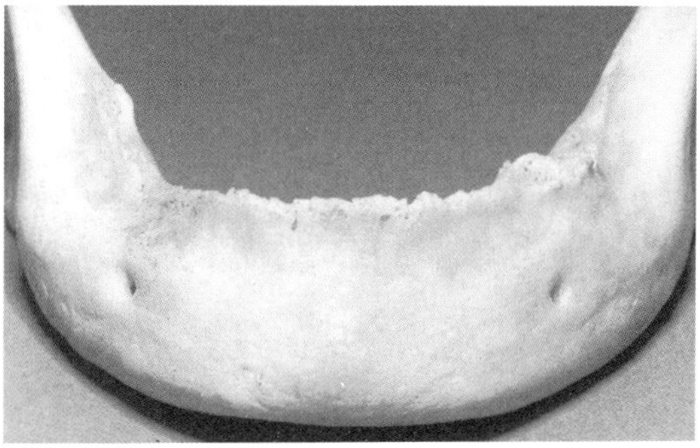

Figure 16.12 Mandible with spiky, irregular bony crest which, if present clinically, is difficult to manage because of the unfavourable support

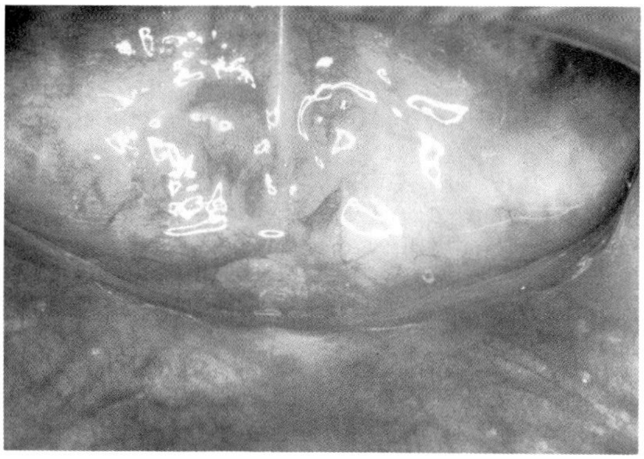

Figure 16.13 Flat lower ridge. The attached mucosa is very narrow and there is no resistance to lateral movement of a denture

Usually the most satisfactory results are obtained after an alveolectomy since this removes the cause. However, when surgical treatment is contraindicated some reduction in the pain and discomfort experienced by the patient may be obtained by relieving the ridge area, thereby placing the greater proportion of the occlusal load on the lateral borders of the ridge but this, occasionally, can be just as painful. A denture constructed with a resilient lining usually reduces the symptoms, but the lining has to be replaced periodically as it deteriorates.

Flat lower ridge

The shape of the ridge provides no resistance to lateral movements of the denture and the actions of the adjacent buccal and lingual musculature are often unfavourable (Figure 16.13).

Treatment: a peripherally adapted impression having adequate extension onto the retromolar pads, and the teeth set up to produce balanced articulation. The prosthetic adage that 'the flatter the ridge, the flatter the teeth' is probably true and so zero-cusp or low-cusp teeth should be used.

High lower anterior ridge

Anterior denture teeth of normal length would present a large surface area for the lip to press against.

A more stable denture is obtained if short anterior teeth are used as lip pressure is then limited to a smaller area and the denture is not so readily displaced backwards. Alveolectomy may permit normal-sized teeth to be used anteriorly but it will result in the loss of very useful ridge support.

Large torus palati

The denture may rock across the midline and eventually fracture, particularly if the occlusion is not balanced. Retention is reduced as the torus prevents the denture bedding into the soft tissue if it is not relieved and the overall support of the denture, when loaded on one side, is also reduced.

Large tuberosity

If the tuberosity is large in a buccal direction then fitting the finished denture requires considerable trimming with loss of peripheral seal.

Treatment should be directed to (a) surgical removal of part of the tuberosity, (b) undercut area blocked out on the cast or (c) denture flange carried only slightly into the undercut area.

The most satisfactory denture is produced if the undercut is eliminated by surgical means as maximum peripheral seal can then be achieved. If the undercut is only blocked out a space will exist, allowing the ingress of air and food between the denture and the tissue in that area, which will have an adverse effect on retention. If the flange is carried only slightly into the undercut area intimate contact between the denture and tissue is maintained, but since the flange does not extend into the full depth of the sulcus the peripheral seal is reduced.

When the tuberosity is fibrous and pendulous it invades the inter-ridge space and not only prevents full base extension of the lower denture, but also presents difficulties in setting the upper teeth with an adequate compensating curve. Alginate impressions are taken and the casts mounted in the retruded jaw relationship. This gives an indication of the amount of tissue that has to be surgically removed. Before doing this a radiograph should be taken to confirm the level of alveolar bone, the position of the maxillary sinus and the possibility of an unerupted tooth. Surgical reduction is by wedge excision.

Abnormal frena

A denture tends to be more easily displaced when frena are attached near to the crest of the ridge and surgical removal should be considered. In the region of the frenum the periphery of the denture should be as broad as elsewhere, although the frenal curve is flatter. Avoid easing the denture in the frenal notch otherwise peripheral seal will be lost.

Variation in tissue compressibility

One of the aims in treatment is to create a stable denture and where the foundation tissues are of uneven compressibility this may be difficult. A compression impression technique and balanced articulation when setting the teeth are essential if the available support is to be correctly utilized. A flabby anterior maxillary ridge is a good example of this problem.

Tight lower lip

Instability of the lower denture due to the backward displacement caused by lip pressure, and vertical lift occurring in the premolar and canine region from the pressure of the modioli, are problems where the ridge is flat and the lip is tight.

Treatment: (a) keep the occlusal plane low thus reducing the contact area with the lip; (b) adequate extension on to the retromolar pads to counteract the lip pressure; (c) keep the denture narrow across the premolar area; (d) upper canines and premolars should be set in their pre-extraction positions to resist the pressure of the modioli on the lower denture; (e) tongue space impression (see next section).

Large tongue

If the tongue is cramped, or the teeth set so that they overhang it, the denture will be moved during function (Figure 16.14).

Treatment: (a) keep the occlusal plane low; (b) provide the maximum intermolar distance by using narrow teeth or grinding away the lingual cusps; (c) anterior teeth should be set slightly forward of the ridge; (d) peripherally trimmed impression technique; (e) remove last molars (Figure 16.15).

Tongue space impression

In a patient with considerable loss of mandibular alveolar bone, an enlarged tongue and a tight lower

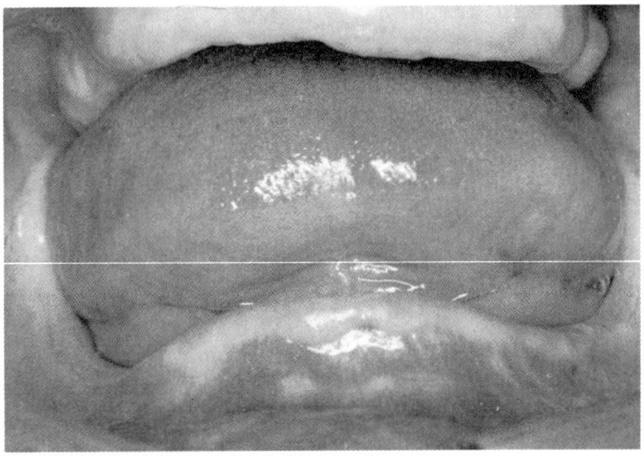

Figure 16.14 Edentulous patient with large tongue. Tooth position on the denture must be correct and the base extension designed accurately

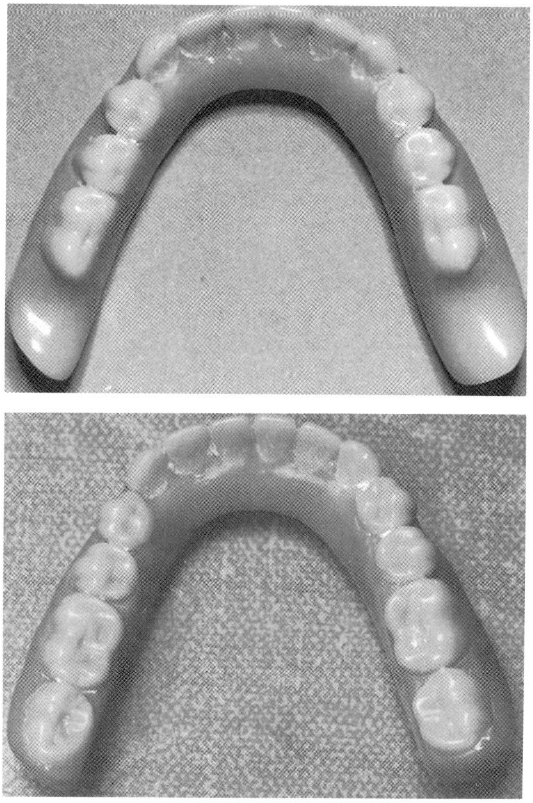

Figure 16.15 Lower denture restricting the tongue space can be improved by removing the last molar and reducing the buccolingual width of the remaining posterior teeth. Note the creation of the posterior lingual shelf

lip, there are difficulties in positioning the lower teeth and defining the tongue space. At the jaw registration stage the wax of the lower occlusion rim is cut out in the incisor region and replaced with soft wax, made of carding wax or a mixture of base-plate wax and petrolatum. Both blocks are inserted and the soft wax is moulded by lip and tongue movements which usually bend the wax forwards to create a labial hollow in which the lip can function. The lower incisors are set to the same inclination as the moulded wax which may be as much as 45° to the vertical plane. This technique is suitable for both aesthetics and function.

Close inter-ridge distance

This is a problem found in Angle class II malocclusion cases and in many groups of the coloured races. It is important to cover the maximum territory with each denture base but thinning of acrylic leads to reduced strength. It is not essential to set the total number of posterior teeth in each quadrant, but a competent intercuspal contact is essential for good function and maintenance of jaw relations. A high impact strength acrylic with acrylic teeth should be used. Metal bases may be considered but the junction between the metal and the acrylic base is a source of weakness.

In extreme cases where the alveolar ridges almost touch in the rest position of the mandible, surgical reduction should be carried out with the study casts mounted to give the surgeon a clear indication of the amount of bone removal required.

The usual fault in these cases is that the lower teeth, because of the reduced space between the crests of the ridges, are set too far buccally and so the denture has the wrong shape. The lower lip easily dislodges it.

Length of time the patient has been endentulous

Patients without teeth, or having had anterior teeth only for many months, develop a habit of protrusive chewing which causes difficulty when recording the position of occlusion. Permanent acrylic bases are made on the master casts with wax occlusion rims. At the time of jaw registration a retruded relation should be made but because of the previous history this may be difficult. Teeth are set, but in the lower posterior quadrants cold-cure acrylic occlusal pivots are made rather than teeth. These give the facility to alter the occlusal position after the dentures have been fitted. When the occlusion is finally stabilized the acrylic pivots are replaced by posterior teeth.

Prominent pre-maxilla

This may cause prominence of the upper lip when a denture possessing a labial flange is fitted but this is usually due to the fact that the flange is too thick or the teeth wrongly positioned. The teeth should be set in their pre-extraction positions, but perhaps at a higher level, and after the denture has been fitted the flange is reduced in thickness from the labial aspect until it is about 1 mm thin (Figure 16.16). If it is made as thin as this in the laboratory it may require easing on the fitting surface at the time of insertion and there would be insufficient acrylic.

Gum-fitted anterior teeth lead to loss of retention, varying in degree according to the shape of the posterior ridges and other factors of retention and, wherever possible, should not be used. Alveolectomy produces a satisfactory result as a labial flange can then be utilized thus providing maximum peripheral seal, but it does have the drawback of removing valuable cortical bone. This can be prevented by using the technique of alveolotomy but if the pre-maxilla is very prominent insufficient space will be gained by this more conservative method of surgery.

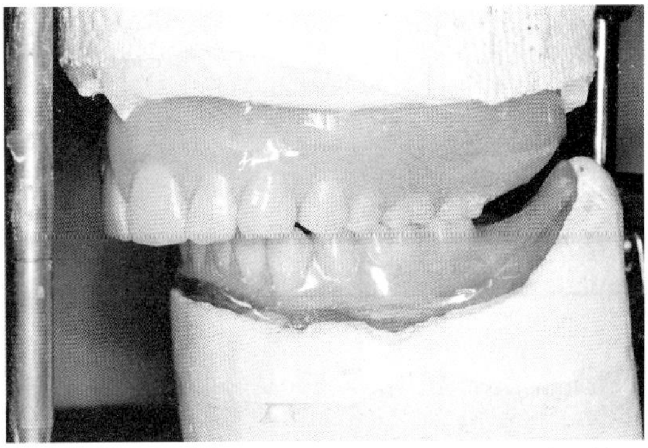

Figure 16.16 Prominent pre-maxilla. Denture made with thin labial flange. Maxillary anterior teeth are set in the pre-extraction position but at a slightly higher level

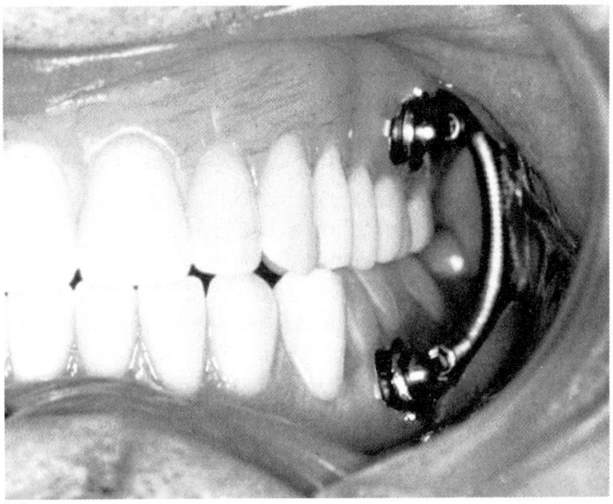

(*a*)

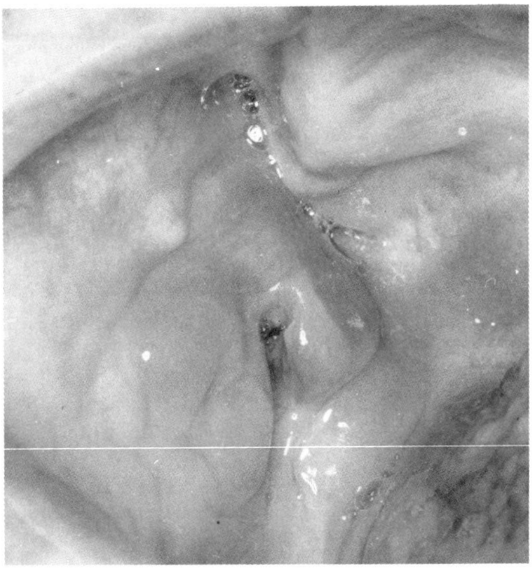

Figure 16.17 (*a*) Complete dentures in occlusion showing springs and swivels on the left side. (*b*) On another patient a view of the right cheek shows damage resulting from wearing dentures fitted with springs and swivels

Aids to retention

There are certain devices which are intended to keep complete dentures in place but their permanent use should only be employed as a last resort, and some not at all.

Springs

These are made of coiled stainless steel, gold-plated base metal or nylon and have their ends attached to swivels in the premolar areas on both sides of the upper and lower dentures. The dentures are thus permanently attached to each other and are held in occlusion for insertion into the mouth: as soon as they are released the dentures are forced apart by the action of the springs and held in place (Figure 16.17).

Disadvantages:

1. The constant pressure may cause mucosal irritation and excessive alveolar resorption.
2. The inner surfaces of the cheeks are frequently injured from frictional contact with the springs (Figure 16.17).
3. Lateral movements are extremely restricted and hence the efficiency of the dentures is impaired.
4. They are generally inefficient and unhygienic.

Denture fixatives

The powder form consists of natural gums such as tragacanth or karaya with cellulose added. It is sprinkled on the moist, fitting surface of the denture which will then usually stick in place for several hours. Gradually the sticky jelly is pressed from underneath the denture or washed away by the saliva, and for this latter reason is rarely of any use for holding lower dentures. Even with prolonged use it does not appear to affect the mucosa. Creams and liquids, containing the same substances as are in artificial saliva, are also available.

Uses

1. To hold the upper record block in position when securing intra-oral records.
2. To prolong the usefulness, for a short time, of an immediate upper denture which is becoming loose through alveolar resorption.
3. To enable a patient to wear an old, ill-fitting upper denture, while a denture in normal use is being repaired.
4. Sometimes used by public speakers, such as actors or clergymen, to give them the assurance that the upper denture will not move while they are addressing their audiences.

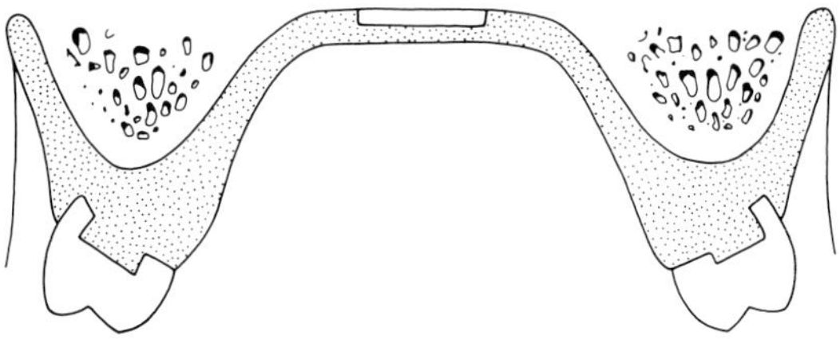

Figure 16.18 Cross-section of an upper denture with a suction chamber. Note the square edges in contact with the palate. This is a damaging technique and should not be used

Disadvantages:

1. It has an unpleasant feel as soon as it is pressed out from beneath the denture.
2. It is only a temporary expedient and the less accurate the fit of the denture the more rapidly is the fixative washed away.
3. It is of little use for retaining lower dentures.

Suction chambers

These often resemble relief areas in shape but differ from them in having a clearly defined outline instead of merging into the surrounding surface (Figure 16.18). When the denture is inserted the patient creates a partial vacuum in this chamber by sucking and swallowing and this small area of reduced pressure helps to keep the denture in place. The mucosa in this area of reduced pressure proliferates to form a mass of denture-induced hyperplasia. For this reason the technique should not be used.

Rubber suction discs (Figure 3.4)

Although these are still used in practice they are only included in this list in order to condemn them. They consist of a rubber disc which is affixed to a stud on the fitting surface of a denture. The partial vacuum created within the perimeter of this disc holds the upper denture suspended from the hard palate. They cause a constant irritation and serve no useful purpose.

Magnets

From time to time the use of small magnets embedded beneath the molar and premolar teeth and arranged with similar poles opposite each other, has been advocated. In theory the repulsion effect will keep both dentures in place but in practice it will be found that, owing to magnetic force being inversely proportional to the square of the distance and also the small size of the magnets which it is possible to fit, the repulsive effect is undetectable when the dentures are separated by more than 1 or 2 mm.

Chapter 17

Appearance

One of the objects in complete denture prosthetics is to produce a harmonious appearance of the denture when in the patient's mouth. Artistic appreciation is a personal appraisement and reaction, however, thus what one person considers to be a pleasing result another may readily find unattractive. For this reason it is difficult to set out hard and fast rules and principles about appearance and aesthetics.

The aim should be to produce dentures which blend in with the patient's general characteristics and which are an unobtrusive part of the general facial appearance. For example, dentures in which the lateral incisors are set to the same occlusal level as the centrals and canines, with all the teeth positioned vertically, and their colour that of the lightest possible hue, will result in an effect which appears obviously artificial.

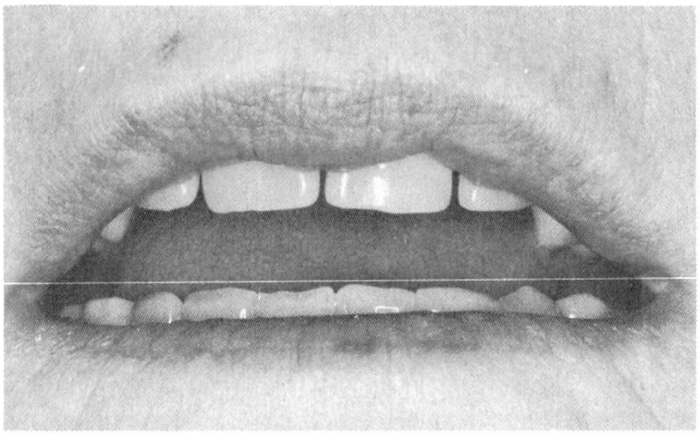

Figure 17.1 During conversation the amount of tooth showing varies. In this complete denture patient note the natural spaces of the upper teeth and the attrition effects of the lower incisal edges

Selection of tooth mould

The most important teeth from the point of view of appearance are the maxillary central incisors as they are generally the teeth most exposed during conversation (Figure 17.1) and usually the focus of attention when an individual smiles or laughs (Figure 17.2). Therefore the selection of the right mould of central incisor is important. Two of the main points to be considered in its selection are the sex and personality of the patient. One associates

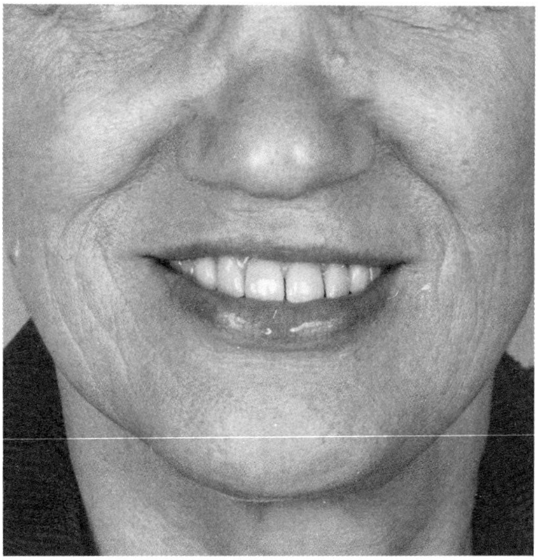

Figure 17.2 Complete denture patient producing a smile. In this case the right side of the face is more active in smiling and so the incisal edges run slightly up to that side to complement the asymmetric muscular activity

the female form with curves, while the male form presents angles and straight lines (Figures 17.3 and 17.4). If this is translated into tooth moulds then a central incisor selected for a female should have a basically curved outline with rounded mesial and distal corners; such an outline is often referred to as the ovoid mould. The basic mould for the male should be a straighter sided tooth with moderately sharp mesial and distal corners: the tapering or square mould (Figure 17.5). This does not mean that all women must have ovoid teeth and all men square or tapering teeth.

The second point, that of personality, should be considered carefully when making the choice of tooth mould. Personality for this purpose is considered from the aspect of the physical and temperamental impression created by the patient. There are two extremes of individuals to be considered, those who fall into the category of healthy, manly and muscular types, classed as a vigorous group, and those who fall into the category of frail and timid individuals, classed as a delicate, group. Ranging between these two groups will be those persons belonging to the average group. The greater proportion of individuals in the delicate group will be female, while those in the vigorous group will be male. There are, however, females ranging from the average group towards the

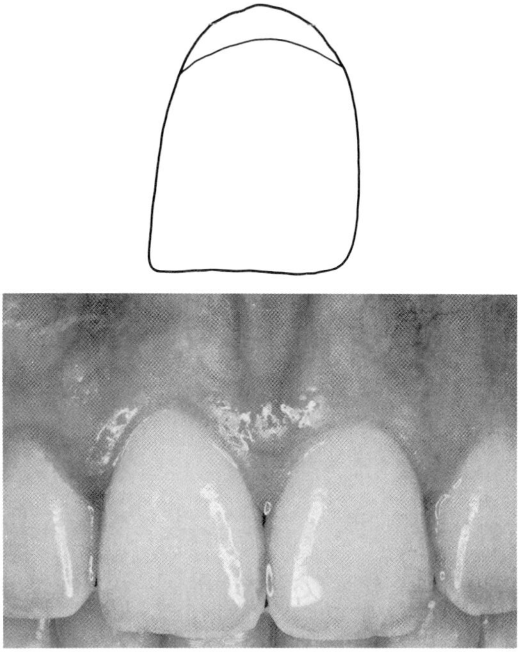

Figure 17.4 The outline of the male figure is more straight lined and angular on contrast to the female form and the basic tooth form should be tapering or square

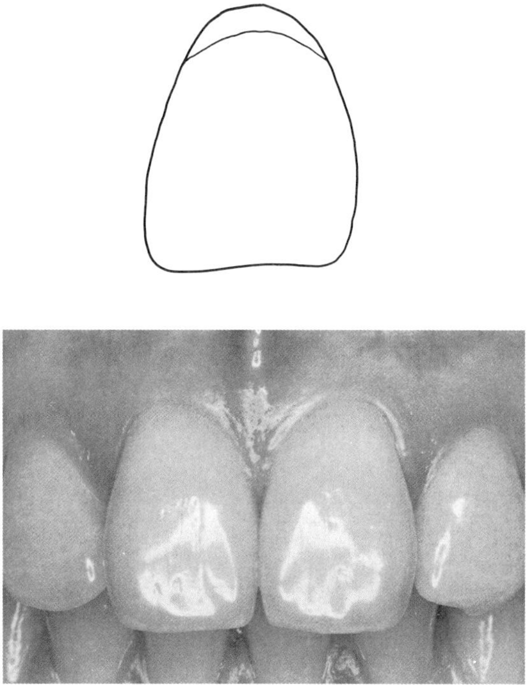

Figure 17.3 The outline of the female form tends to be a series of curves and the basic tooth form should be of the curved or ovoid type

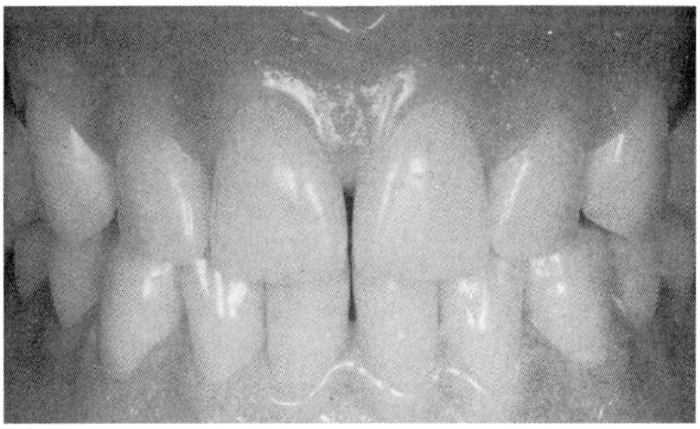

(*a*)

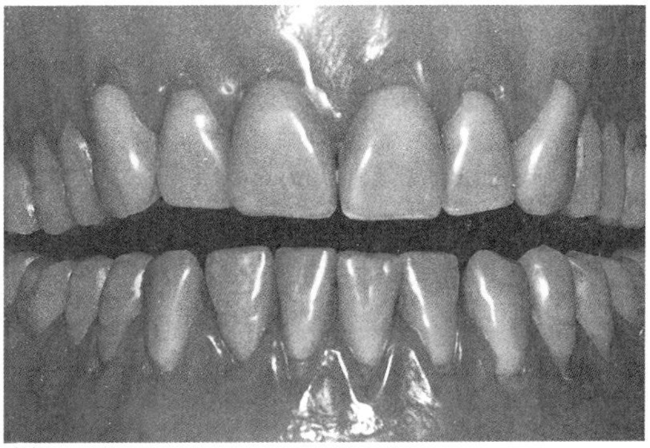

(*b*)

Figure 17.5 (*a*) Complete dentures set for female patient with teeth of more curved outline than (*b*) set for a male patient

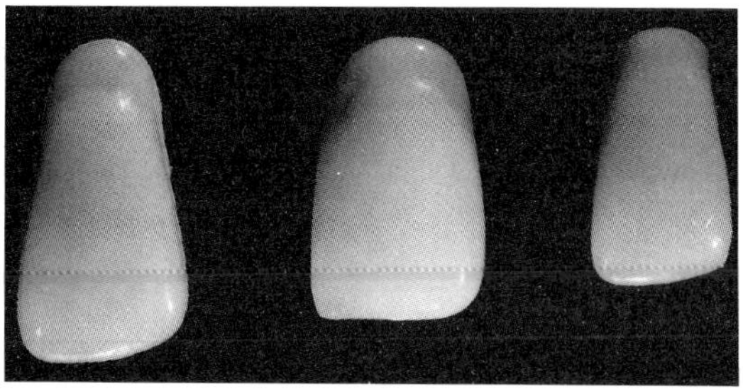

Figure 17.6 Manufactured maxillary lateral incisors vary in shape, size and texture. This gives rise to vigorous effects (centre) and grades of delicacy

vigorous group, such as some business executives, and to a lesser degree males ranging from the average group to the delicate group, for example effeminate types. The average group is by far the largest and the vigorous group is greater than the delicate.

Mould selection based on this grouping means that on the one extreme the tooth should be soft in its outline with curves, no sharp angles and a smooth labial surface, the delicate group, and on the other extreme the tooth should be bold and angular with pronounced labial surface detail of ridges and grooves. If the personality is considered in conjunction with the sex then the vigorous male would be suited best by a bold tapering tooth with sharp angular corners and a prominently contoured labial surface, while a delicate female might best be suited by a thin, ovoid tooth with a smoother surface.

The lateral incisors aid considerably in creating the effect of vigour or delicacy and range from a long, tapering, square-cornered tooth to a small, narrow, round-cornered tooth. The lateral of average length and width and with a rounded distal corner suits the average group of individuals (Figure 17.6).

Tooth size

With the natural dentition there are instances of slightly built individuals having large teeth and heavily built people having small teeth. This is often a conspicuous feature of the person that attracts attention. For this reason, since it is desirable that dentures should be an unobtrusive feature of the patient, it is advisable to select a size of tooth which blends with the general height and build of the patient. The length to breadth ratio of the selected tooth should bear a close relationship to the length to breadth ratio of the person's face. One important factor which must be borne in mind when deciding the size of tooth, and also the level of the incisal edge relation to the lip, is the mobility of the upper lip. Obviously it is desirable to expose as little denture base material as possible when smiling and laughing and therefore a balance often has to be struck between tooth length and incisal edge level in order that the general tooth size may be kept in proportion with the patient's build. A slightly built patient with a very mobile lip may have to have the incisal edge, which would normally have been set 2–3 mm below the lip, raised to lip level in order that a tooth of acceptable length may be used instead of an excessively long tooth. Provided the tooth maintains proportions suitable to the individual the appearance will be best if the tooth fills, or very nearly fills, the space between the resting and smiling positions of the upper lip.

The size of the mouth will control the width of the tooth to a certain extent. It is obviously undesirable to select narrow teeth for a person with a very broad smile which exposes the molar teeth, but it is equally undesirable to select very broad teeth, which will also be proportionate in length, if the sex, personality and physical build of the individual indicates a small mould of tooth. The alternative is to select the appropriate size of tooth and then to space the teeth, without producing an unpleasant appearance, to obtain the maximum width from canine to canine.

Generally, large people require large teeth and small people small teeth. Women usually require smaller teeth than men for relative builds. It is well to remember that the size of the natural teeth does not change throughout life, excluding the effect of attrition, but the body often undergoes considerable alteration and therefore the dimensional changes occurring with age may be misleading when considering the size of teeth.

It is a common failing to select artificial teeth which are too small and this frequently results from the patient influencing the dentist in his choice (Figure 17.7). Patients often imagine their natural

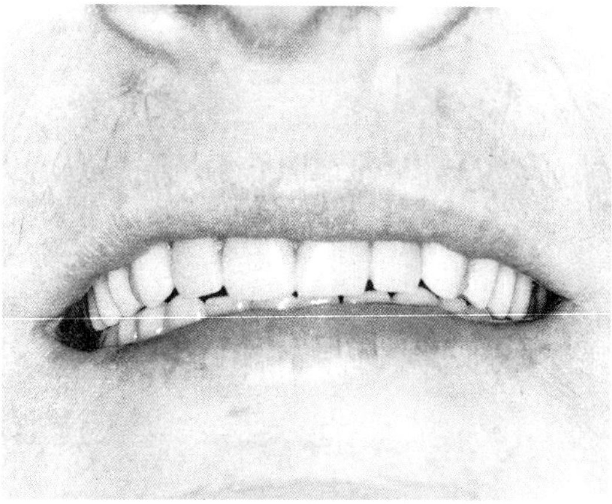

Figure 17.7 Artificial-looking complete denture. Teeth too small, set too far lingually and wrong texture. Sometimes referred to as the '10 tooth smile'

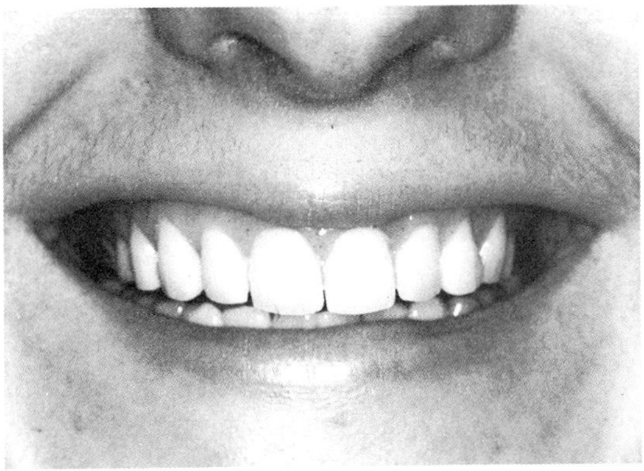

Figure 17.8 In this complete denture the shade is obviously too light and the size of tooth too small. Note the long axis of each central incisor is parallel: the axes should be convergent. The space along the buccal aspect between the denture and the cheek, sometimes referred to as the buccal corridor, gives rise to a pleasing effect

teeth to have been smaller than was actually the case, but it must be pointed out that there is an element of risk in pressing one's own choice of size and mould too strongly. A compromise is sometimes necessary between the choice of the dentist and what the patient desires.

The upper incisors used in complete dentures are often too small and patients and clinicians are both at fault in this respect as the desire to have small white teeth is instilled into us from many sources (Figure 17.8). The mean width of natural upper central incisors is about 9 mm and therefore artificial incisors of less than 8.5 mm should seldom be used (Figure 17.9). An acceptable width of upper central incisor in female patients is 8.5 mm or more, while in males it should be 9 mm or more. If reduction in the total width of the upper six anterior teeth is necessary it may be done by using a narrower lateral incisor but neither the central incisor nor the canine should be reduced in width. The size of the upper lateral incisor varies considerably and often one is different from the other in natural dentitions. The lateral incisors in manufactured teeth are commonly made too large in relation to the central incisor and canine.

Shade of teeth

There is no rule which can be applied to the selection of the correct shade of tooth for an individual. Generally it is a question of trial and error, taking a tooth of one colour from a shade card, placing it in position under the upper lip and assessing its colour tones in relation to the face of the patient. This operation is repeated with different shades until one is found which most satisfactorily blends with the patient's general colouring (Figure 17.10). Blondes with light blue or grey eyes are usually best suited by a light ivory-yellow shade of tooth bordering on the white range. Darker eye colouring may suggest a slightly darker shade of tooth. Brown hair and medium coloured eyes call for the mid range of the biscuit yellow shade, while darker hair and eye tones will require a darker shade of the biscuit yellow range. Occasionally a grey basic tone blends well with the elderly or pale individual, but selection requires careful consideration, as the effect when the patient smiles may be to accentuate the age and debility. Age has an important bearing on colour choice. Natural teeth tend to darken with age and the colour selected for a person of 40 years of age would be too light when that person was 60.

It is not good practice to allow the patient to select the shade as a dry tooth held in the hand is entirely different from a wet tooth under the shadow of the upper lip and set in its correct position.

Shading should be varied in a set of teeth and so mixing of sets of manufactured teeth leads to a more natural effect (Figure 17.11,17.26).

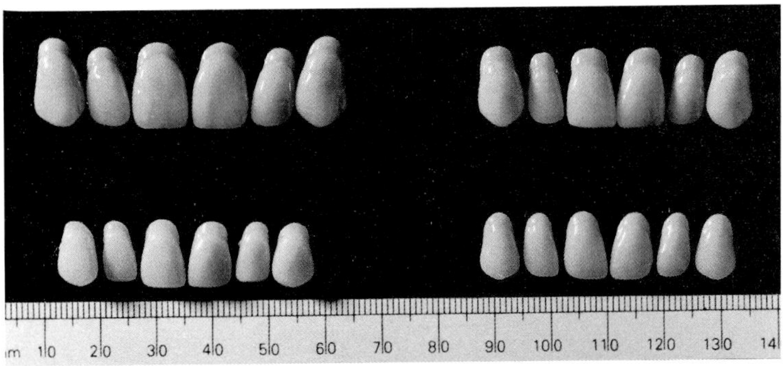

Figure 17.9 Many artificial teeth are too small. Maxillary central incisors of less than 8.5 mm width should seldom be used. Teeth at lower part of the photograph are too small

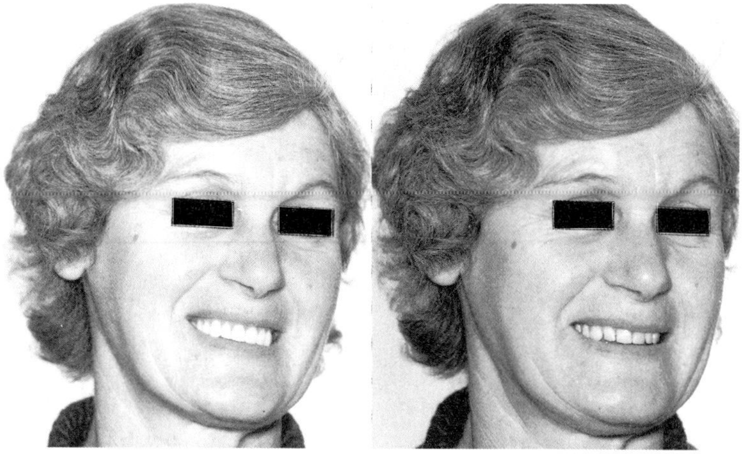

(*a*) (*b*)

Figure 17.10 Complete dentures of (*a*) incorrect and (*b*) correct shade. The maxillary teeth in (*a*) are set too far back and the incisal level is wrong

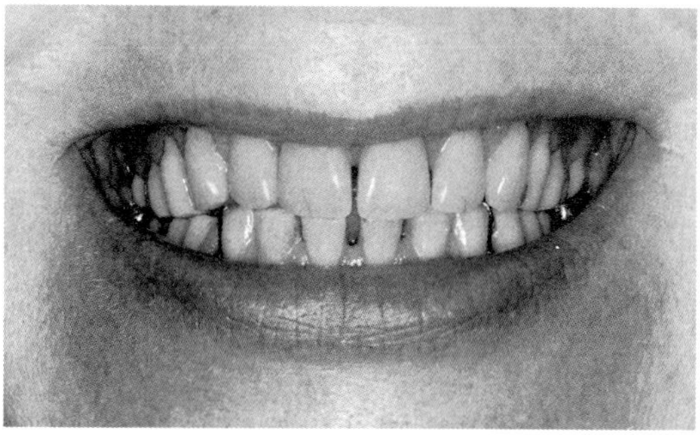

Figure 17.11 Complete maxillary denture; natural lower teeth. A pleasing effect has been achieved by mixing the shades of the maxillary teeth and by complementing the spaces between the mandibular incisors. Note that the length of the first premolars is similar to the canines thus adding to the natural appearance

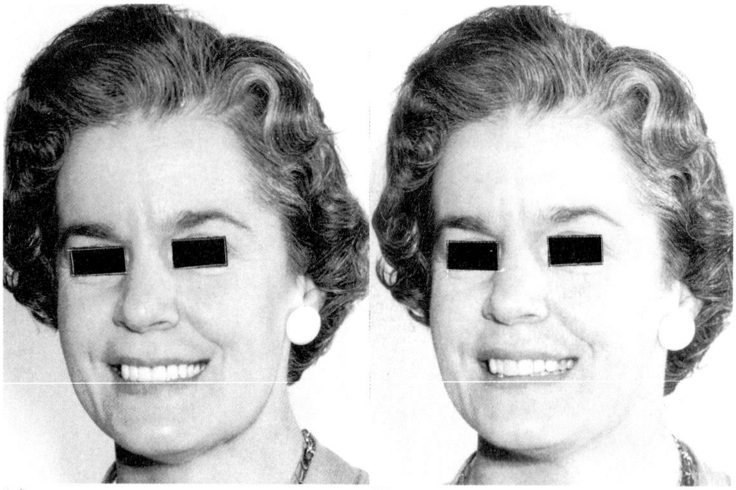

(*a*) (*b*)

Figure 17.12 Edentulous patient with regular and symmetrical features. (*a*) Shade of teeth too light and wrong shape. Incisal edgges too low and teeth set too far lingually (*b*) Complete dentures of correct design with incisors complementing facial shape

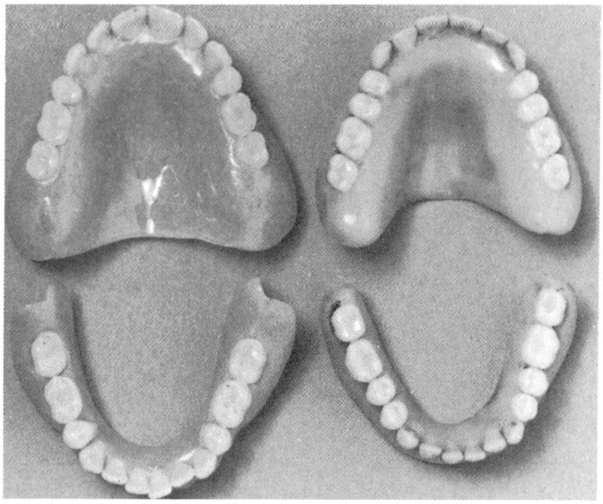

Figure 17.13 A pleasing appearance will never be achieved with complete dentures of the wrong design. The dentures (on the left) made for the same patient restored the facial musculature with correct denture bases and teeth in the pre-extraction position

Position of the teeth

Since the object is to produce a denture which harmonizes with the person's appearance, to present a pleasant effect when smiling or laughing, and to avoid artificiality, the tooth position is important. Basically there are two considerations. The patient who has regular and symmetrical features requires a normal arrangement of tooth position, otherwise their classical qualities will be diminished (Figure 17.12). On the other hand, the rugged type of individual with a degree of facial asymmetry requires irregularity in the positioning of the teeth as otherwise a perfectly normal arrangement of the teeth would contrast with the features and bring the focus of attention on to the denture rather than the face as a whole. Most patients may be placed somewhere between these two extremes and many variations from the normal position of the individual anterior teeth will be found.

Apart from their ability to incise food and aid speech, the anterior teeth form the main feature of the smile and largely influence facial expression (Figure 17.13). In order that they should fulfil these latter two functions satisfactorily, it is important that the teeth should be placed in relation to the alveolar ridge in such a way that adequate support is given to the lip during a smile and that the lip is supported in its natural forward position when it is at rest. Too often artificial upper anterior teeth are set back on the ridge and the lip hangs down vertically or may even fall inwards (Figure 17.14). After the extraction of teeth alveolar resorption of the anterior ridge is upwards and backwards and so the anterior teeth must be positioned forward of the ridge to provide the correct lip support. The degree of this forward placement is directly related to the extent of resorption which has occurred.

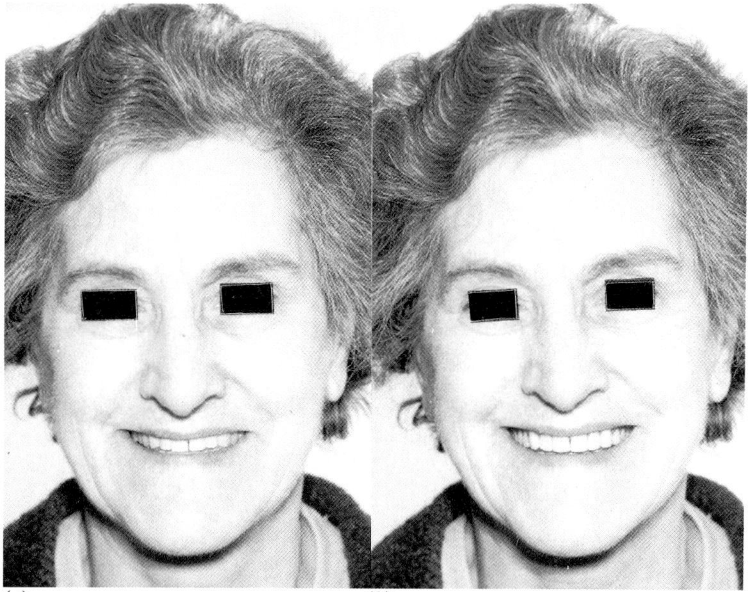

(*a*) (*b*)

Figure 17.14 (*a*) Teeth of complete dentures set on the alveolar ridge; flange of dentures too narrow. (*b*) Teeth set in pre-extraction position and lips correctly restored

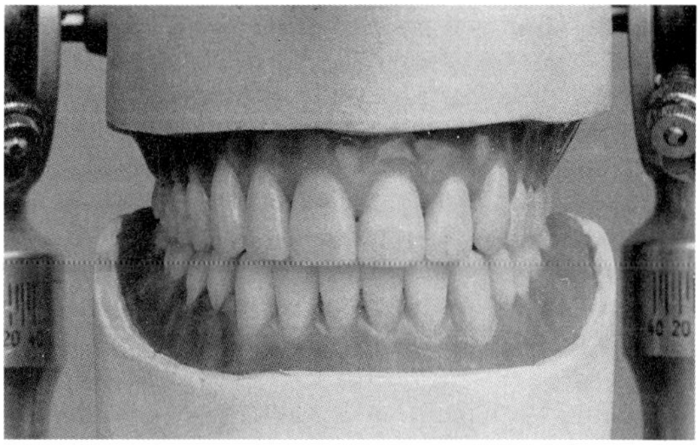

Figure 17.15 Complete denture tooth arrangement without any irregularity ready for trial in the mouth

The central incisor

Keeping both incisors in identically regular positions indicates perfection and would probably only suit those with classical features (Figure 17.15). If one incisor is moved forward of the other at its incisal edge then a somewhat harsher appearance is created while if one tooth is moved out cervically, leaving the incisal edges in line, a softer irregularity is created suitable for use with a female patient. A more vigorous effect can be obtained by bringing one central bodily forward of the other. Further effects of softness or hardness may be brought about by rotating or inclining one or both incisors. Overlapping can be effective, particularly where the canine-to-canine distance requires to be kept small but the tooth size average. In most instances variations of position of the central incisors are acceptable but take care not to make any irregularity so extreme that it becomes immediately obvious.

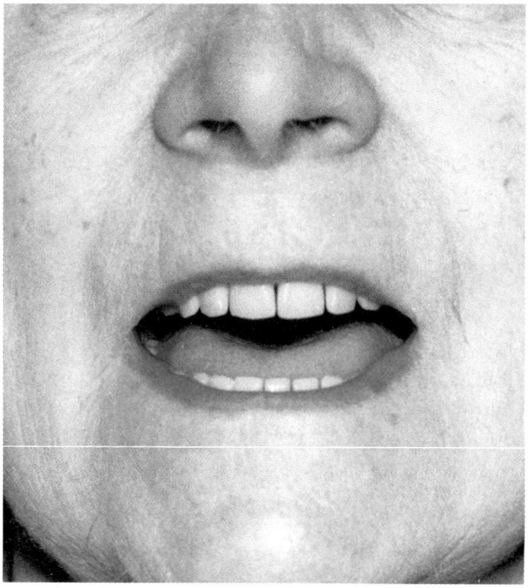

Figure 17.16 Complete denture patient during speech. Note how the maxillary lateral incisors, slightly mesially everted, complement the central incisors

The lateral incisor

Although this is a comparatively small tooth and less apparent than the central it does play an important part in establishing the general composition of the anterior teeth (Figure 17.16). If the lateral incisor is rotated so that the mesial surface is brought forward then the effect of the smile is one of softness; the tooth may even overlap the central. By depressing the mesial edge towards the palate the effect on hardness is obtained. Lateral inclination from the normal vertical axis is an additional variation. One lateral may have a different irregularity than the other and this enhances the natural effect.

The canine

This tooth should be set with the neck more prominent than the incisal tip and its long axis vertical. The more prominent the position of the canine in the arch the more vigorous the smile becomes (Figure 17.17). Similarly the larger the tooth, and the more marked the labial surface detail, the greater the effect of masculinity.

Femininity can be accentuated by setting the anterior teeth with a curvature running from the tips of the central incisors upwards to the canines. This smile curve, formed by the incisal edges, should follow the curve of the smiling lower lip (see Figure 17.28).

Too much symmetry should be avoided when producing irregularities as they frequently increase the appearance of artificiality. On the other hand, over-accentuation of an irregularity is often necessary to be effective and a tooth arrangement which appears somewhat grotesque when set on the articulator becomes pleasantly acceptable when the denture is in the mouth. This emphasizes the effect of environment on the appearance of an object.

Age

Age in relation to appearance should be considered from both the chronological and biological age of the patient. People vary considerably in the effect of age on their physical appearance. Some middle-aged people appear very much older than their chronological age, while some chronologically old people appear young and virile. Tooth selection and arrangement should fit chiefly with the biological age of the patient (Figure 17.18).

A person at the age of 20 years probably has teeth of a uniform colour which still retain the bluish tint of the incisal enamel, but 30 years later these same teeth are likely to have undergone certain changes. They will have darkened slightly, areas of stain will have appeared, and perhaps caries and subsequent fillings will have caused localized colour change.

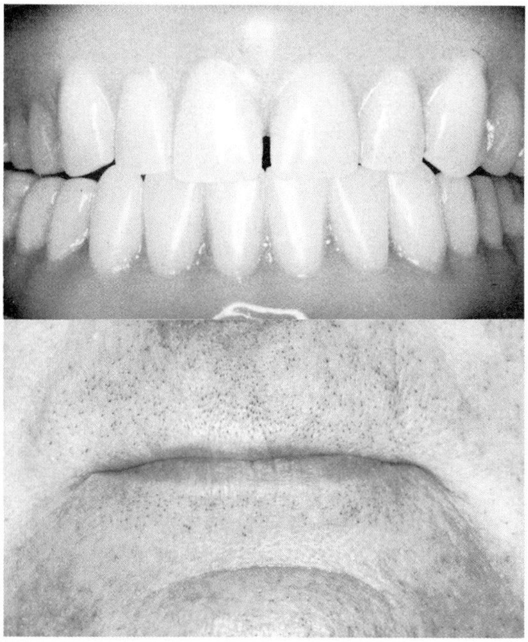

(*a*)

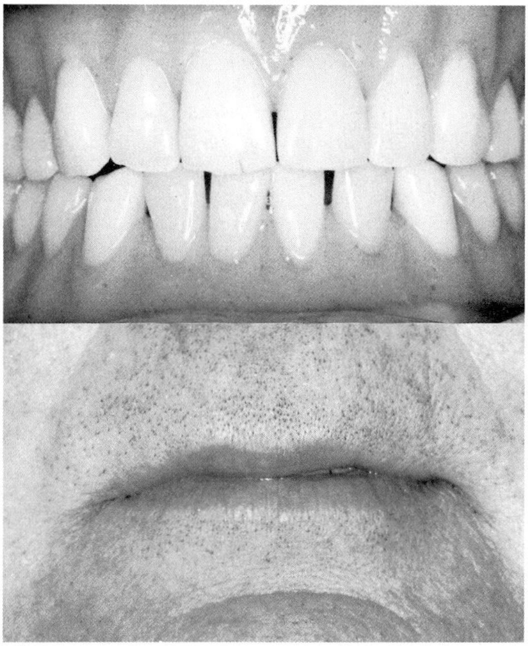

(*b*)

Figure 17.17 (*a*) Unsatisfactory tooth setting and unsupported lip form with dentures *in situ*. (*b*) More vigorous tooth setting and correct peripheral form resulting in better lip form

Gingival recession exposes cementum, and attrition of the incisal edges removes the greater proportion, if not all, of the incisal enamel. It is also to be expected that the surface colour change will be affected by food stains. All this is progressive with age and should be borne in mind when deciding on the colour of the teeth selected for a patient. In certain circumstances, effective results can be obtained by varying the shade of one or two of the anterior teeth (see Figure 17.26) and also by staining individual teeth (see Figure 17.19). More expensive teeth may be purchased from manufacturers with age effects incorporated, sometimes referred to as naturalized or characterized teeth.

Even if such desirable procedures are not adopted the standard set of anterior teeth can be made more in keeping with the patient's age by judicious grinding of the incisal edges, and a study of the attrition of natural incisors will indicate the type of wear which occurs from person to person. Attrition

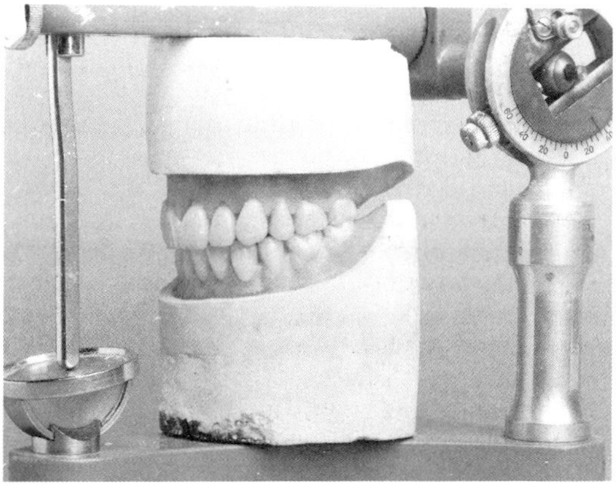

Figure 17.18 Complete dentures being waxed up to complement the age of the patient

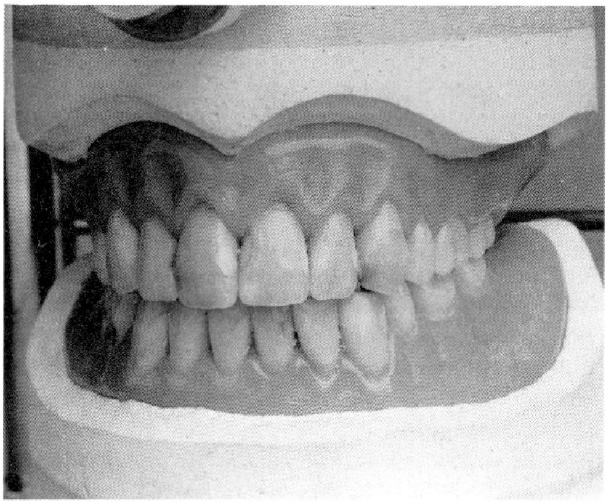

Figure 17.19 Staining individual teeth and introducing interstitial restorations may improve the natural effect of complete dentures

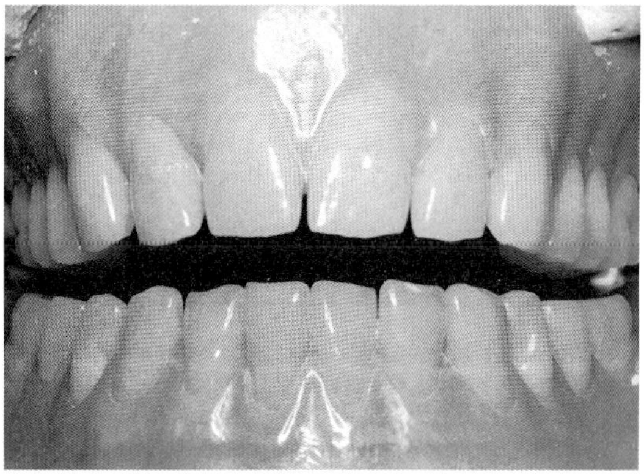

Figure 17.20 Cusps of premolars and incisal edges of incisors ground to produce a more natural appearance. Note the interesting setting of the lower incisors and the texture of the denture bases

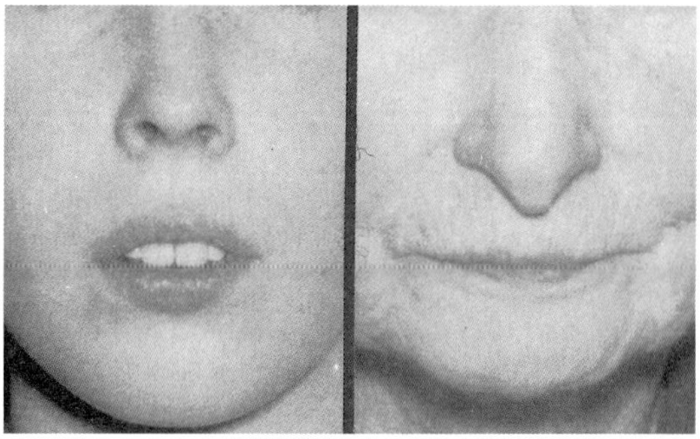

Figure 17.21 Age, lip form and type of nose all affect tooth position in restoration of complete denture patients

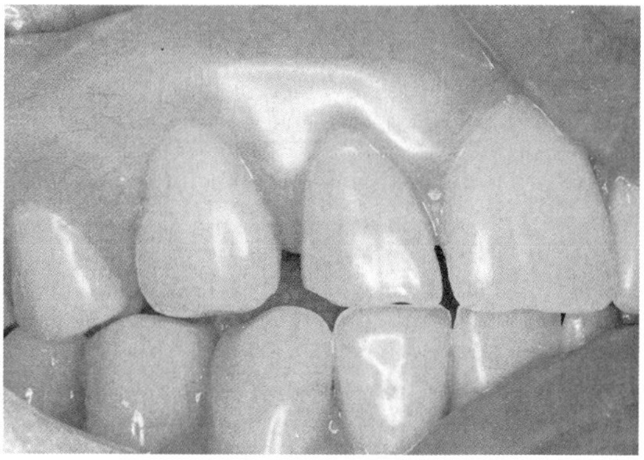

Figure 17.22 In the older patient teeth may be spaced to complement age changes. Note the smooth, glazed surface of this complete denture as part of the ageing process

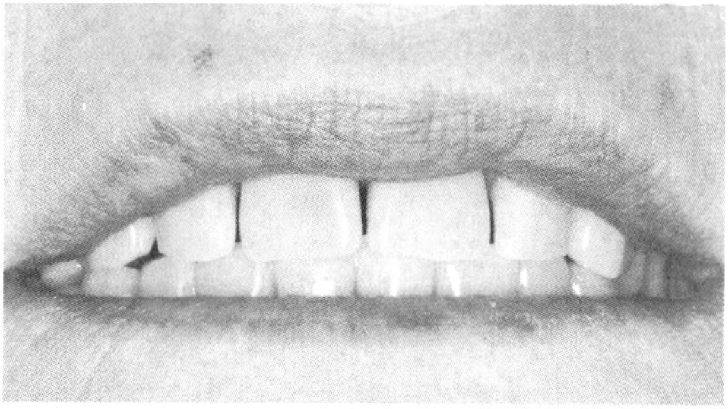

Figure 17.23 Complete dentures with pleasing and natural appearance. Care is needed when setting a diastema as it may have an effect that is not pleasing and may also trap the lip or food

will obviously affect the posterior teeth as well as the anterior teeth, so that if a patient of middle or advanced age is likely to show the premolar teeth when smiling or laughing a more natural effect can be created if the cusps of the premolars are suitably ground and not left in the form of a newly erupted tooth (Figure 17.20).

Age also has a bearing on the position of the anterior teeth (Figure 17.21). Throughout life natural teeth are often being lost for one reason or another and this means that the contact points of the remaining teeth become less firm or even lost, particularly if a partial denture is not fitted. It is not an uncommon state in the middle-aged person, where some posterior teeth have been lost, to find that the contact points of the anterior teeth have parted to the extent that the point of a probe can be passed freely between them, and this fact needs to be considered in relation to the setting of the anterior teeth of a denture. Frequently the appearance of a complete denture constructed for a 60 year-old patient is spoiled by having the teeth set with very tight contact between each tooth, producing an effect which is generally associated with youth. Varying degrees of spacing with either all or one or two of the anterior teeth aids in establishing a natural appearance in relation to age (Figure 17.22). A slight diastema between the centrals is a common occurrence, but caution is necessary in reproducing this state as it is possible that if exaggerated it may appear unpleasant and become a source of amusement to the observer; it may also be an embarrassing food-trap (Figure 17.23). The gingival contouring of a denture should also be related to the age of the patient and is the next consideration.

Just as tightly contacting teeth are predominantly associated with youth so are normal, triangular, sharp-pointed interdental papillae indicative of the young person (see Figure 17.3). Greater harmony in the appearance can be obtained by simulation of some of the changes, which may occur throughout life, in the shape and colour of the interdental papillae and gingival margins. Variation from the normal type papilla suitable in the youngish patient must be made with care, and spaces such as occur between teeth in advanced periodontal disease

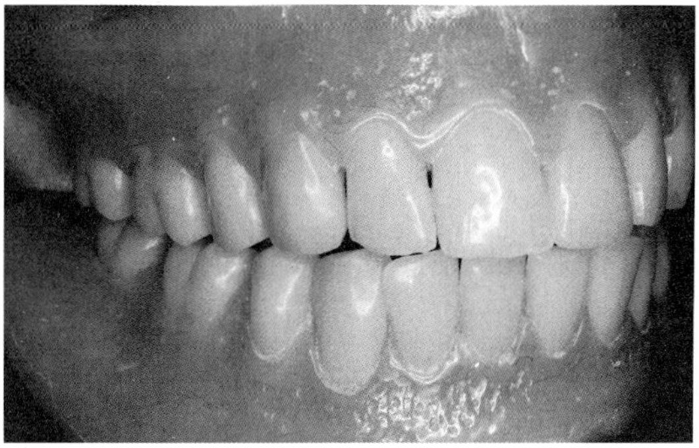

Figure 17.24 Complete dentures showing rolled gingivae, blunt papillae, stippled base acrylic and artificial veins

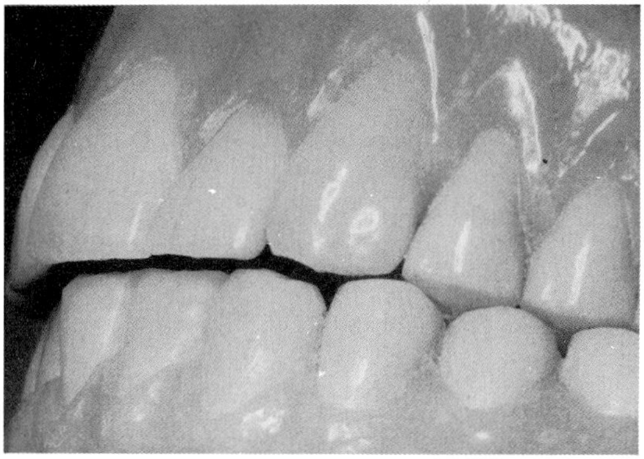

Figure 17.25 Variation in contour of gingivae and tooth length to simulate natural changes

should be avoided. However, the copying of some of the less advanced conditions in which the point of the papilla is rounded instead of pointed, and the base widened to overlap the labial and cervical areas of the tooth to a greater extent than normal, can be most effective, especially if the gingival margin is thickened to form a slight roll (Figure 17.24). Denture base materials having reddish fibres or granules incorporated in them often improve the general effect. A study of natural conditions, as seen on casts of dentate mouths, is of considerable help in gingival design. In the production of such interdental papillae, certain points are important:

1. There should be a variation in the individual length and the degree of simulated change in the tissue from one papilla to the next (Figure 17.25).
2. They must be related to the age of the patient.
3. They should be convex in all directions to avoid food being trapped.
4. They should extend to the contact points of the teeth and fill the interdental space so that food is shed away.

This necessitates care in the selection of the tooth mould in order to avoid those moulds having low contact point areas and therefore excessively long papillae.

Gingival margin and labial surface contour

The gingival margins can be blended to suit the age by thickening or rolling the gingival margin of all or some teeth. In youth the margin is thin and pale pink in colour. In middle age an average appearance would be a slight rolling of the margin with increased red tint in the acrylic and the papillae would be blunter and thicker. In advanced age the gingival tissue would give a characteristic thickened appearance and a deeper red tint, the papillae being broad based with rounded apices. The gingival level of the individual anterior teeth should vary, the central incisor gingiva normally being higher than the lateral incisor, but lower than that of the canine

(*a*)

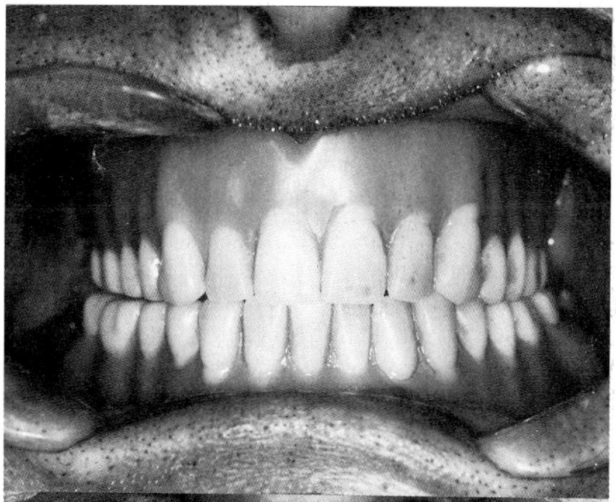

(*b*)

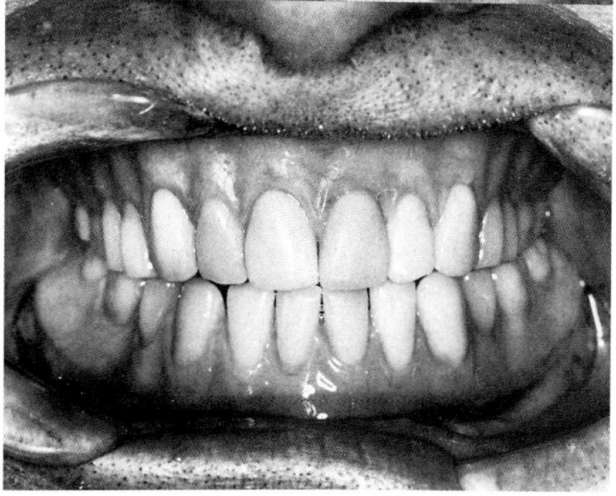

Figure 17.26 (*a*) Complete dentures with little attention paid to aesthetics. (*b*) Tooth setting and shade variation improve the appearance. Note the poor effect of the flat reflection of light in (*a*) compared with the interesting natural contours of (*b*)

(Figure 17.25). Symmetry needs to be avoided and variation in the gingival levels should be the aim. The premolar and molar gingival levels should also vary if a broad smile exists, the first premolar level being below that of the canine, the others being variations of that level. A denture having the gingival margins uniformly shaped and all at the same level with all the teeth set vertically and level with the occlusal plane, creates the impression of a row of acrylic blades, thereby making the denture look artificial.

Another reason for dentures appearing artificial is the manner in which the labial flange is shaped. Often this flange is a flat curved surface from premolar to premolar and when light falls upon it during a smile or laugh it gives a reflection devoid of highlights and shadows (Figure 17.26), which is not the usual occurrence with natural tissues. By contouring the labial flange highlights and shadow effects can be obtained, breaking up the flat reflection of the light falling on the denture (Figure 17.26). To do this, the labial area should be very gently contoured to simulate the prominences caused by the roots of natural teeth. The canine roots are more prominent than the central incisor roots, and the laterals the least of all. When contouring the roots of the teeth the long axes of the crowns must always be followed and anatomical detail copied realistically. Casts taken from natural dentitions as patterns are useful to have at hand when shaping the labial flange.

The finished denture should be lightly stippled, i.e. the reproduction of the matt surface of natural gum tissue which gives it a fine orange peel appearance which breaks up any large zones of light reflection (Figure 17.27). The area covered by the contouring and stippling should be limited to the labial region and that part of the buccal region likely to be exposed when the patient smiles, the reason for this being that a rough and uneven surface tends to collect food particles, whereas a smooth, polished surface is more self-cleansing. The inference is that stippling and gingival contouring should be diminished or possibly avoided in those cases where oral hygiene is poor.

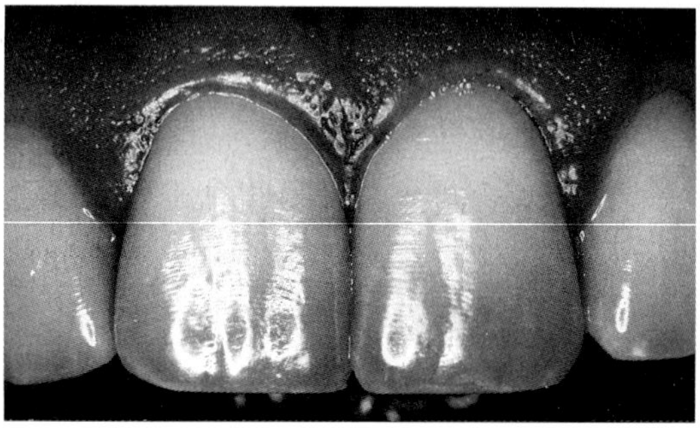

Figure 17.27 Youthful natural gingivae and the typical orange peel texture. Note also the surface texture of natural teeth

The smile curve and arch form

The smile curve related to the setting of the anterior teeth is a line running through the incisal edges of the central incisors, sweeping upwards to the lateral teeth and thence to the tips of the canines (Figure 17.28). This curve tends to follow that of the smiling lower lip and is more accentuated in the young person since there is little attrition of the central incisors. As age and attrition progress the curve flattens. This smile curve is also related to the sex of the patient, bearing in mind the basic curved form associated with femininity.

The amount of tooth showing in the young adult during conversation is 2–3 mm and this diminishes with increasing age. It is sometimes an advantage to show a little more tooth in the female than in the male at the various levels to enhance the quality of femininity (Figure 17.29).

The arch form of the anterior teeth should not be made to coincide with the resorbed alveolar ridge as this may have undergone considerable change. The features of the face should be studied and the arch made to harmonize with them. Generally it will be found that flat, broad-faced individuals are best suited to a square arch and the pointed or sharp-featured person suited to a tapering arch. In between will be the moderate arch curve adopted

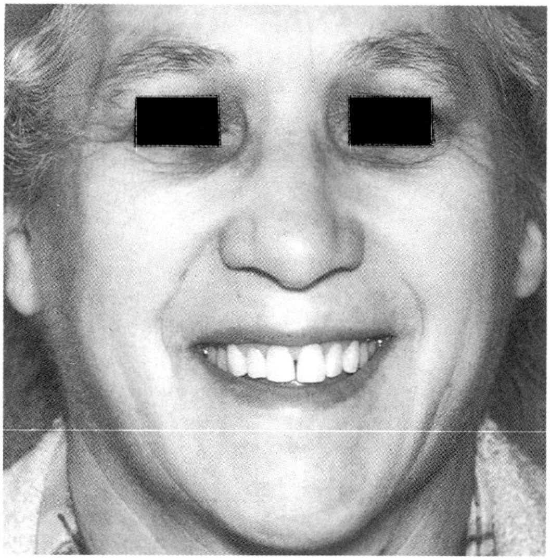

Figure 17.28 Complete dentures. The smile curve is the line of the incisal edges of the maxillary incisors following the contour of the smiling lower lip and gives a very pleasing effect

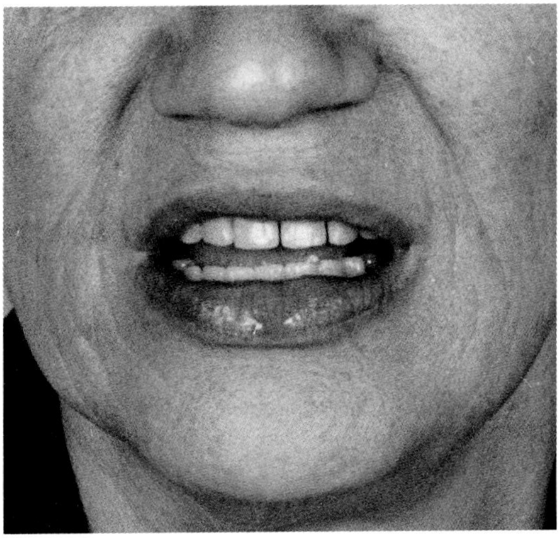

Figure 17.29 Teeth of complete dentures showing during conversation. The relatively horizontal setting of the maxillary incisors was made to harmonize with the horizontal activity of the lower lip

for the majority of individuals. A tapering arch is most adaptable to the overlapping of teeth in the production of irregularities.

Vertical dimension

The restoration of the facial appearance of the edentulous patient requires attention to three points. First, the restoration, by the correct thickness and positioning of the denture matrix and flanges, of the tissue lost during extraction and alveolar resorption (Figure 17.30); second, the correct placing of the anterior teeth; and third, the establishment of the correct vertical dimension of the jaw relationship for the individual. Vertical dimension, from the point of view of appearance, is important as it is related to the establishment of the correct separation of the origins and insertions of the muscles of the facial musculature. If these insertions are brought too close together the muscles will tend to sag and bunch while if they are too far apart the muscles will be stretched to produce a strained appearance. For the muscles to be in their normal relationship the anterior teeth must be correctly positioned and the vertical dimension correct. The modiolus is then in its correct position and so can effectively serve its purpose of acting as an anchor during contractions of certain of the facial muscles associated with expression, speech and eating.

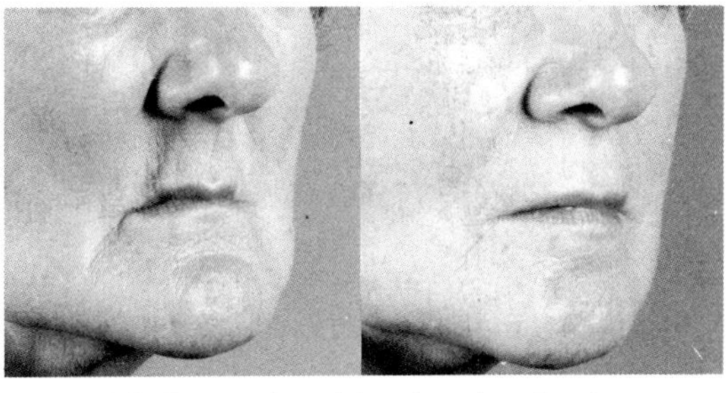

Figure 17.30 Restoration of the edentulous face by complete dentures is an essential prerequisite to good aesthetics

Summary

The final assessment of an appearance at the trial denture stage should always be made with the observer standing away from the dental chair and judgement made at varying distances to obtain the overall effect. Furthermore, a relative or close friend should, if possible, attend at this stage to give a considered opinion. This often saves argument and ill-feeling between the dentist and the patient after dentures have been worn for a few days and criticized by the family and close friends.

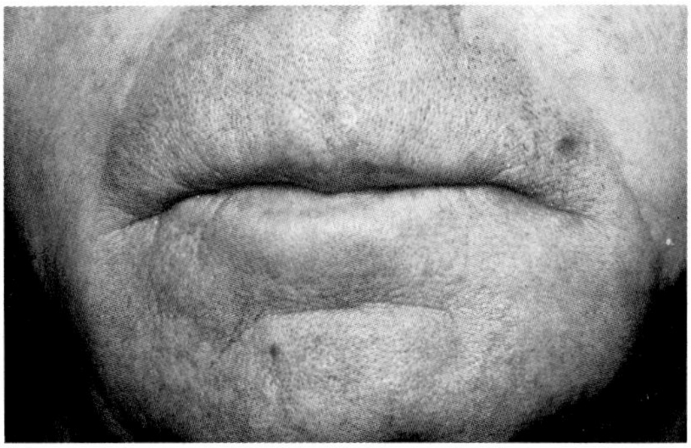

(*a*)

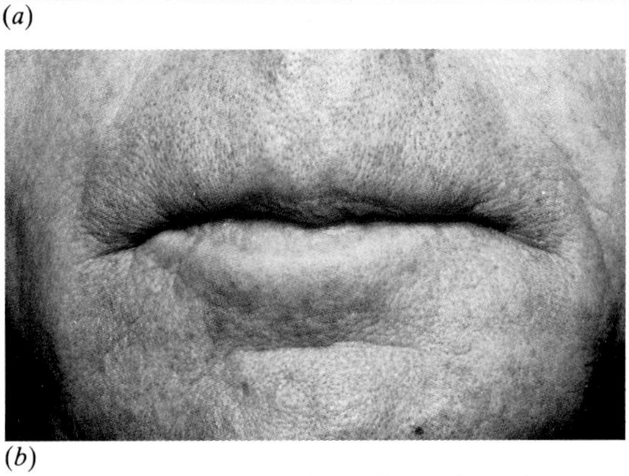

(*b*)

Figure 17.31 Changes following delivery of complete dentures. (*a*) At stage of delivery, the tense activity of the lips leading to a thinning of the borders. (*b*) At 72 hours later, the more relaxed contours of the lips as the patient adapts to the dentures

Change in form of the lips after the loss of teeth is due to the loss of substance and reduction in elastic properties of the connective tissue because of normal age changes and thus there is reduced resistance to the activities of the orbicularis oris and associated muscles. This partly accounts for the change and difference in appearance which takes place from the trial denture stage, the stage of insertion of the dentures and the ensuing follow-up visits (Figure 17.31). Such changes can be very subtle but, in general, one should allow four to six weeks to elapse after insertion of complete dentures before assessing the final appearance of the patient. Every patient should understand this.

Most people dread the thought of losing their teeth and having dentures, one of the reasons being the fear of an artificial appearance. Such people will appreciate the care and thought given to producing a natural appearance and it is therefore wise to have available examples and photographs of the types of natural effects and their appearance when in the mouth. If the patient does not discuss the question of appearance then this question should be raised by the dentist before any natural effects or irregularities are introduced into the denture. Some patients have very definite ideas of a perfect set of teeth, even though they will be obviously artificial.

Chapter 18

Partial dentures

The previous chapters concerned the edentulous patient and those which follow deal with patients who are only partially edentulous, i.e. having one or more teeth missing from the mandible or maxilla or both. Dentures designed for such patients will vary considerably depending upon the number of natural teeth missing from the jaws and will range from those replacing only one tooth to others replacing all but one tooth.

In order to be able to record missing teeth and to make reference to the remaining natural teeth it is necessary to have some easy means of notation. In Zsigmondy's system (also known as Palmer's notation) the mouth is divided into four quadrants by a horizontal line representing the occlusal plane and a vertical line representing the midline. The eight teeth in each quadrant are numbered from the front backwards, commencing with the central incisors, thus:

Patient's right	Patient's left
87654321	12345678
87654321	12345678

A similar plan is used to denote the deciduous teeth, but in this instance letters are used in place of numbers:

edcba	abcde
edcba	abcde

To denote individual teeth this chart is abbreviated by drawing only that quadrant in which the tooth or teeth to be recorded are situated; the upper left second premolar is noted thus $\underline{|5}$, the lower right first molar $\overline{6|}$, the upper right lateral and upper left canine $\underline{2|3}$, and so on.

It does not follow that every patient who loses a natural tooth requires its replacement by means of a removable partial denture. Sometimes a bridge (also known as a fixed partial denture) is a better alternative, and there are instances in which the replacement of lost teeth is considered inadvisable.

Definition of a partial denture

A partial denture is a restoration, removable by the patient, for the replacement of one or more natural teeth in the mandible or maxilla in which one or more natural teeth remain. It occupies more space than did the natural teeth which it replaces and is retained by its intimate contact with the mucosa and remaining natural teeth (Figure 18.1).

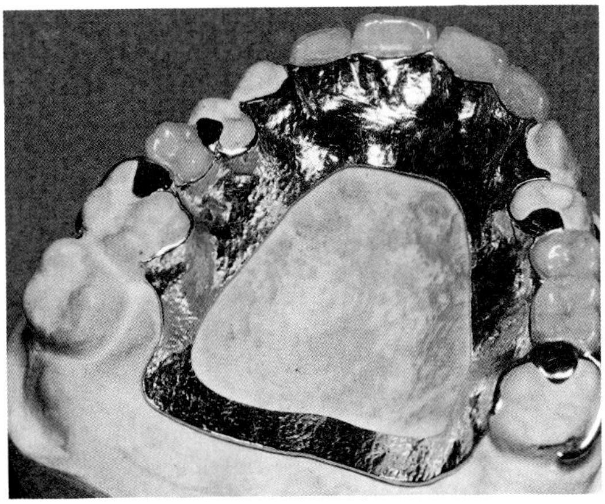

Figure 18.1 A removable partial denture

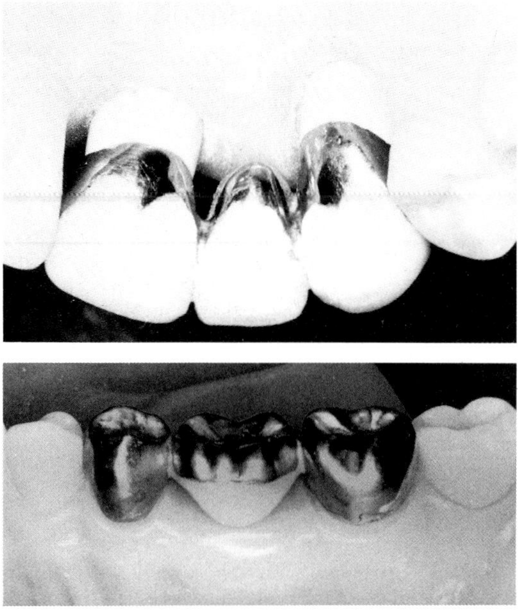

Figure 18.2 Examples of bridges (fixed partial dentures) for the replacement of a maxillary lateral incisor and a mandibular first molar

Definition of a bridge

A bridge is a restoration which is fitted to one or more natural teeth prepared for, and restored by, inlays or crowns. It occupies no more space than did the natural teeth it replaces and is permanently fixed in position (Figure 18.2).

The functions of partial dentures

When a mouth is examined in which some natural teeth are missing a decision has to be reached as to whether the replacement of the lost teeth by artificial substitutes, be it a partial denture or a bridge, will benefit the patient and, if so, what will be the most suitable type of restoration. In each individual case it is necessary to assess the advantages of a partial denture against the disadvantages.

Restoration of masticatory efficiency

While it is an accepted fact that with the more highly civilized healthy peoples, living as they do on soft cooked foods, teeth are not necessary to maintain life, most people consider it essential to have sufficient teeth to be able to masticate normal food with ease. The effect of long-continued inefficient mastication on the alimentary system is difficult to assess, but in persons already suffering from digestive problems, or other debilitating conditions, masticatory efficiency assumes great importance and its restoration is desirable.

Restoration of appearance and speech

The commonest reason for a request by a patient for a partial denture is that of restoration of appearance. Many people will ignore the loss of the majority of their posterior teeth but demand the immediate replacement of a lost upper incisor.

Speech is often affected by the loss of one or more upper incisor teeth.

Prevention of collapse of the dental arch and over-eruption of teeth

When a tooth is extracted from a dental arch the teeth adjacent to it, unless prevented from so doing by the occlusion, tend to drift towards each other, thus reducing the width of the gap made by the extraction. This causes these teeth to lose contact with the teeth adjacent to them and food can then pack between them with consequent gingival damage and increased liability to caries and periodontal disease (Figure 18.3). Loss of occlusion will often cause over-eruption and this, if gross, may mean the loss of that tooth. Thus two or three teeth extracted from different parts of the mouth, if not replaced with a prosthesis, may in a few years lead to complete collapse of the dental arch which rapidly leads to further loss of teeth (Figure 18.4).

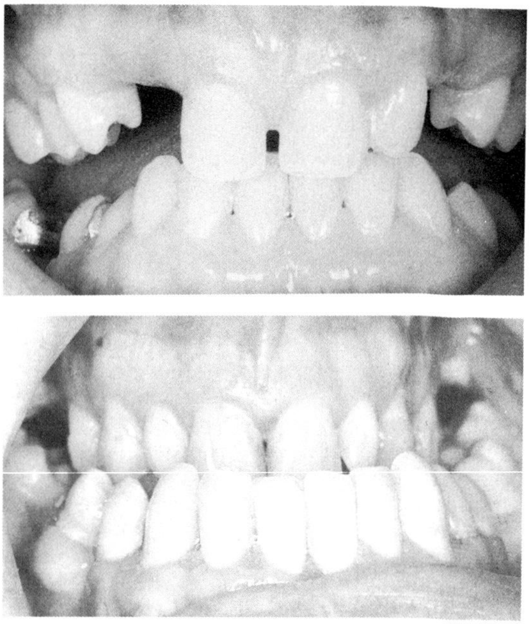

Figure 18.3 Examples of drifting of teeth, closure of spaces and disruption of the occlusion following loss of natural teeth

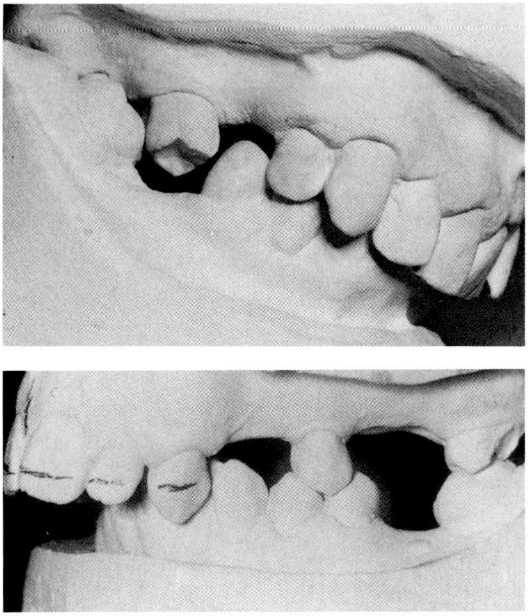

Figure 18.4 Casts showing over-eruption of unopposed teeth, loss of vertical space in saddle areas and malocclusion resulting from extraction of teeth without replacement

The disadvantages of partial dentures

1. They can cause caries.
   By harbouring food debris in close contact with the natural teeth a partial denture may promote caries and gingivitis (Figure 18.5). This will depend on several factors:
   (a) The age of the patient, the younger age group being more susceptible to caries.
   (b) The habits of the patient; if the patient is very assiduous in cleaning his teeth and denture then less damage is likely to occur.
   (c) The design of the denture; this is important because well-designed dentures will cause far less damage to the mouth than .those of careless design and construction (Figure 18.6).
   (d) Regular dental attention; partial denture patients should always be advised of the necessity of regular dental inspection as prevention is better than cure.
2. They can damage the supporting tissues of the teeth (Figure 18.7).
   In a healthy mouth the gingival margins fit closely round the necks of the teeth, rising to a pointed papilla between them; they are firm in texture and pink in colour. Their integrity is usually maintained in a well-developed dentition because:
   (a) Adjacent teeth are firmly in contact mesially and distally and, therefore, food cannot pack

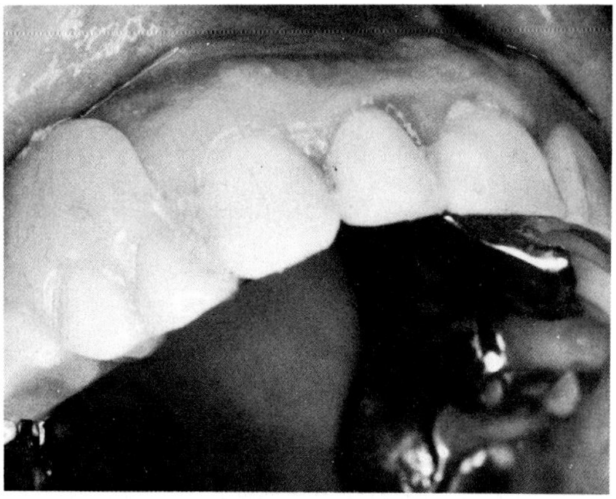

Figure 18.5 Partial denture showing large food trap between the saddle and the natural canine. Note the gingival damage around the incisors caused by the denture and by poor oral hygiene

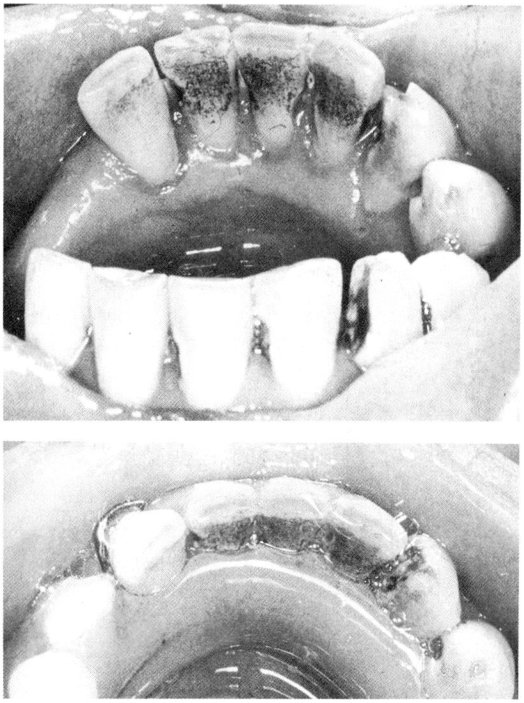

Figure 18.6 Caries and gingivitis caused by faulty design and careless construction of a mandibular partial denture

down between them and traumatize the gingival margins.
   (b) The surfaces of teeth are convex so that food passing over these surfaces strikes the gums below their free margins; any alteration in this arrangement which causes force to be applied directly to the free gingival margin will tend to produce damage.

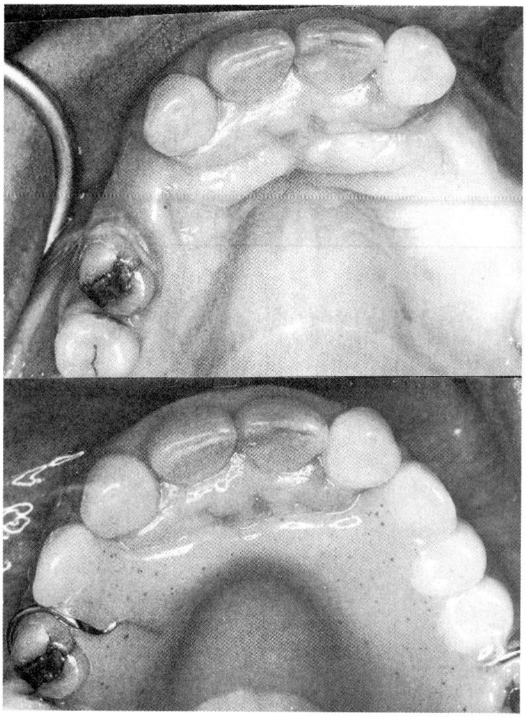

Figure 18.7 Resorption of alveolar bone in the ridges distal to 2/2 caused by a mucosa-borne denture. Note also the mucosal damage in the rugal area and the gingivitis around 4/

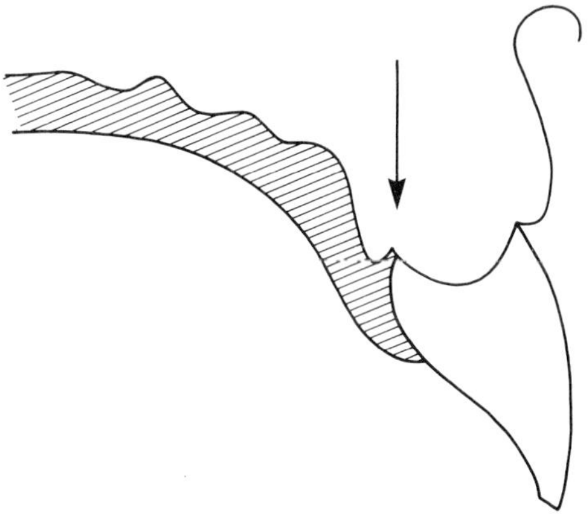

Figure 18.8 Close fit of denture base into gingival margin may lead to damage

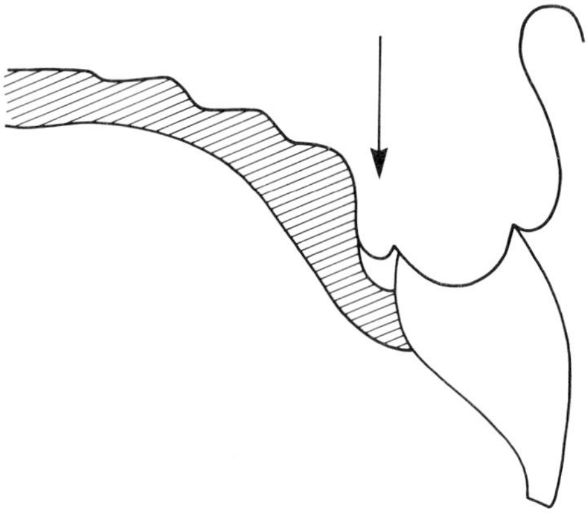

Figure 18.9 Arrow indicates relief of gingival margin, in this case, excessively. A space of this size would probably result in gingival hyperplasia. Relief should only be minimal

Partial dentures may cause damage to the gum margins by:

(a) Fitting too closely into the gingival crevices and causing mechanical injury (Figures 18.8 and 18.9).
(b) Allowing food to pack down between the denture and the teeth. Food packed under pressure against the gingival margins will force them away from the teeth (Figure 18.10) and will also, if allowed to remain in contact with the gingivae for any appreciable time, cause inflammation of the tissues. Such damage to the gingival margins, if untreated, progresses to involve the deeper supporting tissues of the teeth giving rise to periodontal disease and ending with the loss of the teeth.

3. They may loosen the natural teeth by leverage. Clasps wrongly designed or carelessly constructed, or indirect retainers badly placed, may cause excessive stresses on the natural teeth.
4. They can cause traumatic damage to the mucosa. Various types of damage which can be inflicted by a partial denture are hyperaemia, hyperplasia and ulceration (Figure 18.11).

Partial dentures or bridges?

The advantages of removable dentures over bridges are:

1. They can be constructed for any case, while bridges are confined to relatively short spans bounded by healthy teeth and with a fairly normal occlusion.
2. They can be constructed of polymeric materials and therefore are cheaper.
3. They are more easily cleaned as are the natural teeth in contact with them.
4. They are more easily repaired and in many cases can have additions made to them.
5. They do not normally involve much preparation of the natural teeth.

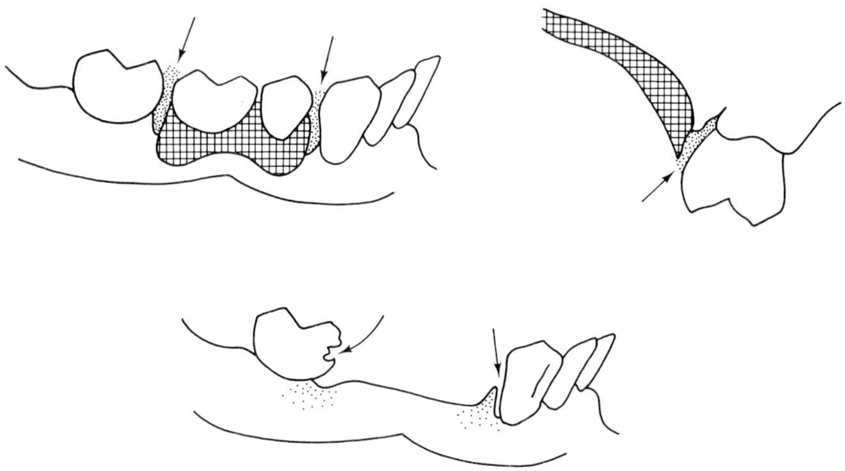

Figure 18.10 Food packing into gaps between denture bases (or pontics) and abutment teeth may lead to caries and gingivitis

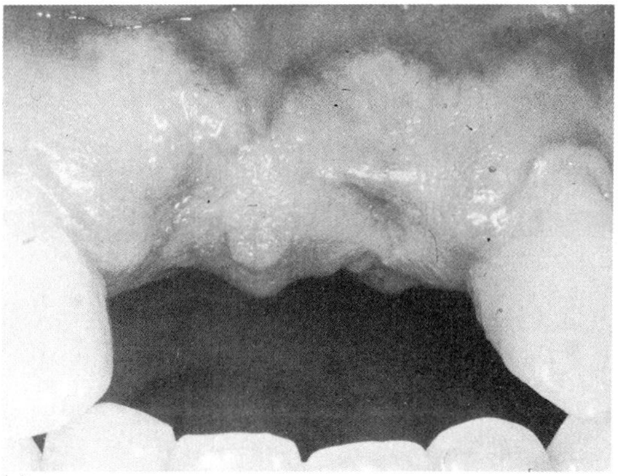

(*a*)

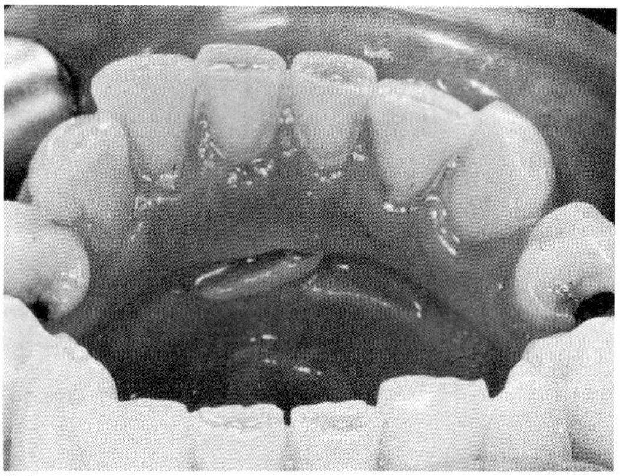

(*b*)

Figure 18.11 (*a*) On the maxillary bounded saddle mucosal hyperplasia caused by a destructive mucosa-borne denture. (*b*) On the lingual mucosa of the mandible a denture-induced flap hyperplasia caused by a lingual bar connector

The advantages of bridges

The selection of the most suitable type of restoration for a patient cannot be fully discussed in a textbook but the following advantages and disadvantages of bridges need consideration when deciding upon the treatment for any partially edentulous patient requiring a prosthesis.

The advantages of bridges over partial dentures are:

1. They require no support from the mucosa and in many instances they are not even in contact with it.
2. They only occupy the same space as the natural teeth which they replace, with the exception of certain designs, and therefore feel more natural in the mouth.
3. They withstand greater masticatory loads than dentures, except when the latter are tooth-borne.
4. Under no conditions is the patient conscious of movement nor can he produce it with his tongue and thus habits of playing with the prosthesis are not formed.
5. Because of the design of the abutment pieces (crowns or inlays), the occlusal loads are transmitted more favourably to the long axes of the abutment teeth.
6. A bridge is *in situ* for 24 h and so the periodontal membrane is not subject to re-adaptation to the temporary removal of a partial denture.

As a result of these advantages a bridge feels more natural in the mouth and the patient more readily becomes accustomed to it.

The disadvantages of bridges over partial dentures:

1. They are confined to short spans bounded by healthy teeth in good positions and alignment while dentures can be constructed for most situations.
2. Their construction is time consuming, requiring great precision, and is therefore expensive compared with the often simpler construction of partial dentures.
3. Since they are fixed they are not so easily cleaned; food debris and plaque tend to lodge between the bridge and the abutment teeth encouraging caries and periodontal disease.
4. If damaged their repair is often difficult and costly.
5. Sound natural teeth have to be prepared for inlays or crowns to act as supports and retainers for the bridge.
6. A natural tooth, lost at a later date, may often be replaced by a simple addition to a partial denture; a bridge can seldom if ever be adapted in this manner.

To make a denture or not?

The decision not to fit a prosthesis when natural teeth are missing is usually a difficult one to make. If such a course is contemplated it is advisable to make a periodic examination of the mouth to ensure that no harmful effects result from the decision not to restore missing teeth.

As a general guide, the following questions should be answered and if these are mainly in the *negative* then the probability is that the patient will be better off without a denture.

1. Is mastication inefficient with the remaining natural teeth?
2. Are appearance and speech adversely affected?
3. Is the occlusion of the teeth such that there is a possibility of over-eruption or tooth drift occurring?
4. Will the benefits of a prosthesis outweigh the possible damage it may cause to the hard and soft tissues?
5. Does the patient maintain a careful oral hygiene, or is he likely to follow hygiene instruction?
6. Is the occlusion unstable?
7. Is the patient's mental attitude to dentures satisfactory?
8. Does the patient's medical history support the wearing of a partial denture?

The answer to this last question may be the sole deciding factor regarding partial denture treatment which may be contraindicated by a history of debilitating illness, age changes, chronic mucosal disease, neuromuscular disorders and similar problems.

Often one is confronted by a patient who has lost one or two posterior teeth in different parts of the mouth some time previously with adjacent teeth having drifted into the resultant spaces. There may have been some over-eruption, tilting, rotation or misplacement. The question that arises is not 'can damage be prevented', since it has already occurred, but whether the damage will worsen if partial dentures are not constructed.

There are not many occasions when a partial denture is not necessary but the final conclusion can be obtained only after carefully weighing up the advantages and disadvantages in each individual case, and with the additional evidence of study casts and radiographs.

Chapter 19

Classification of partial dentures

Before proceeding to the principles of design of partial dentures it is necessary to know the various types of denture which can be constructed so that a correct choice may be made from the information obtained from the clinical examination and case history.

Support classification

One method of dividing partial dentures into basic types is to consider the manner in which the load applied to the occlusal surfaces of the artificial teeth is transmitted to the jaws. The masticatory and clenched loads which are ultimately taken up by the mandible and maxilla when the natural teeth are present is through the medium of the natural teeth, periodontal membrane and alveolar bone. In the case of some partial dentures these structures may still transmit the masticatory loads and the denture is then termed tooth-borne. It is a type which has small projections called occlusal rests, which are placed on the occlusal surfaces of the natural teeth so that the vertical masticatory and clenched load is transmitted via the teeth bearing the rests and not via the mucosa underlying the denture (Figure 19.1). A second way in which the load can be transmitted to the bone is through the interposed layer of mucosa. A denture supported in this manner is termed mucosa-borne and is one in which

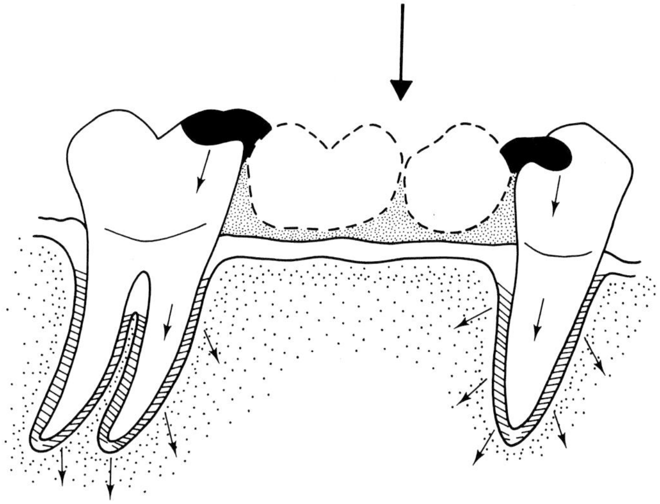

Figure 19.1 Occlusal load being transmitted to the periodontium and bone via the rests and the teeth

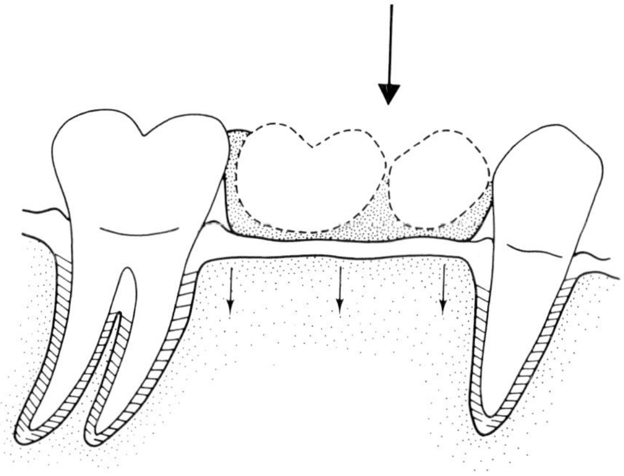

Figure 19.2 Occlusal load being transmitted to the bone via the mucosa

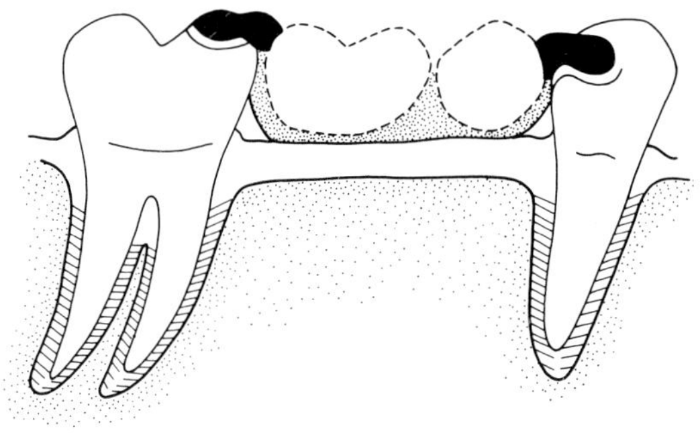

Figure 19.3 In this diagram the fitting surface of the denture saddle is in contact with the mucosa and the fitting surface of the occlusal rests are away from their seats in the teeth. When a load is applied to the denture the rests should be fully in place in their seats when the mucosa is fully compressed

the vertical load is received directly by the mucosa without any assistance from the natural teeth (Figure 19.2), although it may be braced against lateral loads by the natural teeth, which may also be fitted with clasps to aid in the retention of the denture. The vertical load may also be transmitted partly by the teeth and partly by the mucosa, such a denture being referred to as tooth- and mucosa-borne (Figure 19.3). Therefore, a very broad simple division of partial dentures can be based on the tissues which first receive the vertical load of mastication or occlusion contact and they can be classified as:

1. Tooth-borne.
2. Mucosa-borne.
3. Tooth- and mucosa-borne.

The following points should be considered when deciding upon the basic type of denture suitable for a patient:

1. A tooth-borne denture can carry loads nearly equal to those normally imposed on the natural teeth.
2. Sound natural teeth or a tooth-borne denture will impose a greater load on the opposing teeth during mastication than a mucosa-borne denture, as load on the latter is restricted by the pain threshold of the mucosa compressed between the hard surfaces of the bone and the denture base.
3. Occlusal rests must be strong enough to withstand the load applied to the denture but they must never prevent the even occlusion of the teeth. It will frequently be necessary to create a rest or lug seat in the supporting tooth or to grind the opposing tooth, or both, in order to satisfy these two requirements.
4. Only premolar and molar teeth, because of their shape, are suitable to carry occlusal rests. If a canine or incisor tooth is to be equally efficient, preparation may be necessary, even in some cases to the extent of crowning, in order to provide an adequate seat for the rest to resist vertical load.
5. Canines and incisors may sometimes be used to assist in resisting vertical loads, particularly if taken together as a group of three or more teeth.
6. If the resistance is to be through the mucosa, only the saddles are effective in lower dentures; the lingual connectors joining the saddles are usually too vertical to transmit much of the vertical load.
7. A mucosa-borne upper denture can usually spread the vertical load as it covers at least some of the hard palate. A mucosa-borne upper denture which only occludes with a mucosa-borne lower denture does not need to cover any larger area than that covered by the sum of the lower saddles.
8. The larger the area covered by a mucosa-borne denture the smaller the load per unit area for any given load.
9. The pressure required to penetrate food is inversely proportional to the area of the occlusal surface. This means in effect, that the narrower the teeth, buccolingually, the less muscular effort will be required to penetrate the food.

The problem of the tooth and mucosa-borne method of transferring the load is a vexed one and frequently the subject of argument. It is reasonable to assume that it is impossible to construct a denture in such a way that vertical load is evenly distributed between the teeth and the mucosa and, where such an attempt is made, an increasing load is placed on the teeth with the passage of time owing to mucosal changes and alveolar resorption.

Consider the case of the saddle in Figure 19.3. In order to obtain an equal resistance to load by the mucosa as by the teeth the former must be compressed until further alteration in shape ceases and it will then act like a hard tissue and transmit any further load directly to the underlying bone. To obtain this result, a certain load will be required. At this exact load the occlusal rests must be seated on their respective teeth and thereafter any increased pressure will be evenly distributed, but at anything less than this exact pressure the denture will be entirely mucosa-borne. If the occlusal rests are in contact with the teeth before this exact pressure is reached then the teeth are bearing more of the load than the mucosa, a condition which will inevitably arise when the supporting alveolar bone resorbs to the slightest extent. It is extremely unlikely that mucosa will tolerate this degree of load before the threshold of pain is reached, so that the best that can be achieved is that the load is to some extent shared by the mucosa, this share constantly diminishing in amount. Masticatory load is constantly varying and, until this load equals that empirically chosen by the clinician, the denture will be entirely mucosa-borne and the more it exceeds this chosen load the greater the proportion which will be taken by the teeth until the denture becomes virtually tooth-borne.

The few advocates of bounded tooth- and mucosa-borne saddles have never been able to suggest any method by which the optimum pressure for any given case may be assessed nor does it appear possible that such a method could be evolved.

This type of uneven loading is not infrequently seen when an attempt is made to make a free-end saddle tooth- and mucosa-borne. From Figure 19.4 it will be appreciated that the occlusal rest in the distal fossa of the premolar will support the load of the saddle anteriorly while the mucosa in the third molar region will support the load at the other end of the saddle, thus leaving the mucosa along the main length of the saddle with a diminishing load to support. Such a state of affairs will overload the periodontal attachment of the premolar and probably lead to the early loss of this tooth and at the same time cause resorption of the alveolar ridge at the distal end of the saddle. Fuller consideration is given to this problem in the appropriate section on actual design.

Kennedy classification

A further classification of partial dentures in general acceptance throughout the world is that devised by Kennedy in the 1920s and, when used in conjunction with a support classification, enables a fairly clear picture to be formed about the type of denture under consideration during a discussion on partial dentures.

The Kennedy classification is based on the relationship of the saddles to the natural teeth and has four main groups with subdivisions where necessary.

Class I Bilateral free-end saddles posterior to the natural teeth (Figures 19.5 and 19.6).
Class II Unilateral free-end saddle posterior to the natural teeth (Figure 19.7).
Class III A bounded unilateral saddle having natural teeth at each end (Figure 19.8).
Class IV A bounded saddle anterior to the natural teeth (Figure 19.9).

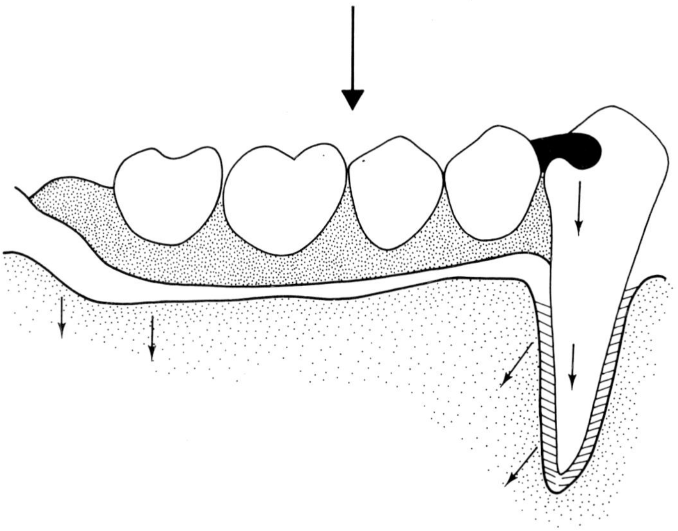

Figure 19.4 The arrows show where the concentrations of stress develop when a free-end saddle is fitted with an occlusal rest

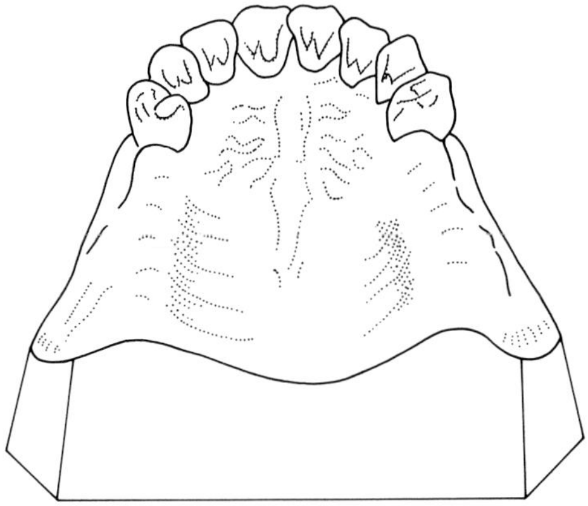

Figure 19.5 Kennedy class I upper

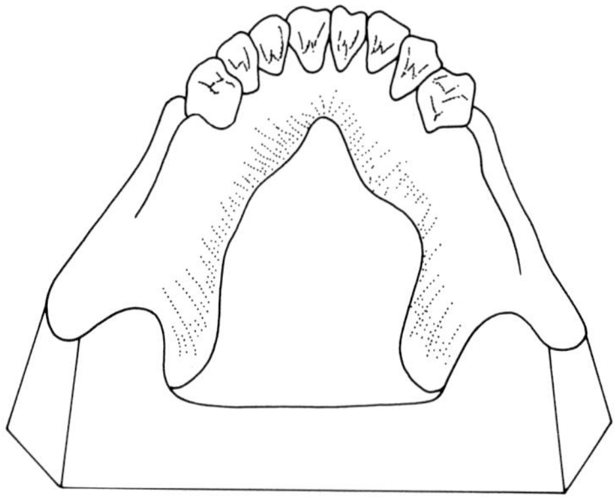

Figure 19.6 Kennedy class I lower

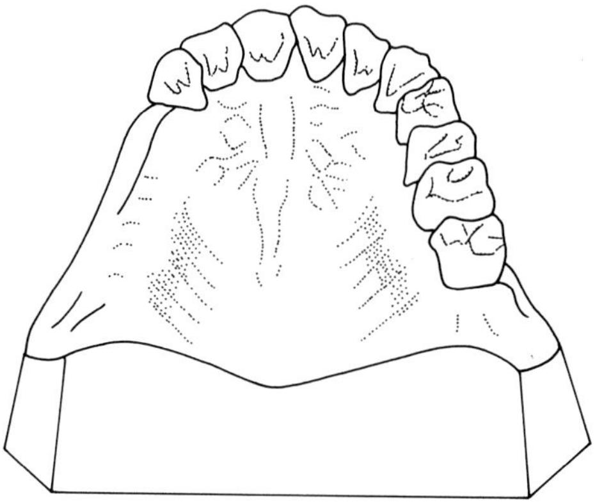

Figure 19.7 Kennedy class II

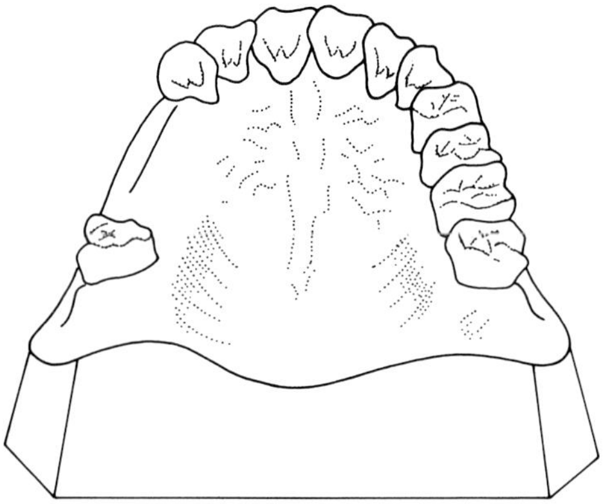

Figure 19.8 Kennedy class III

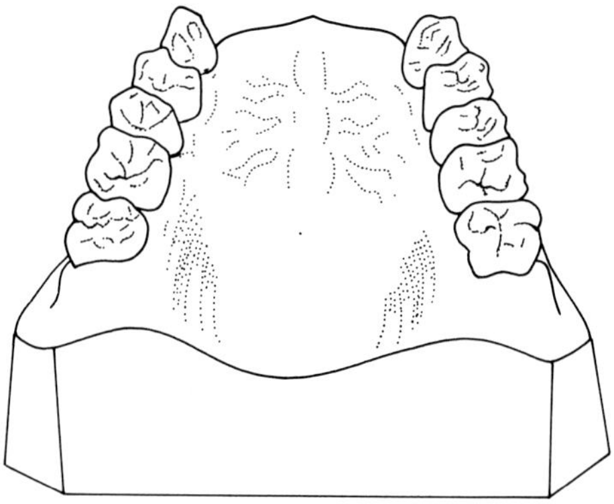

Figure 19.9 Kennedy class IV

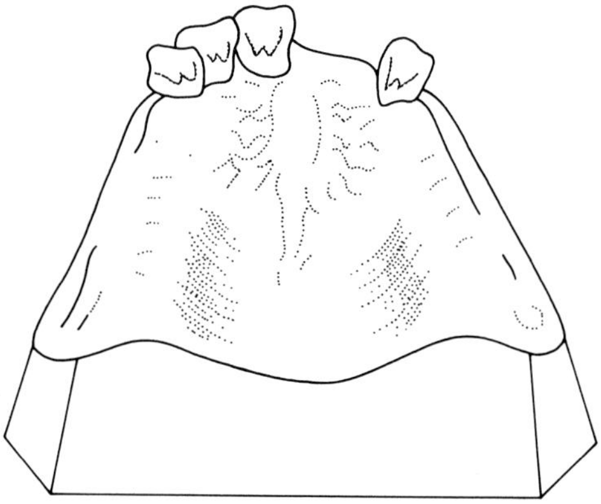

Figure 19.10 Kennedy class I modification 1

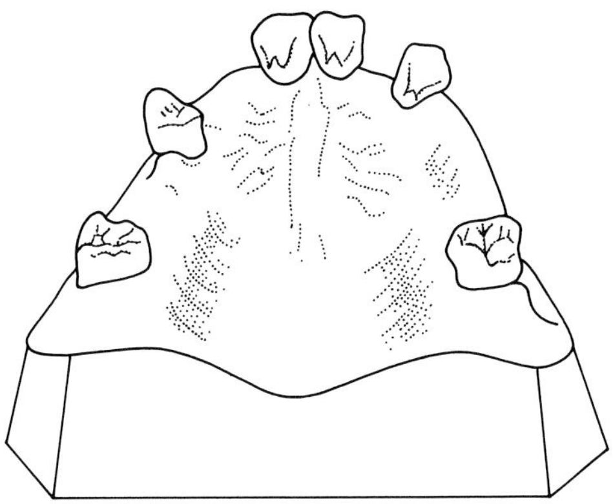

Figure 19.11 Kennedy class III modification 3

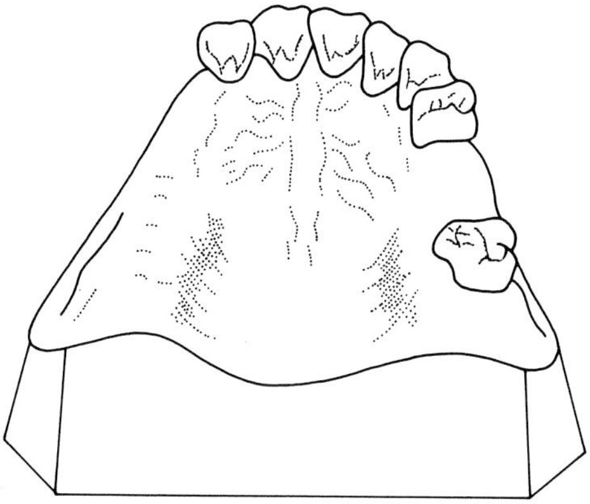

Figure 19.12 Kennedy class II modification 1

All classes, except class IV, are subdivided by modifications, each modification denoting an additional saddle area. Thus an additional saddle area in class I would be designated as class I modification 1 (Figure 19.10) while two additional saddles would constitute modification 2. Class III, modification 3 would be a unilateral bounded saddle with three additional saddles (Figure 19.11), class II modification 1 a unilateral saddle with one additional saddle (Figure 19.12) and so on. Class IV has no modifications since if such occurred then it would fall basically into one of the other classes.

In the Kennedy classification the following points should be noted:

1. The most posterior edentulous area determines the class.
2. The size of the modification is not important.
3. If a third molar is missing, and not to be replaced, it is not considered in determining the class.

Summary

Over the years other classifications of partial dentures, or partially edentulous situations, have been proposed in order to reach a common language among clinicians and technicians when discussing, planning and designing partial dentures. There is no universally accepted classification but the Kennedy classification, and one based on the available supporting tissues, form a sound basis when approaching the problems of partial denture design and treatment.

Chapter 20

Component parts of a partial denture

In order to be able to design a partial denture it is necessary to know the parts from which it is built and the function of each. These parts are:

1. Saddles.
2. Connectors.
3. Direct retainers (clasps).
4. Indirect retainers.
5. Occlusal and incisal rests.

Saddles

A saddle is that part of a denture which carries the artificial teeth. It can be either tooth-borne or mucosa-borne, and different saddles may occur in the same denture (Figure 20.1).

Dentures with tooth-borne saddles are generally made in metallic alloy since a strong material is necessary for the construction of occlusal rests and other fine components; the metal should be capable of being cast so that an accurate fit can be obtained.

Dentures with mucosa-borne saddles may be constructed either of metal or acrylic, but generally the latter for reasons of economy.

The periphery of the denture in the saddle regions should always reach to the functional depth of the sulcus and should be modified only in relation to the appearance when in the mouth.

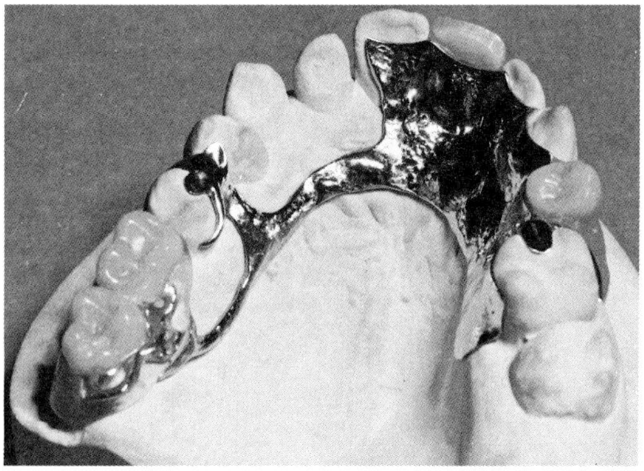

Figure 20.1 Removable partial denture with two tooth-borne saddles and one mucosa-borne saddle

Connectors

A major connector is that part of a denture which joins one saddle to another; a minor connector joins a clasp, rest or indirect retainer to a saddle. Major connectors may be classified as follows:

Palatal plates and bars.
Lingual plates and bars.
Labial plates and bars.

Palatal plates (Figures 20.2 and 20.3)

These should be kept as thin as possible consistent with the required strength and they should be dammed along free anterior and posterior borders in order that:

1. The tongue may pass from mucosa to denture, and vice versa, without encountering an edge.
2. Food particles may not so readily collect under the denture.

This damming must not be too deep or too broad because in many parts of the hard palate the mucosa covering the bone is rather thin.

The advantages of palatal plates as opposed to palatal bars are:

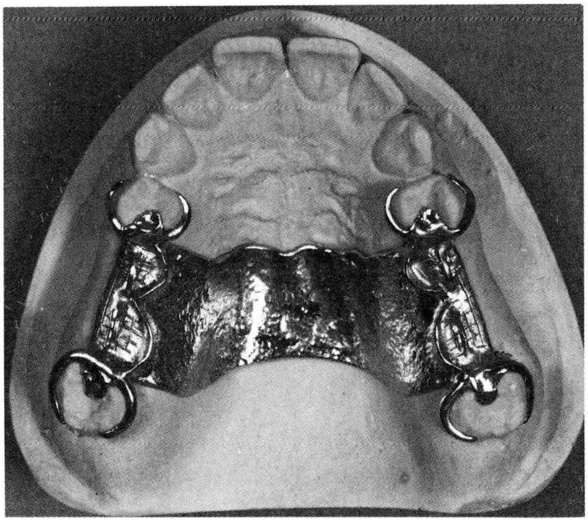

Figure 20.2 A cast palatal plate

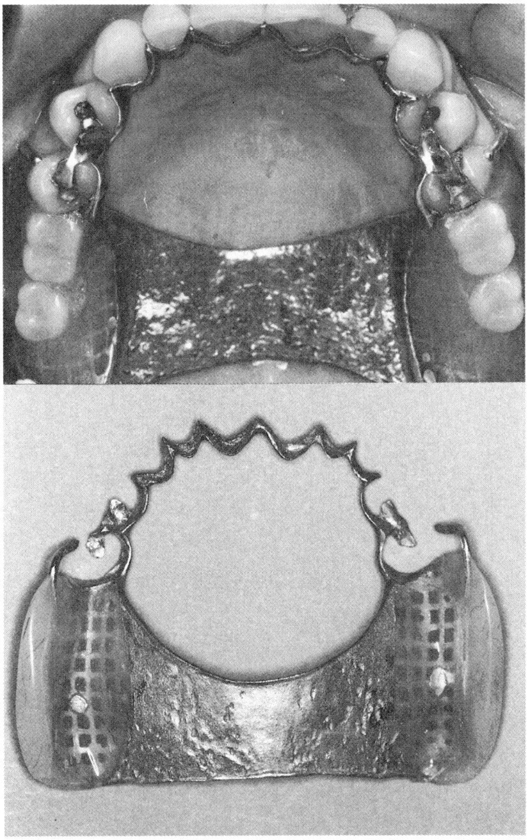

Figure 20.3 A posterior palatal plate and an anterior continuous bar retainer. Note the anterior and posterior dams on the plate

1. They are wider and therefore can be thinner in section than bars.
2. They can transfer some of the occlusal load to the palate.
3. They can be constructed in non-metallic denture base materials when economy is a factor of construction.
4. They do not worry the tongue as much as thicker palatal bars.

The disadvantage of a palatal plate is that it covers more tissue than a bar.

Palatal bars (Figures 20.4, 20.5 and 20.6)

These are always made of alloy and should be as thin as possible commensurate with strength. They must fit the palatal tissue accurately otherwise the patient is conscious of a space existing between the bar and tissue and of food packing in this space. In mucosa-borne dentures it may be necessary to form a relief on the cast where the bar crosses a bony prominence covered by a thin mucosa.

The position of a palatal bar will vary according to the positions of the saddle areas to be connected and will be either in the region of the posterior third of the palate, the middle third, or the anterior third. A posterior palatal bar is the most suitable for the following reasons.

1. Is less conspicuous to the tongue than a middle or anterior bar.
2. Often fulfils the function of an indirect retainer.
3. Is in an area less frequently associated with bony prominences or with thin mucosa.

A middle palatal bar is usually a source of annoyance to the patient as it is positioned in an area where the tongue makes frequent contact with the palate during swallowing and speech. It can seldom act as an indirect retainer.

An anterior palatal bar can be used in conjunction with a posterior bar to increase the rigidity and strength of the denture. It can also act as an indirect retainer and as a link to an anterior saddle from posterior saddles.

When narrow, and therefore thick in cross section, they are not well tolerated by the tongue especially during speech. If a link between bilateral saddles is necessary in the anterior region then the broad bar or plate of thin section is tolerated better, particularly if the free edges are situated in the troughs between the rugae.

Lingual plates (Figures 20.7 and 20.8)

These, sometimes called straps or aprons, may be made of acrylic or alloy. Acrylic is rather bulky and constricts the tongue in many instances, and should be avoided whenever possible. After construction,

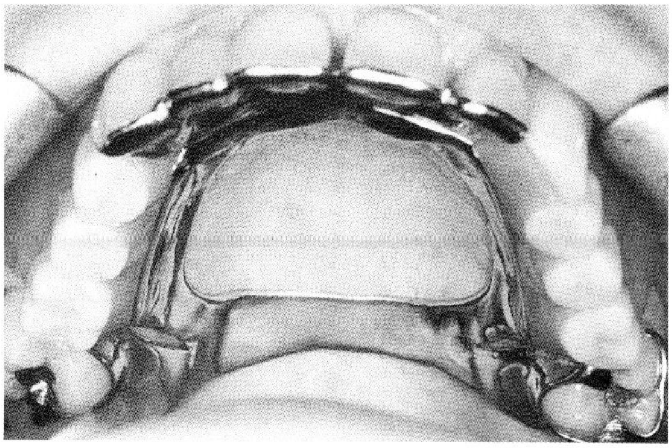

Figure 20.4 Posterior palatal bar

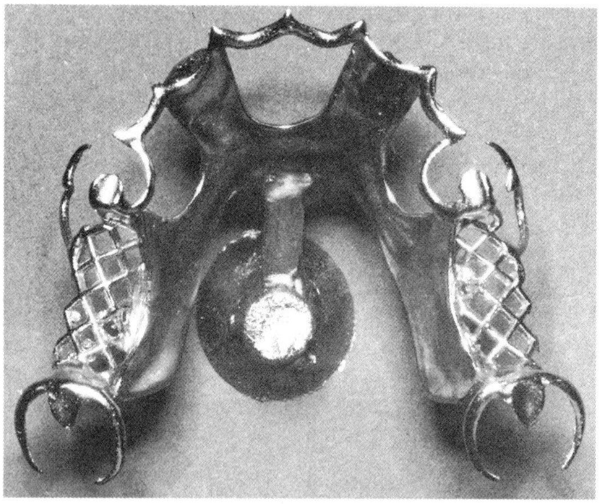

Figure 20.5 Cast cobalt–chromium base after sandblasting showing button and sprue still attached. An anterior palatal bar design

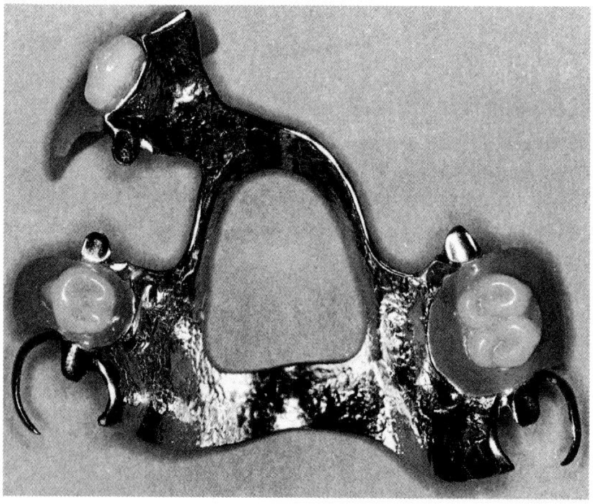

Figure 20.6 A maxillary denture with anterior and posterior palatal bars

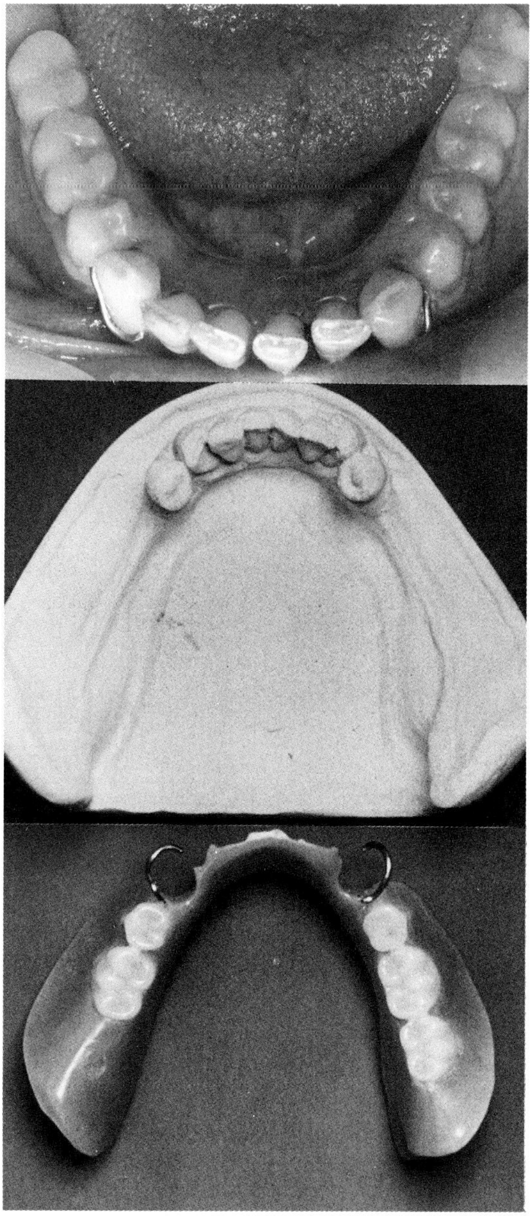

Figure 20.7 Two examples of acrylic lingual plate connectors in mucosa-borne dentures

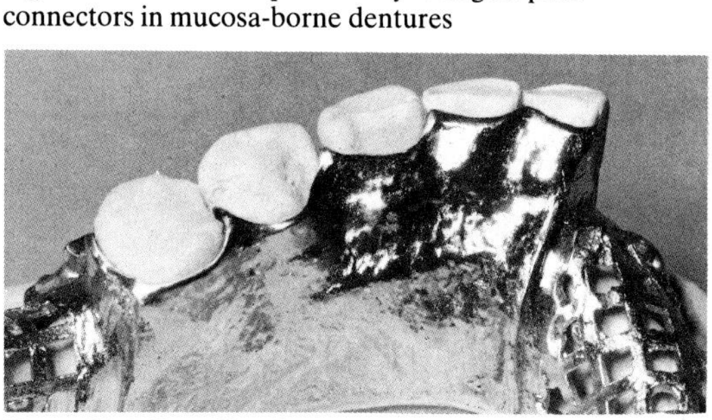

Figure 20.8 Cast alloy lingual plate connector

the gingival margins should be relieved by polishing the projecting ridge of acrylic which is the counterpart of the gingival crevice. Cast alloy plates, provided adequate gingival relief is given, are very satisfactory. They should copy the anatomical form of the lingual surface of the teeth and mucosa and, if made thin, are delightfully smooth to the tongue. Lingual plates, in contacting the teeth, act as indirect retainers and provide good bracing against lateral load. They must fit accurately around the cingulae of the teeth, and between the embrasures, or food will pack down on to the gingival margins and cause damage.

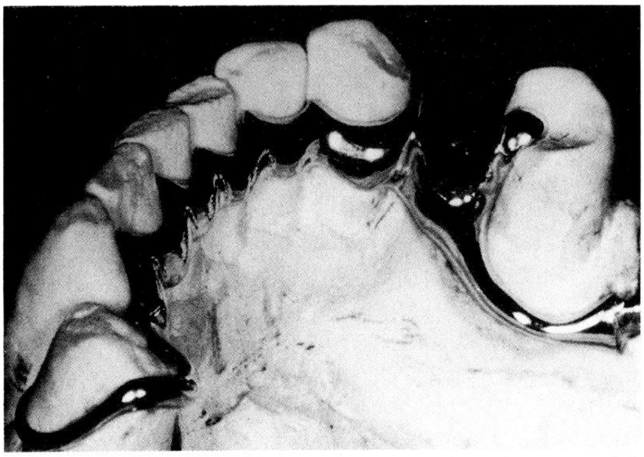

Figure 20.9 A continuous bar connector for a lower partial denture

Lingual bars (Figures 20.9 and 20.10)

These are usually made of metal and are used to connect two lower saddles, or occasionally one lower saddle with a clasp on the opposite side. They should be placed midway between the gingival margins of the teeth and the highest functional position of the floor of the mouth. A cast lingual bar is the most satisfactory type to employ, but if a wrought bar is used then the long axis of the oval cross-section of the bar should be parallel with the underlying mucosal surface; if it stands away on its superior edge food will more readily pack between it and the mucosa while if its inferior edge stands away the tip of the tongue is more likely to catch it and lift the denture. Tissue relief is provided during construction of the bar by swaging metal foil over the surface of the cast. There are contraindications to lingual bars:

1. Lack of space between the functional position of the floor of mouth and gingival margins.
2. Undercut lingual alveolar process.
3. Lingually inclined teeth.

A second connecting bar, termed a continuous clasp (also known as a continuous bar retainer or dental bar), and positioned on the cingulae of the incisor teeth, is sometimes incorporated with a lingual bar to act as an indirect retainer or supplementary rest. It has the advantage of avoiding coverage of gingival margins but usually is not well tolerated by the tongue.

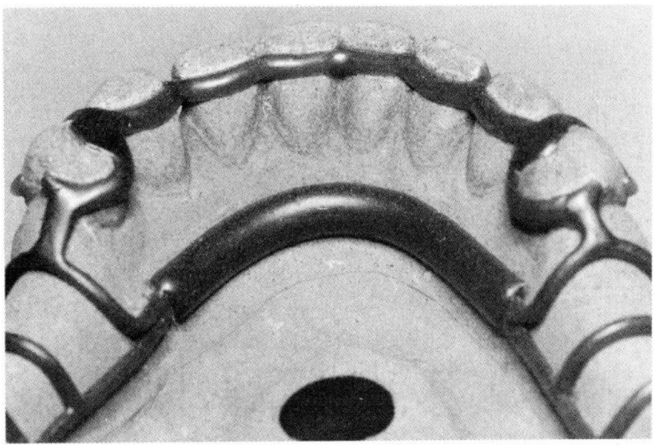

Figure 20.10 Wax pattern on a refractory model showing a lingual bar and continuous bar retainer

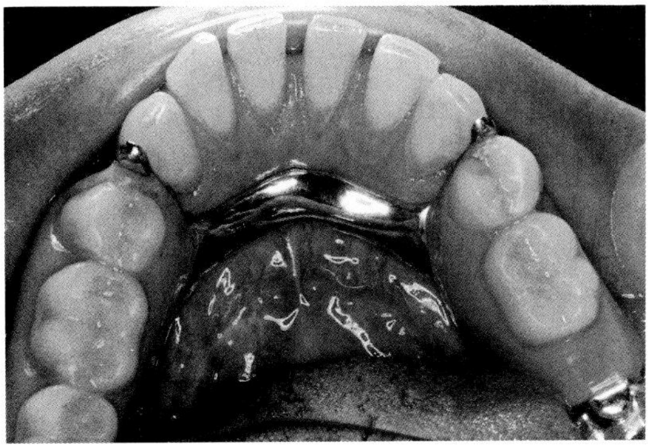

Figure 20.11 A sublingual bar

Sublingual bar (Figure 20.11)

The sublingual bar is an improvement on the lingual bar. It is less obtrusive to the patient because it lies in the anterior lingual sulcus, but is more difficult to make. It is another form of rigid major connector but being situated in the sulcus it has a different cross-section from a lingual bar which is essentially ovoid. The sublingual bar is more kidney-shaped in section but the final shape is particular to each patient. The impression is made with an individual tray whose lingual border is made rather broader than usual and carefully adapted with tracing stick with the tongue elevated forwards. The impression material is one of choice but experience shows that polysulphide rubber is most successful. The master cast may be relieved in the lingual sulcus with 0.06 mm metal foil to avoid any trauma against the lingual tissues.

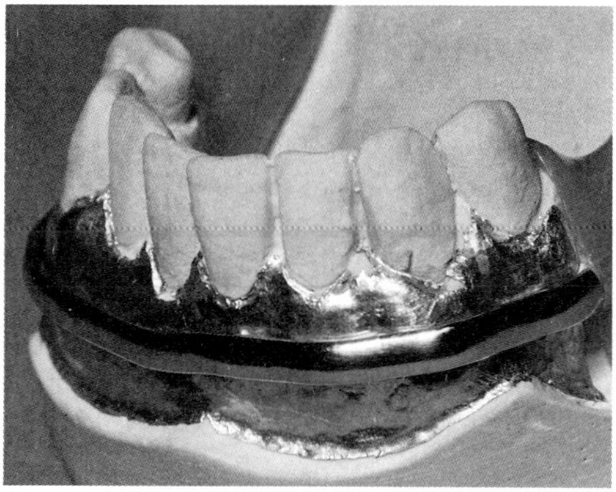

Figure 20.12 A labial bar connector. Note the metal foil used to protect the surface of the stone cast

Labial bars and plates (Figure 20.12)

These are always made of cast alloy but are not used very extensively as they tend to worry the patient's lips. They may be used when lingual connectors are impracticable, due to lingual inclination of the standing teeth, the presence of excessive lingual undercuts or problems such as a torus mandibularis. They should be made as broad and as thin as the sulcus depth and strength of the metal will allow and relief must be provided during their construction to allow for movement during mastication, similar to that for lingual bars. As they are relatively longer than lingual bars they must be greater in cross-sectional area.

Direct retainers

Unlike complete dentures that rely on border seal and selective adhesion to establish retention, partial dentures obtain their retention mainly from clasps attached to the denture which embrace natural teeth and thereby hold the denture in place (Figures 20.2 and 20.5). Adhesion and cohesion, however, do aid slightly in the retention of partial dentures of the Kennedy class I type, particularly in the case of the upper, although this depends on the actual design used. The natural teeth also aid retention by presenting guiding surfaces which offer areas for resistance to movement.

Direct retainers (clasps) can only be planned, designed and fabricated when the shape and relationship of the abutment teeth have been analysed. This involves locating undercuts on the teeth and ridges and different paths of insertion and removal. A cast surveyor (or parallelometer) is used for this.

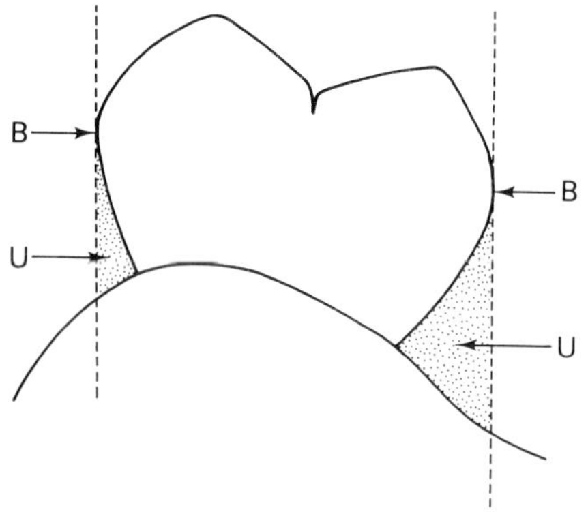

Figure 20.13 Illustrating how the naturally bulbous shape of a tooth produces undercut areas. B, the most bulbous part of the tooth; U, the undercut areas

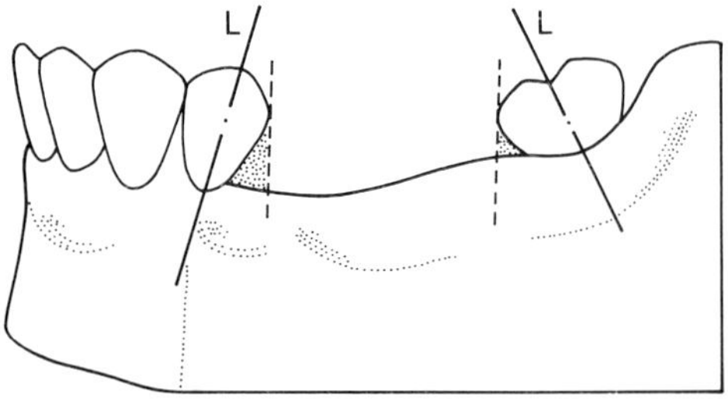

Figure 20.14 Illustrating how a slope of the long axis (L) of a tooth produces an undercut area

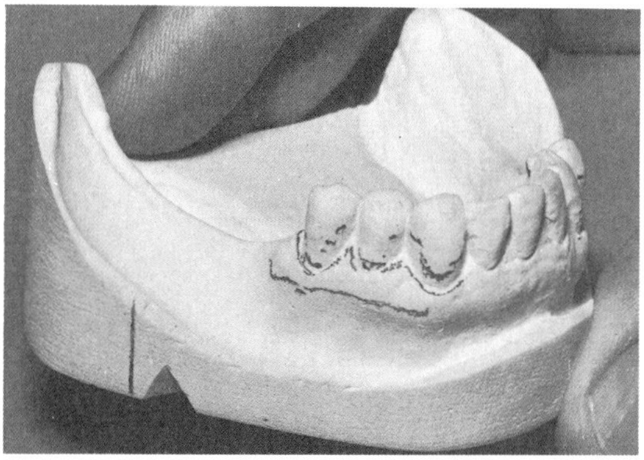

Figure 20.15 Soft tissue undercuts show after surveying at right angles to the occlusal plane (i.e. parallel to mark on side of cast)

Surveying

A partially edentulous mouth has many undercut areas which result from:

1. The naturally bulbous shape of the crowns of the teeth (Figure 20.13).
2. The fact that the long axes of the teeth are frequently inclined at an angle to a vertical taken from the occlusal plane (Figure 20.14).
3. The soft tissue and underlying bone being inclined at an angle to a vertical taken from the occlusal plane (Figure 20.15).

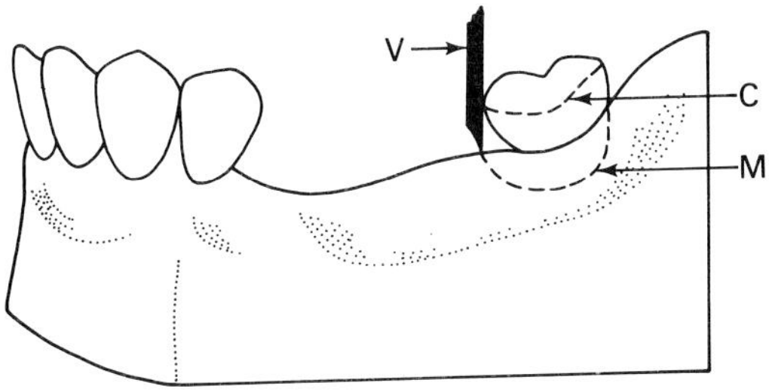

Figure 20.16 The basis of surveying. V, vertical graphite rod; C, the line drawn by the rod on the crown of the tooth; M, the line drawn on the cast

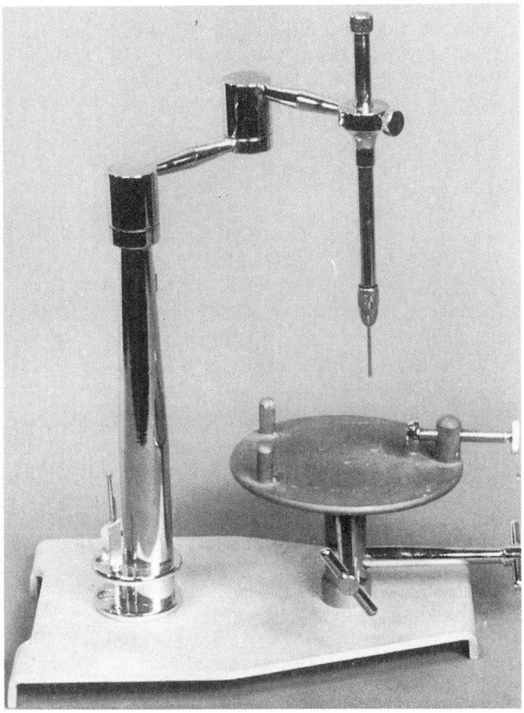

Figure 20.17 A cast surveyor

Rigid denture bases and the rigid parts of clasps will not pass into undercuts. (An undercut may be defined as an area which is out of contact with any vertical dropped from a given horizontal.) Therefore it is essential for the designer of a partial denture to be able to determine these areas on the cast. The technique of this is termed surveying.

Surveying is accomplished by holding a vertical marking edge, such as a graphite rod, in contact with the crown of the tooth and moving either the cast or the rod so that the side of the graphite draws a line around the circumference of the crown and its point draws a line, which is the projection of that on the crown, on to the part of the cast that represents the soft tissues (Figure 20.16). The area enclosed between these two lines is undercut. Similarly, the soft tissue undercuts can be delineated by a line marking the maximum bulge and its vertical projection on to the adjacent soft tissue. Such undercut areas are frequently found in the maxillary labial and tuberosity region, and the lingual alveolar region of the mandible, particularly the molar area. If these soft tissue undercut areas are not delineated, the rigid denture base will not pass over the maximum bulge and enter the undercut, except in cases where the undercut is slight and the mucosa covering the bone is thick and compressible, or where a particular path of insertion is selected for the denture.

Surveyors

Many different instruments are available for surveying but they all work on the principle of the vertical rod or marker. They consist of a firm horizontal base, a mechanism which supports the marking device and enables it to be raised and lowered, and a table to which the cast may be attached, and which may be tilted so as to alter the horizontal axis of the cast. The reason for tilting will become apparent in due course. Such an instrument is shown in Figure 20.17.

The reasons for surveying a cast

Surveying serves six purposes:

1. It enables undercuts to be accurately blocked out on the cast prior to the acrylic processing or alloy casting of the denture, so that the material of the base does not fill the undercuts and prevent the denture from being inserted (Figures 20.18 and 20.19). Two methods are commonly employed for blocking out the undercuts on the cast:
   (a) The area between the survey line on the tooth and that on the mucosa may be filled in with plaster, dental cement, wax, or composition, using the lines drawn by the graphite as guides.

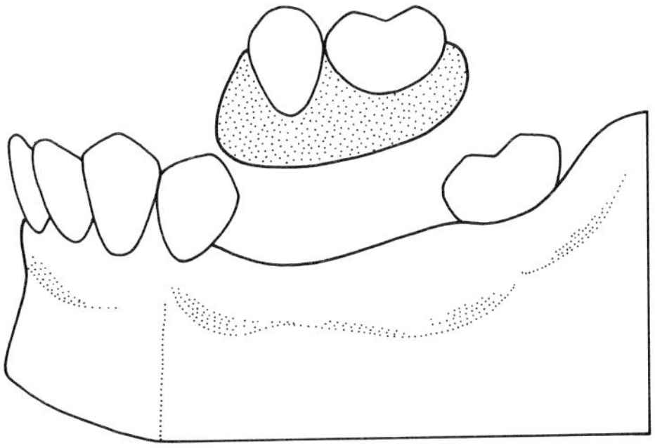

Figure 20.18 A denture made on a cast, the undercuts of which were not blocked out. The denture will not go into place

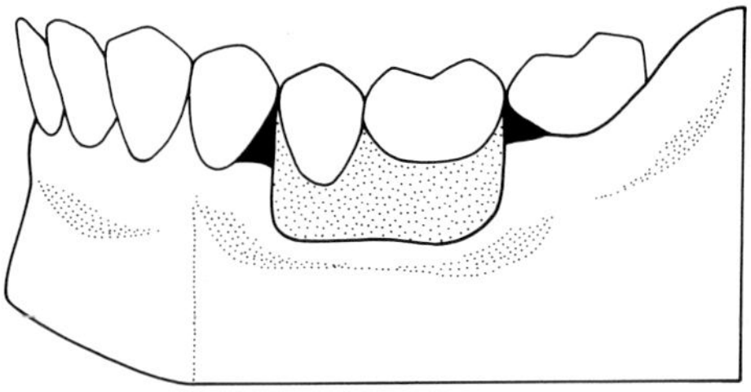

Figure 20.19 Undercuts correctly blocked out and the denture goes into place

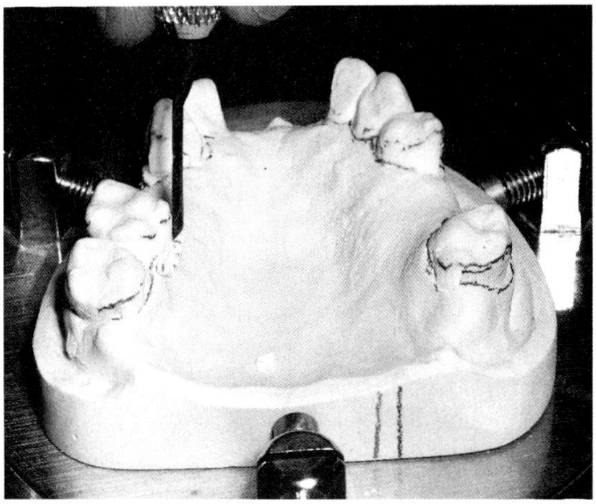

Figure 20.20 Undercuts blocked out and being trimmed with knife on surveyor

(b) The area may be overfilled with hard wax and this may then be trimmed, using a vertical cutting knife on the surveyor instead of a graphite rod (Figure 20.20). This method, which is the more accurate, is used when a duplicate model is to be made for casting an alloy base or processing in acrylic.

2. It marks the most bulbous part of a tooth which is to carry a clasp. This enables the technician to place the rigid part of the clasp above the undercut area, and the flexible arm, which does the work of retaining the denture, into the undercut (Figure 20.21). As will be shown later, tilting of the cast will affect the position of the survey line.
3. It will demonstrate undercut areas which can be used for the retention of the denture. Such utilization of undercuts requires the horizontal axis of the cast to be tilted at an angle which is sufficient to eliminate the undercut in question and bring the side of the tooth adjacent to the undercut parallel with the graphite or analysing rod of the surveyor (Figure 20.22). The line of insertion of the denture is parallel with the side of the tooth adjacent to the undercut, and the denture will only go into place if inserted in this direction because all other undercuts, which develop as a result of tilting the cast, are blocked out parallel with this line. Figures 20.23 and 20.24 illustrate a more complicated case in which tilting the cast has enabled three undercut areas (one mesial to the first molar, one mesial to the first premolar, and the labial undercut of the ridge) to be used for retaining the denture against vertical withdrawal.
4. It enables those parts of the denture base which fit against the crowns of the teeth to be placed above the survey line, and therefore against the teeth. This ensures that the denture fits snugly against the tooth and does not leave a gap into

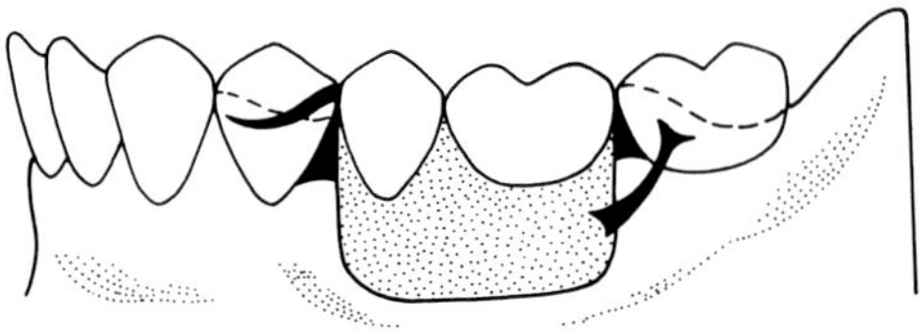

Figure 20.21 Survey lines (broken lines) enable the selection of the correct type of clasp and its accurate position

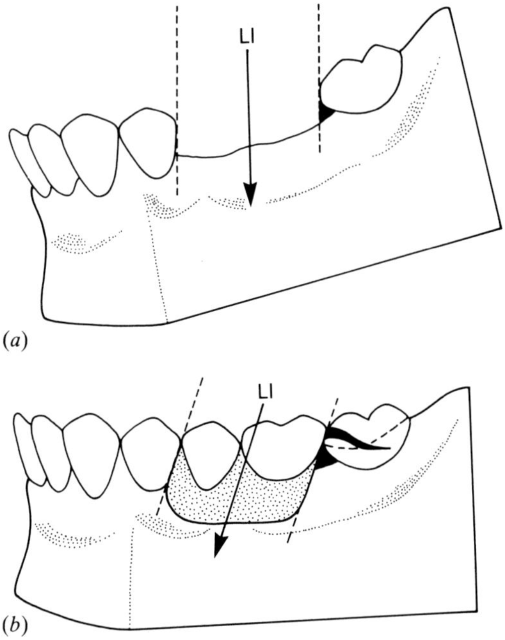

Figure 20.22 (*a*) The cast has been tilted sufficiently to bring the rod of the surveyor parallel to the distal surface of /4, thus eliminating completely the undercut behind this tooth but accentuating the undercut mesial to /7. LI = the line of insertion of the denture. This is parallel with the rod of the surveyor. (*b*) The denture inserted along the direction of LI. It fits into the undercut distal to /4 and will thus resist a vertical withdrawal force. A clasp is necessary, however, on /7

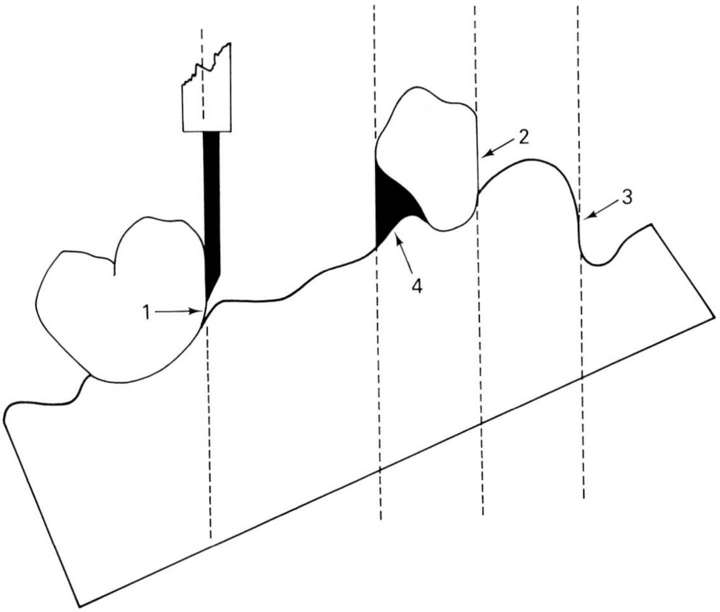

Figure 20.23 Cast tilted to eliminate undercuts. 1, mesial to first molar; 2, mesial to premolar; 3, labial to ridge; 4, is the undercut which needs to be blocked out

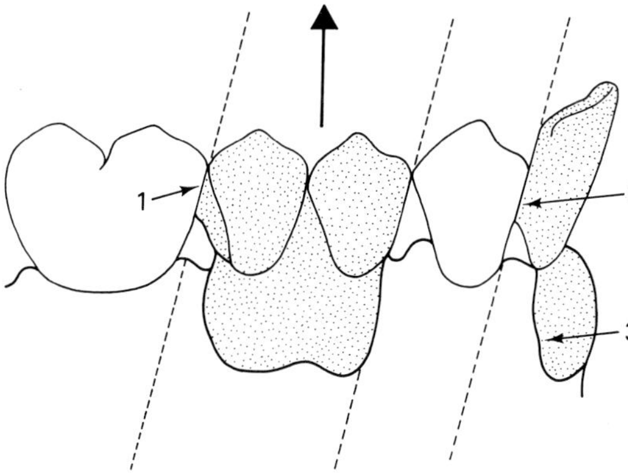

Figure 20.24 Denture fitted to the cast in Figure 20.23 along path of insertion shown by dotted lines will be retained by undercuts against withdrawal along line of arrow

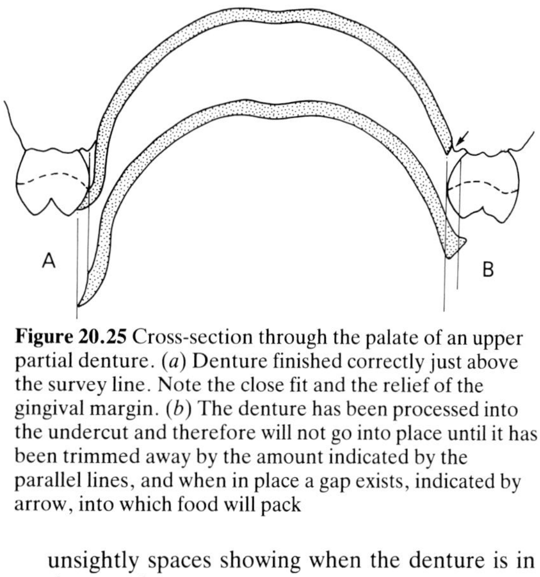

Figure 20.25 Cross-section through the palate of an upper partial denture. (*a*) Denture finished correctly just above the survey line. Note the close fit and the relief of the gingival margin. (*b*) The denture has been processed into the undercut and therefore will not go into place until it has been trimmed away by the amount indicated by the parallel lines, and when in place a gap exists, indicated by arrow, into which food will pack

which food debris may pack, a fault which is commonly seen in dentures which have been relieved empirically without reference to a surveyor (Figure 20.25).

5. It permits the dentist and technician to design a denture with one path of insertion, so that all saddles and clasps are related to this predetermined path, and not as individual units. Frequently a path of insertion is determined by the undercuts revealed during a preliminary survey of the abutment teeth of an anterior saddle. The tilting table often has to be adjusted to obtain the minimal anterior undercut area in order to avoid unsightly spaces showing when the denture is in the mouth.
6. It enables the dentist and technician to measure, with undercut gauges, the horizontal depth of an undercut below the survey line marked on a tooth and thereby determine the type of clasp to be used and the material of which it is constructed. Undercut gauges are usually of three sizes having discs of 10-, 20- and 30-thousanth of an inch or 0.25 mm, 0.50 mm and 0.75 mm respectively (Figure 20.26). They are interchangeable with the vertical surveying rod

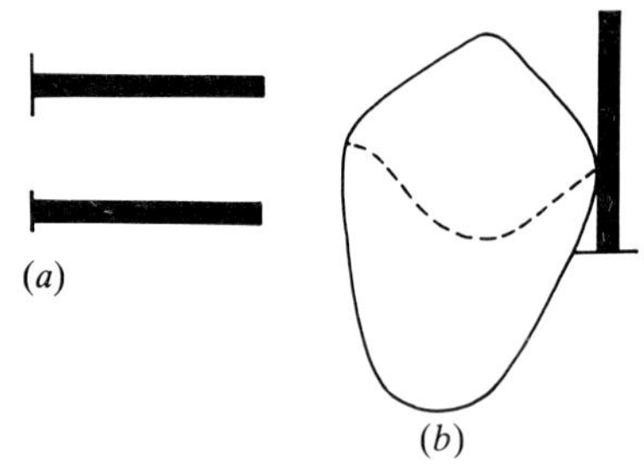

Figure 20.26 Undercut gauges. (*a*) Two sizes of disc; (*b*)the method used to determine the degree of horizontal undercut

and when in use the shank touches the tooth at the survey line and the disc touches the tooth in the undercut. By using the various gauges, the horizontal depth of the undercut can be measured anywhere between the survey line and the gingival margin and the clasp arm can be then placed in a position appropriate to the material and type of clasp. A rigid type of clasp would not need the same depth of undercut that would be required by a more flexible type of clasp.

The technique of surveying

These six functions of surveying have been described separately, for convenience, but in practice all six merge and are closely interrelated. Therefore to show how surveying is carried out, an actual survey is illustrated on an upper cast with the following teeth:

7 4321 / 1234 7

The cast is fixed to the table of the surveyor with the occlusal plane horizontal and the graphite rod moved round 7 4 / 4 7. The lines resulting from this survey are shown in Figure 20.27 and the conclusions drawn are as follows:

1. Undercuts are present mesial to 7 / 7 and the extent of these is shown.
2. The survey lines are very high on the crowns of all the teeth, especially on the proximal surfaces, and therefore no room exists for the rigid bodies of encircling clasps although projection clasps could be used.
3. If projection clasps are used on 4 / 4 and correctly placed just below the survey lines, they will be visible when the patient talks and smiles.
4. No use can be made for purposes of retention of the undercuts mesial to 7 / 7.

A denture could be designed on this cast surveyed horizontally if the undercuts mesial to 7 / 7 are blocked out and all clasps are of the projection type. Even so it would be difficult to fit a reciprocal on the palatal aspect of 7 / because the survey line is so high on the mesiopalatal corner that this part of the reciprocal would have to cross the occlusal surface of the tooth if it is to remain above the survey line at its attachment to the denture.

If, having surveyed the cast horizontally and considered the implications of the lines drawn, they do not appear as satisfactory as could be desired the next step is to survey the cast tilted at various angles, in an effort to develop survey lines which are more suitable for the design of clasps, or which will eliminate undercuts and thus enable them to assist in retention, or both.

In the case illustrated it was considered that a backward tilt of the cast, so that the analysing rod of the surveyor was parallel to the mesial surfaces of 7 / 7, would elminate these undercuts and enable

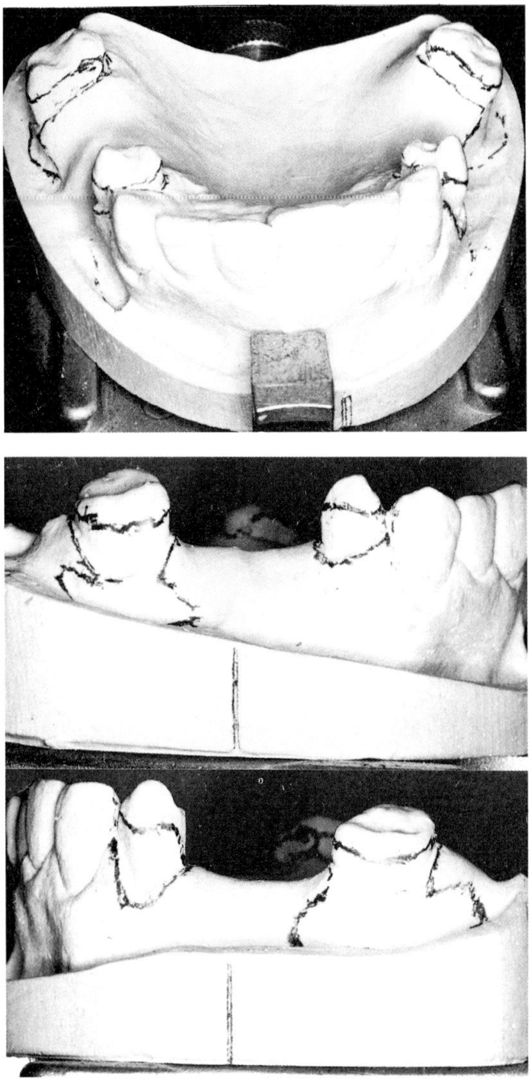

Figure 20.27 Survey with cast horizontal (see text)

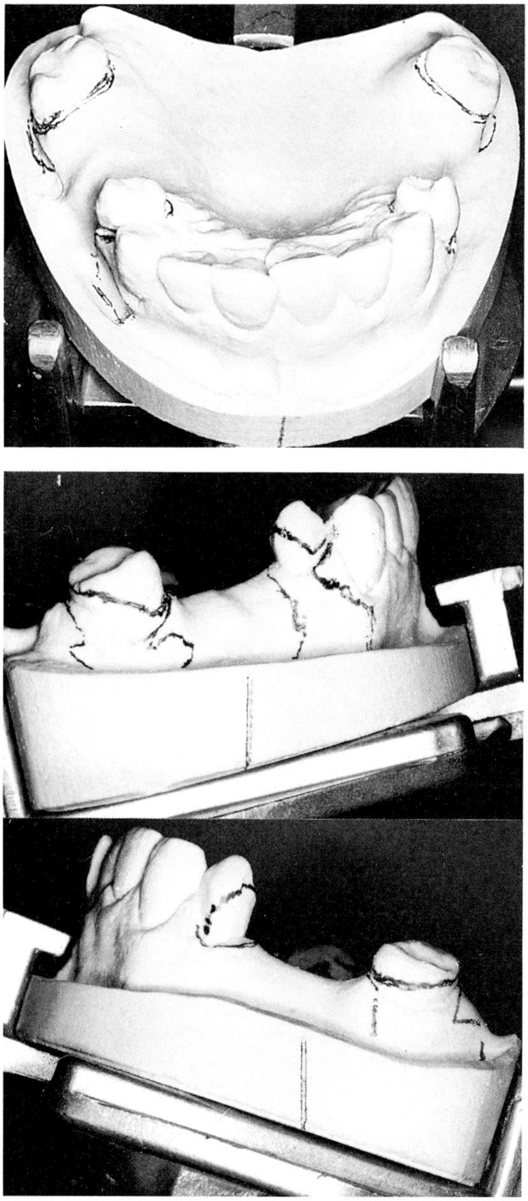

Figure 20.28 Survey with cast tilted (see text)

them to assist in the retention of the denture. The cast was also tilted slightly downwards on the right side to produce more favourable survey lines on 4 / 4. The straight lines drawn on the base of the cast indicate the tilt as these are parallel to the vertical rod of the surveyor.

The lines developed when the cast was surveyed in the position described are illustrated in Figure 20.28.

The conclusions drawn from this survey are as follows:

1. The undercuts mesial to 7 / 7 have been eliminated.
2. Undercuts have developed distal to 4 / 4.
3. The position of all the survey lines has been markedly altered and they are now favourable for the use of encircling clasps with the exception of that on 4 /.
4. The survey line on / 4 has been lowered on the tooth, and an encircling clasp used on this tooth would be almost invisible.
5. The survey line at the mesiolabial aspect of 4 / is also low on the tooth, and a projection clasp correctly positioned here would also be almost invisible.
6. No difficulty now exists in positioning the reciprocals on the molar teeth.

Summary

A denture designed on this cast surveyed with a backward tilt would be superior to that designed on it when surveyed horizontally for the following reasons.

The main retention would be by encircling clasps which collect far less food debris and possess superior bracing properties.

The undercuts mesial to 7 / 7 will also assist in retention as the denture base would lie in them.

The appearance of the patient will not be marred by conspicuous clasps on 4 / 4

The case illustrated is a simple one, but the principles of surveying described hold good for more complex cases. When an anterior tooth or teeth are lost, there is an associated loss of alveolar bone, mucosa and gingival contour. A partial denture should replace all these lost parts and, in order to do this effectively, a wide labial flange should be made. This flange should extend laterally to the apex of the curve of the gingival margins of the natural teeth immediately adjacent to the space, where it should end with a knife-edge finish. In this way the flange will merge with tissue unaffected by the lost tooth or teeth. When an anterior tooth is lost it will be found that, in most cases, an undercut relative to the horizontal occlusal plane exists around the adjacent teeth or mucosa, and it is obvious that if a rigid labial flange is to enter this region, the cast must be tilted until this undercut disappears i.e. an oblique path of insertion must be selected.

Where a mesial or labial undercut is required to provide additional retention against displacememnt, and the retention is to be provided by a rigid portion of the denture base, the cast is tilted to obliterate the undercut and this is indicated by the analysing rod. It should be noted, however, that tilting a cast to make allowances for an anterior flange may present problems if there are also posterior teeth missing. For example, if 1 / 5 6 are missing, the undercuts on distal / 4 and mesial / 7 relative to the occlusal plane may well be about the same degree. The effect of tilting the cast to eliminate the undercuts around 2 / 1 will be to eliminate the undercut on mesial / 7 but at the same time increase the undercut on distal / 4, i.e. the angle of displacement of the posterior saddle is widened and the likelihood of its displacement increased.

Clasps

A clasp consists of a resilient metal projection from the denture which grips the natural tooth and retains that part of the denture, to which it is attached, in its functional position.

The types and designs of clasps are many in number, and some of them are known by the name of their originator. For practical purposes, however, they may be classified into two main types:

1. Encircling or occlusally-approaching clasps.
2. Projection or gingivally-approaching clasps.

Encircling clasps

These consist of two arms which encircle the tooth on opposite sides, and are in contact with it along their whole length, gripping it at their extremities (Figure 20.29). Generally one of the arms is rigid, merely acting as a reciprocal to the force of the other functional arm and so preventing movement of the tooth. If pressure is applied to one side of a tooth only, that tooth will eventually move, irrespective of the patient's age; therefore a clasp should always be envisaged as grasping a tooth, never merely pressing against it. Not infrequently this reciprocal is formed by an extension of the denture base on to the appropriate surface of the tooth. If both arms of the clasp are flexible, each acting as a reciprocal to the other, very careful adjustment of each arm is required because if one presses more strongly on the tooth than the other the tooth will be moved. Each arm may be divided, for descriptive purposes, into the shoulder, root, middle and tip.

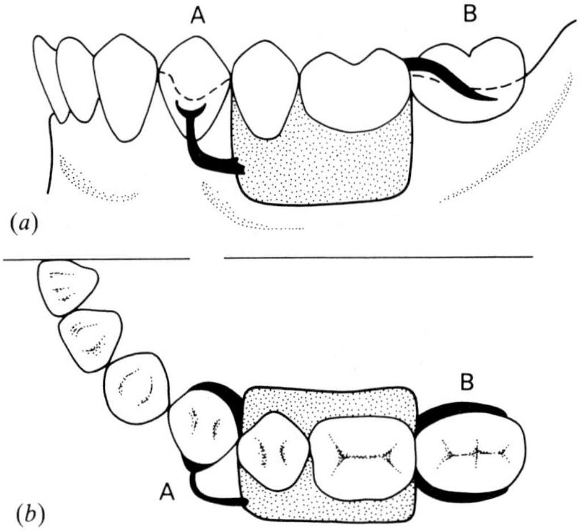

Figure 20.29 A projection clasp shown at A. An encircling clasp shown at B. (*a*) From the buccal aspect; (*b*) occlusal view

Projection clasps

These differ from the encircling type by not being in contact with the tooth along their whole length and by approaching the undercut area from the gingival aspect.

How a clasp functions

Basically, any type of clasp consists of a flexible metal arm attached to the denture. If the arm is flexed, and then prevented from returning to its position of rest, it will possess energy in the form of spring pressure. Thus, if the extremities of a clasp press on an inclined plane the clasp will endeavour to travel down the plane in an effort to release its potential energy.

The basis of correct clasp design, therefore, resolves itself into placing the flexible part of the clasp arm on an inclined plane which is sloping in the right direction. Thus the clasp will retain the denture in place and any force which attempts to withdraw the denture will draw the tip of the clasp up the inclined plane, thus flexing the arm more and increasing its energy to resist the withdrawing force. If, on the other hand, the flexible part of the clasp is placed on an inclined plane which is sloping in the wrong direction, the pressure of the clasp will force the denture out of place.

If a force F (Figure 20.30) which represents the spring pressure of a clasp is applied to an inclined plane AB, it is resolved into two forces, one XY at right angles to the plane and one XZ along the plane. It is the force XZ that retains the denture in

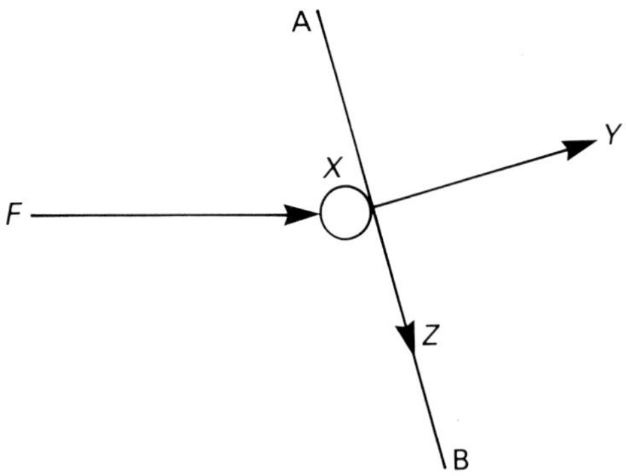

Figure 20.30 How a clasp functions (see text)

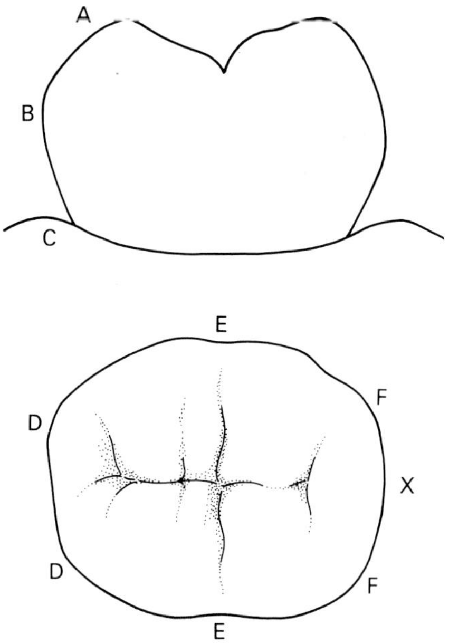

Figure 20.31 Outlines of a natural tooth. Imagine that the clasp is attached on side marked *X* (see text)

place if the plane slopes in the right direction, or expels it if not.

The surfaces of the natural teeth are planes inclined at various angles. This will be clear from Figure 20.31 which shows an average tooth in cross-section and in plan.

If the flexible part of the clasp arm is placed on the inclined planes DE and BC, excellent retention will result. If, however, it is placed on AB or EF, expulsion will ensue. In other words, the flexible part must be placed in an undercut area and the clasp must encircle more than half the circumference of the tooth.

The phrase 'the flexible part of the clasp' has been used deliberately because its flexibility is not uniform throughout its length, for two reasons:

1. Attachment to the denture makes it rigid at one end.
2. Tapering towards its free extremity increases its flexibility out of proportion to its length; a clasp is like a fishing rod, the handle being rigid and unyielding and the tip the most flexible part.

It will also be obvious from Figure 20.31 that the point B represents the most bulbous part of the tooth and that only the flexible part of the clasp will pass over it into the undercut area beneath. Therefore, before the correct type of clasp to be employed on any tooth can be decided upon, the positions of the favourable and unfavourable inclined planes of the tooth must be known. The simplest way of discovering this is to delineate the most bulbous circumference of the tooth, and it then follows that any part of the tooth on the gingival side of this line must slope in a favourable direction for clasp retention, while for any area to the occlusal side of it the converse must hold. This contour line is drawn by means of a clasp surveyor.

Survey lines on teeth vary, and while every effort should be made when surveying to develop lines which will enable an encircling type of clasp to be used, this is not always possible, and it is for these cases that projection clasps are particularly useful.

The reasons why the encircling clasp is superior to the projection type are: (1) the rigid part of the clasp which is in contact with the tooth provides valuable bracing for the denture against lateral movement; (2) it holds the minimum of food debris in contact with the teeth, provided it is highly polished on the fitting surface. This is because it is in close contact with the tooth along its whole length, while the arms of projection clasps are separated from the teeth and soft tissues by 0.5 mm–2 mm and consequently food tends to collect in this space.

The value of projection clasps is considerable, however, because:

1. They can be used in situations unfavourable to the use of encircling clasps.
2. Any degree of flexibility can be obtained by lengthening the arm which passes over soft tissue.
3. They are often less conspicuous.
4. They can be placed in the area of the greatest undercut.
5. They can be used as stress breakers.

Factors in the selection of a clasp

It will be realized that the main factor which guides the selection of clasp form, for any particular situation, is the type of survey line. Other factors do, however, affect this selection.

The position of the tooth

For example the tooth may be adjacent to an edentulous space or it may be separated from it by other teeth or it may lie on the opposite side of the mouth. The tooth may be isolated or have another tooth in contact with it. Clasps will vary in relation to these factors.

The occlusion of the teeth

In some clasps it is necessary to carry an arm across the contact point between two natural teeth. If the occlusion will not allow room for this to be done another clasp may have to be selected, or a space made for the arm by grinding the teeth and this is not always desirable.

The appearance

In the front of the mouth clasps may require to be subservient to the appearance. Retention, however, may often be obtained by adjusting the tilt of the surveying table so that an undercut adjacent to the anterior abutment tooth can be engaged by the denture base.

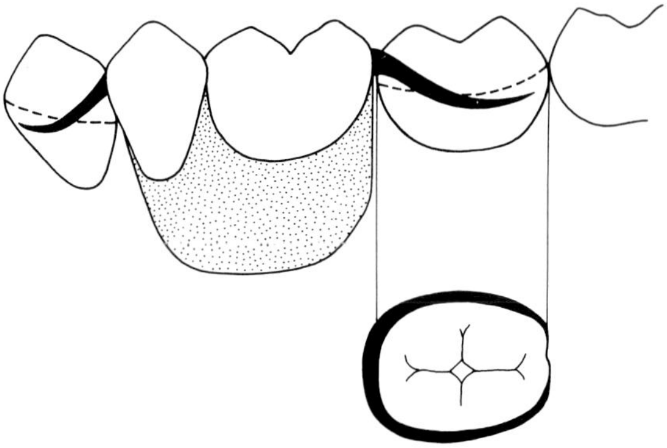

Figure 20.32 Two-arm encircling clasp from the buccal and occlusal view

Types of clasps

It is intended to illustrate the various types of clasp primarily in relation to the types of survey line, and the other factors will be mentioned when they have a bearing. Eleven types of clasp are described as they are most commonly used. These eleven forms are far from being exhaustive of the clasps available but they point to the basic principles of clasp design and if these are grasped the usefulness of other forms may be assessed.

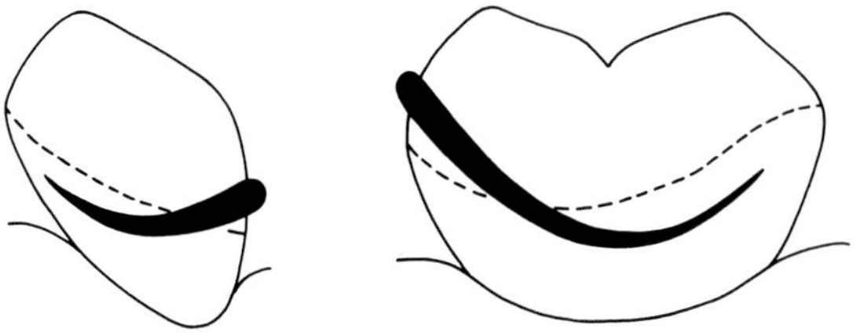

Figure 20.33 Two-arm encircling clasp. The tip should travel in the undercut area for as long a distance as possible

Encircling clasps

Two-arm encircling clasp

The *normal arm* (Figure 20.32) is a useful clasp which can be employed whenever the tooth to be clasped is adjacent to an edentulous space, and the survey line on that part of the tooth nearest to the space allows room for the rigid part of the clasp. The design of the arms should be such that the flexible terminals of the clasp travel for as long a distance as possible in the undercut area (Figure 20.33).

In the *recurved arm* clasp the length of the arm is increased by curving in on itself as shown in Figure 20.34.

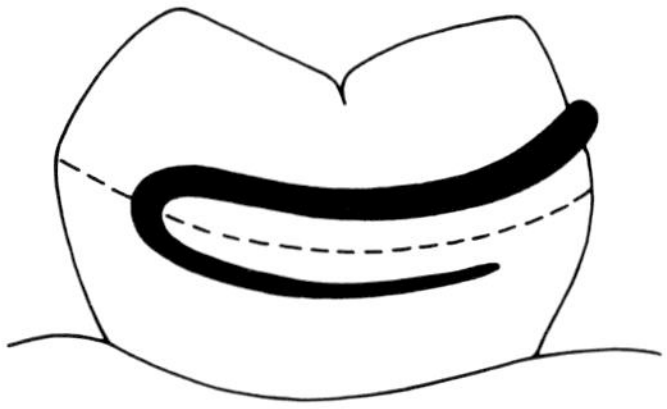

Figure 20.34 Recurved arm encircling clasp

It can be employed in situations similar to those suitable for the normal form but it requires a fairly large area of tooth above the survey line to allow room for the rigid part of the clasp. It has the disadvantage that food tends to pack in the space where the arm recurves.

The advantage of an arm of this shape is that it allows the length of the retentive terminal to be increased and brings it nearer to the denture so providing superior retention. This is because the distance over which leverage is effective is reduced (Figure 20.35). The length of the rigid part is also increased and so provides excellent bracing.

One-arm form

This type of clasp is similar in every way to the two-arm variety, except that only one arm is flexible, the other arm, or reciprocal, being formed by an extension of the denture (Figure 20.36). The form of the single arm may be normal or recurved.

This type of clasp does not provide such good retention as the two-armed clasp because there is only one flexible terminal. The lateral bracing is good, however, being provided by the unyielding reciprocal. This type of clasp is easy to make and is commonly employed with acrylic-based dentures.

Circumferential form (ring clasp) (Figure 20.37).

In this type of clasp the flexible arm is an extension of the reciprocal. It is usually employed on isolated teeth, e.g. lower molars exhibiting a survey line which allows plenty of room for the long rigid part. It provides excellent bracing, and like the recurved encircling clasp brings the flexible terminal near the denture, so reducing leverage.

Back action form (Figure 20.38)

This is very similar to the ring clasp except that it is attached to the denture by means of a strut placed anterior or posterior to the saddle on the lingual or

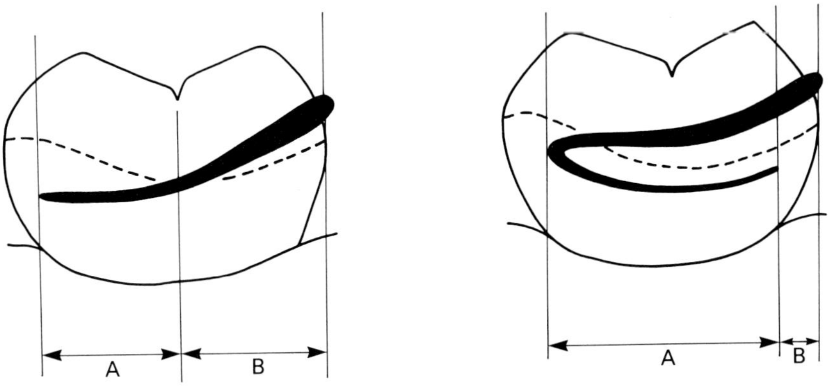

Figure 20.35 A = length of retentive terminal. B = distance from the denture to any part of the retentive terminal

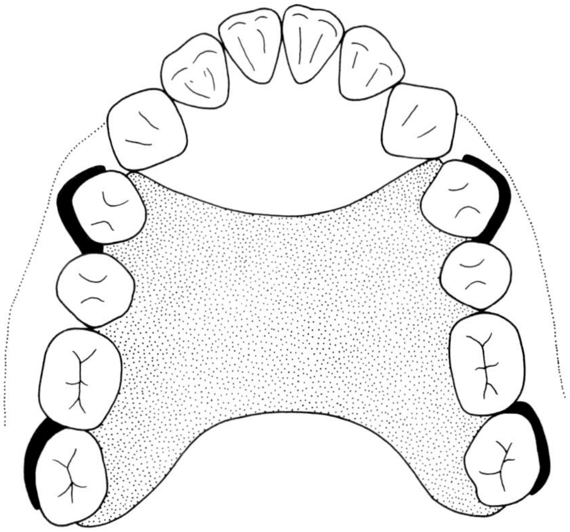

Figure 20.36 One-arm clasps reciprocated by mucosa-borne denture base

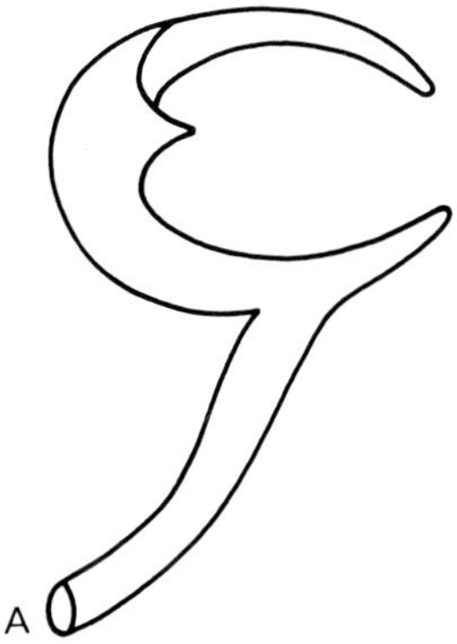

Figure 20.38 Back action clasp with occlusal rest. Clasp is attached to denture at A

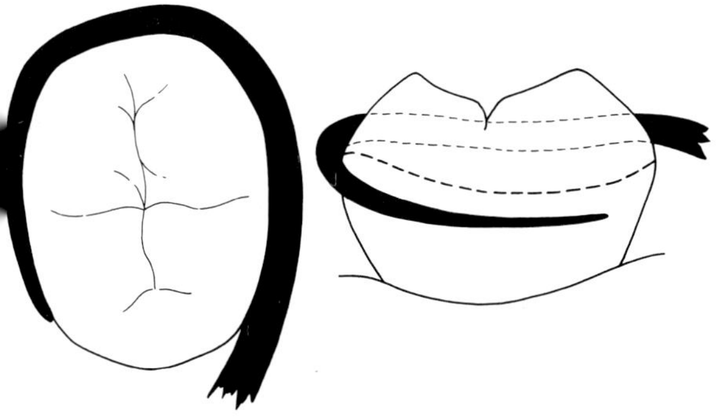

Figure 20.37 Ring clasp

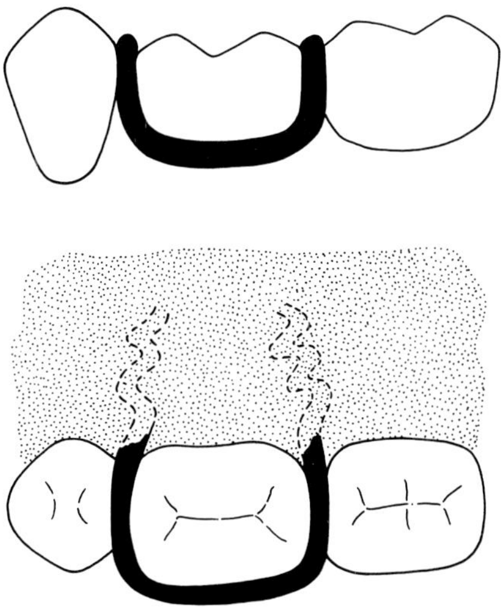

Figure 20.39 Diagram of Jackson crib clasp reciprocated by denture base

palatal side; if placed on the buccal side it is called a reverse back action clasp.

Jackson crib

This is a completely encircling clasp with no free flexible terminal. It provides retention because those parts of the clasp which are situated on the proximal embrasures of the tooth are springy and grip the undercuts which exist in these areas (Figure 20.39). This clasp is valuable when no edentulous space exists on either side of the tooth to be clasped. Room must exist, or be made by grinding, for those parts of the clasp crossing the occlusal surface.

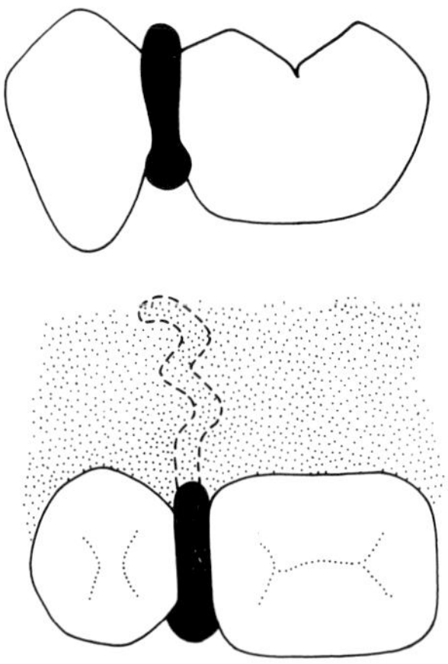

Interdental (Figures 20.40 and 20.41)

This clasp has two forms. The first consists of a round wire which has been fused at the end to form a ball. The wire is carried across the occlusal surface at the contact point of the teeth, and the ball fits into the undercut area between the embrasures.

The second, which is usually cast, substitutes a small triangular wedge or two clasp arms in place of the ball.

Interdental clasps are employed when no edentulous gap exists between the teeth. Space must exist or be made for the arm which crosses the occlusal surface.

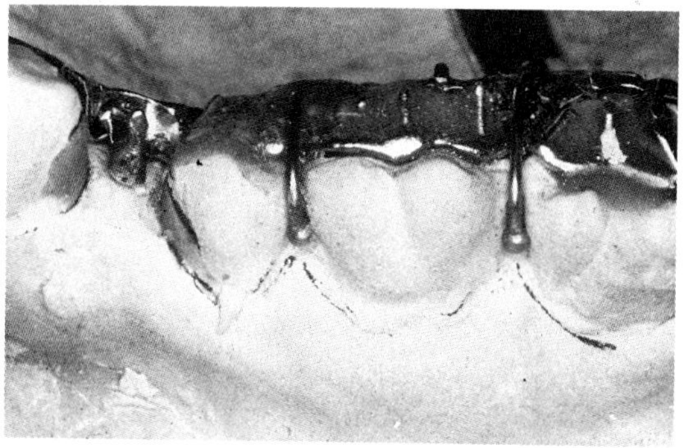

Figure 20.40 Ball-ended interdental clasp, usually made of wrought alloy

Projection clasps

T-shaped (Figure 20.42)

This is a useful clasp form to employ when the survey line indicates that no room exists for the rigid part of an encircling clasp and yet there is a large undercut area.

The length of both the arm and the part which makes contact with the tooth may be varied to suit the requirements of retention and flexibility. This clasp is usually made with rigid reciprocation.

This clasp is valuable for use on canine and incisor teeth with the added advantage that it is the least conspicuous type because it approaches from the back and not the occlusal surface (Figure 20.43).

U-shaped (Figure 20.44)

This clasp is useful when the survey line dips to the gingival margin on the buccal aspect of the tooth, a common finding on molars because of their anatomy.

L-shaped (Figure 20.45)

This type of clasp is usually employed on premolar or canine teeth when the area gingival to the survey line is extremely small and where no other type of clasp can be used.

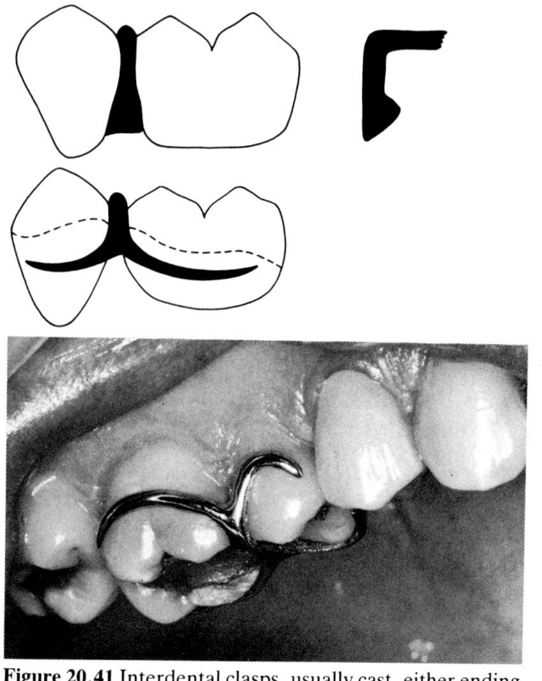

Figure 20.41 Interdental clasps, usually cast, either ending in a wedge or spreading into two buccal arms

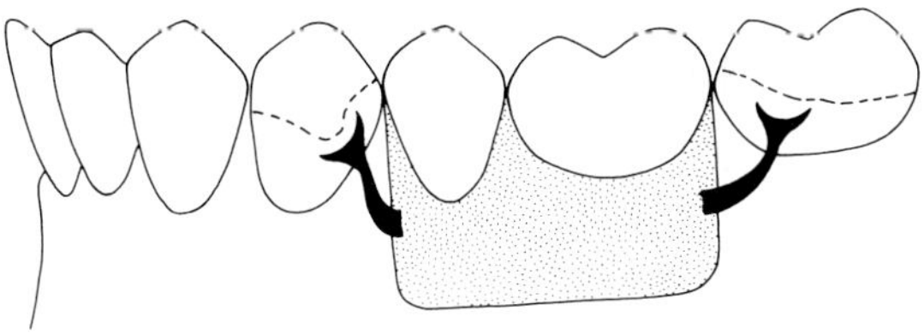

Figure 20.42 T-shaped projection (gingivally-approaching) clasps

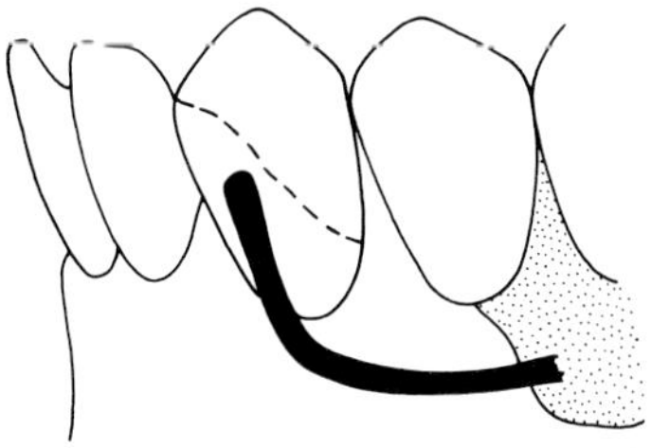

Figure 20.45 L-shaped projection clasp

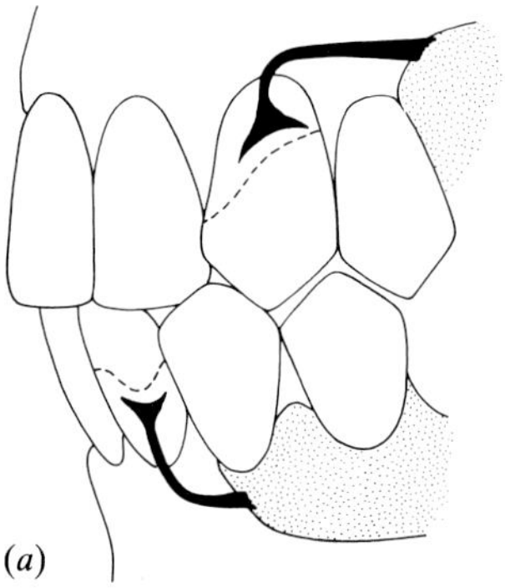

(*a*)

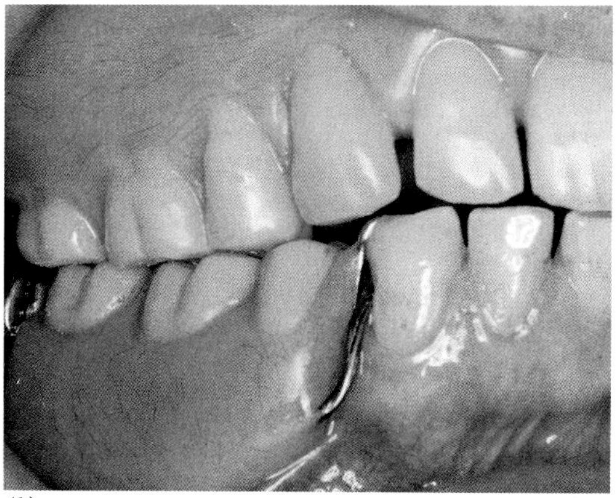

(*b*)

Figure 20.43 (*a*) T-shaped projection clasps on anterior teeth (diagrammatic). (*b*) In actual practice the clasp arm should be much nearer the denture base and is then less obtrusive

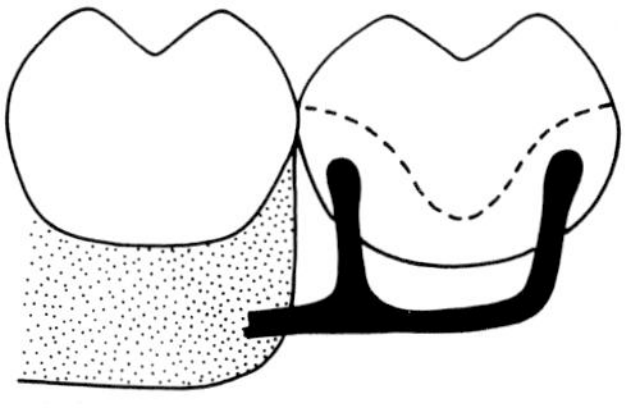

Figure 20.44 U-shaped projection clasp

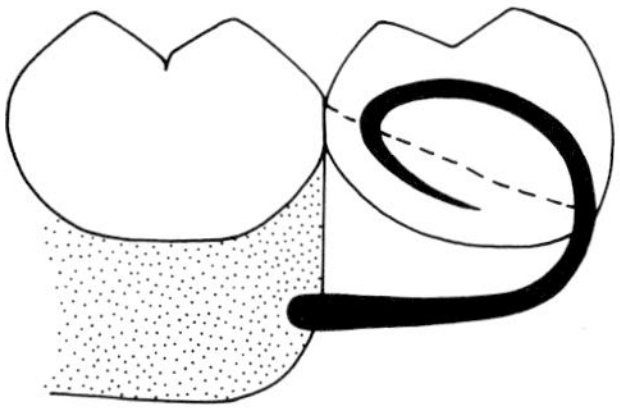

Figure 20.46 C-shaped projection clasp

C-shaped (Figure 20.46)

This type of clasp is almost exclusively reserved for use when a tooth exhibits only a small undercut area mesially or distally. The long curved arm increases the flexibility and thus enables the terminal portion to be placed in the undercut area. It also provides some lateral bracing.

Ball and socket (Figure 20.47)

This type of clasp is invaluable when the slope of the tooth surface is such that no undercut area exists. A round platinized gold wire, which has been fused to form a ball at one end, is constructed to terminate on the buccal surface of the tooth, at which point a gold inlay is made. When the denture is fitted, thin marking paper is inserted between the ball and the inlay, and the ball given a smart tap. When the denture and paper are removed a small blue spot will be found on the surface of the inlay which coincides with the ball when in position. At this point a cup-shaped hollow is drilled in the inlay with a round bur, and the clasp arm bent slightly inwards so that when the denture is inserted the ball of the clasp clicks into the hollow. This clasp gives a very positive retention and need not be restricted to teeth which exhibit no survey line.

Location of clasps

A clasp will retain only that part of the denture to which it is attached. Clasps should thus be located as regularly as the case requires round the periphery of the denture, so that the resultant of their several forces falls as near the centre of gravity of the denture as possible (Figure 20.48).

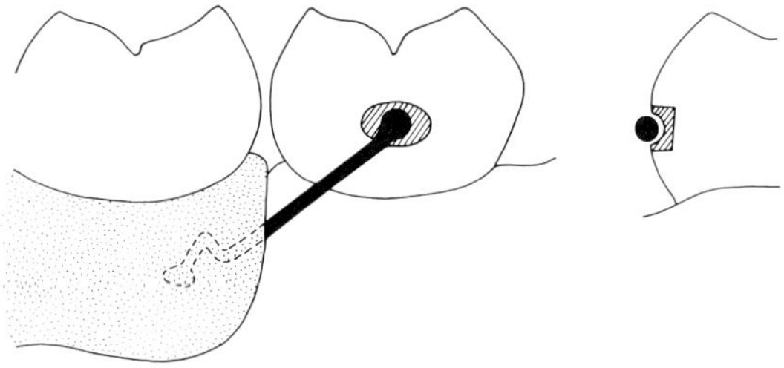

(*a*)

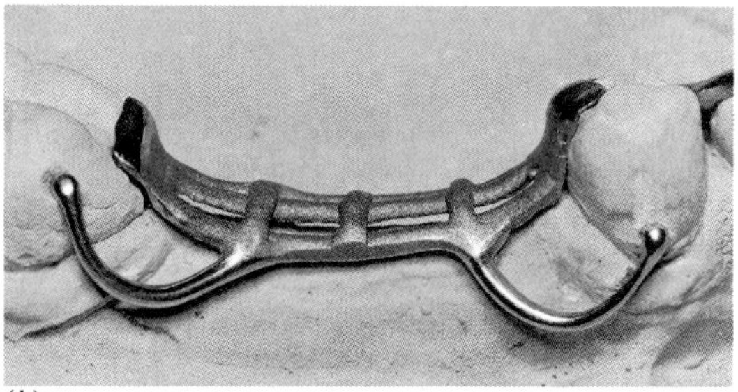

(*b*)

Figure 20.47 (*a*) Ball and socket projection clasp. (*b*) Cast cobalt–chromium alloy

In such a case as that depicted in Figure 20.49, in addition to direct retention, indirect retention is required to retain the back of the denture. This is discussed later in this chapter.

While it is impossible to lay down hard and fast rules about the number of clasps required, the following precepts are broadly applicable to most cases:

1. Tooth-borne dentures require clasps at the ends of all saddles.
2. When only two clasps are used, a straight line joining them should bisect the denture as nearly as possible.
3. If a denture would tend to rock about a line joining two clasps, then a third clasp should be added and the farther it is away from the other two the better.

Which teeth to clasp?

The following list gives the teeth in order of suitability for clasping from the point of view of shape, strength and size, assuming normal, healthy teeth in normal relation to each other in every case:

1. Molars.
2. Premolars.
3. Canines.
4. Incisors are unsuitable.

When the location and type of clasp to be used have been decided, there still remains the question of the type of material to be employed in their construction. In order to be able to select intelligently a material for making a clasp, a knowledge of the mechanical properties required is important.

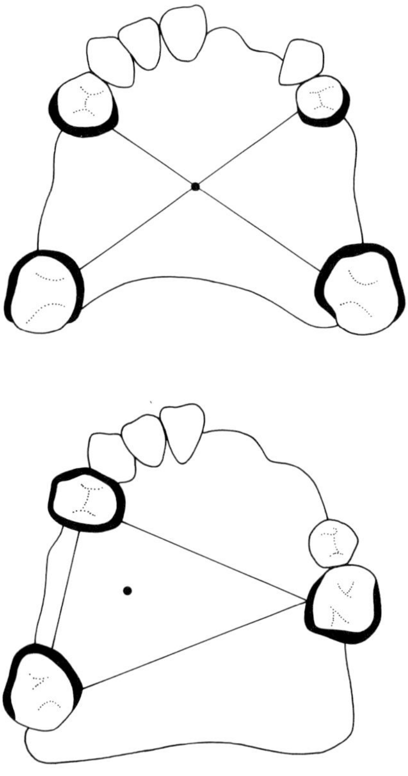

Figure 20.48 Location of clasps (see text)

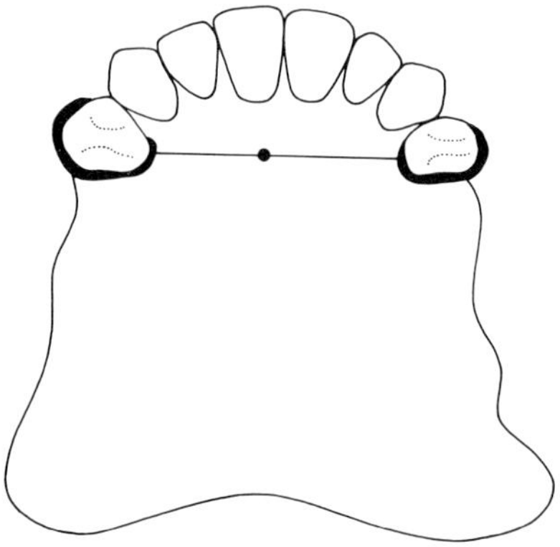

Figure 20.49 Location of clasps: Kennedy class I upper (see text)

The principles of clasp design

The main principles of clasp design are enumerated below for easy reference:

1. The rigid portion must be on the occlusal side of the survey line.
2. At least part of the flexible portion must rest in an undercut area.
3. The flexible portion must not fit more deeply into an undercut area than its elastic or proportional limit will permit.
4. The tip of the clasp must remain in contact with the tooth.
5. Any pressure must be opposed by equal and opposite pressure or by some unyielding part of the denture, i.e. a clasp must never press on one side only of an unsupported tooth.
6. The clasp, together with its rigid opponent or reciprocal, if it is of the single arm type, must embrace more than half the circumference of the tooth.
7. Unless fitted with an occlusal rest the clasp must not rest too near the gingival margin.

Mechanical properties of clasp alloys

Clasps require to be strong enough to resist permanent distortion in the mouth, elastic enough to regain their original shape when flexed, flexible enough to spring over the bulbous parts of the teeth, and springy enough to apply the force required to hold the denture in place. Such terms as these, however, are loose and as expressed lack definite meaning and cannot be accurately assessed. If, however, they are defined and the implications of the definitions grasped, the correct selection of a material for any given clasp is simplified.

Specifications issued by manufacturers of alloys suitable for clasps and denture bases usually quote figures for certain mechanical properties.

Proportional limit

This may be defined as the greatest stress to which a material may be subjected without becoming permanently deformed. Sometimes the figures for elastic limit or yield point are given instead of the proportional limit, and for practical purposes all three may be taken to correspond. Proportional limit is the criterion of useful strength of the material, and in a clasp this property requires to be high, otherwise the clasp may bend during use and no longer function as a clasp. The proportional limit varies in heat-treatable materials, being higher in the hardened than in the softened state. A figure of 300 MN/m^2 in the hardened condition is the minimum acceptable figure for proportional limit, and figures of 500 MN/m^2 and over are desirable.

Modulus of elasticity

This is computed from the formula, stress divided by strain. Therefore the greater the stress and the smaller the strain, up to the proportional limit, the larger will be the figure for the modulus and vice versa. It may be taken therefore as the criterion of stiffness. A material with a high figure for the modulus of elasticity will be stiff, and one with a low modulus, flexible. Figures for the modulus of elasticity vary from about 100 GN/m^2 in some of the gold alloys, to 250 GN/m^2 in the cobalt–chromium alloys and some of the stainless steels.

The arm of a clasp acting as a reciprocal or bracing element requires to be stiff and unyielding, and therefore should be made of a material with a high modulus of elasticity. The functional arm of a clasp, on the other hand, requires to be flexible and ideally should be made of a material with a low modulus of elasticity.

Percentage elongation

During fabrication and later at the final fitting and adjustment of a denture, clasps require to be bent or plastically deformed. If the material from which they are constructed is highly ductile they will withstand considerable adjustment without developing weakness or breaking. If, however, they are not ductile, a slight adjustment may fracture them. Percentage elongation is a measure of the ductility of a material or the degree of adjustment to which it may be subjected. It varies in heat-treatable alloys, being much greater in the softened than the hardened state.

A figure of 10% or above in the softened state is desirable, and this should not fall to less than 2% in the hardened state.

Resistance to fatigue, by the repetitive application of a load, and creep, the slow deformation under constant stress, are properties which should be highly developed in materials for clasp construction. Unfortunately, little information is available on these properties in relation to clasp alloys. The only guide is the higher the proportional limit, the higher the resistance to fatigue is likely to be.

Before these facts can be applied to clasp design the relationship of them to the dimensions and form of the material must be known.

Resistance to permanent or plastic deformation

This varies directly with the cross-sectional area of the material.

If cast clasps are to be used the dimensions should be related to both the proportional limit and the stress to which the clasp is likely to be subjected. Unfortunately reliable data available on this matter are limited, except clinical experience. It is probably true, however, that clasps are as frequently deformed out of the mouth than in.

Stiffness and flexibility

These vary with the square of the cross-sectional area. This means that if the cross-sectional area of a clasp is doubled the stiffness will be increased four times and the flexibility reduced four times. The critical feature is the thickness of the clasp arm (i.e. the buccolingual direction) rather than the width (i.e. the occlusal-gingival direction), and as the deflection varies inversely as the cube of the thickness and only directly as the width, the width/thickness ratio should be 2 or above.

The practical application of these facts may be summarized as follows:

1. A highly platinized wrought gold alloy is the best material available for constructing a clasp, because it develops to the highest degree the desirable mechanical properties. It is essential that it is correctly heat treated to develop these properties to the full.
2. If a high degree of flexibility is required in the terminal third, while preserving rigidity in the body of the clasp, the arms should taper towards their tips (see Figure 20.33).
3. If it is desired to carry the tip of a clasp deeply into an undercut to provide better retention, a material with a high proportional limit and a low modulus of elasticity must be chosen or the distance which the clasp arm is required to travel may cause its plastic deformation (Figure 20.50).
4. If great stiffness is required in the reciprocal or bracing part of a clasp, and yet it is required to keep the dimensions small, a material with a high modulus of elasticity must be chosen.
5. If the clasp arm has to be long the modulus of elasticity should be high or the tip of the clasp may be too flexible and therefore provide insufficient retentive force.

The physical form of clasps

It is generally accepted that the retention of plaque and minute particles of food in contact with the enamel is a predisposing cause of dental caries, and so it must be accepted that any form of clasp is potentially dangerous to the health of a clasped tooth. It follows, therefore, that any form of clasp should be self-cleansing and streamlined, although it is impossible for any clasp to fit so closely to the tooth as to prevent saliva laden with minute particles of food from lodging between it and the surface of the tooth; the smaller the surface area the less dangerous the clasp. Further, it is most important that the inner surface of clasps should be smooth and polished. This is particularly important in cast clasps for if the inner surface is left rough it will attract plaque and is difficult for the patient to clean. Round wire, making as it does only a line contact, is a clean form of clasp as is half-round wire. This line contact is often a disadvantage since it allows a rotation about that line, and unless there is a fair degree of undercut, a round wire may be unsuitable because of lack of surface friction. Cast materials are dependent on their surface area which varies according to design and technical competence.

Wrought wire

1. Clean.
2. Minimum friction.
3. Highly flexible.
4. Easily constructed.
5. Suitable for cases requiring several clasps (especially if the denture base is acrylic)
6. Does not transmit every movement of the denture to the tooth, i.e. it possesses stress-breaking properties.

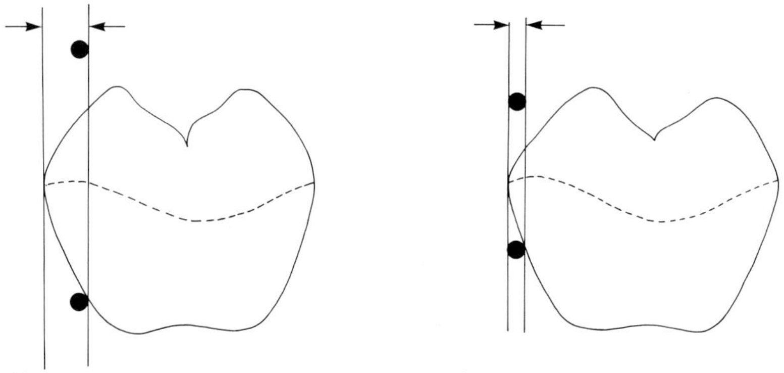

(*a*) (*b*)

Figure 20.50 Illustrating the amount which a clasp must deform as the denture is inserted, if placed: (*a*) a long way below the survey line; (*b*) only just below the survey line

Cast alloy

1. Accurately fitting.
2. Easily varied in thickness, form and taper i.e. versatile design.
3. Easily formed to act as a rigid bracing or reciprocal element.
4. Can easily include an occlusal rest.
5. Can be cast as an integral part of a gold alloy or cobalt–chromium denture base.

Indirect retainers

An indirect retainer is so called because it retains in position some part of a denture remote from itself. It works on the principle of the counter balance. In Figure 20.51, AB represents a bar suspended off centre at C. Point B will drop and A will rise until equilibrium is attained. If point A is prevented from rising by placing an immovable block D above it then point B cannot drop. This principle can be employed in partial dentures whenever a free-end saddle is present and cannot be retained adequately by the clasp fitted to the abutment tooth. A typical example is shown in Figure 20.52. The denture is retained directly by clasps C, the free-end saddles tending to fall away from the tuberosities as the denture rotates round the fulcrum through the clasp tips. In addition, the clasps exert leverage on the premolar teeth. If an extension A of the saddles of the denture is made on the opposite side of the line joining the clasps, and this extension rests on the palatal surfaces of the canines and incisors, then provided that the retention supplied by the clasps is adequate to retain the denture against normal dislodging forces, the saddles cannot drop unless the indirect retainer (A) forces the incisor and canine teeth out of position.

Indirect retainers are best made of cast alloy so that they fit the teeth accurately and appear as unobtrusive as possible. They should be placed as

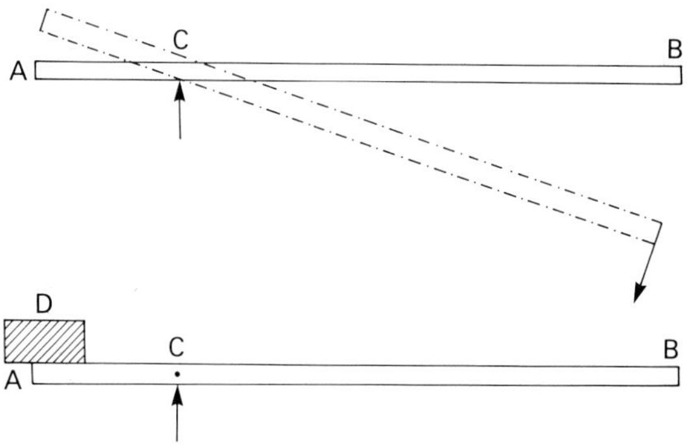

Figure 20.51 Indirect retainers work on the principle of a counter balance (see text)

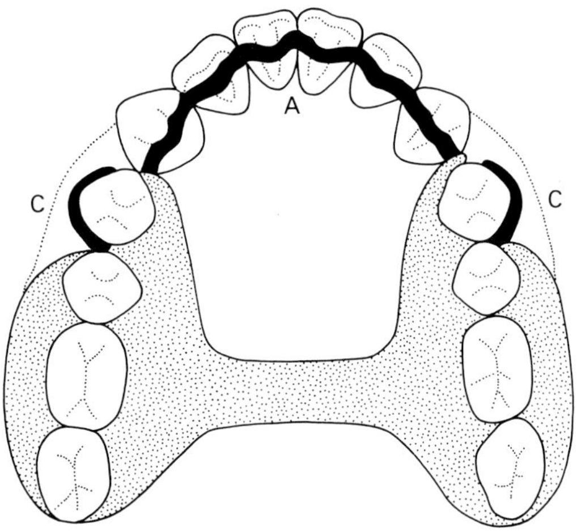

Figure 20.52 Denture retained by clasps C, C. Extension A rests on the lingual surfaces of the upper anterior teeth and therefore prevents the free-end saddles dropping (see Figure 20.3)

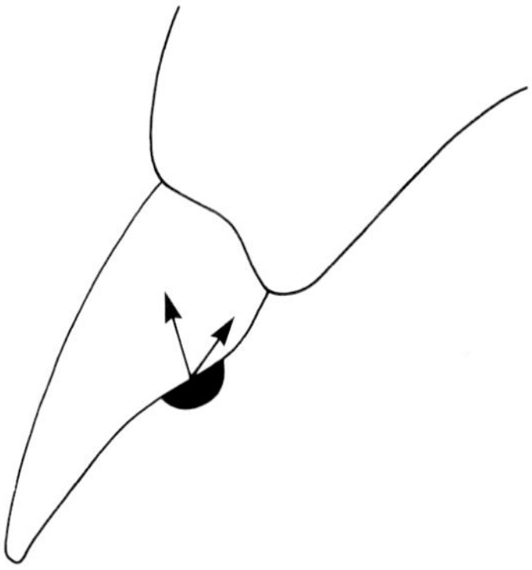

Figure 20.53 Position of indirect retainer on incisor

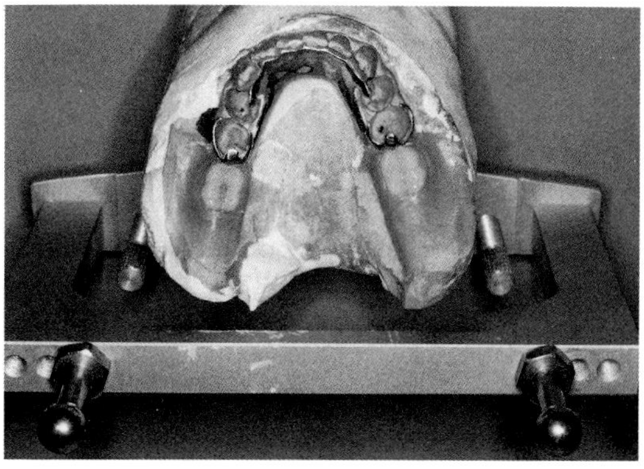

Figure 20.54 Partial lower denture deflasked and remounted. The lingual plate (major connector) will act as an indirect retainer when the free-end saddles tend to rise in the mouth

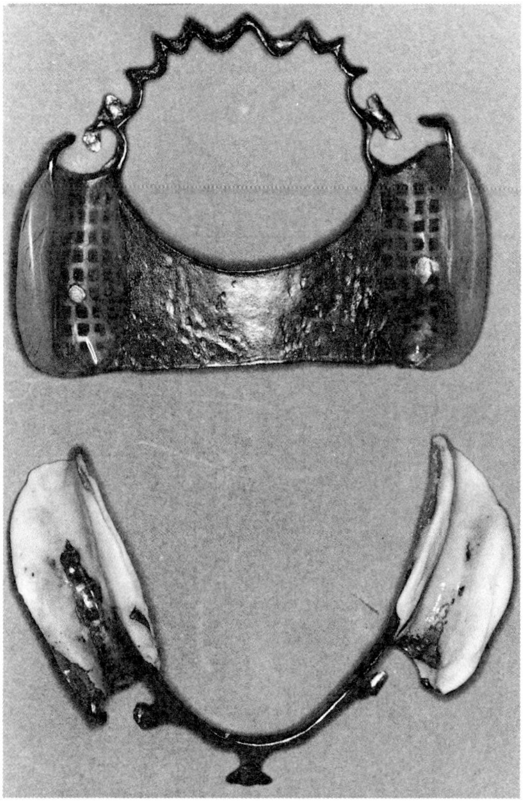

Figure 20.55 Indirect retainers. In the maxillary denture the continuous bar retainer lying on the anterior teeth resists dropping of the bilateral free-end saddles. On the mandibular denture an indirect retainer projects from the lingual bar to lie on the lingual surfaces of the central incisors to resist upward movement of the saddles. (Saddles temporarily rebased with tissue conditioner)

shown in Figure 20.53. In this position they are low enough on the tooth to prevent excessive leverage developing, and any tendency for the retainer to slide down the tooth is resisted by its cingulum.

Indirect retainers may be made of alloy as part of a major connector as illustrated in Figure 20.54.

An occlusal or incisal rest, a connector or a saddle may act as an indirect retainer provided its position is such that it is on the opposite side of the line or lines joining the direct retainers or clasps to that part which requires to be retained. Figure 20.55 illustrates how various parts of a denture may act as an indirect retainer. The more remote the position of an indirect retainer from the line joining the points of direct retention the more efficient it becomes.

The points to bear in mind regarding indirect retainers are these:

1. They should be used only on peridontally sound teeth.
2. They should contact as many teeth as possible to reduce the possibility of moving teeth by the application of excessive force.
3. Extensions of the denture base on mucosa are effective provided the mucosa is firm.
4. They can only function in conjunction with direct retainers (clasps) i.e. an indirect retainer by itself does not provide retention.

Occlusal rests

Partial denture support

The forces acting on the occlusal surface of a partial denture must ultimately be absorbed by the alveolar bone. If the area of mucosa covered by the denture is sufficiently large, these forces will be absorbed by the soft tissues and transmitted to the bone in the same way as occurs with complete dentures. However, if the area of a partial denture is small, as often happens, the force applied to unit area of the soft tissue will be above its tolerance, and pain and ulceration will ensue with ultimate destruction of hard and soft tissues. In these cases, therefore, other means of transferring the occlusal loads to the bone are required. This is achieved by supporting the denture either wholly or partly on the natural teeth which, being designed to transmit forces of high magnitude to the bone, suffer no damage if their supporting tissues are sound and the denture properly designed. The parts of the denture which transmit the loads to the teeth are called supporting elements or rests. The main function of rests is to transfer some or all of the clenched and masticatory loads to the natural teeth. In addition they may serve four other important functions:

1. They act as contact points and thus prevent food packing between the denture and the natural tooth.
2. They maintain clasps in their correct position and prevent them sinking and pressing into the gingival tissues.
3. They often act as indirect retainers.
4. They assist in bracing against lateral movements.

Rests are of three types: occlusal, cingulum, and incisal.

Occlusal rests (Figure 20.56)

These are made to fit into a mesial or distal fossa on the occlusal surface of a tooth and to be satisfactory they must comply with the following requirements:

1. They must fit the tooth accurately in order to minimize the collection of food debris beneath them and also to locate them correctly in relation to the tooth.

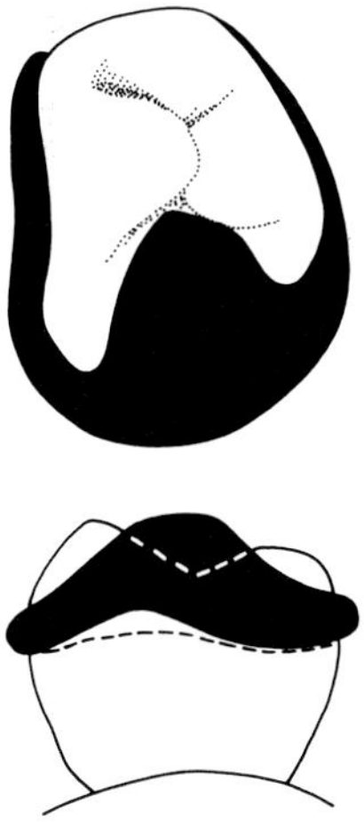

Figure 20.56 An occlusal rest forming the supporting element of a 3-arm clasp

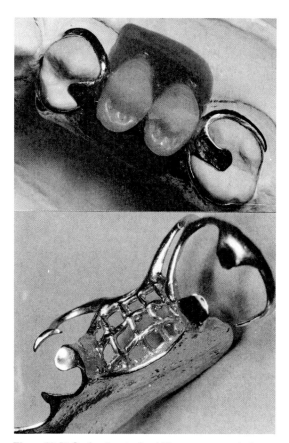

Figure 20.57 Occlusal rests should have an anatomical form to merge with the abutment tooth rest seat. Occlusion with opposing teeth should be checked in all mandibular positions

2. They must be strong enough to bear all normal masticatory and clenched loads without deformation.
3. They must not interfere with the occlusion; in the majority of cases a certain amount of preparation of the tooth surface is necessary in order that room may be made for the rest and the shape of the occlusal surface made favourable for it (Figure 20.57); this preparation is carried out with carborundum stones or diamond points without penetration of the enamel; if such penetration is necessary an inlay or filling must be made to accommodate the rest or caries will occur; if an opposing cusp is ground to make room for a rest make sure there is still sufficient occlusal contact otherwise the opposing tooth will shift before the denture is fitted.
4. They must transmit the stress down the long axis of the tooth as this is the only direction in which the load can be increased without damage to the periodontal membrane.
5. They must be at right angles or less to the long axis of the tooth otherwise the pressures of mastication will tend to force the denture away from the tooth or vice versa; an undue load will be placed on the resilient portion of a clasp which is made in conjunction with an obtuse angled occlusal rest.

Cingulum rests (Figure 20.58)

These are made to lie on the palatal or lingual surface of anterior teeth. They are often unsatisfactory because the shape of the palatal surfaces of most teeth are not suitable to carry a rest. This will be appreciated from a study of Figure 20.59. If an occlusal load A is transmitted to the rest it will in

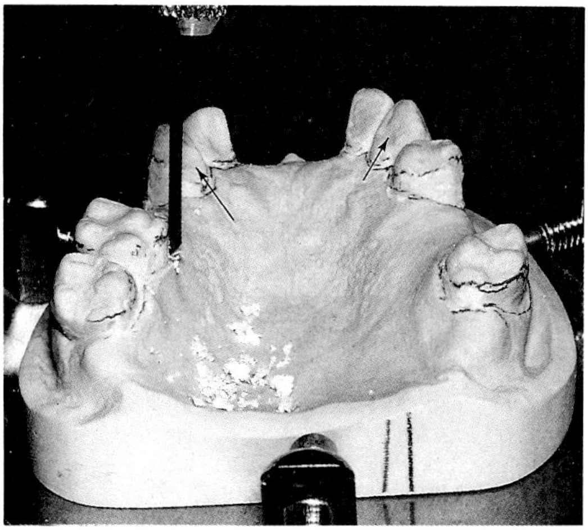

Figure 20.58 Cingulum rest seats prepared in canines (arrowed)

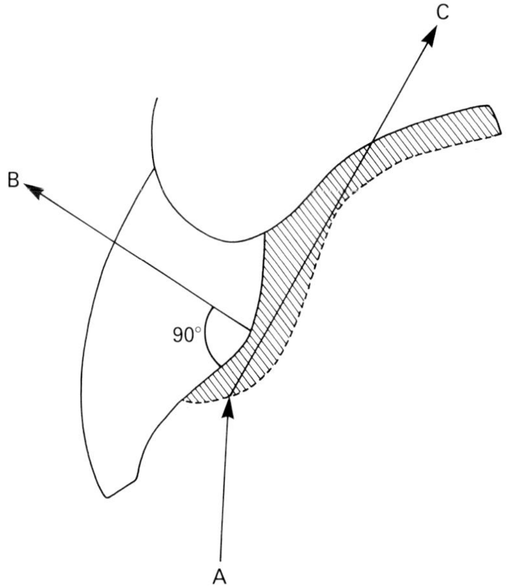

Figure 20.59 Cingulum rest. Resolution of forces (see text)

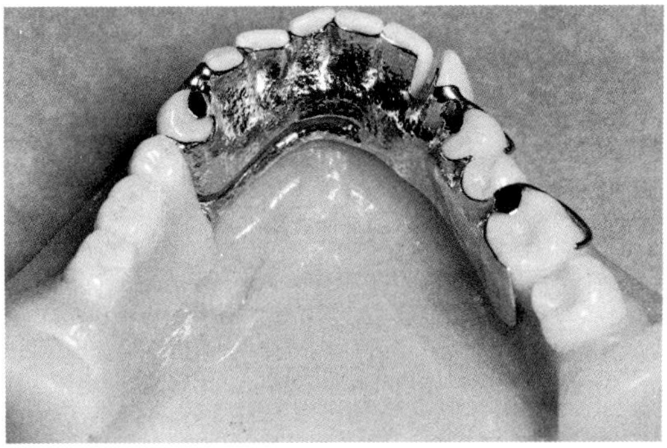

Figure 20.60 Incisal rests on distal canines and distal left lateral incisor as extensions from the cast major connector

turn transmit it to the tooth. This load will then be resolved into two loads, B broadly at right angles to the rest, and C broadly parallel to it. It will be appreciated that at least half the load which the rest is supposed to transmit to the tooth is actually devoted to forcing the rest down the tooth and must be absorbed by the underlying soft tissue.

In order to counter this problem rest seats (sometimes called lug seats) must be prepared in most anterior teeth. These should have a flat floor but must be sufficiently deep otherwise they are ineffective and care must be taken that the alloy or the acrylic fits accurately into the prepared seat. The rest must not interfere with the occlusion, particularly in lateral and protrusive positions.

Incisal rests (Figure 20.60)

Cingulum rests can be used on maxillary canines or central incisors and on some mandibular canines. The shape of most incisors, however, is such that incisal rests have to be used. Rest seats on anterior teeth may be cut on the incisal edges. These are best made semilunar in shape, occupying only the lingual part of the incisal edge. In this way the tooth is weakened only minimally and the incisal rest is not seen. Another method of deriving support is to chamfer the incisal edge and drape the cast alloy over the whole incisal edge surface, making sure the alloy is as thin as possible (see Figure 20.4). On maxillary laterals, and most mandibular incisors, where the incisal edges are thin, effective support is gained by notching the mesial or distal corner to create a rest seat about 1 mm wide and 1 mm deep. Provided the resultant denture base fits snugly into this preparation the appearance is good and produces no problems for the patient. Like all rests, care must be taken to avoid occlusal interference.

Chapter 21

Materials for partial denture bases

Design of a partial denture is greatly influenced by the material of which the denture is made and so a knowledge of the various materials and their properties is essential. The bases for partial dentures may be made of either polymeric materials or metal alloys.

For a long time, gold alloys have been first in swaged and later in cast form, the material of choice for the construction of a large majority of partial dentures, but unfortunately, its present high cost now seriously limits its use.

More recently, the introduction of base metal alloys, in particular cobalt–chromium, has provided an alternative to gold and these materials will be compared for their suitability for the construction of partial dentures.

Polymeric materials

In the past many polymeric materials have been used for dentures and most of them have been discarded as their unsuitability for this purpose became apparent. Celluloid, phenolformaldehyde, epoxy resin, vinyl polymers, polycarbonate and nylon are examples. At the present time only polymethyl methacrylate (acrylic resin) is in general use.

Advantages for acrylic resin

1. Simulates the appearance of natural mucosa and gingivae.
2. Technique is reasonably simple and requires little special apparatus.
3. Can be used for all cases although it is not necessarily the best material for the majority.
4. Can be used for the whole denture including the teeth.
5. Forms a chemical union with acrylic teeth thus giving a very strong attachment.
6. Repairs and additions can easily be made.
7. Light in weight.
8. Easy to keep clean.
9. Insoluble and inert in oral fluids.

Disadvantages of acrylic resin

1. The design of dentures is greatly limited by the weakness of the material.
2. Its resistance to fatigue is low, and it frequently fractures after a few months in the mouth.
3. Has a tendency to warp during deflasking, as the stresses induced in the material during processing are released; this may lead to inaccuracy of fit; it also warps when re-cured for repairing.
4. Its abrasion resistance is low and leads to rapid wear when used for posterior teeth; it is also easily abraded by cleaning with a stiff brush.
5. Residual monomer, which weakens acrylic and makes it more flexible, may be present (monomer may also irritate oral mucosa).
6. Subject to porosity which affects strength, surface polish and water absorption.
7. Water absorption and drying lead to dimensional changes.
8. Subject to crazing which weakens the material, although cross-linked polymers are less prone to this.
9. Radiolucent, a problem if part of an acrylic denture is inhaled or swallowed when detection by radiograph is impossible.

Recent improvements

1. High impact polymethyl methacrylates, in the form of rubber modified resins, have better fatigue and impact properties.

2. Strength and rigidity may be improved by the addition of carbon fibres although the black colour is a distinct drawback.
3. Barium sulphate may be added to acrylic to make it radiopaque but as this additive weakens the material it is often best to use high impact acrylics, especially where there is a likelihood of fracture taking place.

Metal alloys

The modern dental techniques of casting alloys have almost completely supplanted other means of constructing denture bases. The construction outside the mouth of metal parts of a denture can be traced back to the earliest history of dentistry, and gold alloys have long played an important part. This is due to two factors: the ease with which they may be fabricated, and their chemical inertness. Gold alloys fall into two categories: those supplied in the wrought form, and those intended for casting. Their physical properties, such as strength, hardness and ductility are subject to considerable variation according to the type of alloy used.

The earliest method of working gold alloys was by heating, bending and shaping, and even today this method is still used to a limited extent. Modern methods of casting by the lost wax process have proved superior in every way and this is now the accepted technique. Although gold has been the metal of choice for dental restorations for many years, its cost has risen to a figure which prohibits its use in many cases. However, cost alone does not justify the substitution of a base metal alloy where a noble one might give more satisfactory service, but when a base metal alloy has been shown to have equal or superior properties there should be no hesitancy in using it.

In an effort to reduce cost, there has been an increasing use of palladium in dental alloys. This is the cheapest of the platinum group of metals which, besides having a lower specific gravity, has a whitening effect on gold when present in the proportion of only 5–6%. These alloys containing palladium and known as 'white golds', were formerly in common use for casting denture bases. They vary widely in their composition and consequently in their physical properties and cost. A few, in fact, contain no gold at all.

Advantages of metals

1. Their superior physical properties enable them to be used in thin section and this factor allows great latitude in the design of the denture. It is also appreciated by the patient, as partial metal dentures take up little space in the mouth.
2. Their resistance to fatigue is great and fracture in the mouth is uncommon.
3. Their high thermal conductivity enables normal sensations of heat and cold to be appreciated.

Disadvantages of metals

1. The techniques of their fabrication are time-consuming, require a high degree of skill, and need special apparatus.
2. Their appearance does not simulate the natural mucosa.
3. Additions and repairs cannot be performed easily because these operations entail either soldering or welding and, in the majority of cases, before either can be performed the teeth need to be removed from the denture.
4. They may cause electrolytic action if the denture is in contact with a dissimilar metal filling.

Yellow gold alloy

Type IV alloy is an excellent material for constructing any type of partial denture. Its good features are:

1. If cast into an investment which gives compensatory thermal expansion for the casting shrinkage, the final denture is accurate.
2. Due to the fact that all properly constituted gold alloys contain from 12–15% of copper, they are susceptible to heat treatment. The value of this is that the casting may be softened for the final adjustment of clasps, and then given the hardening heat treatment to produce:
   (a) a high proportional limit, thus enabling it to resist all normal stresses in and out of the mouth.
   (b) a modulus of elasticity sufficiently high to allow the connectors to be made thin, but not so high as to deprive the clasps of adequate flexibility.
3. Any additions, such as wrought clasps or metal backings for porcelain teeth, may easily be soldered to the main base.

The only true disadvantage of yellow gold is its high cost, although some consider its colour and weight to be disadvantages.

Silver–palladium alloys (white golds)

Advantages:

1. They produce accurately fitting dentures.
2. They are susceptible to heat treatment but the final mechanical properties are not so satisfactory as yellow gold alloys.
3. They can be added to by soldering.
4. Cheaper than yellow gold, although the cost is still considerable.

Disadvantages:

1. Alloys containing a high silver content tend to tarnish in use due to the formation of silver sulphide.
2. The alloy tends to be sluggish and difficult to cast.
3. The high rates of occlusion and dissolution of oxygen tends to produce porosity.
4. Care must be taken, and the manufacturers' instructions rigidly adhered to, when heat treating these alloys or brittleness will result as the percentage elongation is reduced.
5. The proportional limit and ultimate tensile strength are less than yellow gold alloys.

Cobalt–chromium alloys

Constituents

As is the case with gold alloys the individual alloys on the market differ slightly from each other but their general composition is roughly within the range of either:

(a)	chromium	30%	or (b)	chromium	30%
	cobalt	60%		cobalt	30%
	molybdenum	5%		nickel	30%
				molybdenum	5%

The main constituents of these alloys are cobalt and chromium in the approximate proportions of cobalt 60% and chromium 30%. The chromium content ensures that the alloy is corrosion resistant while cobalt gives strength and hardness. Nickel may be partially substituted for cobalt and this results in a reduction in tensile strength but an increase in ductility.

The other 5% constituents present, and which control the physical properties of these alloys, are listed below.

Molybdenum: this prevents intragranular corrosion and surface pitting and promotes homogeneity of the alloy. The normal molybdenum content is about 5% and contributes strength.

Tungsten: this is an occasional substitute for molybdenum as it conveys the same benefits but it causes a slight reduction in elongation.

Carbon: carbon is always present in the form of chromium carbide and improves the strength; up to 0.2% increases hardness and strength. When present in amounts greater than 0.25% it has a definite tendency to cause brittleness by the formation of excessive metallic carbides.

Manganese: this acts as a flux and scavenger, combining with the sulphur and oxygen while the alloy is molten and increases the fluidity and 'castability'.

Silicon: this softens the alloy indirectly by its action on carbon, but by its own effect it hardens it, and makes a denser casting and also increases fluidity and 'castability'.

Aluminium: this forms a compound of nickel and aluminium which increases the ultimate tensile strength and yield strength of the alloy.

Mechanical Properties

Specific gravity

This property is defined as the ratio of the weight of a body to the weight of another body of equal volume taken as a standard, and this standard for solids is generally water. The higher the figure, the heavier the comparative weight. This property is important in alloy restorations, particularly in the upper jaw. Gold has the highest specific gravity (16–17) of any of the metals used in the mouth, and this property can be a serious disadvantage if castings are large and bulky. The specific gravity of cobalt–chromium alloys (7–9) is approximately half that of gold alloys and this, coupled with the fact that its greater rigidity allows thinner sections to be employed, results in a lighter denture base.

Hardness

When metals are tested for hardness they can be either hard or soft according to the type of heat treatment to which they have been subjected. Softening and hardening heat treatments are a necessary procedure in the manipulation of gold alloys but cobalt–chromium alloys are worked in the 'as cast' condition after a period of slow cooling and removal from the investment. Cobalt–chromium alloys are considerably harder than gold alloys, only stainless steel having a higher Brinell hardness number. The advantage of the greater hardness of a cobalt–chromium alloy is that it maintains its high polish indefinitely and is, therefore, more hygienic under mouth conditions. A disadvantage is that trimming and polishing a cobalt–chromium appliance is a longer procedure and requires considerably greater speeds.

Tensile strength

The ultimate strength is the greatest stress that can be induced in a body without rupture. Fracture under tension is called ultimate tensile strength. In this respect cobalt–chromium alloys have very similar properties to cast gold alloys. Fractures do occur with most materials at some time or another, especially in clasp arms which engage undercuts, but the reason, in most instances, can be attributed to faulty design. Experience has shown that where the design and construction have been correctly carried out, the incidence of fracture of components of partial denture bases constructed in cobalt–chromium is low.

Yield point

Yield strength is an indication of the minimum stress required to deform a material to such an extent that it will not return to its original shape. This property is important in denture bases where there is a liability to deformation in use and during insertion and removal of the denture. Displacement of the clasp arms away from the tooth would, for example, render the clasp ineffective in its retentive and stabilizing functions. The figures for this property show that cobalt–chromium alloys have slightly lower yield points than gold alloys, but this factor is related to the flexibility of the material and this must be taken into consideration.

Elongation

Ductility is described as the ability of a material to withstand permanent deformation under a tensile load without rupture. Wrought alloys have a high degree of ductility which enables them to be worked satisfactorily, but this property is not so important in casting alloys.

One of the methods of measuring ductility is to compare the increase in length after rupture to the original gauge length. This ratio, expressed as per cent, is known as elongation. The figures obtained indicate that the cobalt–chromium alloys have a higher degree of ductility than has casting gold.

Modulus of elasticity

The modulus of elasticity may be defined as the load required to effect unit strain. In other words, if we take two wires of equal size and different composition and bend them the same amount, we shall probably find that a greater amount of force will be required to bend one or the other. This indicates that one material is stiffer than the other, and this property can be expressed numerically and is measured in terms of force per unit area. This means that a material having a higher modulus of elasticity will be stiffer and will require more force to effect the same bending than would be the case in a substance of lower modulus.

The figures for the modulus of elasticity of cobalt–chromium alloys indicate that a large force is required to produce a small deformation of the material; in other words it is stiff. Such a property is desirable in such parts of a partial denture as connectors, rests and indirect retainers. Taken together with the proportional limit, however, it means that the alloy possesses a low flexibility which is a disadvantage in clasps.

Modifications of the retentive components of partial dentures must also be made in view of the importance of the distribution of load between the abutment teeth and the saddle areas. There is considerable difference of opinion among prosthodontists as to how the vertical and lateral loads occurring during mastication and clenching should be shared between the mucosa and the natural teeth. In general it is true that the greater part of the load should be borne by the healthy standing teeth and the share taken by any single tooth should be reduced by distributing both lateral and vertical loads over the largest number of teeth. Therefore, if a clasp made in cobalt–chromium is to transfer the same amount of lateral load to the abutment tooth as a gold alloy clasp, a reduction in the section of the clasp arms may be made, owing to the relative stiffness of the alloy. Gingivally approaching clasps are often more flexible than occlusally approaching clasps, owing to the greater length of the arms and may, therefore, engage more deeply into undercuts. Irrespective of the type of clasp, however, one made in cobalt–chromium alloy should always engage less horizontal undercut than the same type made in gold alloy.

$$\text{Modulus of elasticity} = \frac{\text{stress}}{\text{strain}}$$

and is a constant for any metal or alloy. If the modulus of elasticity is low the alloy will flex easily. The modulus of elasticity for cast gold alloys is considerably lower than that for cobalt–chromium and therefore a cobalt–chromium clasp, made in the same dimensions as a gold alloy clasp, is very much stiffer and a greater force is required to bend the clasp into, and out of, an undercut. The elastic limit of cobalt–chromium is, however, about the same as gold alloy and so the clasp is liable to be deformed under the load required to deflect it. Fracture of the clasp arm is also liable to occur.

General points to note about clasps

1. Use a thinner section of arm when designing cobalt–chromium clasps. Pre-formed wax patterns are essential since it is almost impossible to obtain an accurate and uniform cross section if the wax is applied freehand.
2. Engage in less undercut in the abutment tooth (added advantage that more types of teeth can be clasped). Gold alloy: horizontal undercut usually 0.75 mm; cobalt–chromium: usually 0.25 mm. Where the undercuts are greater than 0.25 mm, gold alloy or stainless steel wire should be used. As an alternative a wrought cobalt–chromium wire may be used with cast cobalt–chromium bases. It is supplied in a ‘half hard’ condition and when cold worked with pliers becomes ‘spring hard’. It can then be soldered to the cast base in this condition without its resilience being impaired.
3. The retentive part of the arm should be at some distance from the body or point of attachment to

the denture base to allow greater flexibility (this applies especially to premolars).

4. Use gingivally approaching clasps whenever possible as these clasps apply less lateral load to the abutment tooth (this might be excessive due to the high modulus of elasticity).
5. Because the percentage elongation is insufficient, cobalt–chromium cast clasps cannot be adjusted after the casting is complete otherwise fracture may occur. Consequently extreme accuracy is essential in the making of these clasps.

Application of properties to design

1. The cross-sectional area of connectors such as lingual bars, palatal bars and continuous clasps may be less than that usually employed when using a gold alloy. This is due to the greater stiffness of the material and not to its greater strength.
2. The dimensions of clasps should be as small as possible and taper towards their tips. The reasons for this are:
   (a) The flexibility of the material is low and its stiffness high. These factors vary with the square of the cross-sectional area and if this is kept as low as possible and further reduced by tapering the tip of the clasp less force is required to insert and remove the denture and the tooth will not be gripped too rigidly.
   (b) If the clasp arm is placed too deeply into a severe undercut it will have to travel outwards a great distance to pass over the most bulbous part of the tooth and then a corresponding distance inwards to grip the tooth. As the flexibility is so low, the force required to drive the arm outwards this distance may be greater than the proportional limit of the material will withstand and consequently it will distort.
3. Clasps must be accurately positioned and accurately cast because the percentage elongation is insufficient to allow much adjustment.

Wrought alloys

Gold alloys and stainless steel can be fashioned into partial dentures by swaging between dies and counter dies.

Since the mechanical properties of wrought metals are superior to those of cast, due to the difference in grain structure, swaged dentures can be made even thinner than those which are cast. However, the main disadvantages of wrought metal denture bases are:

1. The fit is far less accurate than with castings, particularly adjacent to abutment teeth.
2. Skeleton dentures are very difficult, if not impossible, to fabricate.
3. Strengthening of individual areas can only be done by soldering or welding on an extra thickness of metal.

Stainless steel for many years has been the main wrought alloy used in dentistry but its use for partial dentures is greatly limited by the exacting technique of hydraulic swaging together with the difficulties of adding components by welding and soldering which affect the mechanical properties of the alloy.

As a general rule, metallic partial denture bases should always be cast although clasps may be fabricated in wrought alloy.

Chapter 22

Principles of partial denture design

Requirements

The requirements of a partial denture may be summarized as follows:

1. It must spread the forces which will act on it evenly over the supporting tissues to a degree within their physiological limit and be adequately retained in position in the mouth during all normal functional movements.
2. It must prevent the dental arch from collapsing by preventing the teeth from drifting or tilting into edentulous spaces. It must also cause the minimum amount of damage to either soft or hard tissues.
3. It must maintain the health of previously unopposed teeth by restoring their function and preventing their over-eruption.
4. It must restore masticatory efficiency and appearance and be comfortable to wear.

To satisfy all the above requirements it will be apparent that the designer of a partial denture must take into account many details, satisfy many needs and solve many problems. The group of problems which it is intended to deal with here is restricted, for simplicity of explanation, to the method of designing a denture so that it may satisfactorily transmit to the supporting tissues the loads which will be applied to it in function in such a manner that the tissues themselves do not have to bear loads above their tolerance and the denture itself will remain stable under all normal conditions.

Vertical loads

When deciding whether a particular denture is to be tooth-borne, mucosa-borne or tooth- and mucosa-borne the following points should be kept in mind.

1. A tooth-borne denture will resist the greatest clenched loads and provide the most efficient mastication.
2. If the denture is opposed by natural teeth, tooth-borne support is desirable because under these circumstances the load applied to the denture will be at the maximum.
3. A denture can only be fully tooth-borne by teeth with sound and well-formed roots whose long axes are almost vertical and are embedded for an adequate distance in healthy bone (the information to enable one to make a decision on this aspect will be available from the clinical and radiographic examination). Canines and incisors alone cannot provide sufficient support for a tooth-borne saddle, due to the inclination of their palatal or lingual surfaces, unless suitable restorations are made with cingulum or incisal rest seats prepared in them. Taken together as a group of three or more teeth, however, they may be able to support a denture without the necessity of tooth preparation.
4. If occlusal rests are to transmit the loads imposed on the denture effectively to the abutment teeth there must be sufficient space for them to be adequately seated. Study casts will show if there is sufficient space for the rests with the teeth in occlusion and if there is not space it can frequently be made by grinding the opposing tooth. The rest seat should always be restricted to the enamel of the tooth and if the dentine is involved a restoration must be made for the tooth and the seat cut in that. Obviously any such preparation must be completed prior to the master impressions.
5. If the saddle areas are extensive, i.e. where more than three natural teeth are missing from any saddle area, it may be necessary to design the

denture so that the loads applied to it are transmitted via the soft tissues. Under these circumstances as great an area as possible must be covered so as to reduce the load applied per unit area. The reason for considering mucosal support in such circumstances is that a long tooth-borne beam might place excessive load on the abutment teeth simply by nature of the beam length. If the denture-bearing area of the mucosa-borne denture is considered inadequate to withstand the anticipated vertical load, as in some instances of a Kennedy class I lower in which there is a narrow ridge with shallow sulci, it helps to reduce the vertical load applied during mastication by:

(a) reducing the buccolingual width of the denture teeth
(b) omitting the last tooth from the saddle.

The problem of the tooth- and mucosa-borne method of transferring the load is a vexed one and frequently the subject of misconception and this question has been discussed in Chapter 19.

A few examples of individual cases will be given to illustrate how a decision is arrived at with regard to resistance to vertical loads.

Figure 22.1 represents a partially edentulous maxilla of the Kennedy class III type with 6 5 / 5 6 missing. It is opposed by a full natural lower dentition. The crowns of 7 4 / 4 7 are sound (the word 'sound' as used means that the crown of the tooth is either caries free or has been satisfactorily conserved) and the roots are supported for more than two-thirds of their length by bone.

In a case of this type the choice of method for supporting the vertical loads is by occlusal rests on 7 4 / 4 7. A tooth-borne denture will enable the patient to chew normally, it will not tend to sink nor be forced into the mucosa, and the rests themselves will prevent food being packed down between the denture and the abutment teeth on to the gingival margins. Before a final decision can be made that occlusal rests can be used in this case the casts must be examined in occlusion to see either that space exists for the rests or that it can be provided by limited grinding of the teeth. Rest seats should be prepared in the fossae of the teeth carrying the rests.

If the alveolar bone in a case of this type is considered on examination of the radiographs to preclude the additional load of the denture, i.e. if the roots of the abutment teeth, or any one of them, are supported for less than one-half of its length by bone, or if the radiographs show that the bone is undergoing rapid resorption, then the saddles may have to be mucosa-borne. In that case they should be outlined on the casts to cover as large an area as possible so that the vertical load applied to the denture is spread widely.

In a case such as this, mucosa-borne saddles as a means of transmitting the vertical load are definitely inferior to occlusal rests as will be appreciated by studying Table 22.1, which shows a comparison between the surface area of the periodontal membranes of / 4 7 available to support a tooth-borne saddle and the surface area of the mucosa which will support a mucosa-borne saddle. In addition, the mucosa in function will distort unevenly and therefore only some of its surface will actually transmit the load and later resorption of the ridge will further upset the equilibrium.

Nevertheless, in many cases of this kind, mucosa-borne saddles do provide a satisfactory foundation for transmitting the vertical load and such dentures are frequently worn for many years with satisfactory results although they are more damaging, less efficient and less comfortable than tooth-borne dentures.

Figure 22.2 illustrates a case similar to that in Figure 22.1 with more extensive bounded saddles, 6 5 4 / 4 5 6 being missing. Here the decision between tooth-borne and mucosa-borne saddles is not quite so simple to make. The 7 / 7 can certainly carry rests, but with three teeth on each saddle

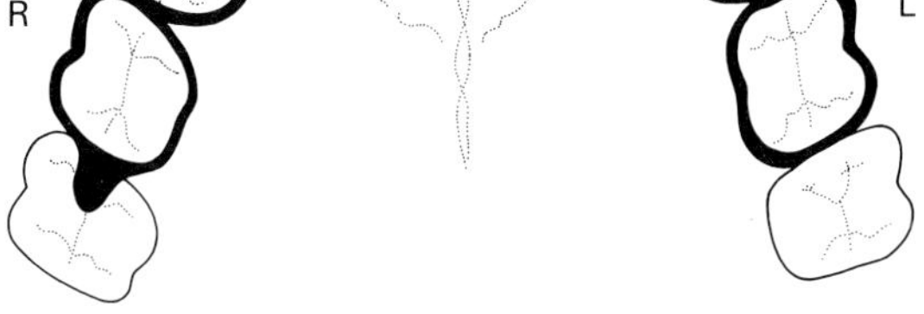

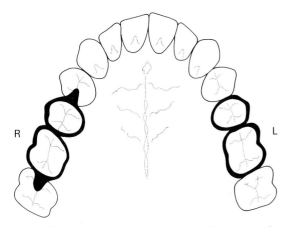

Figure 22.1 On the patient's right the approximate area of the periodontal membrane available for supporting the occlusal loads is 640 mm^2. Compare this with the area available on the patient's left if mucosal support only is enlisted (200 mm^3.) See text and Table 22.1. Note: in this Figure, and in the following Figures, missing teeth are outlined heavily in black

Table 22.1 The deficit of supporting tissue is very marked when the periodontal area of abutment teeth is compared with the saddle area of the gap between them

Periodontal area	Saddle area
/4 = 220	
/7 = 420	
640 mm^2	200 mm^2
Difference = 440 mm^2 which is the *support deficit*	

instead of two, as in Figure 22.1, the extra load which the 7 / 7 can be called upon to accept will be proportionately heavier and unless the roots of these teeth are long and very well supported in dense bone such extra load is likely to cause loosening and tilting of the teeth. The canines are not suitable teeth for carrying rests because the palatal and cingular slopes of these teeth form an inclined plane, and reference to Figure 20.59 shows that a vertical load applied through a rest to such a surface is resolved into a force along the surface and one at right angles to it and, if the angle of inclination of the palatal surface is steep, then most of the occlusal load is converted into a force tending to drive the rest off the tooth. If, as in a case like this, the posterior movement of the saddle which such a force will cause is resisted by the buttressing effect of the mesial surfaces of the upper second molars then an additional and unfavourable backward load is applied to these already overloaded teeth. If it is decided that the canines must carry rests then proper preparations must be made in them with rest seats designed to transmit the vertical loads straight up the long axes of the canines. In saddles of the length of that shown in Figure 22.2, therefore, adequate support would be provided by the molars and canines and so the denture would be tooth-borne.

If the six anterior teeth in this case are considered as a group, and the denture carried up on the cingulum of each tooth as shown in Figure 22.3 in the form of a continuous clasp but without any tooth preparation, then probably sufficient resistance to occlusal load would be provided to make the saddles tooth-borne. If the slope of the palatal surfaces of these teeth is steep, however, a backward thrust of the denture is likely to result. In addition, a continuous clasp of this type may impinge on the palatal gingival margins of these teeth and be detrimental to the health of these tissues. A narrow bar can be used to overcome this difficulty but patients frequently dislike the feeling which such a bar presents to the tongue and also a large majority of patients will present such a deep vertical overlap that space is rarely available for such connectors.

From the foregoing considerations it will be obvious that in the majority of cases a tooth-borne denture would be the method of choice, while a mucosa-borne design might be considered if the abutment teeth were not periodontally sound.

Figure 22.4 illustrates, in the lower jaw, a similar case to Figure 22.2. The main differences are that the size of the saddle area is much less because in the lower jaw the buccal and lingual slopes are almost vertical but, in addition, the lower molars tend to tilt mesially and so reduce the potential saddle coverage. Therefore, this case should be made tooth-borne although the remarks regarding the effect of a continuous clasp on the inclined lingual surfaces of

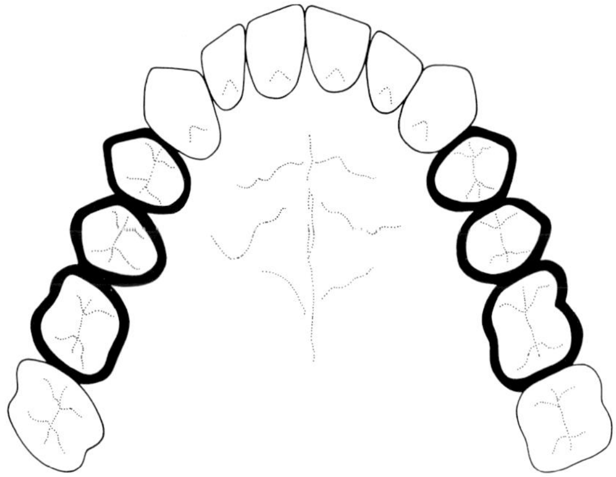

Figure 22.2 Maxillary arch with 654/456 missing. Mucosal support would be limited approximatly to the area of the ridges and tooth support is therefore advisable (see text)

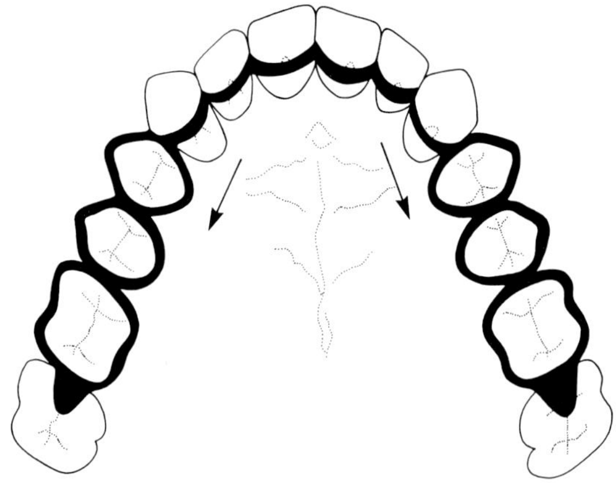

Figure 22.3 Maxillary arch with 654/456 missing. If the palatal slopes of the incisors are unfavourable the denture may thrust backwards as indicated by the arrows (see text)

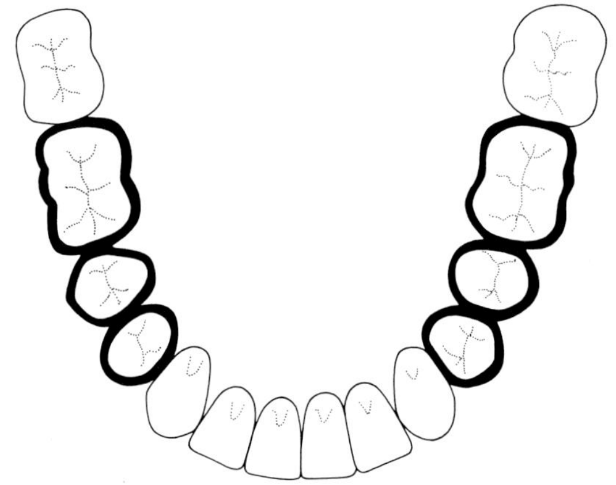

Figure 22.4 Mandibular arch with 654/456 missing. A partial denture for this case should always be made tooth-borne (see text)

the lower anterior teeth apply even more because the angulation of the inclines of these teeth is steeper as a general rule than those of the upper teeth.

Figure 22.5 illustrates a case with three saddles in which the choice of support of vertical load is complex. Following the above reasoning the right free-end or distal extension saddle carrying 7 6 5 4 / should be mucosa-borne, while the anterior saddle should be tooth-borne with proper rest seat preparation of 3 / 1. The left bounded saddle carrying / 5 6, and having as abutments / 4 7, should also be tooth-borne.

Thus there are two tooth-borne saddles and one mucosa-borne saddle and because of the different forms of support, consideration should be given to the method of connecting the saddles. When a natural tooth is loaded vertically it can be intruded into the alveolus by about 20 μm but under similar conditions mucosa can be displaced up to 500 μm and this different behaviour of these different tissues has a profound effect on the design of connectors between saddles of partial dentures.

In Figures 22.6 and 22.7 are illustrated cases where the number of teeth missing is so great and the bounded saddles of such a length that mucosal support is the design of choice in both upper and lower dentures. If tooth support were used in the upper, then 4 / 1 7 would be overloaded although additional support from 3 2 1 / would help to spread the load. In the lower denture tooth support on 6 / 4 would probably lead to periodontal breakdown of these teeth, particularly / 4 because of its small periodontal area compared to 6 /; the problem would also be compounded by the fact that the saddle is curved and so it would be difficult to direct loads down the long axes of the abutment teeth.

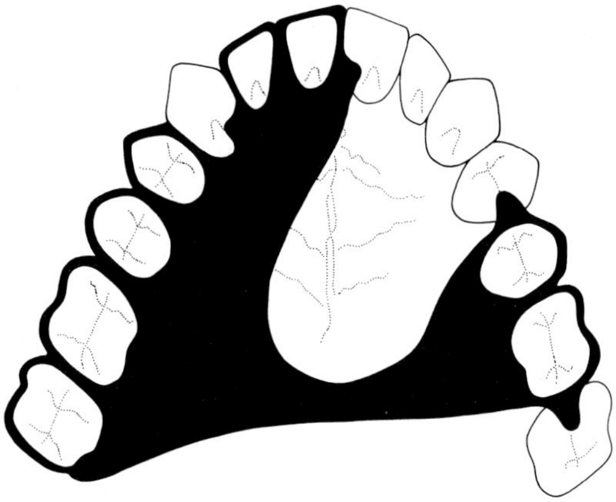

Figure 22.5 Maxillary arch with 87654 21/56 missing Saddles on 21/ and \56 are tooth-borne while the free-end saddle is mucosa-borne. Connection is the difficult design feature (see text)

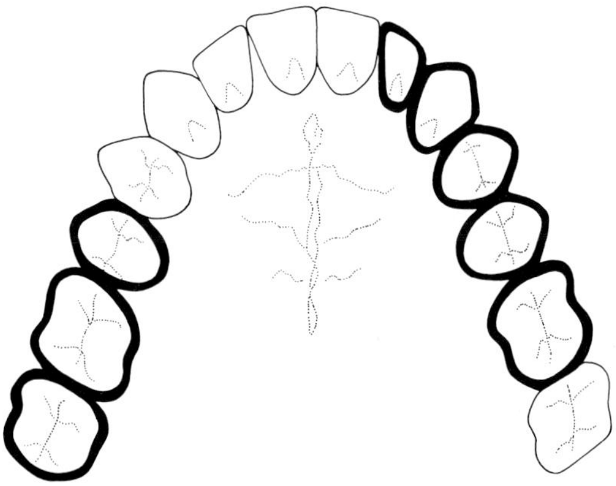

Figure 22.6 Maxillary arch with 8765/23456 missing (see text)

Lateral loads

These loads are imposed during lateral movements of the mandible with the teeth in contact and also during normal mastication; they can be varied by tooth form, tooth area and the design of the occlusion, but they cannot be eliminated. Even if the teeth are left out of any possible contact a lateral load can still be applied through the medium of intervening food. The greatest lateral stresses arise where there is cuspal interference and when this is absent the lateral stress is proportional to the occlusal area.

The tissues which resist the lateral movements of the denture and transmit them to the underlying bone are the lingual and palatal surfaces of the teeth and also their buccal surfaces if clasps incorporating bracing elements in the functional arms are fitted. The lingual, palatal and buccal surfaces of the ridges also provide a considerable surface area for resisting

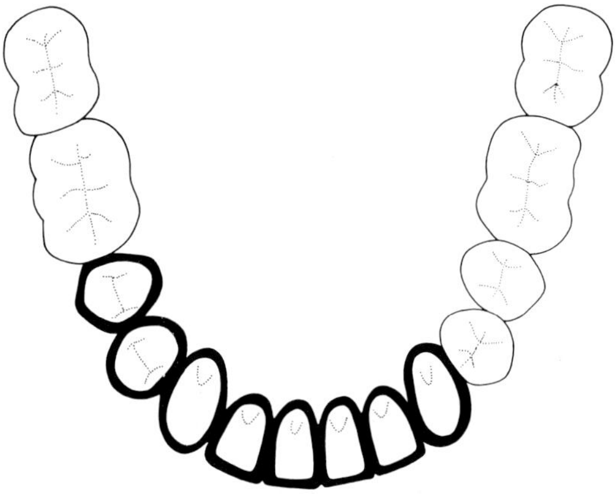

Figure 22.7 Mandibular arch with 54321/123 missing (see text)

the lateral loads applied to a denture. If, however, both teeth and soft tissues are used to resist lateral movements, then, for the same reasons as given in the section on occlusal loads, it is likely to be the abutment teeth which will carry the major portion of the load. This should always be kept in mind when designing a denture.

To illustrate this question of resistance to lateral loading, and to enable the designer to understand the method of deciding how the denture in question is to be planned to resist the lateral loads which are applied to it, three examples will be considered.

Figure 22.8 represents a Kennedy class I upper with well-formed ridges, deep sulci and a high, broad palate. The observations made when studying such a case would be that the well-developed ridges of the saddle areas could provide good resistance to lateral movement of a denture during occlusal contact or mastication to either the right or left sides. Therefore it would be unnecessary to utilize the standing teeth to resist lateral movement provided there was adequate mucosal coverage of the denture.

Figure 22.9 represents a Kennedy class I upper with poor, atrophic ridges, shallow sulci and a broad, flat palate. The inference from this example is that there is little resistance to lateral movement from the buccal and palatal surfaces of the ridges and therefore the natural teeth would need to be utilized for such resistance. The denture outline to resist lateral movement in this case might be as shown in Figure 22.10. In Figure 22.9 the denture makes no contact with the palatal aspects of the teeth but relies entirely on the ridges for support against lateral movement, whereas in Figure 22.10 all the palatal surfaces of the teeth are covered by the denture to brace it against lateral movement. Additional bracing is also obtained from the rigid parts of the clasp arms.

Figure 22.11 represents a Kennedy Class III modification 1 case, either upper or lower, with first molars and second premolars missing. The abutment teeth are sound and well supported by dense bone. Under these circumstances, with the occlusal load being supported by rests, lateral loads can safely be accepted by these teeth and resistance to lateral movement can be gained by carrying clasps and reciprocals on the buccal and palatal aspects. In addition, of course, the occlusal rests, being seated in rest seats in the teeth, provide a marked degree of resistance to lateral loads.

If, in a case such as this, the abutment teeth are periodontally involved and not well supported by bone, it may be necessary to transmit the lateral load entirely by means of the palatal and buccal slopes of the ridges and a decision will have to be made on whether the resistance offered by these surfaces is adequate to provide sufficient resistance to lateral movement in the same way as the decision

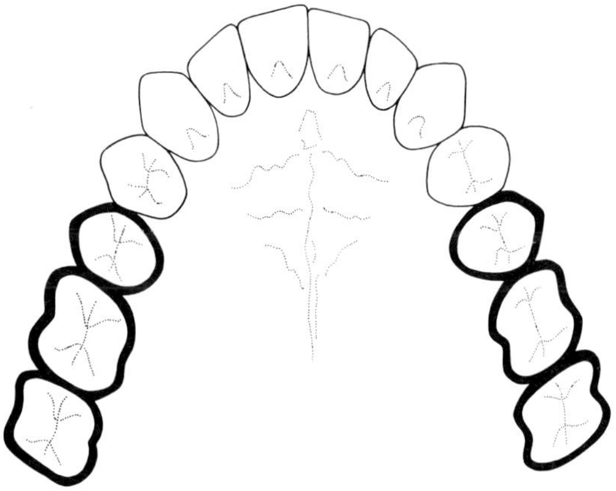

Figure 22.8 In this Kennedy class I upper, lateral resistance offered by the well-formed alveolar ridges is favourable to a mucosa-borne denture

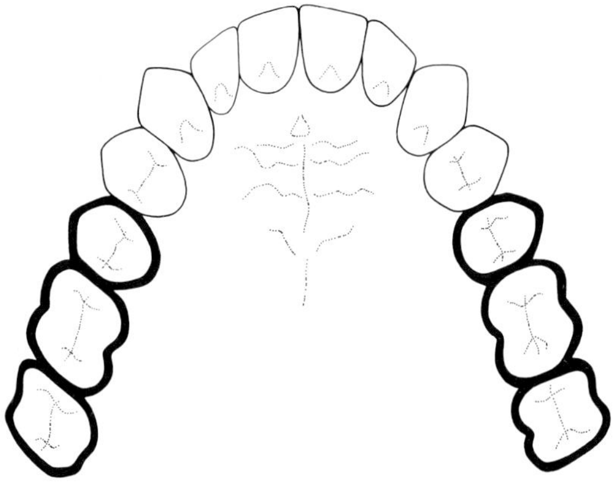

Figure 22.9 Similar case to Figure 22.8 except that the residual alveolar ridges are resorbed and the palate is flat (see text)

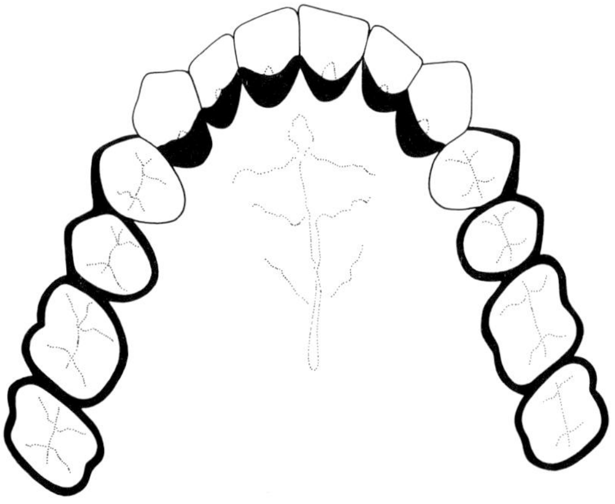

Figure 22.10 Kennedy class I with 8765/5678 missing, atrophic ridges and flat palate. Lateral resistance is provided by carrying the denture base round the anterior teeth and using buccal arms on 4/4

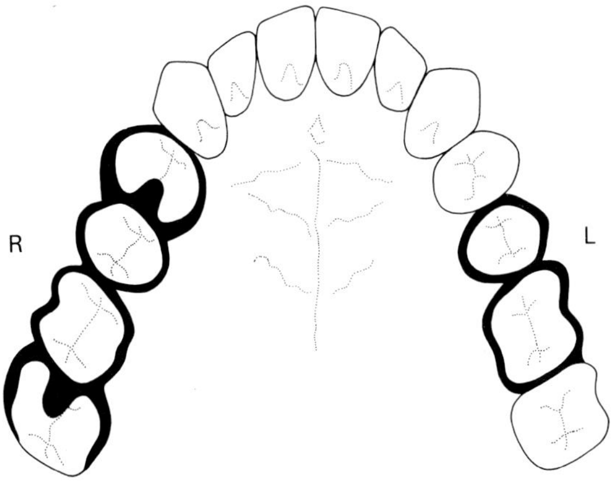

Figure 22.11 In a patient with both first molars and second premolars missing tooth support of the saddle, combined with clasps and reciprocals, is a much more efficient way of restoring the gap (right) than a mucosa-borne saddle on the left

was made in the cases illustrated in Figures 22.8 and 22.9. If the ridges are capable of resisting the load then a possible outline might be broad coverage of the lateral slopes of the ridges. If the buccal and palatal slopes of the ridges are considered inadequate to provide sufficient resistance to lateral loads then it may be necessary to carry the denture round the palatal aspects of all the standing teeth to gain sufficient resistance as illustrated in Figure 22.10.

In some cases where there is doubt about whether the buccal and palatal slopes of the ridges are adequate to resist lateral movement, and yet it seems unnecessary to carry the denture round all the standing teeth, a compromise may be made by carrying the denture round some of the standing teeth and sharing the load between the slopes of the ridges and the teeth, as illustrated in Figure 22.12.

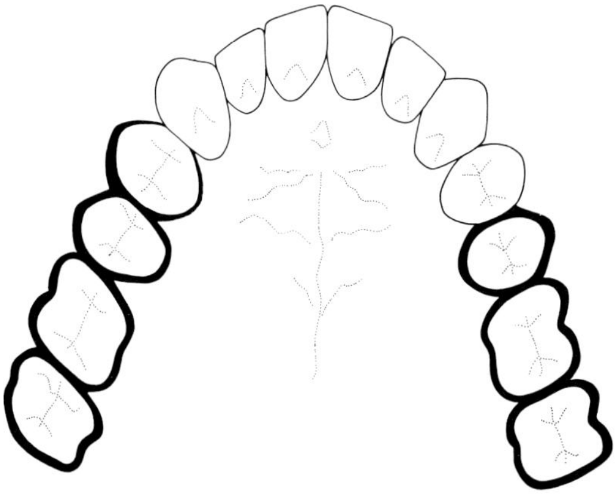

Figure 22.12 Where maxillary posterior teeth are missing, and the ridges are not suitable for resisting lateral load, clasps may be added to the mucosa-borne saddle as shown on $\underline{4}$/

All that has been said about these maxillary designs is, of course, applicable to mandibular cases of similar type, in these instances the lingual and buccal surfaces of the ridges being the tissue surfaces capable of resisting lateral movement of the denture. Frequently, however, in mandibular cases it is found that the ridges are less well developed than maxillary and so greater lateral support must be enlisted from the standing teeth.

When designing a denture to resist lateral movement, care must be taken that no individual abutment tooth is subjected to too much load either in a direct lateral direction or in the form of a rotary one.

The case illustrated in Figure 22.13 is an example of how this possibility may develop: a Kennedy class I modification 1 lower with bilateral free-end saddles, a short bounded saddle and an isolated lower second premolar. The ridges are resorbed and the sulci are shallow and, if the denture is designed with a lingual bar as illustrated, then the tendency of

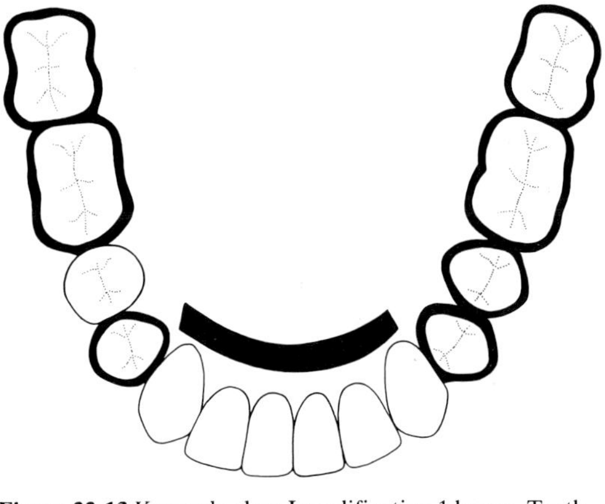

Figure 22.13 Kennedy class I modification 1 lower. Teeth missing outlined in black. Major connector lingual bar (see text)

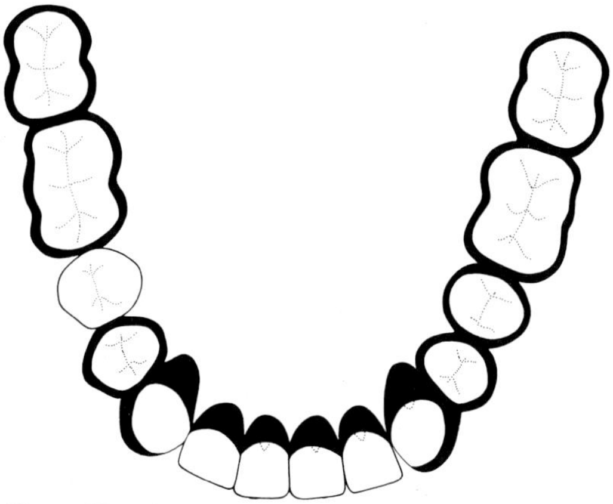

Figure 22.14 An alternative method of treating the case in Figure 22.13 (see text)

the denture to move sideways is resisted almost entirely by its contact with the isolated premolar. In addition there is a tendency for the left saddle to move backwards during occlusal contact and mastication and to inflict a torsional strain on this isolated tooth. In such a case the resistance to lateral movement must be increased by carrying the rigid connector around the lingual aspects of all the lower anterior teeth, as illustrated in Figure 22.14, and also by placing a bracing type of clasp on each lower canine.

One of the most effective methods of resisting horizontal loads is to prepare guiding surfaces or guide planes on the proximal and lingual aspects of the abutment teeth. These are particularly effective in the prevention of rotational movements of dentures.

Anteroposterior loads

These, like lateral loads, are best resisted by the remaining natural teeth, though they may be resisted by the soft tissues via a large labial flange or, less satisfactorily, an extension of a lower denture on to the anterior slope of the ascending ramus. Groups of teeth provide the most satisfactory resistance to anteroposterior loads applied to a denture because they give mutual support to one another. An isolated tooth is rarely satisfactory to resist these loads, with the possible exception of a sound, well-rooted canine or molar. It must be remembered that the tooth immediately anterior to a free-end saddle is an isolated tooth if it is clasped to resist a backward load, although it may still be one of a group of teeth capable of resisting a forward load.

The use of illustrations will clarify this question of the resistance to anteroposterior loads. Figure 22.15 represents a Kennedy class III modification 1 case in which there are two bounded saddles. The resistance to anterior movement of this denture is provided by the distal surfaces of the canines, which themselves are reinforced by the four incisors, and provided these teeth are adequately supported by bone they are quite capable of resisting all the anterior loads likely to be applied to this denture during function. Posteriorly-directed loads are similarly resisted by the mesial surfaces of the first molars, which are buttressed by the second molars. In this type of case no real problem arises with regard to the anteroposterior type of movement.

The main problems of designing a denture to resist anteroposterior movement are concerned chiefly with Kennedy class I free-end saddle dentures and Kennedy Class IV anterior saddle dentures. Figure 22.16 illustrates a Kennedy class I lower. Resistance to anterior movement of the saddles is provided by the distal surfaces of the canines which, as in Figure 22.15, are well buttressed by the other natural teeth. The resistance to posterior movement, however, can only be achieved by carrying the distal extension of the saddles as high up the ascending rami as the case will allow. Figure 22.17 shows how finishing the saddle

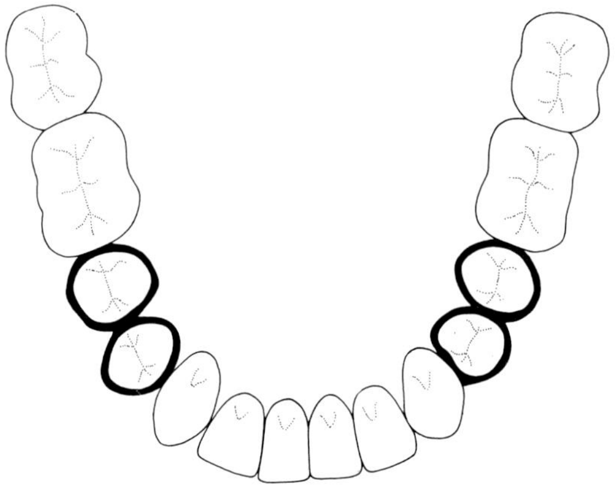

Figure 22.15 Resistance to anteroposterior loads when all four lower premolars are missing is offered by all the remaining teeth

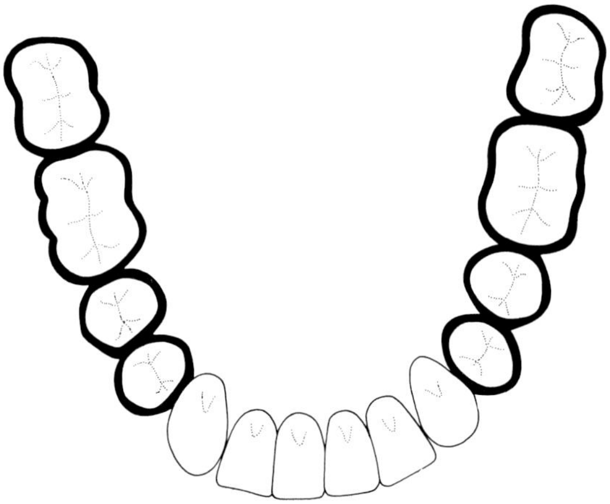

Figure 22.16 Bilateral lower free-end saddles. Resistance to anterior movement is provided by canines

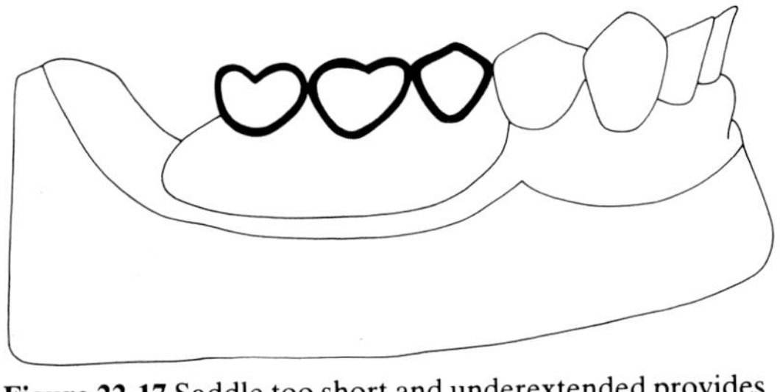

Figure 22.17 Saddle too short and underextended provides no resistance to posterior movement

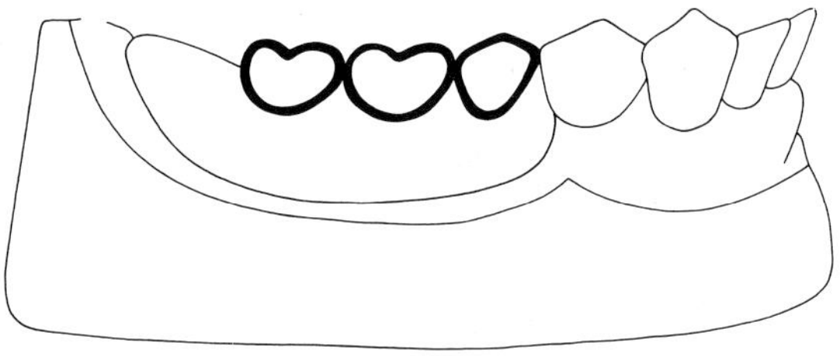

Figure 22.18 Correctly extended saddle provides resistance to posterior movement

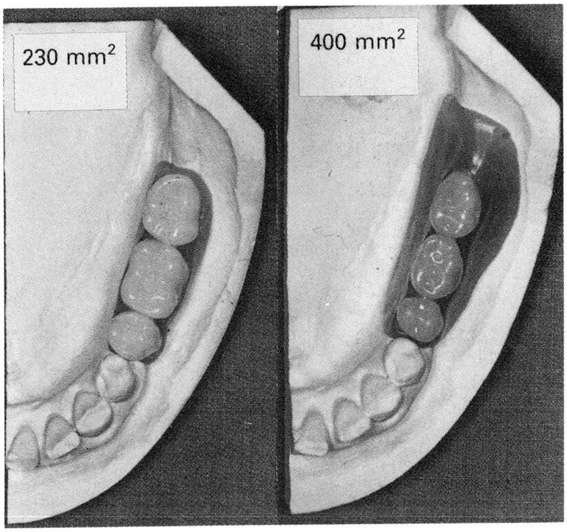

Figure 22.19 Extending free-end saddles provides greater coverage of supporting tissue and reduces load per unit area

short distally provides no resistance to posterior movement, whereas Figure 22.18 shows how the extension of the saddle towards the ascending ramus and on to the pear-shaped pad will provide a resistance to posterior movement (Figure 22.19). If, in addition, clasps are fitted to the lower canines with satisfactory bracing action, these also will provide additional resistance to posterior movement. Care must be taken, however, that these clasps are not so rigid that they tend to place abnormally high loads on these teeth and, of course, the appearance has also to be considered.

In Kennedy class I maxillary dentures there is no anterior slope of the ascending ramus such as exists in the lower to buttress the denture against posterior movement. A well-defined tuberosity and hamular notch both help to resist backward movement but, if either of these is absent, then buccal arms on the canines may be necessary. Fortunately, however, most of the loads applied to an upper denture during mastication and occlusal contact are in a forward direction due to the upward and forward movement of the lower jaw and the inclines of the cusps, and so the distal surfaces of the canine teeth and the anterior slope of the palate provide adequate resistance to anterior movement.

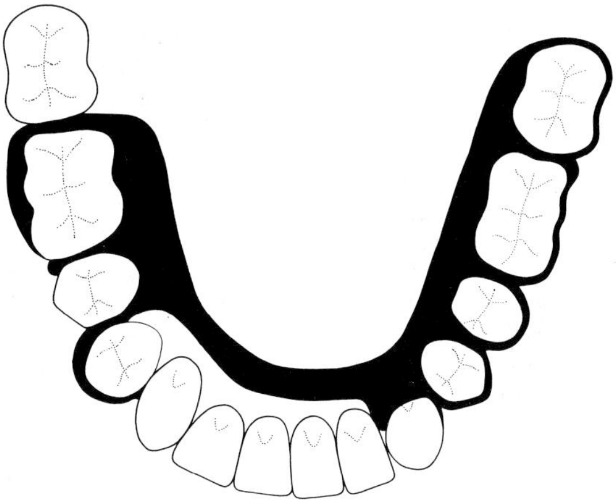

Figure 22.20 Lower unilateral free-end /45678 missing (see text)

The Kennedy class II case (Figure 22.20) sometimes presents considerable problems in relation to resistance to posterior movement and here it is necessary to provide bracing by carrying a rigid connector to the other side of the mouth and firmly clasping the teeth on that side. This may produce a torsional movement of these teeth but provided they are well-rooted, and two or sometimes three of them are clasped, they are usually capable of resisting the torsional load applied to them. If, in addition, the lower canine on the side of the free-end saddle is also clasped and the denture carried round it and up its lingual surface, and the posterior aspect of the saddle is carried on to the ascending ramus, adequate resistance to posterior movement can be provided. The carrying of the rigid connector, such as a sublingual bar, or lingual plate, round to the opposite side of the mouth also provides considerable resistance to lateral movements applied to this denture.

Kennedy class IV cases present one or two special problems. In the case illustrated in Figure 22.21 posterior movement, which is slight, can be adequately resisted by a labial flange on the mesial surfaces of the upper canines while the anterior movement of the denture can be resisted by the slope of the palate and by carrying the denture around the palatal aspects of the canines. Pure anteroposterior movements, however, are not the only ones to which this type of denture is subjected, because when food is incised there is an oblique load applied to the denture and, if the saddle is not tooth-supported, the anterior ridge and some of the surface of the palate act as a fulcrum. This action frequently produces considerable damage to the ridge and anterior surface of the palate, producing

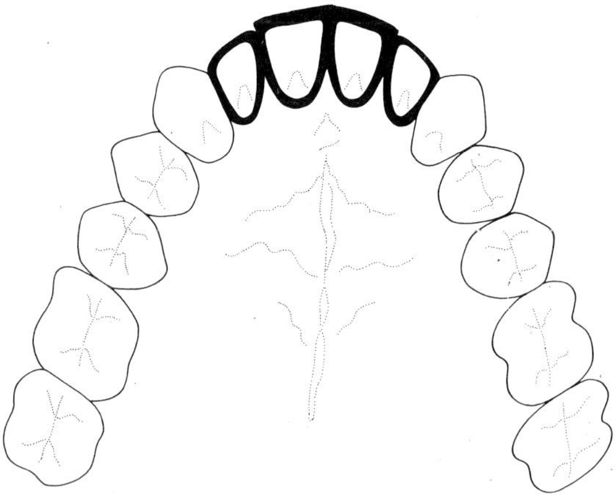

Figure 22.21 Kennedy class IV upper (see text)

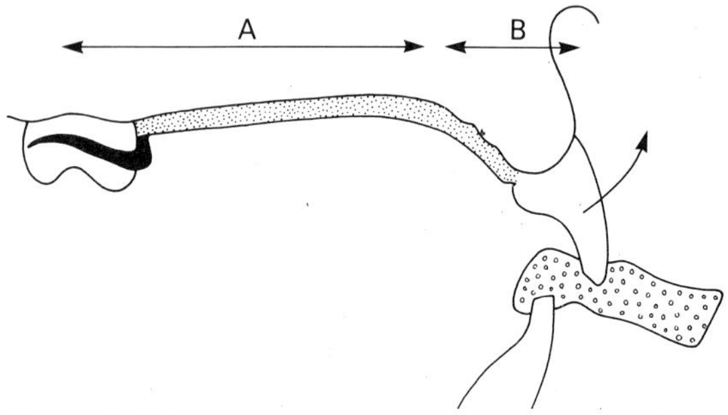

Figure 22.22 Incision of food. If a posterior tooth on either side of the mouth is clasped the area available for resisting the incising load is greatly increased. The further back in the mouth the clasped teeth are the greater the mechanical advantage because the fulcrum is in the area of the anterior ridge and the palate and the distance A is much longer than B (curved arrow indicates incising load)

quite rapidly an inflamed mucosa and loss of alveolar bone. It is, therefore, particularly important that some means of spreading this load is incorporated in the design of the denture. The use of a labial flange will do much to reduce stress by providing a broad bearing surface anteriorly and thus helping to resist the tilting load applied to the denture. Further resistance may be gained by clasping the last molar teeth which are situated some distance from the fulcrum and therefore the mechanical advantage is great (Figure 22.22). In some cases it is impossible to put a labial flange on this type of case and then clasps must be fitted as far posteriorly as possible in order to resist torsional movement.

Vertical dislodging forces

Forces which tend to dislodge a denture are:

1. Gravity, applying to upper dentures only.
2. Sticky foods, applying to both upper and lower dentures.
3. The tongue, more applicable to the lower denture but may apply to either if the patient has formed a habit of playing with the denture.
4. Part of the lateral and anteroposterior loads will be resolved into torquing stresses.

Peripheral seal plays no part in retaining partial dentures because, even if the periphery is located for a considerable part of its length in the sulcus or postdam region, its seal is broken wherever it makes contact with a natural tooth. Adhesion and cohesion play a small part, being proportional to the area of the tissue covered by the denture, but this will only be effective if a large area of the palate is covered; these surface forces play practically no part in the retention of lower dentures. Muscular control acts in the same way as it does with complete dentures and is proportional to the size of the denture: the more the denture fills the denture space the more effective will muscular control become. The use of undercuts, as described in the chapter on surveying, plays an important part in the retention of partial dentures, as does the selection and preparation of guiding surfaces and the fit of the denture against the natural teeth. The use of friction to assist retention must be employed with great care and the limitations of its use fully appreciated. It can be used only when there are teeth anterior and posterior to a saddle and the denture is then made to fit closely to these adjacent teeth. If this is excessive a wedging action results and the periodontal membrane of the tooth may be damaged while, on the other hand, insufficient pressure will reduce friction to a minimum. Retention by friction is soon reduced in time because the constant pressure from the denture acts like an orthodontic appliance and the teeth will move slightly apart as a result. Repeated insertion and removal of the denture will cause wear of the saddle where it fits most closely and this also reduces the frictional effect.

The main methods, therefore, of retaining a partial denture against withdrawal forces is the use of guiding surfaces and clasps. The selection and design of the latter is fully discussed in Chapter 20.

Thus, when the retention of a partial denture is under consideration, careful thought must be given to the following:

1. The use of clasps (direct retainers).
2. The material from which these clasps are to be made and the dimensions in relation to the physical properties which each material can be expected to produce in function.
3. The use of undercuts which, if they do not exist naturally, may be created by the fabrication of crowns or inlays or the addition of light-cured composite (Figure 22.23).
4. Guiding surfaces (or guide planes) and the friction which is likely to be obtained by contact between the denture and the abutment teeth.

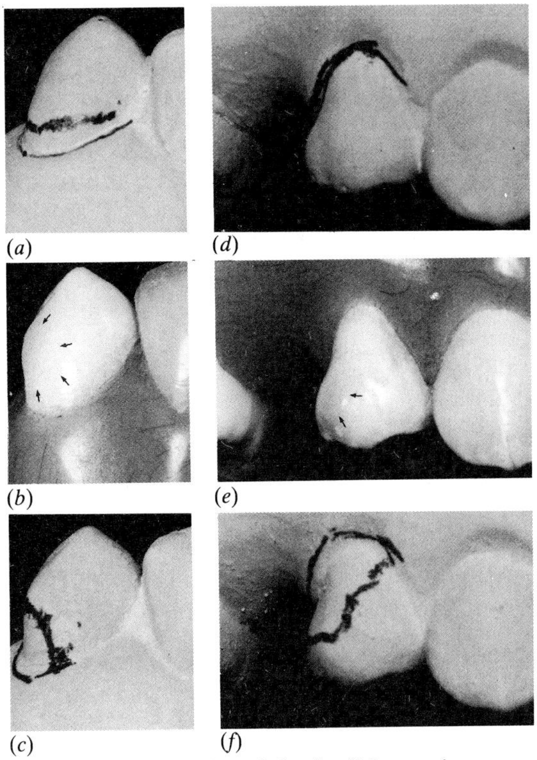

Figure 22.23 The addition of ultrafine light-cured composite alters the position of the survey line and provides undercuts for retention. (*a*), (*b*), (*c*) mandibular first premolar; (*d*), (*e*), (*f*) maxillary first premolar

5. Adhesion and cohesion, increased in mucosa-borne dentures by covering as large an area as possible.
6. Gravity, although of little importance in comparison to the amount of dislodging vertical force.
7. Indirect retainers.

While considering the problem of designing a denture to resist withdrawal, thought should also be given to the design of the occlusion, because if there are occlusal errors the load applied to the denture will probably be greater than the method of retaining it will withstand. Every effort should be made when setting the teeth for a partial denture that the occlusion of the natural teeth is stabilized before making the denture and that after delivery of the denture the teeth, both natural and artificial, share equally in accepting clenched as well as masticatory loads.

Preservation of tissue health

The health of the tissues covered by a denture will not maintain the same level that might be expected if no dentures were fitted.

This is because: (1) the denture holds food debris and plaque in contact with the tissues and constitutes an irritant; (2) by covering the tissues the frictional stimulation and cleansing from the surface of the tongue and fibrous foods, which maintain a healthy keratinization, is prevented from occurring; (3) the movement of the denture, although slight, tends to produce trauma; (4) the oral ecology changes in a patient wearing a partial denture.

A denture may cause damage to the following tissues:

1. The mucosa generally.
2. The gingival margins specifically, leading in time to severe damage to the supporting structures of the teeth.
3. The bone of the edentulous alveolar ridge.
4. The remaining natural teeth.

All mucosa-borne dentures transmit the load to the bone via the mucosa during clenching and mastication and damage can be inflicted to this tissue:

1. By failing to cover a sufficiently large area of the supporting tissues and thus overloading the area which is covered.
2. By fitting a denture which has insufficient lateral bracing against the natural teeth or slopes of the ridges, and which therefore moves from side to side or backwards and forwards and causes trauma of the mucosa by friction. This is especialy so in a case which presents deep, convoluted surfaces of the palate and for which the impression has been taken in an alginate impression material which faithfully copies those deep convolutions. This produces a denture with a fitting surface which has a roughness comparable to that of sandpaper. This often results in a granular type of hyperplasia in which clinically the tissues are red and inflamed, a condition often misdiagnosed as sensitivity to polymethyl methacrylate.
3. By fitting a denture which accepts the first occlusal contact on closing, the entire load is taken on the denture but little or none on the natural teeth, with the consequence that a severe overload is placed on the mucosa and underlying alveolar bone. Frequently the damage remains confined for some time to the mucosa, showing as a localized or generalized inflammation, but often the consequences of the excess load result in resorption of the alveolar ridge leading to an inaccurate fit of the denture base, a worsening of the condition and loss of a stable and efficient occlusion.
4. By gross cuspal interference and locking of the occlusion resulting in the denture being dragged across the mucosa.

Any or all of the above-mentioned conditions may also cause damage to the gingival margins, but in addition there are damaging factors which are specific.

If a denture is made to fit the gingival margins accurately, its every movement will cause that part of it which fits the gingival crevice to press or drag with consequent injury, and any settling of the denture (a mucosa-borne denture is bound to change its position slightly because of mucosal compression) will tend to cause the fitting part of the denture to cut into the margin.

Figure 18.8 illustrates a sharp damaging denture margin, and indicates how it will fit against the gingival tissues in the mouth and force the gingival margin away from the tooth with any movement of the denture. These sharp margins should either be trimmed and polished before the denture is fitted or the cast surface covered with 0.06 mm metal foil to produce a smooth, atraumatic, slightly relieved fitting surface. Figure 18.9 shows how a denture, trimmed and polished, will be free of the gingival margin.

Any failure of fit of the denture around a natural tooth will leave a space down which food will be forced directly on to the gingival margin. Such a denture might in fact be thought to have been designed specifically to direct food on to the margin. Figure 18.10 illustrates this condition and Figure 20.25 shows in cross-section on the right side how a space between the tooth and the denture, made either by careless surveying and blocking out or by incorrect easing when inserting the denture, leaves a gap. The left side of Figure 20.25 illustrates the correct manner in which a denture should fit in close contact with the tooth just on or above the survey line, thus directing food from the occlusal surface of the tooth on to the polished surface of the denture.

Caries may be caused either by food being held in contact with the teeth due to a poorly fitting denture or to roughness of its surface.

The supporting tissues of the teeth may be damaged by excessive lateral or anteroposterior load being applied to them by the dentures or by using the teeth for lateral or anteroposterior bracing where the periodontal attachment is inadequate to withstand the load.

Wearing a removable partial denture (RPD) increases plaque scores and the degree of tissue damage is related to the number of hours a denture is in the mouth in any given week. The dilemma here is that if the denture is in the mouth damage to hard and soft tissues is likely; if the denture is not in the mouth then the remaining teeth are liable to shift position, even in minute amounts, and this will have a detrimental effect on the occlusion; furthermore, when the denture is again inserted, the periodontum will have to re-adapt to the denture. This constant re-adaptation is one of the main causes for gradual destruction of hard and soft tissues.

Although emphasis has been placed on the damage which may result from partial dentures, careful design can generally reduce the damage to a minimum and the advantages of making good partial dentures always outweigh the disadvantages. In many cases the partial denture prolongs the life of the remaining natural teeth by supporting them and reducing the clenched and masticatory loads placed on them. It also prevents drift and over-eruption of natural teeth.

The basic principles of partial denture design have now been considered individually, but in practice they are obviously inter-related and considered together. In order to illustrate how a partial denture should be designed one or two examples of the method will be given.

The economic position

The cost of partial denture treatment is important and in most cases the designer of a denture is faced with the problem of producing a design and using a material which will confer the maximum benefit on the patient at reasonable cost.

When designing dentures it is helpful to use a diagram of the outline of the upper and lower teeth as illustrated in Figure 22.24. The shape and extent of the various parts of the denture can be drawn on this diagram. As the design of the denture proceeds its ability to resist each of the component forces should become clear if the design is planned in a logical sequence. It is generally best to plan the support first, then the major connectors between the various components, and finally the retention. After these basic features consideration is given to axes of rotation, indirect retention, minor connectors, lateral and anteroposterior bracing, indirect support, occlusion, patient comfort, materials to be used and aesthetics. The advantage of sketching out the design is that each of these factors is continually being considered as each is usually dependent on the others. The following examples should help to make the meaning of this paragraph quite clear.

Example of the technique of designing

An upper dentition is a Kennedy class II modification 2 with $\underline{8765|12458}$ missing opposed by a lower dentition of Kennedy class II modification 1 with $\overline{865|5678}$ missing (Figure 22.24). The technique of designing dentures for this case is as follows:

1. The clinical examination shows that $\underline{|6}$ and $\overline{|4}$ have sound amalgam restorations; $\underline{1|}$ has a class IV mesial synthetic restoration; $\underline{4|}$ has a mesio-occlusal amalgam and lower $\overline{74|}$ have occlusal amalgams. The mucosa of the ridges and palate is healthy and firm, but the lower left

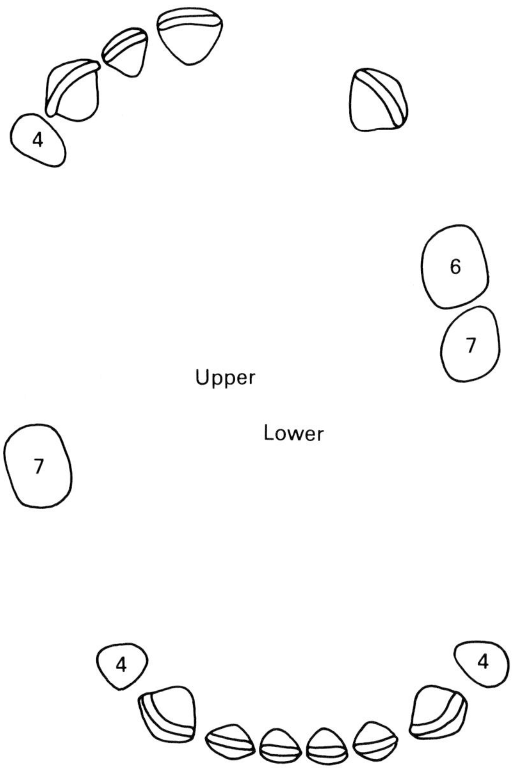

Figure 22.24 Chart of existing teeth in a partially edentulous patient (see text)

free-end saddle is extremely resorbed and the mylohyoid ridge is prominent. There is mild pocketing around most of the gingival margins of the teeth, but it is not severe, with the exception of the palatal aspects of 3 2 1/.

2. The radiographic examination shows that all teeth are supported for more than two-thirds of their length by normal dense bone.
3. The female patient, aged 30, is wearing acrylic partial dentures made 6 years previously.
4. The economic position in this case is that these dentures should be constructed relatively inexpensively.

Decision one

The first problem is to decide how vertical occlusal loads are to be supported. On the mounted casts it is seen that 7/7 will occlude with the upper denture and that /6 7 will occlude with the lower denture. This means that the load applied to these saddles will be greater than if they were opposed by artificial teeth. The question therefore arises: can either of these saddles be made toothborne to resist this extra load better than if they were mucosa-borne?

Both these saddles are free-ended with no posterior abutment tooth, so no effective tooth support against vertical loads can be used. The decision with regard to these saddles, therefore, is that they must be mucosa-borne and cover as wide an area as possible so as to resist occlusal loads and the first stage of the design is to outline the area of these saddles.

The next consideration is the question of vertical load in relation to the lower right saddle. This saddle could be tooth-borne because it is abutted posteriorly by a sound molar tooth and anteriorly by a premolar, both of which could support rests. To make this saddle tooth-borne, however, might be a bad decision for three reasons:

1. If tooth-borne it will be capable of applying greater vertical loads to the opposing saddle of the upper denture which, as has already been decided, is to be mucosa-borne.
2. If this saddle is made tooth-borne, and the free-end saddle on the opposite side of the lower denture is to be mucosa-borne, then a flexible or movable connector may be required to join the two saddles because they are dissimilarly supported.
3. As the load-bearing capacity of the upper mucosa-borne saddle is the limiting factor in the power with which the patient will be able to chew on the right side nothing much will be gained from making this saddle tooth-borne.

The next consideration is the question of the vertical load in relation to the upper left saddle. Here the same remarks apply in relation to making the saddle tooth-borne as applied to the lower right saddle, with the additional fact that the palatal surface of the canine in this case is unsuitable for supporting a rest.

The final saddle requiring consideration in relation to vertical load is the anterior saddle of the upper denture, carrying /1 2. This should also be a mucosa-borne saddle because of the decision about the other two saddles. Here the question of the tilting load applied when the patient incises also requires to be considered and a decision must be made as to whether a labial flange is to be fitted for appearance and to assist in resisting this tilt and whether 4 / 7 are to be clasped to provide resistance against the tilting force. In almost every case where anterior teeth have been lost there is an associated loss of alveolar bone and gingival contour. For this reason a labial flange should be used in this case.

Decision two

A decision is now made about providing adequate resistance to the lateral movement of the dentures. In the lower denture the resistance to be gained from the slopes of the ridges is poor, and because of the prominent left mylohyoid ridge no use can be made of the lingual surface of the ridge in this area. In addition, as the left saddle of the lower denture occludes with / 6 7, the lateral loads applied to this saddle are likely to be great. The flanges of these saddles will need to be carried as deeply into the sulci as muscular function will allow, but no coverage of the mylohyoid ridge should be attempted. As the area of the saddles for ridge resistance to lateral movement is poor it will be necessary to ensure that adequate resistance to lateral movement is gained from the standing teeth. What possibilities do these offer?

The denture can be carried round the lingual surfaces of 7 4 / 4 and this will provide resistance to movement towards the right, but resistance to movement towards the left will fall entirely on / 4 which would overload this tooth. Carrying the denture round the lingual surfaces of 3 2 1 / 1 2 3 would produce some extra stability against movement towards the right and left by the impingement of the denture against the lingual surfaces and embrasures of these teeth, but the additional resistance to lateral movement of the left would be outweighed by covering the gingival margins of these teeth. A better method might be to use bracing clasps on the buccal surfaces of 7 4 / if the survey lines of these teeth allowed such clasps to be designed. If these teeth had unsuitable survey lines, however, the only course would be to carry the major connector round the lingual surfaces of 3 2 1 / 1 2 3.

In the upper denture resistance to lateral movement is not so difficult because this case has a deep palate and well formed ridges and so soft tissue resistance to lateral movement is good. As the upper right saddle is opposed by 7 /, and greater lateral loads will be applied by this tooth than if the saddle were opposed by artificial teeth only, it would be best to gain extra resistance to lateral movement by carrying the denture round the palatal surfaces of 4 / 6. Resistance to lateral loads will be gained by the contact of the denture against the mesial surfaces of 1 / 3.

Decision three

Resistance to anteroposterior loads now need to be considered. In the lower denture the right saddle presents no problem because it is buttressed against forward movement by the distal surface of 4 /, which is itself aided by 3 2 /, and against distal movement by the mesial surface of 7 /. This is a solitary tooth but has a large periodontal area and is adequately supported by bone.

The resistance to forward movement of the left saddle is provided by the distal surface of / 4 but the resistance to posterior movement of this saddle is a problem. It will gain some from the keying effect of the right saddle between 7 4 /, but the torquing action occurring through the long lever arm of the connector will place a considerable strain on these teeth and additional resistance should be provided by extending the saddle up to the ascending ramus and placing a clasp around / 4 This will probably produce a reasonable resistance to posterior movement for this saddle but a note should be made that the cusps of the teeth on this saddle should be low so as to reduce its tendency to be thrust distally.

The anteroposterior movement of the upper denture is now considered. The left saddle is adequately braced between / 3 6 and the mesial surface of / 3 will also resist posterior movement to some extent. The distal surface of 4 / will resist forward movement of the saddle on that side and is aided by 3 2 1 / and the anterior slope of the palate.

In this case the resistance to backward movement of the right saddle is questionable but there is a keying effect provided by the anterior and the left bounded saddles and, taking into account the fact that the tendency of an upper denture to move backwards is less than a lower, such keying effect would be considered adequate. It is still advisable, however, to make a note that the cusps of the teeth of this saddle should be low in order not to provide inclined surfaces for the development of posterior forces.

Decision four

The question of resistance to withdrawal forces now needs to be considered. In the lower denture clasps have been placed on 7 4 / 4 for their bracing action against lateral movement. These clasps will also provide retention of the denture. The centre of their retentive action will fall much nearer the right saddle than the left, however, and the resistance to withdrawal of the distal end of the left saddle, which is a long one, is not good. If the major connector is made in the form of a lingual plate, however, it will act as an indirect retainer to resist this movement.

The resistance to withdrawal of the upper denture is simpler. There is considerable friction gained by the close fit of the denture against mesial surface of 1 / 3 and / 3 6 and, in addition, a large area of the palate is being covered by the denture base to resist lateral and anteroposterior movement and therefore adhesion and tongue control will markedly assist retention. It is therefore not considered necessary to put clasps on this denture.

Decison five

The final decision is to produce the complete outline of the dentures in relation to the types of connectors and the coverage or freeing of the gingival margins. In the lower denture the major connector between the two saddles may be a cast lingual bar and indirect retainer that leaves the gingival margins uncovered or an acrylic plate carried round and up the lingual aspects of the anterior teeth. In the upper denture the acrylic of the palate may be carried round all the teeth or leave the gingival margins free.

The need to secure firm resistance to lateral movement and adequate indirect retention of the left saddle dictates the use of a lingual plate as the lower major connector. The question of cost decides that it shall be made of acrylic. In the upper 3 2 1/ 7 may be left uncovered by the denture because they show evidence of gingival damage.

General comment

In any particular case the choice of design depends on:

Position and number of missing teeth.
Health of remaining tissues.
Periodontal areas of remaining teeth.
Degree of bone loss.
Nature of supporting bone.
Size and number of the abutment teeth.
Size and relative position of saddles.
Position, direction, magnitude and duration of loads.
Position, dimension and material of major connectors.
Position, size, number and dimension of occlusal rests.
Position, number and dimension of retainers.
Properties of materials used.
The philosophy and design of stress-breakers.
The type of occlusion and jaw movement.

Stress-breakers

Stress-breaking is based on the belief that the action of certain parts can be separated from the movement of free-end (distal extension) saddles of partial dentures. Thus, when the term stress-breaker is used it is generally applied to a device that allows some movement between the mucosa-borne saddle and the rigid framework with its retainers and occlusal rests.

A stress-breaker can be defined as a 'device intended to relieve abutment teeth of load' or a 'device which relieves the abutment teeth of all or part of the occlusal forces'.

Aims

Five purposes or aims of stress-breaking may be listed:

1. To direct occlusal forces in the long axes of the abutment teeth.
2. To prevent harmful loads being applied to the remaining natural teeth.
3. To share loads as evenly as possible between the natural teeth and saddle areas according to the ability of these different tissues to accept the loads.
4. To ensure that the part of the load applied to the saddle area is distributed as evenly as possible over the whole mucosal surface.
5. To provide greater comfort for the patient.

Methods

A number of methods have evolved over the years to manage the problem.

1. Mechanical devices e.g. flexible connectors, hinges, or movable joints, are located between the free-end saddle and the tooth-supported part of the denture (Figure 22.25). The recovery of mucosa after load is viscoelastic in nature and compared with the periodontal membrane round the teeth it takes longer to recover its original position than the teeth and this is bound to affect the mutual relationship. The amount of displacement of mucosa can be up to twenty times more than that of teeth and if the saddle coverage is too small there is a greater intrusion into the mucosa than with large saddles. Throughout a saddle area the thickness of mucosa is variable and the difference in compressibility between the anterior and posterior parts of a saddle area affects the rotation of the saddle when under load. For example, if the anterior end is less compressible than the posterior end the whole denture rotates away from the anterior teeth, and vice versa.
2. Functional impression or tissue displacement techniques are used to compress the mucosa of the free-end saddle area so that the displacement of the mucosa relates to that of the periodontium

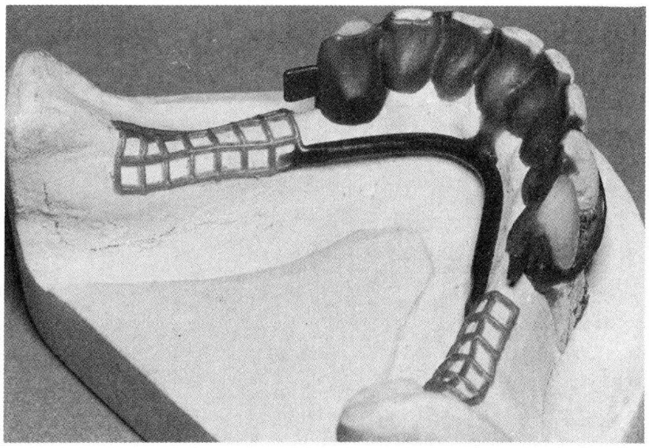

Figure 22.25 Flexible connection between tooth-borne element and mucosa-borne saddles in a case with bilateral lower free-end saddle areas. This is a diagnostic wax-up to demonstrate the use of cantilever canines and vertical fins

when the denture is under masticatory or clenched load. Impression wax is used in the altered cast technique or the supporting tissues may be equilibrated by rebasing the finished denture, either at the time of delivery or after it has been worn for a few weeks.

3. Dentures designed with an RPI (Rest, Plate, I-bar) clasping system are rigid but are intended to pivot around the abutment teeth without damaging the teeth or the mucosa (see Figure 22.44). This system comprises an occlusal rest (placed mesially on the abutment tooth), a proximal plate (contacting a distal guiding surface) and a gingivally-approaching clasp (the I-bar).

Comment on stress-breakers

Many stress-broken designs are theoretically unsound. Hinges are commonly used but they have the drawback of preventing an even load to the whole saddle area and also, because of wear, an excessive lateral movement of the saddle. The term stress-breaker is not a particularly good one and other terms used are stress distributor, stress spreader, stress equalizer or stress director. Designs with stress-breakers need good retention in order to provide the necessary indirect support because without retention the dentures behave in the same way as rigid designs (Figure 22.26). Indirect support means that the retainer on one side of the fulcrum axis through occlusal rests can provide indirect support for the part of the denture on the opposite side of the rests and this is an important principle that many clinicians using stress-breakers fail to recognize. In actual practice, however, indirect support is not fully effective in removable dentures since it is seldom possible to make the clasping system sufficiently retentive to provide it. This is

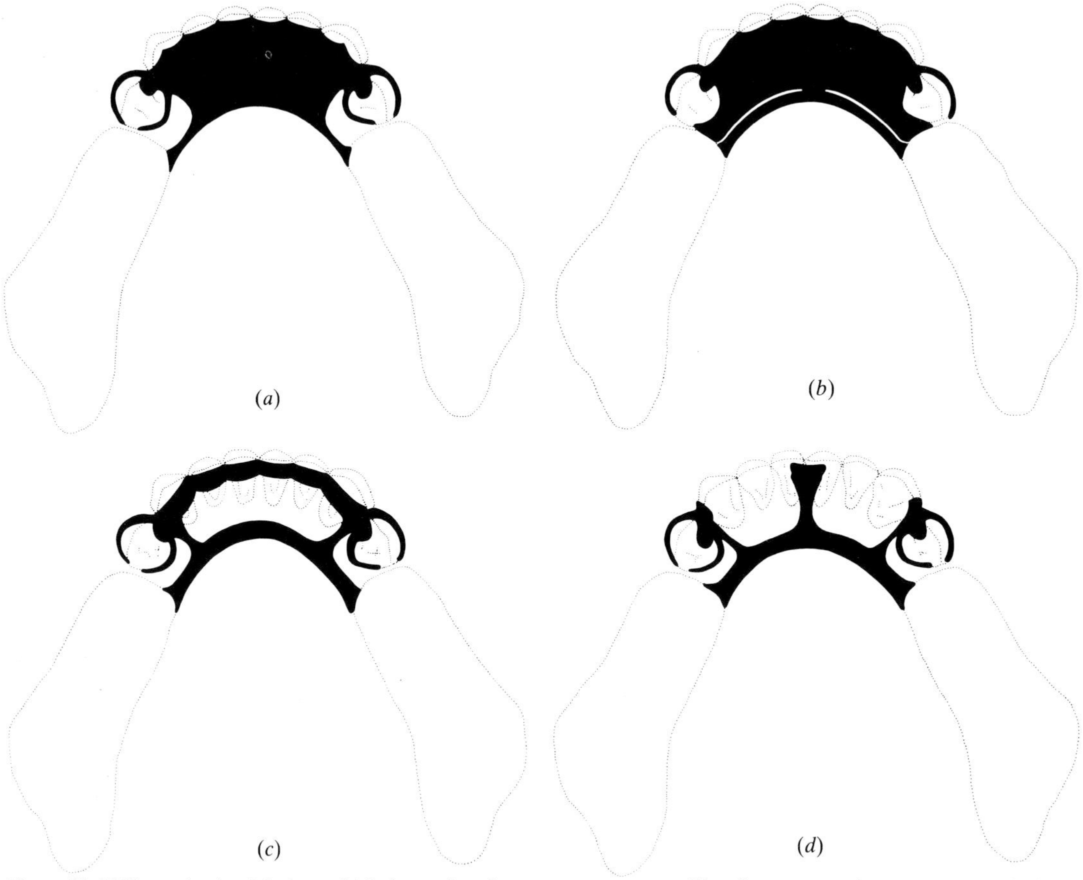

Figure 22.26 'Stress-broken' designs which do not function as expected because, when the saddles are loaded, the denture rotates round the fulcrum axis through the occlusal rests. The distally-facing clasps do not prevent this rotation. Thus the dentures behave as if they were rigid. (*a*) Cast lingual major connector with semi-flexible connectors; (*b*) split connector (one-piece casting); (*c*) one-piece casting with lingual bar connector, continuous 'clasp' (indirect retainer), semi-flexible connectors; (*d*) identical to (*c*) but with continuous 'clasp' replaced by anterior indirect retainer to reduce bulk

one of the reasons that the principle of indirect support is more effective in fixed partial dentures (bridges) than removable.

There are two useful designs that incorporate stress-breakers:

1. Dimple-hinge denture (see Figure 22.34) in which the anterior tooth-supported casting is linked to the mucosa-borne saddles (connected by a rigid bar) by a transverse hinge placed anterior to the fulcrum axis. Because the hinge is placed at the lower edge of the tooth-borne part, and provided the latter is adequately retained, then some load is accepted by the teeth as well as the mucosa.
2. Disjunct denture (see Figure 22.35) in which the only connection between the differently supported parts of the denture is by means of horizontal pins at the ends of the stiff buccal bars located at the middle of each free-end saddle. This complete disjunction eliminates harmful loads being applied to the remaining natural teeth.

Disjunct and dimple hinge dentures, if they are correctly made, are comfortable as they avoid the 'tugging' effect of rigid constructions, although the RPI clasping system, along with an altered cast technique, is a most successful design.

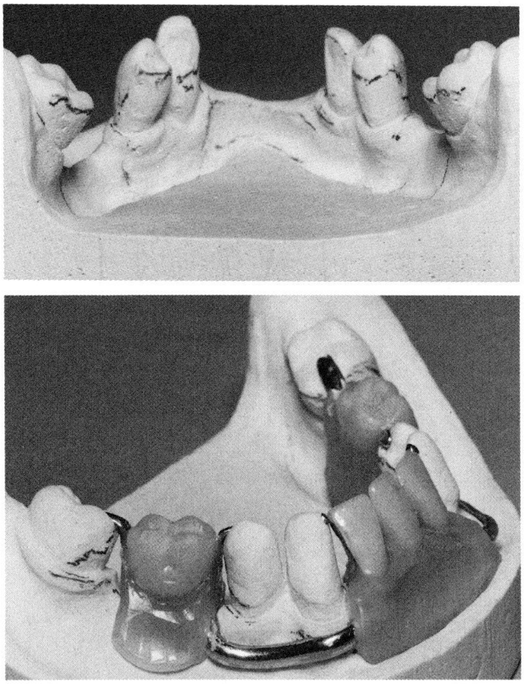

Figure 22.27 Design 1 (see text)

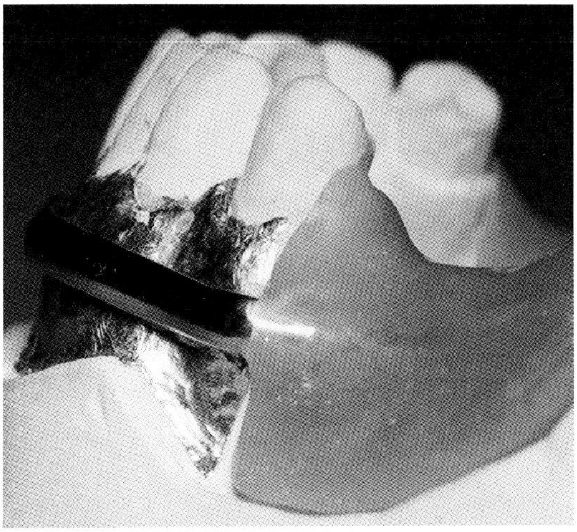

Figure 22.28 Design 1. Wrought labial bar where the incisors are inclined lingually

Examples of designs

It is useful to illustrate a variety of partial denture designs based on the principles discussed in this chapter, together with additional features in particular cases.

Design 1

The important feature of this case (Figure 22.27) is the lingual inclination of the six remaining abutment teeth. This not only reduces the saddle areas but also presents difficulty in insertion. Four of the teeth, i.e. canines and second molars have large areas of periodontal membrane and so the best method of support of the dentures is by rests on these teeth, together with additional support on the premolars. Rest seats are prepared in the mesio-incisal edges of the canines while the marginal ridges are reduced slightly on the posterior teeth to receive occlusal rests.

Connecting the three tooth-borne saddles is a problem, partly because of the lingual inclination and partly because of the need to avoid damage to the gingival tissues which might arise if the major connector covered them. For these reasons a buccal bar has been used in this one-piece cast cobalt–chromium denture. In actual practice the undercuts mesial and distal to each abutment tooth would be blocked out so that, in the finished denture, spaces would result. These spaces, although unsightly, are self-cleansing and so help to avoid damage and minimize plaque around the gingivae.

In this illustration the teeth are mounted in wax. Retainers would have to be added in order to resist upward movement of the denture but have been intentionally omitted to simplify the design principles. Wrought wire clasps would be the material of choice but care would be needed to avoid interfering with the self-cleansing embrasures.

In Figure 22.28, another example of a labial or buccal bar is shown for a case where the anterior teeth are lingually inclined. This bar is made of wrought stainless steel and, because the arc made by a labial bar is longer than a lingual bar for the same case, the labial bar is liable to be too flexible and easily distorted. The cast surface, as seen in Figure 22.28, is protected with thin metal foil during shaping of the bar.

Design 2

Figures 22.29 and 22.30 show two designs for the same case and both have faults. In Figure 22.29 the cast cobalt–chromium base covers all the gingival margins and although the base is tooth-borne such a practice is not good. Even if the hygiene were perfect, plaque deposit and lack of normal frictional effects would produce, at least, a marginal gingivitis.

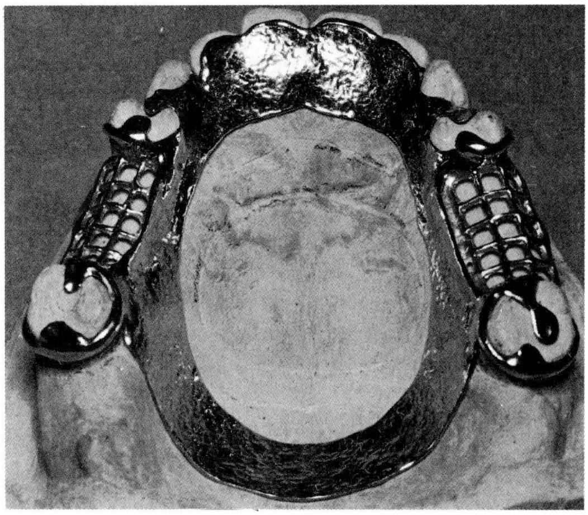

Figure 22.29 Design 2 (see text)

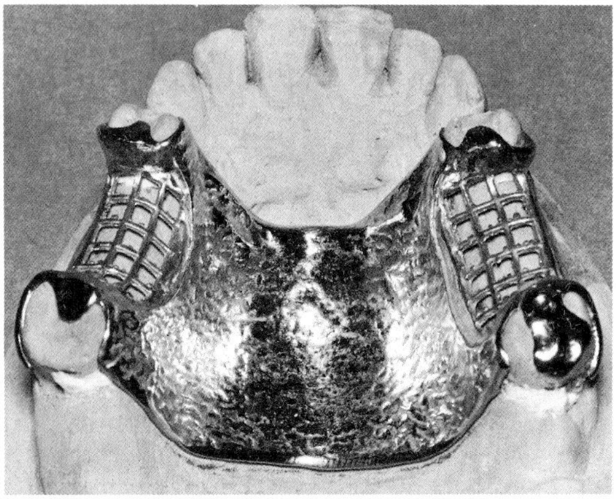

Figure 22.30 Design 2 (see text)

This is a very rigid base and resistance to lateral movement is considerable because of the 'ring' design of the connector together with the heavy clasping of the four abutment teeth.

The broad, flat posterior palatal connector is correctly positioned and in this situation would be well-tolerated by the patient. It is sufficiently rigid and offers a small amount of indirect retention to possible displacement of the anterior part of the denture.

The anterior major connector may be used to provide an incisal platform for the opposing lower incisors while at the same time protecting the upper incisors from an unfavourable occlusion. It may be considered as a form of periodontal splint. It is important to mount the refractory model on the articulator so that the casting wax may be built in harmony with closed lateral and protrusive mandibular movements.

The only benefit of four clasps is the resistance to lateral movement, a property particular to this case as the clasps are excessively thick in section.

In the other design (Figure 22.30) the connector is a palatal strap and is sufficiently, if not excessively, rigid. This particular casting is very thick as can be seen at the posterior edge. It would occupy too much space in the mouth and would interfere with function, especially speech.

The four buccal arms are reciprocated by the rigid base extended on the palatal surfaces of the teeth. This makes a more streamlined effect and one that feels better to the patient as compared to lingual clasp arms. On the other hand, extending the base as in Figure 22.30 leads to damage of the palatal gingivae and plaque deposits on the covered teeth.

The occlusal rests are made in conventional positions but lack the contour usually necessary to oppose mandibular holding cusps (occlusal stops). Note the shape and extension of the rest on ⌊7 which was made as a partial overlay to restore occlusion against the opposing tooth.

This cast base is excessively heavy and bulky for the replacement of four maxillary teeth especially when compared with fixed restorations which is the treatment of choice in such a case, provided other factors are favourable.

Note in Figures 22.29 and 22.30 the use of palatal stops to contain the acrylic of each saddle so that when the denture is finished the palatal surface feels smooth and uninterrupted in the mouth.

Design 3

Figure 22.31 shows different designs for similar maxillary partial dentures. All have short bounded saddles and so have been made tooth-borne by occlusal rests on the mesial and distal fossae. In (*a*) a canine is the anterior abutment and a cingulum seat has been prepared to receive the rest. The main

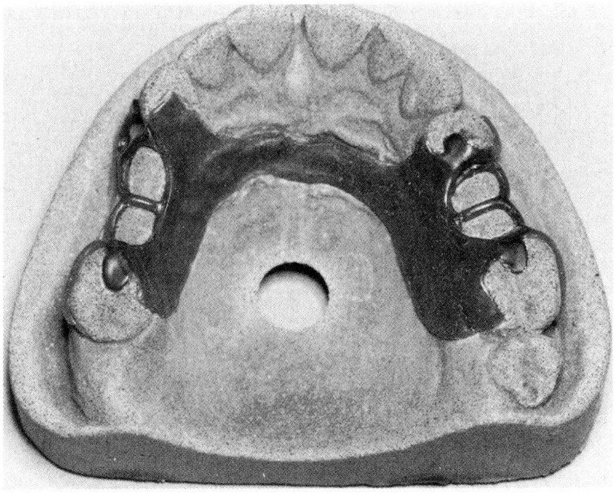

(*a*)

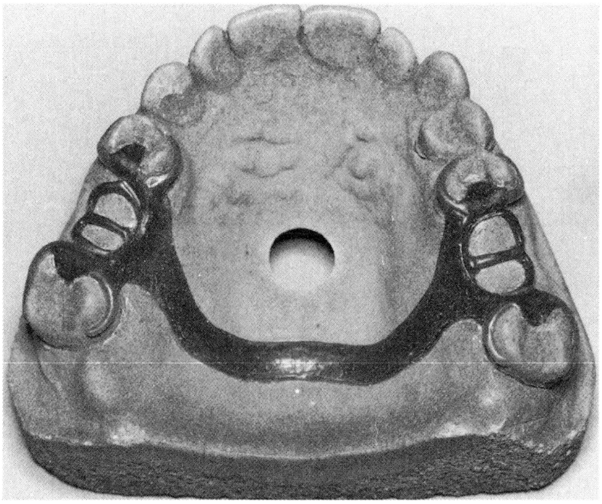

(*b*)

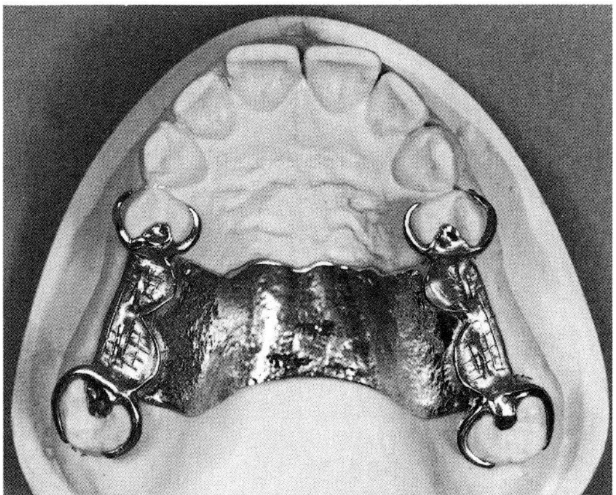

(*c*)

Figure 22.31 Design 3. (*a*) Anterior palatal bar; (*b*) posterior palatal bar; (*c*) palatal strap or plate. (Note (*a*) and (*b*) are wax patterns on refractory investment models)

variation in the designs lies in the different major connectors. In (*b*) the connector is a posterior bar in a good position as the patient would find it relatively unobtrusive, although it may interfere with food being passed backwards across the palate. However, in its simplicity the design is not good as the denture would be weak and easily distorted, especially when out of the mouth. The same criticism may be made about the design in (*a*), in which the anterior palatal bar has been made flatter to fit neatly into the palatal rugae but its transverse strength would be insufficient to resist distortion. Note in this design the bracing of the clasps is derived from extensions of the palatal base and these elements may cause gingival damage. The bracing on $\underline{7|}$ is intentionally short so as to fit into the palatal fissure on that abutment.

The design in (*c*) is an improvement on the other two designs in the sense that the major connector takes the form of a palatal strap which is more rigid than the other two connectors. The only criticism is its comparative bulk. Note that the four clasps are designed to keep the gingival margins free of denture base coverage. These, however, are not in any way self-cleansing, and particularly vulnerable areas for collecting food are the angled junctions between the palatal arms and the major connector. The occlusal rests are broad and resistant to load, and contoured to continue the anatomical shape of the abutment teeth. The palatal stops are a particularly neat feature of this base and are made to receive the pontic teeth of the saddles. Four clasps are perhaps rather excessive in this design and three, or even two, may be sufficient; on the other hand, the use of four provides good retention, bracing and symmetry.

Design 4

This is an Every denture named after the clinician who proposed the design (Figure 22.32). It is mucosa-borne and is suited to maxillary arches where there are a number of saddles and where the remaining teeth are of doubtful prognosis. Resistance to vertical load is partly shared by the wide palatal coverage, lateral load by the flanges and rigid palatal structure, and anteroposterior load by the contact of each saddle against the abutment teeth bounding each saddle. Retention is gained partly by adhesive and cohesive forces between the palate of the denture and the mucosa and partly by the frictional contact between the end of each saddle against the abutment teeth. In order to maintain this intimate contact against the abutment teeth the denture base is extended to the distal surface of the last-standing tooth on each side and this prevents distal migration of the teeth which otherwise would cause loosening of the denture. It is usual to place round or half-round wrought wires in these acrylic

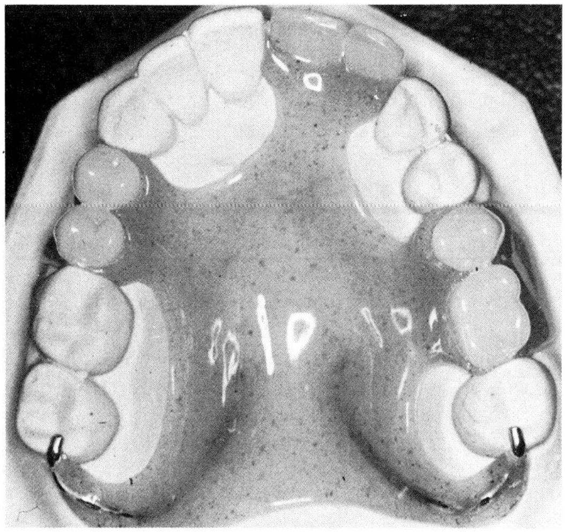

Figure 22.32 Design 4. Every design (see text)

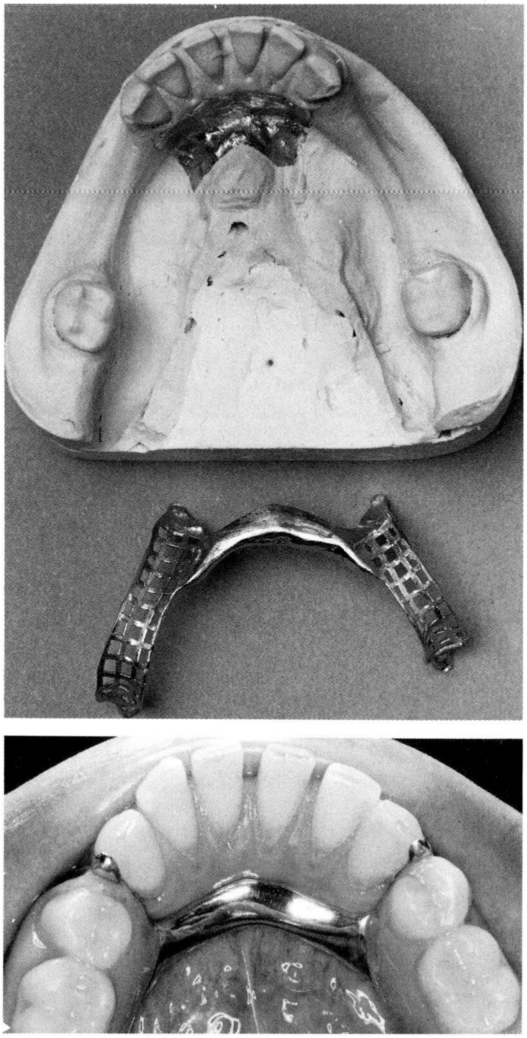

Figure 22.33 Design 5. Sublingual bar (see text)

extensions as these are more permanent than acrylic. In some cases the wire is extended on to the occlusal surface of each tooth, as in Figure 22.32, partly to support the posterior part of the denture and partly to provide indirect retention for possible dislodgement of the anterior saddle.

It is important to make a point contact between the saddle and the abutment tooth just above the survey line as this is not only more self-cleansing but also tends to spread some occlusal load on the saddle in a mesiodistal direction rather than a lateral direction which would occur if the contact area was too wide. The contact is best developed by using porcelain teeth in the denture because these do not wear so readily as acrylic teeth or denture base acrylic. The acrylic should leave each saddle on the palatal aspect at right angles to the curve of the gingival margin, thus providing a self-cleansing area rather than an acute angled food trap. A shallow dam is cut on the cast surface around the intended perimeter of the palatal connector. This ensures an intimate fit between denture and mucosa and, when the denture is fitted, the edge should be lightly chamfered to make the palate/denture junction as imperceptible as possible. For the same reason, the palate should be very thin.

If the technical work is of a high standard, and the oral hygiene is good, an Every denture is often very successful but, because it is basically mucosa-borne, there are limitations in the clenched load and damaging effects on the mucosa, gingivae and underlying alveolar bone.

Design 5

The sublingual bar (Figure 22.33) is an improvement on the orthodox lingual bar as it is less obtrusive to the patient because it lies in the anterior lingual sulcus. On the other hand, it is more difficult to make. It is another form of rigid major connector but, being situated in the sulcus, it has a different cross-section from a lingual bar which is essentially ovoid. The sublingual bar is more kidney-shaped in section but the final shape is particular to each patient. The impression is made with an individual tray whose lingual border is made rather broader than usual and carefully adapted with tracing stick with the tongue elevated forwards. The impression material is one of choice but experience shows that polysulphide rubber is most successful, although it has to be said that this type of impression material can behave with uncertainty in the wet floor of the mouth during setting. The master cast may be relieved in the lingual sulcus with 0.06 mm metal foil to supply a modicum of relief to avoid any trauma against the lingual tissues.

This bilateral bounded saddle case has rest seats prepared on distal canines and mesial second molars which have been prepared with full veneer gold alloy crowns. The molars were previously mesially tilted (a common finding with isolated posterior teeth) and the crowns have been made with mesial guiding surfaces parallel with the distal surfaces of the canines.

Note the use of broad denturc tccth in this case as, in general, patients prefer teeth approximately the same buccolingual size as natural teeth. The similarity in width feels more natural.

Design 6

The dimple hinge (Figure 22.34) is a stress-breaking design that incorporates a movable joint rather than flexible connectors. The joint is made up in the

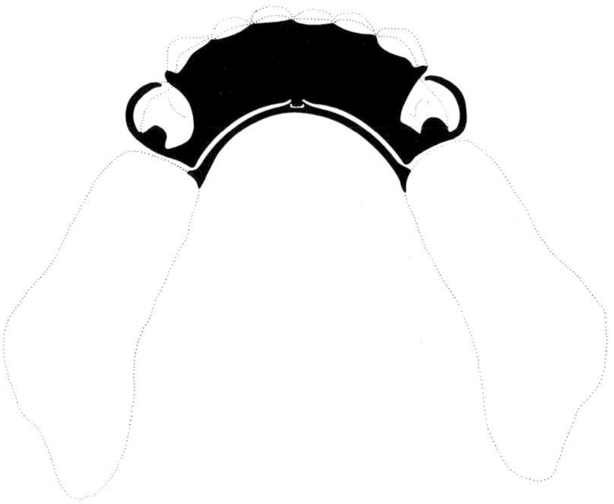

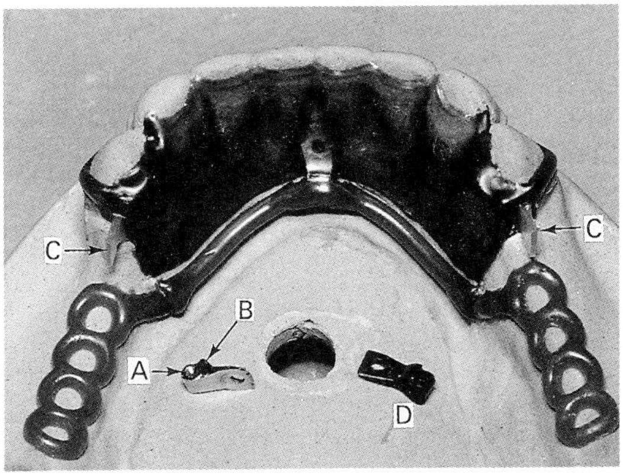

Figure 22.34 Design 6. Dimple hinge wax pattern on refractory model showing: (*a*) semi-circular dimple in pre-cast part of the hinge attachment; (*b*) ridge or stop to prevent upward movement of lingual bar; (*c*)vertical fins to resist lateral movement of saddles; (*d*) wax pattern of pre-cast part of the hinge attachment (shown for illustration only)

dental laboratory. The denture has a rigid transverse axis so that when one side is loaded the other saddle is also depressed into the mucosa, provided the anterior tooth-borne part is adequately retained. Another advantage is that the location of the hinge at the lower edge of the tooth-borne component and in front of the fulcrum axis means that load is spread between mucosa and anterior natural teeth. This distribution of load, and the absence of any tugging effect on abutment teeth, are reasons why this design is very comfortable for patients.

The centre part of the dimple hinge is precast. The melting range of the alloy used should be higher than that used to cast the dentures to which they are attached. This attachment is cheap and not difficult to make in the dental laboratory by using profile wax or a plastic sprue of 2 mm diameter and approximately 2.5 mm long. With a no. 4 round bur a semicircular dimple is cut into both ends ensuring that they are diametrically opposed. A piece of 0.5 mm sheet casting wax is attached to form a tag and blue inlay wax added to form a ridge or stop. This will prevent any upward movement of the saddles in the eventual denture. When completed, this wax pattern is carefully sprued, invested and cast to provide an alloy master hinge. A mould can be made from this and any number of hinges produced from it in wax. These can be cast in batches and kept until required.

Design 7

The disjunct design (Figure 22.35) is one in which the tooth-borne part and the mucosa-borne part are completely disjoined or separated so that loads on the free-end saddles do not place unfavourable loads on the remaining natural teeth. In other words, it is ideal in those cases where the periodontal prognosis of the remaining teeth is not good. An additional benefit is the resistance to lateral movement offered by the stiff buccal bars and so it is a useful design where the saddle areas are flat and atrophic. The design demands good retention of the anterior component to provide indirect support when the saddles are loaded but, in spite of the obtrusive retainers, and the apparent complexity of the denture as a whole, disjunct dentures are extremely comfortable. In cases where they are not comfortable the explanation usually lies in careless technology. Other features that should be noted are:

1. The skirt of alloy to protect the distal gingival tissues of the abutment teeth.
2. The pin at the end of the buccal bar lies midway along the length of the saddle to act as a fulcrum.
3. The slot to receive the pin is lined with stainless steel tape to prevent wear.
4. The denture is easily disassembled by the patient for cleaning.

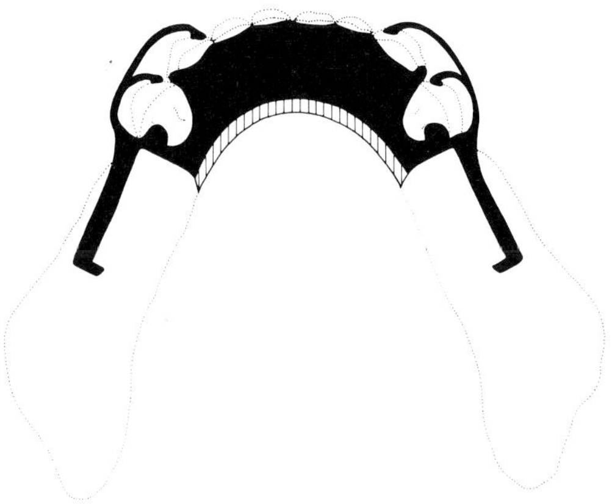

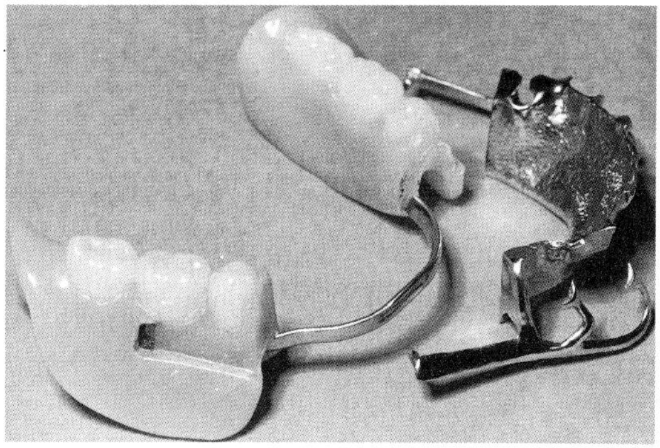

Figure 22.35 Design 7. Disjunct denture (see text)

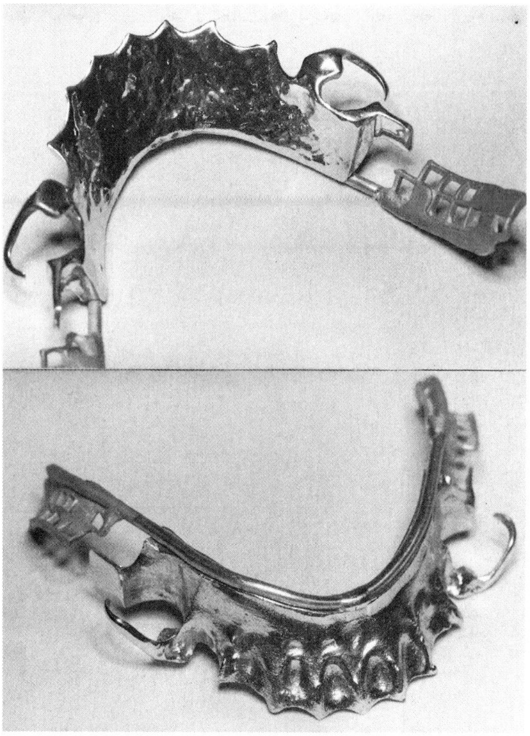

Figure 22.36 Design 8. Cast cobalt–chromium framework with wrought wire stress-breaker soldered in midline (see text)

5. The anterior part must be tooth-supported otherwise the remaining teeth and gingivae will be seriously damaged.
6. Good oral hygiene of the denture and tissues is essential.

Design 8

Flexible connectors (see Figures 22.25 and 22.26) are used in partial dentures in order to relieve the abutment teeth of harmful loads or to separate the load as evenly as possible between the mucosa and the remaining natural teeth. This is the basis of so-called stress-breaking, but many of these designs are unsuccessful and the one shown in Figure 22.36 would not work as a stress-breaking denture because the clasps do not prevent the rotation of the denture through the fulcrum axis when the saddles are loaded. This denture, therefore, acts in the same way as a rigid design. The weakness of this design is that the anterior part of the lingual plate is not firmly retained and so moves when the saddles are loaded. The only way the flexible connectors can act as stress-breakers is if the anterior lingual plate is firmly retained. This is the basis of the concept of indirect support and many so-called stress-breaking dentures fail to utilize this. The vertical fins at the distal ends of the anterior tooth-borne lingual plate are designed to resist lateral movement of the free-end saddles because with flexible connectors lateral movement is a considerable problem, particularly when the ridges are atrophic. Undoubtedly this denture yields readily to loads in the mouth and in that sense is more comfortable than a rigid design but it is no less harmful. If stress-breaking is desired in a situation like this then other designs such as the disjunct or dimple hinge should be considered.

Design 9

A lingual plate (sometimes called a strap or apron) is a major connector often used with bilateral free-end (distal extension) saddles. The simplest is where acrylic is used (Figure 22.37). The saddles cover a wide area to reduce the load per unit area and zero-cusp teeth are used to reduce occlusal trauma. The denture is retained with wrought wire clasps on the first premolars and these clasps also prevent distal movement of the denture. The denture is entirely mucosa-borne and, while the

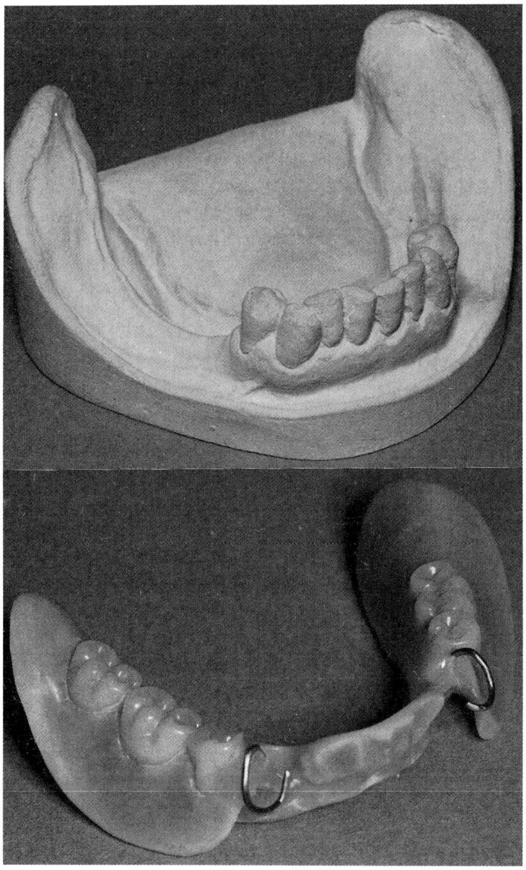

Figure 22.37 Design 9. Acrylic denture for bilateral free-end saddles (see text)

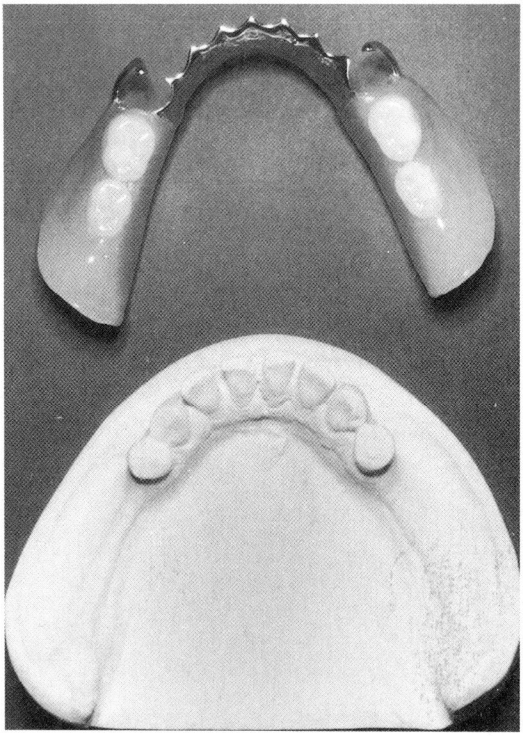

Figure 22.38 Design 9 (see text)

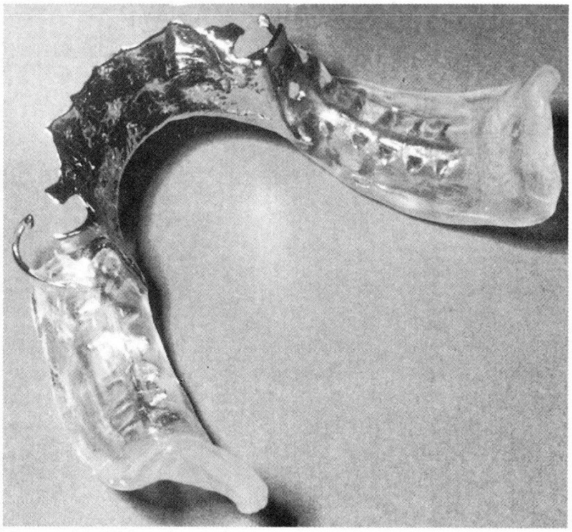

Figure 22.39 Design 9 (see text). Cast cobalt–chromium framework with temporary acrylic saddles added for an altered cast technique with impression wax

acrylic lingual plate lies against the lower anterior teeth, very little tooth support is derived from this source. This design is potentially damaging to the gingivae of the anterior teeth and especially to the distal gingival margins of $\overline{4 | 4}$. It also tends to sink out of occlusion as mucosal changes on the free-end saddle areas occur, followed by alveolar resorption. It is a very good transitional denture but its comfort in most cases masks its damaging features.

In Figure 22.38 a similar design is shown, the main differences being that the lingual plate and clasps are made of cast cobalt–chromium alloy. This is of little consequence in the overall support of the denture which is entirely mucosa-borne. The only benefits in using alloy are its greater transverse strength and its thinner bulk.

In Figure 22.39 an improvement has been incorporated as the mesial rests on the first premolars provide valuable tooth support. Any tendency for the distal part of the saddles to rise will result in a fulcrum action across a line joining these occlusal rests but the movement will be resisted by the lingual plate acting as an indirect retainer against the lower incisors.

The rigidity of lingual plates offers much resistance to lateral movement of the saddles, a common problem in any free-end saddle situation, particularly when there is marked atrophy of the supporting tissues.

Design 10

Lingual bars are another form of rigid major connector and can be used in a number of different situations in mandibular partial dentures.

In Figure 22.40 indirect retention is supplied by the extension from the midline contacting lower central incisors and the main advantage is that the gingival margins are free of coverage. Reciprocation to the distal-facing occlusally-approaching clasps is supplied by a plate extension of the lingual bar as it runs up to the combined occlusal rest on distal canine and mesial premolar. The axis of rotation is through the occlusal rests. Increased retention could be obtained by clasps on the molars but these would add complications to the denture and make it less acceptable to the patient.

In Figure 22.41 a wrought bar is used as a rigid connector between mucosa-borne saddles, a conventional design of limited use. The problem with this design is lack of indirect retention and little resistance to the pivoting movement in the mouth. Even when the clasps are added to engage $\overline{5 | 4}$ the denture is essentially uncomfortable and limited in function. Its main virtue is the freedom it offers to the gingival margins. Important features of the saddles in such a case are posterior coverage, buccal extension, narrow teeth and a lingual shelf of sufficient length distal to the last molar to allow control by the tongue.

Figures 22.42 shows other uses for rigid lingual bars, e.g. as part of two stress-broken designs for free-end saddles similar in principle to Design 8. In one, the bar is joined by minor flexible connectors to the clasps but because the clasps face distally this design would behave as a rigid design. The indirect retainer prevents upward movement of the free-end saddles. Lack of coverage of lingual gingival margins is a good feature. In another, the design is improved as the mesial facing clasps provide some indirect support for the free-end saddles as the tooth-borne

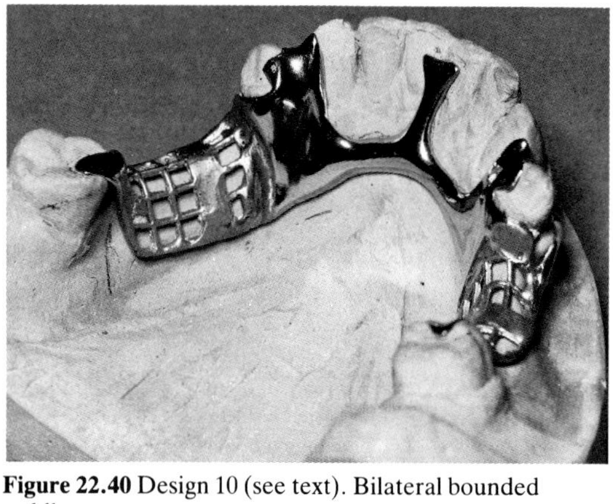

Figure 22.40 Design 10 (see text). Bilateral bounded saddles

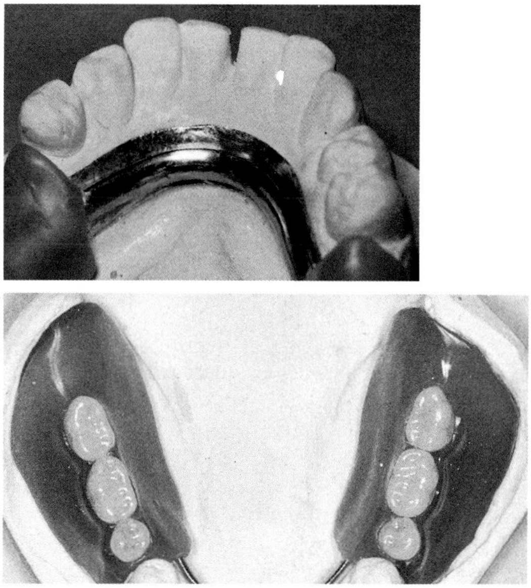

Figure 22.41 Design 10 (see text). Lingual bar in mandibular bilateral free-end saddles. Note the metal foil protection of the cast surface during fabrication of the wrought stainless steel bar

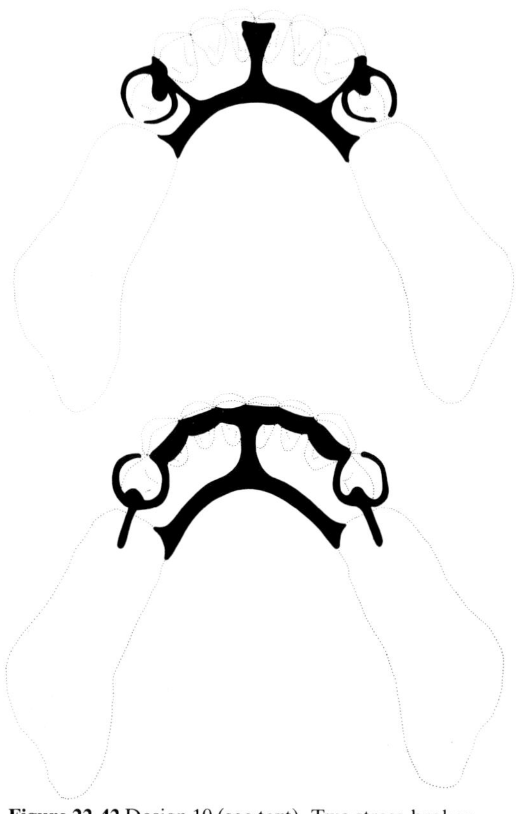

Figure 22.42 Design 10 (see text). Two stress-broken designs

element tends to rise on load being applied to the denture. The continuous clasp (or dental bar) provides connection between the clasps and indirect retention. The vertical fins provide lateral bracing for the saddles, a particularly useful addition when the saddles are long and the ridges are flat and atrophic (see Design 8).

Design 11

It often happens when an incisor is lost that the resulting gap reduces in size by movement of the adjacent teeth. If a partial denture is made it is usually impossible to use a replacement tooth of the correct size. In the case of a maxillary central incisor it is very important that the space is adequate to receive a tooth the same width as its natural counterpart, particularly at the level of the gingival papilla.

A useful design is a temporary partial denture which incorporates finger springs to move the adjacent teeth to an acceptable position. In Figure 22.43 the acrylic overlay design has an Adams clasp on 6/, an Adams clasp with accessory arrowhead on /5 6 and finger springs with double guide on 21/. Such an appliance has a rapid action and the more permanent denture with the correct size /1 acts as a retainer to prevent relapse of the space.

Obviously many other designs may be used as orthodontic appliances as part of the prosthodontic programme of treatment.

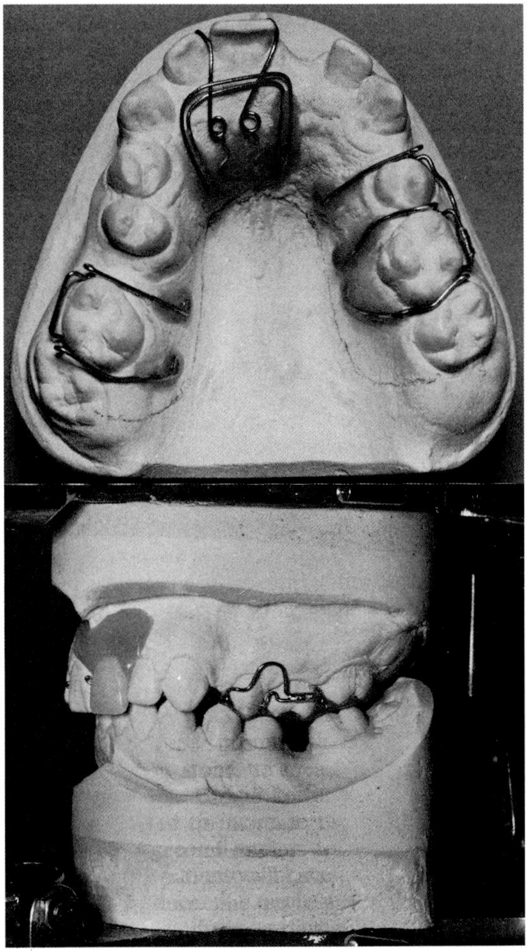

Figure 22.43 Design 11 (see text). Note use of wide flange around /1 to ensure replacement of lost tissue

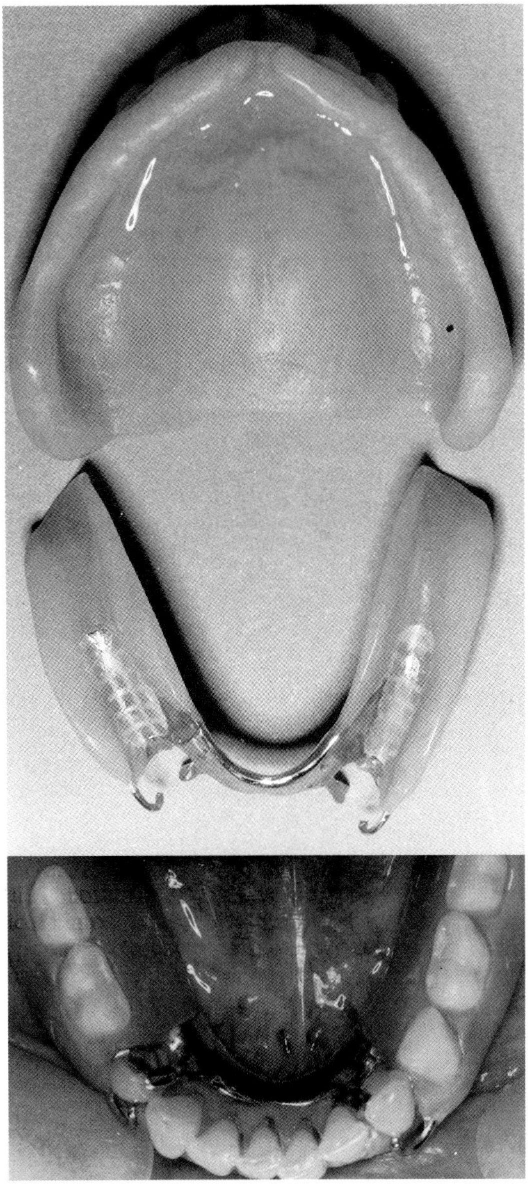

Figure 22.44 Design 12. The RPI design (see text). The major connector is a sublingual bar

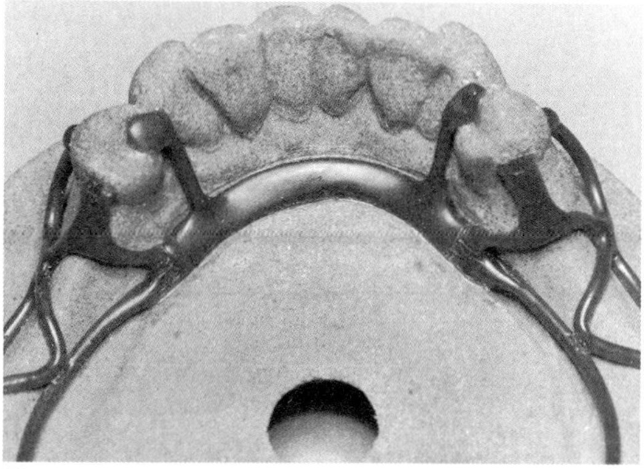

Figure 22.45 Design 12. The RPI design. Wax pattern on refractory investment model

Design 12

The RPI system is a method of clasping used in free-end saddle dentures (Figures 22.44 and 22.45). The clasps are designed to avoid damage to the abutment teeth.

Vertical force on the distal base causes the I-bar to move mesiogingivally away from the tooth while the plate at the back of the abutment teeth moves further into the undercut. In this way both the I-bar and plate disengage the tooth and thus reduce the torquing effect on the abutment. Distal load produces rotation which occurs round a fulcrum line passing through the mesial rests. The location of the minor connector running up to the occlusal rest, the proximal plate and the I-bar should provide for more than 180° encirclement.

One of the features of the I-bar is that it is less conspicuous than many other types of clasp and provides good retention due to its 'tripping' action if the denture tends to rise. In addition, there is minimum contact between the clasp and tooth and thus less potential damage to the enamel through caries. There is also minimal interference with the gingival margin.

There is some danger from the minor connector running up to the occlusal rest as it may place undue force on the mesial aspect of the abutment tooth when load is applied to the distal extension base because, of course, the design is essentially rigid. For this reason the contact surface of the minor connector should be painted with disclosing wax or pressure-indicating paste when the alloy base is first checked in the mouth. Any areas of 'wipe-off' can be eased, leaving the occlusal rest as the only contact on that part of the tooth.

This design is a rigid one but takes into account the fact that the compressible saddle mucosa means denture base movement but such movement is not harmful to the abutment teeth. The RPI denture is usually combined with an altered cast technique to equilibrate as far as possible the differences between mucosa and periodontium when these tissues are subject to load. R = rest on mesial fossa; P = plate on prepared distal surface; I = I-bar, a gingivally-approaching clasp shaped like a lower-case i.

Chapter 23

Partial dentures in relation to the treatment of the mouth as a whole

Treatment planning

In order to coordinate the treatment of a patient requiring a partial denture it is advisable to formulate a plan which may be used as a routine at the initial examination.

1. History
   (a) Previous partial denture experience:
      (i) satisfactory.
      (ii) unsatisfactory.
      (iii) none.
   (b) What are the patient's reasons for requesting a denture?
      (i) for restoration of appearance.
      (ii) for improvement in mastication.
      (iii) old denture now ill-fitting or broken.
2. Clinical examination
   (a) Condition of remaining natural teeth:
      (i) carious.
      (ii) periodontally involved.
   (b) Condition of mucosa.
   (c) Type of ridge in the edentulous areas.
   (d) Occlusion of the natural teeth.
3. Radiographic examination
   (a) For caries undiscovered at the clinical examination.
   (b) For the condition of the bone surrounding the natural teeth and that of the saddle areas.
   (c) For unerupted teeth, retained roots or any evidence of pathology.
4. Study casts

Examination of patient

There are many factors presented by each individual patient which may influence partial denture design:

1. Health and attitude of the patient.
2. Condition of remaining natural teeth and periodontal tissues.
3. Number of remaining natural teeth.
4. Distribution in the arch of remaining natural teeth.
5. Probable life of remaining natural teeth.
6. Distribution and extent of edentulous areas.
7. Condition of mucosa, especially over edentulous areas.
8. Form of edentulous areas.
9. Relation of opposing arches.
10. Nature of existing occlusion.
11. Position of occlusal plane.
12. Appearance, especially the extent to which teeth and gingivae show during function.
13. Shape and contours of remaining natural teeth.
14. Long axis inclination of abutment teeth in relation to other teeth in the same arch.
15. Occlusal surface morphology of natural teeth.
16. Extent of intermaxillary space at the accepted occlusal face height.
17. Clarity of speech and speaking space.
18. Support available for partial dentures.
19. Economic factors.
20. Materials and technical facilities available.

These factors are assessed by clinical and radiographic examination and then in more detail on study casts mounted on an articulator.

The remaining natural teeth

Included in the initial examination of the patient a decision may have to be made about restoration or extraction of teeth prior to partial denture treatment. The following list (not necessarily in order of importance) should be considered when making a treatment plan:

1. Lack of oral hygiene.
2. Gross caries.
3. Multiple fillings or crowns beyond normal restorative treatment.
4. Reduced crown height: tooth surface loss affecting crown form.
5. Reduced crown height with pain or sensitivity.
6. Recent or old fracture of teeth.
7. Failed endodontics.
8. Apical lesion or pathology.
9. Root resorption: crown/root ratio.
10. Superficial or deep periodontal disease.
11. Narrow attached mucosa: extraction may lead to reduced sulcus depth and problems around the periphery of a denture.
12. Tight lower lip: similar result as 11.
13. Fremitus of some or all teeth.
14. Mobility of some or all teeth.
15. Pain or discomfort on percussion of teeth or palpation of mucosa.
16. Proclination of teeth.
17. Over-eruption of teeth.
18. Retroinclination of teeth.
19. Over-eruption of canines.

(16–19: position may prevent development of a balanced occlusion against a complete denture in the opposing jaw.)

20. Atrophy of alveolus of free-end saddle area.
21. Atrophy or age change of mucosa in edentulous area.
22. Obtuse angle between horizontal and vertical ramus means lack of posterior stop.
23. Non-existence of pear-shaped pad produces lack of posterior stop.
24. Sharp mylohyoid ridges: support problem in lower denture.
25. Patient never worn any denture: avoiding extraction will allow a transitional partial denture to be made.
26. Facial deformity, e.g. cleft, post-surgical defect, traumatic injury, gross malocclusion, etc., leading to prosthetic difficulty.
27. General medical state, e.g. parkinsonism, bulbar palsy, epilepsy, etc., leading to general prosthetic difficulty.
28. Age and/or physical condition of patient.
29. Inability or unwillingness by clinician to make a denture of the correct design because of, for example, cost or lack of adequate technical services.
30. Attitude of patient.

History

This information is extremely useful. A patient not wearing a denture may have had one previously but discarded it because it was painful, moved during mastication or was a general source of annoyance (Figures 23.1 and 23.2). An examination of such a denture, if available, may lead to the discovery of a basic error of design or construction or, by questioning the patient further, some aspect of the design which the patient found irritating, thus providing the dentist with valuable information when designing the new denture. For example, on the basis of this information, the retention of the new denture may be increased or its support improved to overcome movement during mastication and speech, or the position or shape of connectors may be changed to overcome irritation to the tongue.

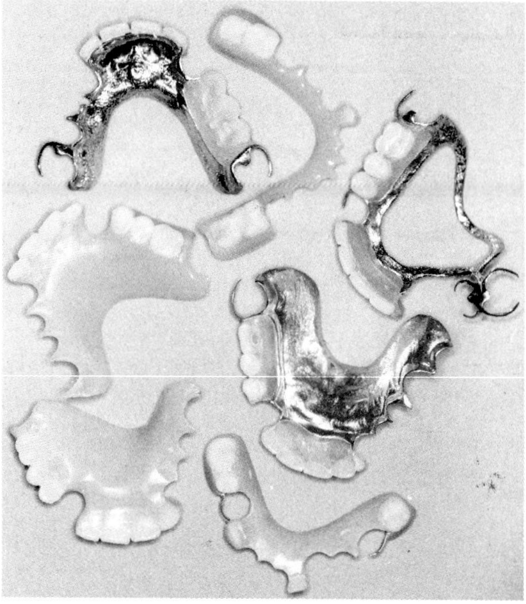

Figure 23.1 Collection of dentures, none of which was comfortable, produced by a patient at the time of examination (see Figure 23.2)

The reasons why a patient requests a denture may be an inability to chew food adequately or to the fact that lost anterior teeth have spoilt his appearance and speech. Information on these points provides the dentist with knowledge of the aspect of the denture with which the patient is most concerned and therefore how criticism may develop once the denture is fitted. Treatment and denture design can then be planned accordingly.

Clinical examination

The delivery of partial dentures should be the last stage in a course of treatment designed to render a person dentally fit. It may appear obvious and therefore unnecessary to stress that all extractions, fillings and periodontal treatment should be completed prior to making partial dentures. Such pre-prosthetic treatment must be coordinated as a

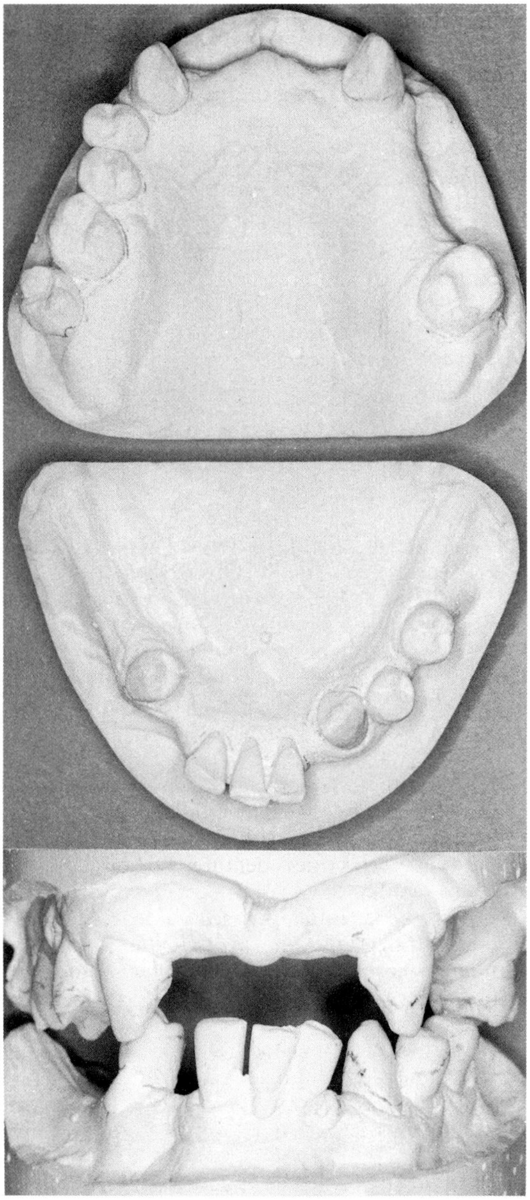

Figure 23.2 Casts of patient who presented with collection of dentures (shown in Figure 23.1). Note the malpositioned teeth and the gingival state

plan and not performed as isolated operations. The consideration of the need for a denture, therefore, should not be left to the end of the treatment but should be planned at the patient's first visit so that the mouth may be suitably prepared.

At the initial examination carious teeth are noted and a decision made regarding their restoration or extraction. It is irresponsible to plan treatment, design a partial denture, discuss the case with the patient and then be faced with the extraction of a tooth at a later date and the possible need to re-design the denture. Teeth which require treatment may require a particular type of restoration to match the denture design, e.g. a gold inlay or a full veneer crown, and for this reason the restorative treatment and denture design must be coordinated. Details of the gingival and periodontal condition are recorded so that this information is at hand during the study of the radiographs.

The mucosa is examined and any areas of inflammation or colour alteration noted. Assessment of the health of the mucosa is based largely on its colour and texture. Redness is a sign of reaction to irritation which may be mechanical, chemical, bacterial or systemic, but whatever the cause it should receive attention before the tissue is covered by a denture. Although redness is the commonest change in colour to be noted, whitish patches or localized areas are frequently seen, and the cause of any variation from the normal colour must be diagnosed and, if necessary, treated. The texture is assessed by palpation and the ideal is an even thickness of firm mucosa neither thin nor pendulous and lubricated by a normal flow of saliva.

The form of the edentulous ridge should be noted, as in edentulous patients, as hard and well-shaped, knife-edged or flat. This information when considered in conjunction with radiographs will enable an assessment to be made of the load which the saddle areas may be expected to withstand and the denture design related to it.

The functional depth of the sulci should be examined. A clinical estimation of their depth is important since study casts poured from impressions taken in stock trays may produce an inaccurate picture of the true depth of the sulci because of over- or under-extension of the stock tray. This may result in an inaccurate design of the dentures on the study casts, the error only being discoverd when the working casts, poured from functionally trimmed impressions, are to hand.

The teeth in occlusion should be observed as part of the examination and any teeth which are considerably over-erupted noted for possible extraction. In cases with a deep vertical overlap and pronounced upper incisors, the lower teeth may be in contact with the palatal mucosa (Figure 23.3). Such cases may require modification of the incisors to create space so that a partial denture may be fitted later. This may consist of a very thin stainless steel or cobalt–chromium base on the denture if the lower incisors are not quite in contact with the mucosa of the palate. If they are in contact then the attachment of the teeth to the denture may have to be by a buccal bar approaching from the buccal side and not from the palate. In certain cases the vertical dimension (occlusal face height) may have to be increased by an overlay denture.

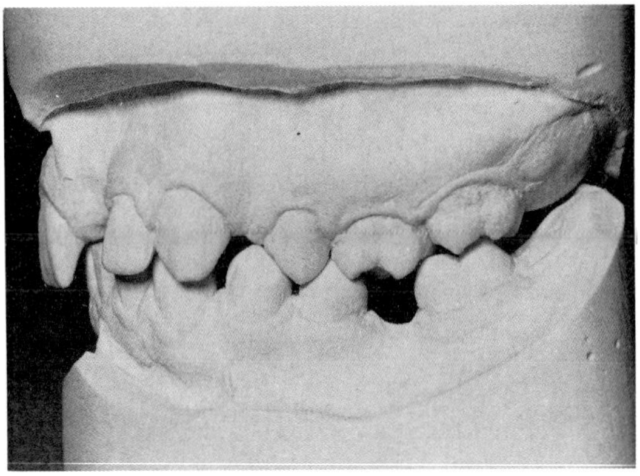

Figure 23.3 Study casts showing deep vertical overlap (see text)

The teeth should also be examined when sliding from a retruded position to lateral occlusion. If good tooth contact is maintained on the working side with disclusion on the non-working side during these excursions the dentures should be made to follow this occlusal design. This will require the use of an adjustable articulator and a face-bow mounting so that the denture teeth may be set in balance with the natural teeth.

In many instances, however, only a limited occlusion occurs in lateral movements before posterior tooth contact is lost because of the deep anterior vertical overlap which may cover half or more of the labial surface of the lower incisors so that when the anterior teeth are brought into edge-to-edge contact the posterior teeth are completely out of occlusion. Dentures in these cases are unlikely to result in cuspal interference posteriorly and can therefore be made on a more simple articulator, any slight cuspal interference being reduced by the careful use of marking paper and stones. Obviously such deep overlaps cannot be eliminated by modifying the natural anterior teeth to bring the posterior teeth into contact without drastic loss of tooth substance. Such a course is not justified.

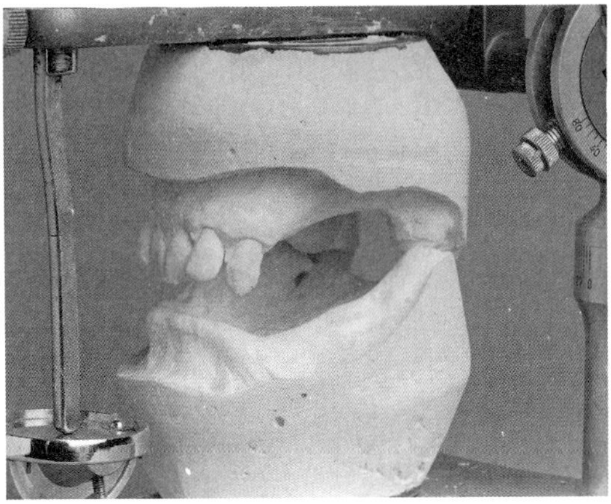

Figure 23.4 Study casts mounted on articulator show the lack of inter-ridge space because of the very prominent left tuberosity. When this was surgically reduced satisfactory dentures were made

Factors likely to unstabilize a partial denture are noted so that the denture design may be developed and planned to overcome them. Such factors may be jaw relationship, disparity in the relative size of the maxilla to the mandible, tongue size, frenal attachments, abutment tooth size and position, edentulous ridge atrophy, and similar findings (Figure 23.4).

Radiographic examination

Bite-wing films are desirable for the diagnosis of caries either interstitially or under existing fillings and full mouth radiographs may be required in order to estimate the extent of alveolar changes associated with any existing periodontal lesions. The condition and extent of the bone surrounding the natural teeth will give an indication of the probable load to which a given tooth may be subjected without rapid deterioration of its supporting structures. In a similar way, the radiographic appearance of the bone structure in the saddle areas may indicate the likelihood of changes occurring in the bone when a clenched load is applied through a denture. Poorly formed bone will obviously not withstand the same load by a denture that would be tolerated by dense, well-formed bone with a good trabecular pattern.

This information, coupled with that of the history and clinical examination and used in conjunction with study casts, gives the clinician a sound basis on which to plan the denture design.

Study casts

These are casts of the mouth poured from hydrocolloid impressions and mounted on an articulator either by using the interdigitation of the teeth as a guide to occlusion, or by using a wax record made at the same time as the impressions. A wax record is taken by placing a D-shaped piece of base-plate wax on the occlusal surfaces of the maxillary teeth and inducing the patient to close the teeth on the wax, care being taken to see that the teeth are in occlusion. It is then chilled and removed.

Examination of study casts

The casts are examined in occlusion and the following points observed.

1. Over-erupted teeth (see Figure 18.4). The presence of such teeth may make a partial denture difficult or impossible and consideration must be given either to the extraction of the offending tooth or teeth if the over-eruption is gross, or modification of the occlusal surface if it is only slight.
2. The closeness of the occlusion. In the incisor region the lower teeth may occlude either with the palatal mucosa or be so close to it that not more than 1 mm space exists. In such cases it must be decided whether the vertical height has closed and should be restored as part of the treatment or whether a thin metal base or other technique should be used in the denture design.
3. Close interdigitation of the teeth. If partial dentures are to be tooth-borne, rests will have to fit selected natural teeth. Rests take up space and those teeth which are to carry them frequently require either preparing or restoring to provide this space. In addition, part of the tooth which opposes the occlusal rest may have to be ground. The study casts will show if space for rests exists or where tooth preparation will be required.

The casts are then examined separately and the dentures tentatively designed on paper. As this is done the value of any isolated tooth may be assessed and a decision reached whether such a tooth will assist in the support, bracing or retention of the denture or make its construction less satisfactory and thus might be better extracted. Teeth which show exaggerated inclinations, and which would make the insertion of a denture difficult, should at the same time be noted and an estimation made regarding the value to be gained by retaining such a tooth. If there is no advantage in retaining the tooth then it may be best to extract it.

The following cases illustrate how study casts are used.

Patient A (Figure 23.5)

/5 was over-erupted and almost in contact with the lower free-end mucosa but it was decided to retain the tooth and modify it to serve as an intermediate abutment in a saddle bounded by a lateral incisor and a third molar, both teeth with relatively small periodontal areas.

/45 were sound premolars but the amalgam restorations were old and had rounded, worn contours. New restorations were planned with appropriate rest seats.

87/ was lingually inclined with a deep mesial undercut. Retention of this tooth avoided a free-end saddle and so it was prepared for a full veneer crown with a mesial surface parallel to 47/ distal surface to provide favourable guide planes. It also had a mesial rest seat and an undercut to receive a buccal retainer.

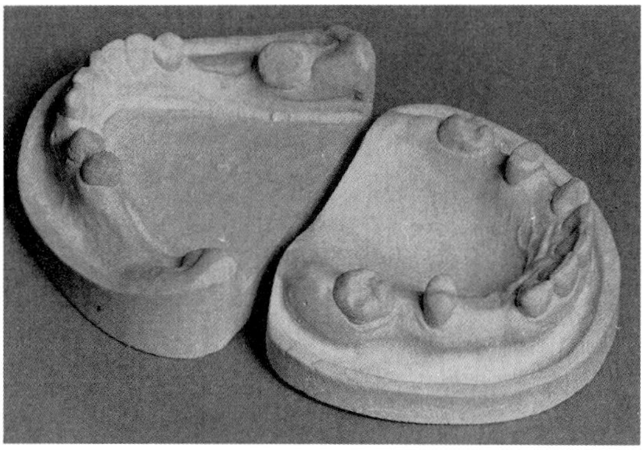

Figure 23.5 Patient A. Study casts (see text)

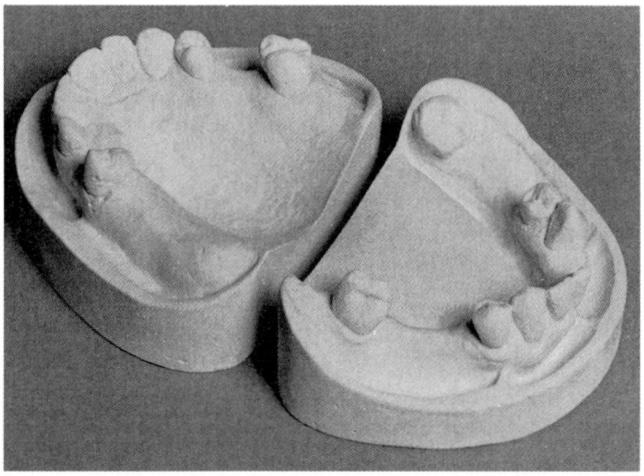

Figure 23.6 Patient B. Study casts (see text)

Patient B (Figure 23.6)

/8 was over-erupted and not in occlusion with any mandibular tooth; radiograph showed mesial bone loss. Taking into account that the right quadrant was a free-end saddle it was decided to extract this tooth, thus simplifying the design of the upper denture.

87/ had a marked mesial undercut and 47/ a distal undercut. These had the effect of reducing the size of the saddle that could be inserted and so increasing the food traps. Both teeth were prepared with restorations to provide parallel guide surfaces for better retention and rest seats for tooth support.

Patient C (Figure 23.7)

This patient was wearing a mucosa-borne upper acrylic denture. The standard of hygiene was excellent and the health of the tissues good. 77/ was almost in contact with the opposing maxillary free-end mucosa. /58 were inclined to produce contrary undercuts thus effectively reducing the size of the saddle. Because of the favourable supporting tissue it was decided to restore the lower arch by bridges on 757/ and /358; the upper arch was

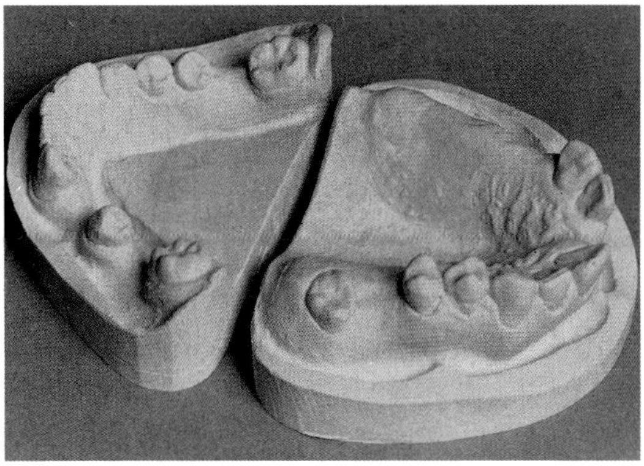

Figure 23.7 Patient C. Study casts (see text)

restored by a partial denture with tooth-support on 3 2 / 1 5 8 and mucosa-support on the right free-end saddle area.

These three cases illustrate some of the points that may be considered with study casts. In actual practice the casts would be mounted on an articulator so that the occlusal relations could be examined. It should also be noted that the casts are neatly prepared and as accurate as possible. It is less than satisfactory to make study casts deficient in detail and carelessly trimmed.

Damage produced by partial dentures

Caries

Predisposing causes:

1. Lack of oral hygiene in patients wearing partial dentures.
2. Faulty denture design; dentures which cover large areas of tooth surface or have food retentive areas which are difficult to clean increase the caries risk, or damage the periodontal tissues.

Preventive measures:

1. Instructing the patient in general oral hygiene especially with regard to cleaning the denture; he should be told to rinse his mouth and wash his denture after every meal; he should be taught how to clean the insides of clasps and those parts of the denture which fit round the teeth by using a small test-tube brush or an interspace toothbrush.
2. Partial dentures should be designed so that they cover as little tooth surface as possible and are completely free from rough, food-retentive areas; the fit must also be extremely accurate.

Periodontal damage

In partial denture cases more teeth are probably lost through destruction of the periodontium and surrounding alveolar bone than by caries.

There are, of course, a number of local and general causes of periodontal disease but, in partial denture cases, we find two kinds of lesion. These occur in different ways but may be present together in the same patient.

Superficial lesion

This starts as a marginal gingivitis and is due to trauma of the gingival margins by food impaction, clasp arms or the denture edge. It may progress to destruction of the periodontium. Marginal gingivitis, however, is always present from the start and is related to the area of trauma.

Deep lesion

This starts as destruction of the periodontal membrane or resorption of the alveolar bone. It is caused by excessive vertical, lateral or torsional loads on the natural teeth or residual alveolar ridges. The first symptom may be pain or looseness of the teeth and there is often little sign of inflammation at the gingival margin.

Mucosal damage

Damage to the mucosa will result from:

1. Excessive load caused by:
   (a) Inadequate extension of saddle area.
   (b) Unequal distribution of load.
   (c) Lack of relief, e.g. torus palati.
   (d) Occlusal trauma.
   (e) Excessive denture base movement, as in mucosa-borne dentures.
2. Lack of oral hygiene.
3. Laboratory faults, e.g. rough cast surface, edge of relief area, careless postdam preparation and unpolished edges.

Appearance

The general principles of dental and facial restoration which apply to complete dentures apply also to partial dentures but the presence of natural teeth for comparison often demands more exacting standards. The aim should be to restore the lost tissues with an artificial replacement which matches the form, colour and texture as exactly as possible.

When a single tooth is lost a change of the adjacent interdental papillae occurs as well as a loss of alveolar bone. These losses cannot be replaced by simply 'gum-fitting' a tooth in the space. It is necessary to restore the lost gingival contour with carefully matched acrylic which has been shaped and stippled to imitate the papillae. The acrylic flange should be translucent and should taper to a knife edge at its margins which lie on the attached alveolar

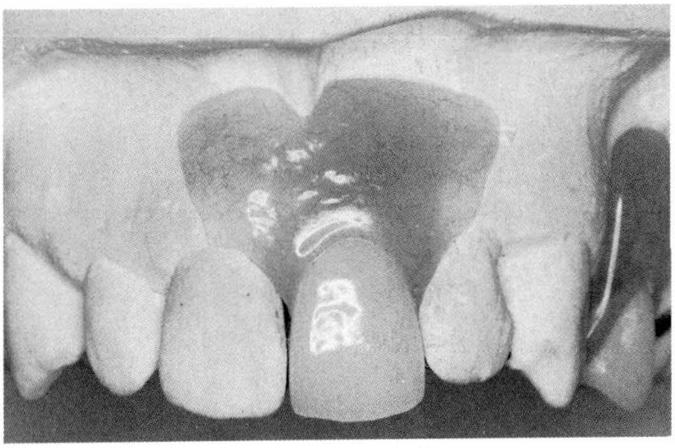

Figure 23.8 Replacement of maxillary central incisor and lost mucosal contour with wide labial flange

mucosa (Figure 23.8). Stippling can be done with a fine offset round bur rubbed lightly in small circles over the acrylic which is then lightly polished.

When fitting a denture with an acrylic flange wide enough to restore the interdental papillae, difficulty will be encountered unless a path of insertion has been chosen which eliminates the undercuts on the labial sides of the anterior teeth. This is done by tilting the cast on the surveying table until the marking edge can touch the labial gingivae without touching any other part of the anterior teeth (Figure 23.9).

In the selection and placement of the teeth themselves the following points should be noted.

Size

The upper central incisor is about one-and-a-half times the breadth of the lower central incisor. This proportion should always be kept in mind and small centrals should not be used. Even if a space appears to be too small it is possible in most cases to fit correctly sized central incisors by setting them further forward and overlapping them slightly.

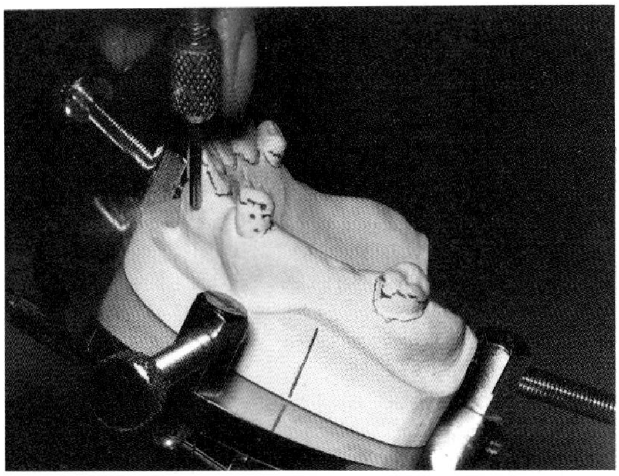

Figure 23.9 Tilting of cast until the vertical rod touches the labial gingivae when planning a path of insertion

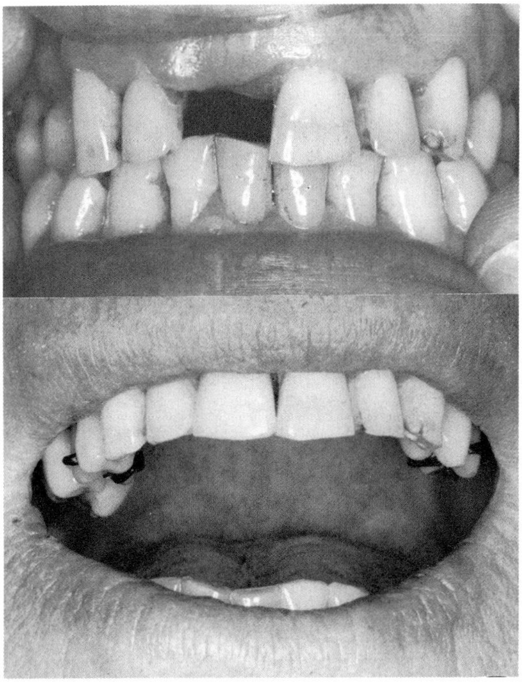

Figure 23.10 Restoration of right maxillary central incisor. Note the simulation of the enamel hypoplasia and trimmed incisal edge on the denture tooth

If a central incisor is missing on one side only, its artificial replacement should always be the same size as the natural tooth. If the space has closed it is usually possible to get the same breadth of tooth in by rotating it but, if not, orthodontic treatment should be started to gain space (see Figure 22.43). Nothing makes a denture look more artificial than artificial teeth which are smaller than their natural counterparts. A very important measurement is the width of the tooth at the horizontal level of the gingival papillae, and many artificial teeth are too narrow at this point (Figure 23.10).

Shape

Manufacturers tend to concentrate too much attention on the outline form of the teeth, but it is just as important to select teeth which have the correct three-dimensional form. It is common to see artificial teeth which have a correct outline but incorrect body contour which highlights their artificiality. Many moulds are too flat and it is sometimes necessary to select a larger tooth so that it provides enough bulk to allow shaping to the correct contour.

Texture

The texture of artificial teeth should be carefully matched with that of the adjacent natural ones.

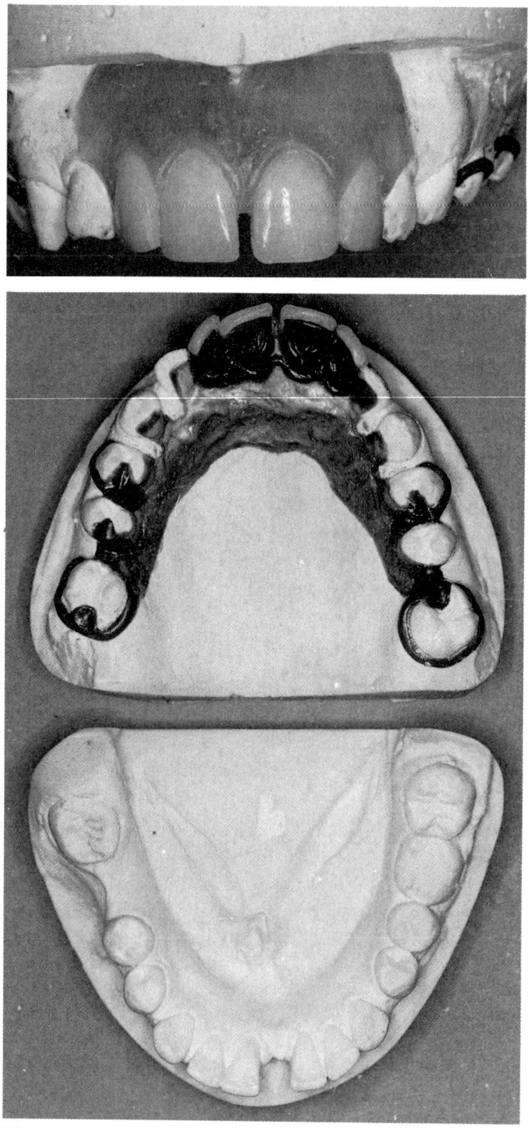

Figure 23.11 Tooth-borne RPD replacing maxillary incisors with median diastema. The incisors have been set in the pre-extraction position and a wide flange is used to replace lost tissue

Correct surface texture is as important as shade. A tooth of the correct texture but the wrong shade tends to look more natural than one with the correct shade but the wrong texture.

Position

The guides to tooth position applicable to complete dentures should be used when positioning anterior teeth on partial dentures. As a rule, owing to loss of alveolar bone, it is necessary to set the teeth anterior

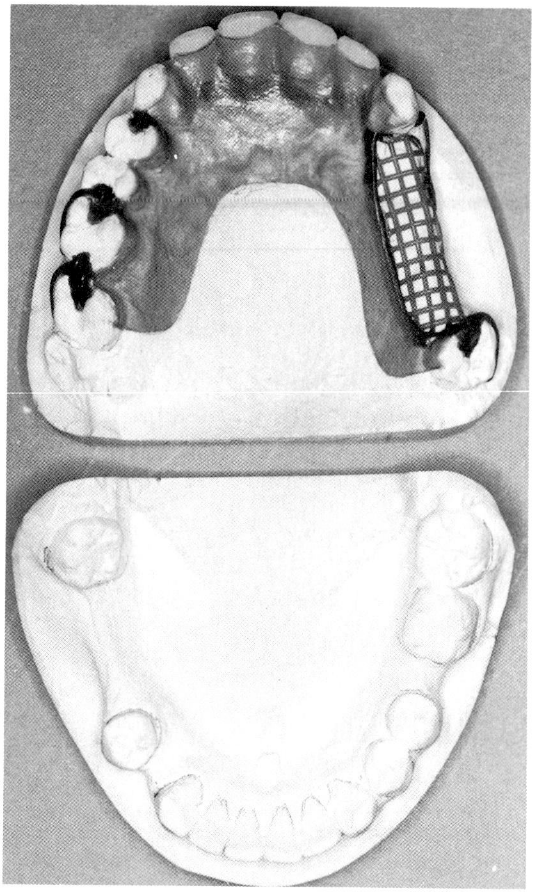

Figure 23.12 Tooth-borne RPD showing incisors of the correct size forming an arc with the teeth in the pre-extraction position

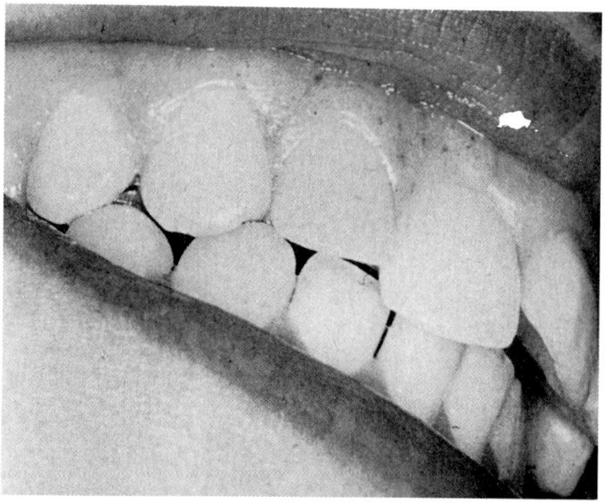

Figure 23.13 Partial denture replacing maxillary right lateral incisor with wide acrylic flange to replace lost tissue. The final appearance in this case is spoilt by use of mottled acrylic

to the alveolar ridge (Figure 23.11). 'Gum-fitting' is never justified except possibly in a few single-tooth restorations and, where two or more anterior teeth are missing and alveolar resorption has taken place, it is impossible to obtain the best effect if the teeth are fitted to the mucosa. In most cases like this it is also impossible to fit teeth of the correct size if they are fitted to the mucosa because the arc which the natural teeth formerly occupied is much wider than that of the residual alveolar ridge (Figure 23.12).

Shade

Because the tendency is to select too light a tooth it is always better to start at the dark end of the shade guide. The teeth should be viewed from several angles and with a different incidence of light before the final decision is made. More natural effects can be obtained as in complete dentures by mixing sets of different teeth rather than by using the teeth from one manufactured shade.

Denture acrylic

The colour of the mucosa should be matched against discs of different mixtures of acrylic at the same time as the tooth shade is selected. There are many different types of pink, clear, mottled and veined acrylics which can be mixed together in different proportions to produce almost any shade one is likely to require for patients (Figure 23.13). Additional shades can be added for the coloured races.

Chapter 24

Impressions for partial dentures

All the materials commonly used for making impressions and their methods of preparation have been fully described in the section on complete dentures. It is only intended therefore to describe here the essential points in their application to the making of partial impressions.

Trays for partial impressions

The type of tray required for an impression will vary in relation to the number of natural teeth. If the majority of natural teeth are present, a stock or standard box tray may be used (Figure 24.1) and in some cases no master impression in an individual tray will be required. If extensive edentulous spaces exist, a preliminary impression in a stock tray will be required to produce a cast on which an individual tray may be made for the final working impression. The reason for this difference is that dentures replacing a few isolated teeth will not be carried deeply into the sulci and therefore an accurate impression of the functional depth of this region is unimportant. Where large edentulous spaces exist, however, the denture will be carried into the sulci and the only means of obtaining an accurate impression of them in their functional position is by using an individual tray (Figures 24.2 and 24.3).

Adapting a stock tray

Mouths containing both extensive edentulous areas and a group of natural teeth are frequently encountered. In such cases a partially edentulous tray is useful but a box tray may be successfully adapted to fit the mouth and thus allow an accurate impression of the functional sulci bounding the edentulous area to be made. The tray is adapted by filling that part of it which will cover the edentulous area with softened impression compound and then

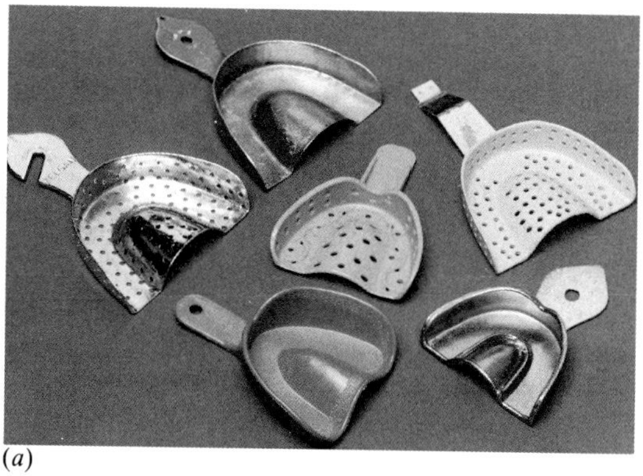

(*a*)

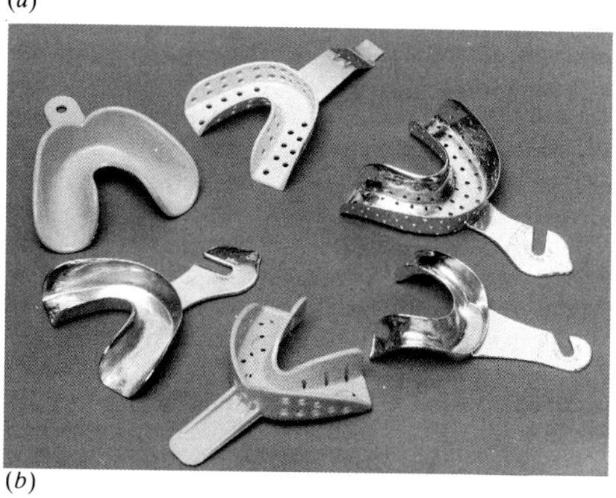

(*b*)

Figure 24.1 (*a*) Maxillary and (*b*) mandibular box trays for recording impressions of patients with natural teeth present

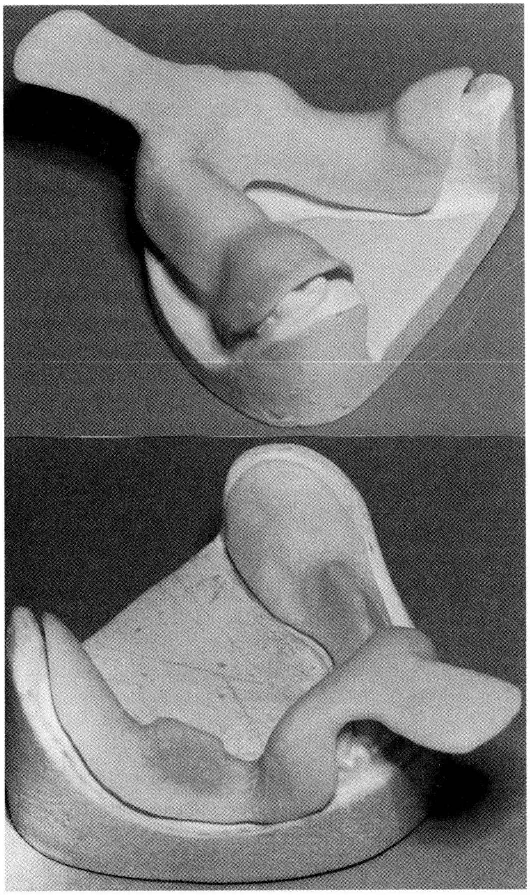

Figure 24.2 Cold-cure acrylic individual trays for partially edentulous arch. In some cases the labial flange is cut away in the region of the standing teeth to avoid distortion of the sulcus in the anterior part of the saddle area. Note the addition of finger stands in the lower photograph

inserting the tray; when the tray is in place the cheek is manipulated so as to trim the compound in the sulcus. The tray is removed and the compound impression of the edentulous ridge widened and deepened slightly with the finger to allow room for the material to be used for the final impression.

The problem of producing an accurate cast of a partially edentulous mouth is due to the fact that natural teeth are normally undercut and are composed of unyielding tissue. Many techniques have been evolved, employing many different materials, in attempts to gain accuracy but alginates and elastomers have generally superseded such techniques as the reversible hydrocolloid impression since alginates and elastomers are both accurate and straightforward to use, provided that the manufacturers' instructions are followed.

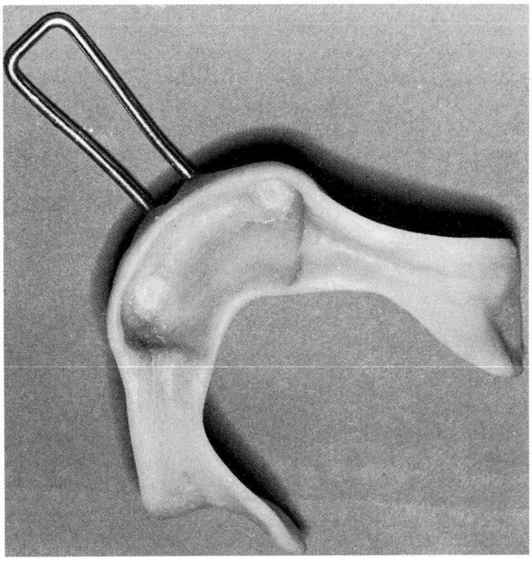

Figure 24.3 Lower acrylic individual tray for case with bilateral free-end saddles. A wire handle, emitting the mouth at the level of the oral commissure, is often preferred. Note the stops located over the canines to stabilize the tray during the setting of the impression material

Impression materials

Alginates

To produce an accurate impression of the hard and soft tissues of the mouth it is necessary that this material be used in a rigid type of tray which will not be distorted during the working period, particularly the moment of withdrawal from the mouth when considerable force is often employed. This is extremely important when a cast is required for the construction of a metal casting in which the slightest distortion in an impression becomes obvious when the casting is tried in the mouth. For such an impression a rigid tray is essential, made either as an individual tray in cold-cure or heat-cure acrylic or a standard metal box tray adapted with impression compound. In the latter case it is desirable when taking an upper impression to postdam the tray with compound and insert the tray so that this compound is first seated in close contact with the tissues; this will prevent the impression material escaping posteriorly, which is desirable both from the point of view of the comfort of the patient and also because a mass of alginate unsupported by the tray will tend to pull away from the palate and distort the impression material further forward.

An individual tray made in thermoplastic shellac or thermoformed polymer may be used satisfactorily where extensive saddle areas are present requiring the denture periphery to be placed accurately at the functional level of the various sulci, since extensive saddles indicate only a few natural teeth standing. These do not usually restrict the easy removal of such an impression and therefore there is less chance of distorting the impression tray.

Alginate should be placed with the finger in those areas of the mouth where it is anticipated that air may be trapped prior to the insertion of the filled tray to avoid small bubbles and surface deficiencies which may otherwise occur in the impression. Such areas are the palatal vault and the occlusal pits and fissures of the natural teeth.

Only those areas of the mouth required for the construction of the denture should be included in the master impression because alginate distorts easily, and to make an impression with a large excess of material with wide and deep peripheral over-extensions is both undesirable and unnecessary, and is also very unpleasant for the patient.

Inaccuracy of alginate impressions

Inaccuracy can be caused in the following ways:

1. Failure to follow closely the manufacturers' instructions with regard to mixing.
2. Inadequate preparation of the tray. It is necessary to use impression compound on the upper tray to prevent alginate from falling away from the palate in the postdam region. Spray adhesive is necessary to ensure adherence of the impression material to the tray and left long enough to reach maximum adhesiveness. It is also very important to spray on the buccal and lingual aspects of the tray since if the alginate tears away from the tray at any point a major inaccuracy will result.
3. Alginate in contact with mucosa sets first, that in contact with teeth next, followed by the material nearest the tray. Varying pressure on the tray and movement during gelation of the alginate in the mouth causes a build up of stresses within the material during setting and when the impression is removed the release of strain causes distortion.
4. Presence of plaque on teeth, especially near the gingival margin, will affect the setting and sharpness of the alginate gel and therefore teeth should be polished before impressions are made.
5. Faulty removal of the impression. Alginate impressions should be removed with a quick pull after the peripheral seal has been released. The impression should never be eased slowly out of the mouth since alginate is much less resistant to a force slowly applied than to one applied rapidly and is apt to tear and distort on slow removal. Sudden displacement ensures the best elastic behaviour.
6. Isolated teeth tend to resist removal of the set alginate, particularly as they are often tilted lingually or mesially. The alginate therefore becomes displaced from the tray without being noticed. This tooth on the resultant cast lies below the correct occlusal plane so that when the denture is inserted it stands off the tooth although it fits perfectly on the anterior teeth. This problem can be solved by selecting a path of withdrawal of the impression.
7. Failure to pour the impression as soon as it has been made. Alginate impressions rapidly lose water and shrink. The amount of shrinkage is reduced if they are kept in an atmosphere of 100% humidity but a certain amount of distortion is still apt to take place. It is therefore wise to pour them immediately but if this is not possible they should be wrapped in a piece of damp gauze and poured within 15 minutes.
8. Careless handling and pouring of the impression. Alginate impressions should never be laid on a bench since the heels of the impressions will be distorted by the weight of the impression. They should be propped or hung up so that the weight is taken by the tray itself. This sort of distortion, and distortion caused by forcing the impression down into a thick mix of stone during pouring, are perhaps the commonest causes of major inaccuracies.

Elastomers

These materials, polysulphides (thiokol rubber, mercaptan rubber or rubber-base materials) and silicones (siloxane polymer or silicone rubber), have already been referred to in Chapter 5 for use as impression materials for edentulous patients. Two types of silicone rubber material are available: condensation-curing and addition-curing, the latter being the type more useful for partial denture impressions.

A fourth elastomer, polyether impression rubber, is occasionally used but it has a number of drawbacks. It is very stiff when polymerized which makes withdrawal from the mouth rather hazardous if undercuts are deep or divergent or if one or two teeth are slightly mobile. This stiffness is also a problem in the laboratory when the impression has to be separated from the set stone cast as teeth may be fractured. After the impression has been made it must be kept dry as the dimensional stability is affected by moisture. The material absorbs water and swells.

Polysulphides are used in rigid individual trays and either medium-bodied or light-bodied varieties are best. Heavy-bodied are too viscous. Rubber adhesive is applied to the tray, ahead of mixing equal ropes of base and activator, in order to derive maximum adhesion between tray and impression material. Polysulphides, like all elastomers, are hydrophobic so that faults and deficiencies may occur in areas where there is moisture. In the large expanse of the partially edentulous mouth there are bound to be areas where moisture lies, for example around gingival margins, even if the mouth is dried before inserting the impression tray. The problem is that the material may slump away from wet areas without the fault being recognized on removal from the mouth. In spite of that drawback, however, many clinicians prefer the dimensional accuracy of elastomers which is more reliable than that of alginates.

When using addition-cured silicones the best method is to mix the wash and syringe it around the teeth, add the putty to the tray, seat it in the mouth and allow the two materials to set in the mouth.

With condensation-curing silicones the putty is added to the tray, seated in the mouth and allowed to set. The tray is removed, putty cut away from undercuts, newly-mixed wash added to the putty and the whole re-seated to allow the wash to set. An alternative is to place a spacer of thin polythene over the teeth before the putty is seated and, before the putty has set, the tray is rocked to ensure enough space between the putty and teeth. A wash is then applied to complete the impression.

All elastomeric materials have good elasticity and adequate tear strength and are ideal for recording undercut areas although heavy-bodied materials may prevent easy withdrawal if undercuts are severe. The hydrophobic problem has already been mentioned.

Occasionally air may be trapped in elastomeric materials and in alginates in such a way that it is covered by a very thin skin of impression material. On inspection of the impression the fault is not noticed but when the impression is poured in the laboratory the dental stone, which is fairly viscous if mixed correctly, distorts and bulges the skin to produce rounded protuberances on the cast surface. These may appear to be anatomical oddities but, of course, they are impression faults.

Choice of impression material

When a relatively simple acrylic partial denture is planned, perhaps of a transitional or temporary nature, alginate in a stock tray, suitably modified with impression compound, is adequate. Any alginate of choice may be used, although some of these materials with a free-flowing, low viscosity have a poor tear strength and this may produce problems if undercuts are deep or if the tray does not fit the mouth with sufficient accuracy. One of the problems with using a stock or standard tray is that the impression compound modification takes up too much space and so the alginate, especially if it has a low viscosity, takes the form of a wash. In this form alginate is not accurate and also tends to tear away from the compound. Inaccuracy is bound to follow.

In more difficult partial dentures the choice lies between high viscosity alginates and any of the elastomers. Individual trays are usually recommended and these should be rigid. In very wet mouths alginate, because it is a hydrocolloid, is the material of choice as it is in mouths where there are severe undercuts and mobile teeth. If cost is a consideration then alginates are cheaper but this must be weighed against the cost of making the denture, particularly if it has a cast alloy base when extreme accuracy is important.

Compression impression

In certain cases it may be desirable to compress the mucosa of a free-end saddle area in order to equilibrate the reaction of the tissue in relation to the much less compressible periodontium of the natural teeth. Some clinicians prefer to do this at the master impression stage while others prefer to wait until the cast alloy framework has been made and then equilibrate the mucosa with impression wax on a temporary, close-fitting acrylic saddle after which a new cast is poured by the altered cast technique.

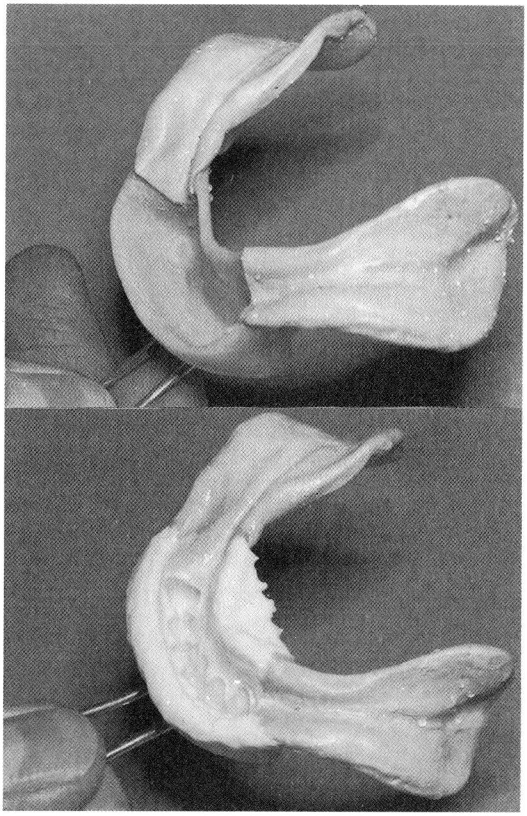

Figure 24.4 Compression impression technique with bilateral mandibular free-end saddles (see text)

Others prefer to wait until the finished partial denture has been in the mouth for a few weeks and then rebase the saddle in order to compress the mucosa under occlusal conditions.

Technique (Figure 24.4)

1. Place soft impression compound in the individual tray opposite the free-end saddle areas.
2. Insert and seat the tray with gentle pressure making sure that the tray does not contact the standing teeth.
3. Remove the tray and chill.
4. Trim away any compound which has flowed beyond the limits of the saddle areas.
5. Reinsert the tray with firm pressure on the saddle areas.
6. Remove the tray and ask the patient if he could feel the tray contacting the teeth when the pressure was applied. If he did feel a contact add more compound and repeat the procedure until no contact of tray and teeth is felt even on the application of very heavy pressure.
7. Apply adhesive to the empty portions of the tray i.e. opposite the standing teeth.
8. Make mixes of impression paste and alginate (or elastomer). Apply very little paste to the compound overlying the saddle areas, and alginate (or elastomer) to the rest of the tray.
9. Insert the tray and seat with heavy pressure on the saddle areas.
10. Maintain an even, heavy pressure until the impression materials set.
11. Remove the impression and pour it in dental stone.
12. Note that more compression can be obtained by omitting the impression paste wash. In such a case the impression compound must be used at the correct temperature to obtain good surface detail and chilled correctly in the mouth to reduce thermal contraction.

Oral health

Apart from obvious mouth preparations before partial dentures are made, such as periodontal treatment, extractions, elimination and treatment of caries, modification of abutments and stabilization of occlusion, master impressions should not be recorded until the mucosa is healthy. If the patient is wearing a partial denture and the mucosa is oedematous or inflamed, the state of the mucosa can be improved either by leaving the denture out for a few days, or by lining the partial denture with a tissue conditioner which is changed every seven days until the mucosa is improved. Tissue conditioners vary in their composition but in general they comprise polyethyl methacrylate powder and a liquid consisting of an aromatic ester (often butyl phthalyl butyl glycolate) and ethyl alcohol. These materials form a gel, the ethyl alcohol having great affinity for the polymer.

Casts

Although satisfactory study or preliminary casts may be made from plaster and some artificial stones, only a hard, accurate, dental stone, mixed under vacuum at the correct water–powder ratio, should be used for partial denture work, for two reasons:

1. All partial dentures have some contact with the natural teeth, as distinct from complete dentures which are only in contact with mucosa, and as the teeth are rigid, or at least must be treated as such, the greatest possible accuracy is required.
2. A considerable amount of technical work will have to be carried out on the cast, and unless the cast surface is hard, the resultant wear is bound to spoil the fit of the denture made on it.

Chapter 25

Occlusion in partially edentulous patients

Mandibular positions

When natural teeth are present in both arches it is important to determine whether the tooth position (intercuspal position) coincides with the retruded contact position (RCP) of the jaws. If there is a discrepancy, a decision must be made as to whether the occlusion should be adjusted. If so, the adjustments must be made before master impressions are taken. When there are opposing natural teeth with interceptive or deflective occlusal contacts, occlusal adjustment is usually indicated. When only a few teeth are to be replaced, adjustments are not usually necessary unless there is obvious periodontal damage or joint symptoms due to the occlusion.

In general, therefore, partial denture occlusion will conform to the tooth position (intercuspal position) of the patient. This means, in most cases, that tooth contact will occur in the intercuspal position (which may or may not coincide with RCP) and also in working occlusion; there will be no contact on the non-working (balancing) side. There should be no interruption to the movement from intercuspal to working positions. This is sometimes referred to as unilateral balance, segmental balance or group function and is an acceptable occlusion when restoring with partial dentures. In other cases the only contact in eccentric positions is on the upper and lower canines, the remaining teeth being disoccluded or discluded during these movements. This canine guidance or rise is also acceptable.

The danger of bilateral balance, such as we make in complete dentures, is that the constant load on saddles and abutment teeth might be detrimental to these tissues and contacts on the non-working side tends to produce harmful parafunctions and temporomandibular joint problems. Nevertheless, when a partial denture has to be made opposing a complete denture then bilateral balance is necessary otherwise the complete denture will be unsatisfactory. In many cases the partial denture may have to incorporate an overlay design in order to achieve a satisfactory balanced occlusion.

Recording retruded contact position

In recording RCP in the partially edentulous patient one should recognize that the patient may be in an unstable position or habitual occlusion. This can be eliminated by making an acrylic occlusal splint which the patient wears for a number of weeks. The splint is made for the maxillary arch and covers all posterior occlusal surfaces and, in most cases, the incisal edges of the incisors. The occlusal surface is flat except for canine guidances, has no indentations of the lower teeth and should be worn 24 h per day. The occlusal surface can be modified by grinding or adding cold-cure acrylic as the jaw position alters.

After a splint has been worn for some time the patient's jaw may be guided into RCP along the terminal hinge axis. A check record is made at a pre-contact position with a D-shaped softened wax wafer on the maxillary teeth. Only one record is usually necessary but the method is liable to error because of movement in the wax and difficulty of transferring the record to casts and articulator. It is best, therefore, to make another check record after the casts have been mounted to verify the accuracy of the relationship.

Natural teeth in occlusion

Frequently, the occlusion is sufficiently stable to enable the intercuspal position to be accurately determined by the interdigitation of the teeth when the casts are occluded.

If any doubt exists, however, as to the exact jaw relationship a wax record, adapted to the maxillary teeth, should be made and the casts mounted with it.

Large edentulous spaces

In cases presenting extensive edentulous areas the casts cannot be accurately related by the interdigitation of the natural teeth and so it is necessary to record the retruded contact position. Record blocks are made in a manner identical with that employed for edentulous cases, the only difference being that the rims are not continuous but merely fill the edentulous spaces. Sometimes it is only necessary to make a record block for one jaw if sufficient natural teeth exist in the opposing jaw. The relationship and interdigitation, if any, of the mandibular and maxillary teeth should be examined and noted before the record blocks are inserted in the mouth. In the majority of partial cases both the vertical and anteroposterior dimensions are indicated by the interdigitation of the remaining natural teeth. All that the dentist is required to do, therefore, is to trim the occlusal surfaces of the rims until they just fail to occlude when the natural teeth are fully in occlusion.

Localization grooves are then cut in the rims and a mix of registration paste or plaster placed on the surface of the lower rim. The record blocks are inserted in the mouth and the patient requested to close the teeth together. The dentist should watch carefully to ensure that the natural teeth are fully in occlusion and interdigitating. The blocks are then removed from the mouth, casts placed in them and the occlusion of the casts checked.

The firm occlusion and interdigitation of the natural teeth is emphasized because a very common source of trouble with partial dentures is that when they are finally delivered to the mouth they are found to hold the occlusion open from the natural teeth thus defeating one of the main purposes of partial denture treatment which is to restore the occlusion.

A contributory cause of this trouble is undoubtedly failure on the part of some technicians to pay sufficient attention to the elementary rules of flasking and packing acrylic, thereby altering the tooth/cast relationship. The main cause is usually traceable, however, to the fact that the casts were mounted with the natural teeth slightly out of occlusion.

It sometimes happens that when the record blocks are in the mouth and the natural teeth are in full occlusion, when the blocks are removed from the mouth and the casts located in them the teeth are slightly separated. The cause can be traced to the fact that the rims of the blocks were not trimmed so as to allow a small space to exist between the occlusal surfaces when the natural teeth were in full occlusion. This has resulted in compression of the soft tissues by the record blocks and compression of the resilient wax rims of the blocks, thus allowing the natural teeth to come into occlusion. When the record blocks are placed on the cast, however, the stone representing the soft tissues will not compress and consequently the natural teeth are held out of occlusion. Theoretically if partial dentures are set and finished to a record obtained under such circumstances the dentures should compress the soft tissues when the jaws are closed and allow the natural teeth to occlude; in practice, however, this is not borne out and if this error of recording is made, considerable occlusal errors result. This points to the resilient nature of some dental waxes and to the distortion of record blocks.

Tooth-borne dentures

Where a cast alloy base has been constructed for a tooth-borne partial denture it is advisable to check the jaw relations with wax rims attached to the base so that RCP is recorded under conditions similar to that occurring at the finished stage of the denture. It is easy to overlook faulty occlusion of the natural teeth due to premature contact against an occlusal rest or part of the cast alloy base.

Where the natural teeth do not occlude

In these cases the vertical and horizontal occlusal relations are assessed in the same way as if the patient were edentulous but determination of the occlusal plane, free-way space and speaking space are all made easier by the presence of the remaining natural teeth. The essential difference between partial and edentulous cases is in the adjustment of the incisal guidance table of the articulator. In partial cases the natural teeth provide the guidance (assuming anterior teeth are present) and the table should be set so as to allow these teeth to remain in occlusion when lateral and protrusive movements are made.

Trial stage

The main considerations at this stage are the verification of jaw relations, the testing of the stability and retention of the denture and the approval of the appearance by the patient.

The occlusion of the artificial and natural teeth is checked with mylar tape (shimstock) for evenness of pressure. It is important that the pressure is no heavier on the artificial teeth than it is on the natural teeth, the ideal being equal pressure on both. Clasps are assessed for their position and their relationship to the soft tissues, the gingival margins in the case of encircling clasps, the sulcus and attached mucosa in the case of projection clasps.

The artificial teeth are observed for mould and shade, and any alterations of position and angulation of such teeth carried out at the chairside to produce harmony with the natural teeth. Anterior teeth of a trial denture may be left very slightly longer than the neighbouring natural teeth in order to allow for any incisal adjustment to produce a more natural appearance of the anterior teeth in the finished denture.

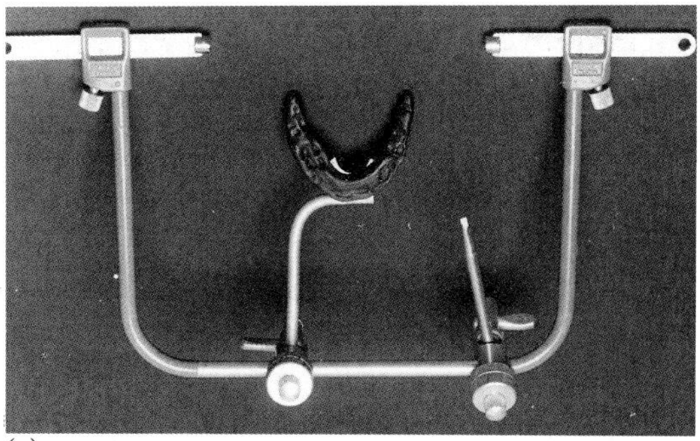

(*a*)

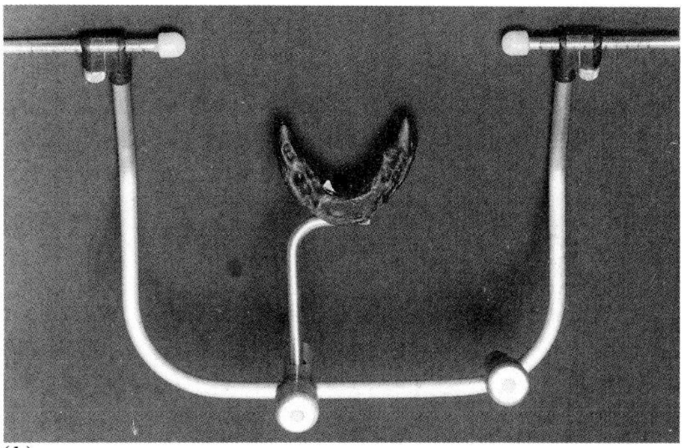

(*b*)

Figure 25.1 Mounting partially edentulous casts. Facebow assembly with compound indentations of maxillary teeth. (*a*) Condylar rods adjusted to landmarks on the lateral aspect of the face. (*b*) In this earpiece facebow the rods relate the terminal hinge axis to the external auditory meatus of the ears and is more stable on the patient's head. Note: the use of the orbital rod is optional

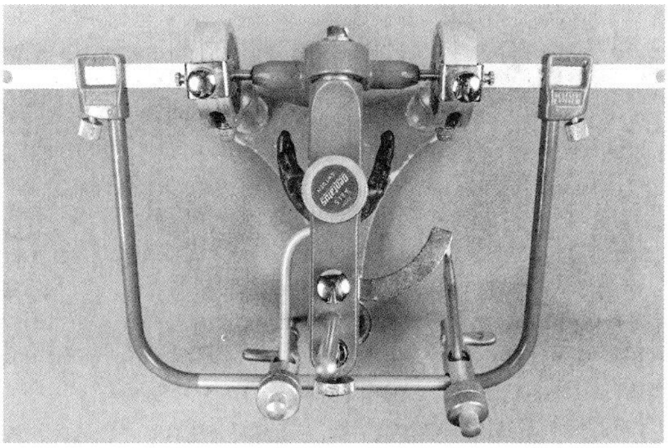

Figure 25.2 The facebow assembly located on the articulator. The readings on the condylar rods are adjusted to be the same on both sides to centre the assembly and the orbital rod contacts the orbital flag to adjust the angle of orientation of the maxillary occlusal plane to the Frankfort plane

Delivering partial dentures

If the cast has been accurately surveyed and the denture properly designed, the finished denture should fit the mouth easily and accurately. It is frequently discovered, however, especially when acrylic is the base material, that the denture binds slightly on the natural teeth and will not go fully into place. If the surveying and blocking out of undercuts has been carried out carefully, the commonest cause is that the teeth on the cast have been rubbed and worn during the fabrication of the denture. In order to insert such a denture the acrylic round the teeth must be eased slightly and to do this accurately careful observation is necessary. The denture should be coaxed into place as far as it will go easily. Use a mouth mirror to check where the denture is in contact with the natural teeth. Remove the denture from the mouth and ease the acrylic on the fitting surface, but not the polished surface or the final contact will be disturbed. This process must be repeated until the denture slips into place. Under no circumstances should the denture be forced because if this is done it will be found extremely difficult to remove.

If the exact area of hard resistance cannot be discovered by observation use disclosing wax or pressure-indicating paste on the surface of the denture against the suspect tooth and the denture inserted as far as it will go. On removal the wax or paste will be found to have been squeezed from the area of hard contact which may then be eased accurately.

It is emphasized that easing a partial denture into place requires care and patience because if material is removed from the wrong area, or an excessive amount of material removed, the fit of the denture may be ruined. Such easing should be unnecessary and is best avoided by a careful and exact technique at the chairside and in the laboratory.

Adjusting the occlusion

Inaccuracy in occlusion is an ever present problem in partial denture prosthetics. The causes of this may be of clinical or technical origin and all too frequently the technician is blamed for such an occurrence resulting from failure of the clinician to obtain the correct occlusion in the first place.

Clinical causes of errors

In cases where the edentulous areas are few and many natural teeth are present and the occlusion is stable, all that is usually required is to mount the casts in the intercuspal position on the articulator. It is important, however, to check the occlusion of the casts against the patient's intercuspal occlusion and to ensure that their relations are identical because it is possible to occlude the casts in a slightly incorrect position with disastrous results. In most cases, a moving-condyle articulator should be used, the upper cast mounted with a facebow and the lower cast related to the upper by means of a thin D-shaped wax record located on the maxillary teeth (Figures 25.1, 25.2 and 25.3).

Those cases requiring wax record blocks to register the position of occlusion are the ones in which clinical errors cause faults. The record blocks are trimmed until the upper and lower rims just occlude when the natural teeth are in occlusion; soft wax may then be interposed between the blocks and the patient instructed to close. What occurs then is one of two things. The clinician fails to check that the natural teeth are in occlusion. Often the anterior teeth are slightly out of occlusion, but this frequently escapes notice as it is masked by a deep vertical overlap when viewed from the front. Alternatively, the wax blocks compress and distort

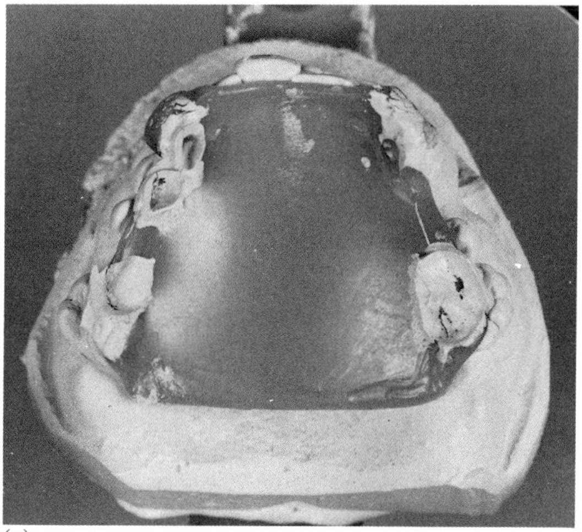

(*a*)

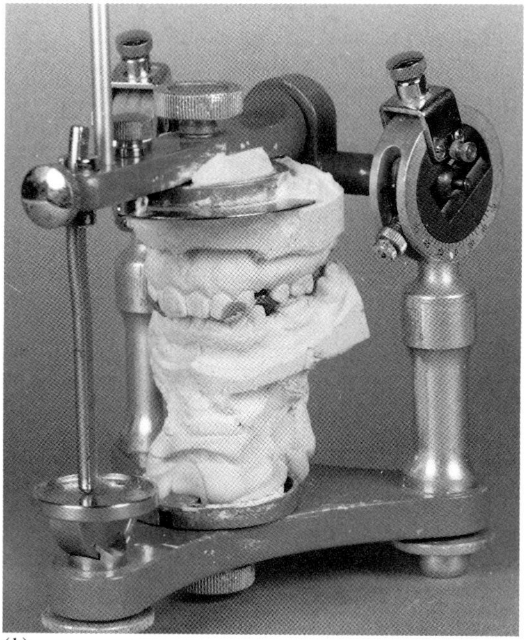

(*b*)

Figure 25.3 (*a*) A retruded contact position (RCP) record is made with a D-shaped wax wafer adapted to the maxillary teeth (the centre of the D is rigid and so the wafer does not distort). A quick-setting zinc oxide–eugenol (ZOE) completes the accuracy of the record. (*b*) The mandibular cast is mounted on the articulator against the record

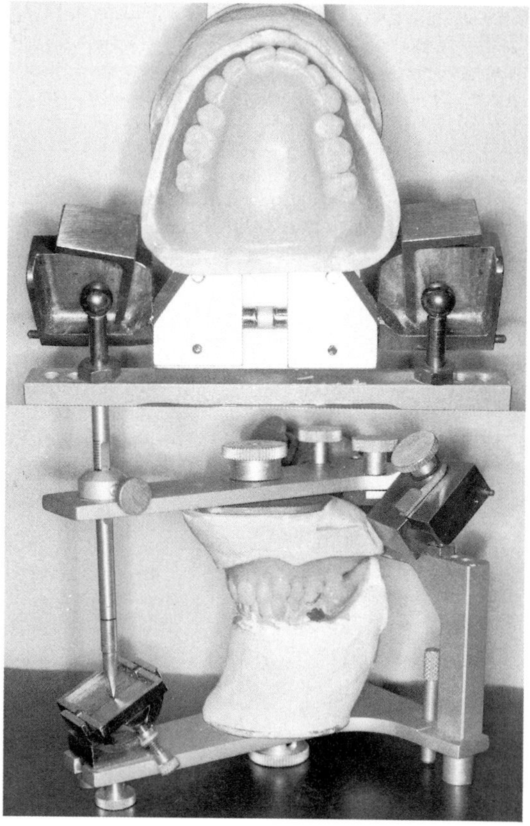

Figure 25.4 Remounting after deflasking is important to verify and correct the occlusion. Complete upper and partial lower denture on a semi-adjustable articulator

under the force of occlusion and then elastically recoil when the teeth are parted. In either case when the casts are located against the record blocks prior to mounting them, the teeth on the casts will be slightly out of occlusion and unless very careful comparison is made with the position of occlusion of the natural teeth the error passes unnoticed. Frequently this cause escapes notice at the trial stage because again the wax around the teeth will compress on occlusion. When the unyielding dentures are fitted, however, the error will become obvious and either a lot of occlusal grinding will have to be done or, alternatively, the patient will be instructed to wear the denture for a few days in the hope that they will 'settle'. If they do, it will be at the expense of the stable natural occlusion, the periodontium, the gingival margins and soft tissues. These are not uncommon causes of damage by removable partial dentures.

Technical causes of errors

The first of these is a continuation of the fault already mentioned, i.e. failure to occlude the casts so that they truly represent the occlusal relationship of the natural teeth. If the location of the casts is left to the technician such things as wax recoil, excess of wax, warping of wax and rubbing of plaster teeth may all contribute to this error, and it is strongly advised that the luting of casts should be made at the chairside by the clinician.

The second and very common technical error is the gradual introduction of occlusal faults as the denture teeth are set in position. Frequently in partial cases the vertical or interalveolar space for a tooth is limited. The tooth is ground, but not sufficiently, the articulator is closed and the opposing tooth rubbed. The vertical dimension is thus opened slightly. The posterior teeth are usually involved and if such a case is observed critically it will be seen that the anterior teeth are often more than a millimetre out of occlusion, but this is frequently masked by the vertical overlap. When such a case is tried in the mouth the elasticity of the wax and the normally slack fit of the trial bases often allow these errors to pass unnoticed and they only become apparent when the unyielding finished denture is being fitted.

Other causes of occlusal errors are processing faults:

1. Failure of the two halves of the flask to meet due to the extrusion of acrylic flash.
2. The denture teeth are driven into the investing plaster containing them, either as a result of excessive pressure applied through the acrylic, or due to weakness of the investment.
3. Errors in the method of flasking the particular case.
4. Failure to remount the case on the articulator after deflasking in order to refine the occlusion before removing the denture from its cast (Figure 25.4).

Chapter 26

Immediate dentures

Definition

A denture constructed before the extraction of the teeth which it replaces and fitted immediately after the teeth are extracted.

Advantages

1. The edentulous period is eliminated and this has a great social and psychological significance.
2. A very natural and functional result can be obtained as the lip position, occlusal plane, vertical height and occlusion can all be exactly reproduced, although the occlusion may be unstable because of a slight malocclusion and may require altering in the denture.
3. Function of mastication is maintained.
4. There is little interference with speech.
5. There is little interference with the temporomandibular joint and its function.
6. Facial contour and tone of facial muscles is maintained.
7. Change in tongue shape is prevented.
8. No unnatural mandibular movements will develop.
9. Little interference with diet.
10. Size, shape, shade and position of teeth can be accurately reproduced.
11. Resorption of alveolar bone is lessened due to maintenance of function.
12. Sockets are protected and healing is quickened.
13. Patients fear the edentulous state and immediate dentures will encourage them to lose 'diseased' teeth they might otherwise wish to retain.

Disadvantages

1. If the natural teeth are maloccluded then accurate reproduction is not possible otherwise a prosthetic malocclusion will result, e.g. deep vertical overlap, extreme rotation, tilting or migration.
2. Additional expense and time.
3. General health may not permit multiple extractions
4. Cannot be made for all types of patients as some are irresponsible and wear immediate dentures for excessively long periods and give rise to oral damage.
5. Gross oral sepsis and other pathology.

Main types

With anterior teeth socketed (open face design)

Advantages

1. Very natural appearance.
2. Easy to insert.
3. Exact reproduction of tooth position.
4. Easier to set teeth in laboratory.
5. No interference with lip musculature.

Disadvantages

1. Poor retention and inadequate support.
2. Natural appearance is not long maintained.
3. Denture has short life.
4. Slightly more difficult to rebase.
5. Irregularities of anterior ridge may develop (spiky alveolus, flabby mucosa) (Figure 26.1).
6. Sockets and gingivae must not be traumatized during surgery (Figure 26.2).

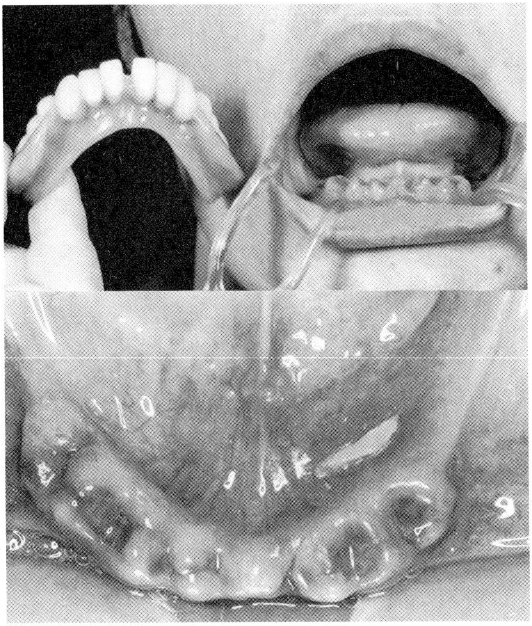

Figure 26.1 Mandibular immediate denture with anterior teeth socketed. This design should not be used as the supporting tissues are always damaged

Labial flange without alveolectomy

Advantages

1. Good retention and support.
2. Rapid healing with smooth ridges (Figure 26.3).
3. Ease of rebasing.
4. Stronger denture.

Disadvantages

1. Poor appearance owing to labial fullness.
2. Difficult in case of undercuts.
3. Lack of space around necks of teeth and so denture teeth are often shortened after final waxing and finishing

A variation of this type of immediate denture is where the anterior labial flange ends as a knife-edge between the gingival margin and the vestibular sulcus. It therefore blends with the surrounding mucosa, somewhere near the mucogingival junction, and eliminates the disadvantage of fullness as the lip position is not changed; if undercuts are present then the knife-edge of acrylic can finish at the crest of the convexity. This thin labial flange, however, is often very weak and the knife-edge may traumatize the mucosa.

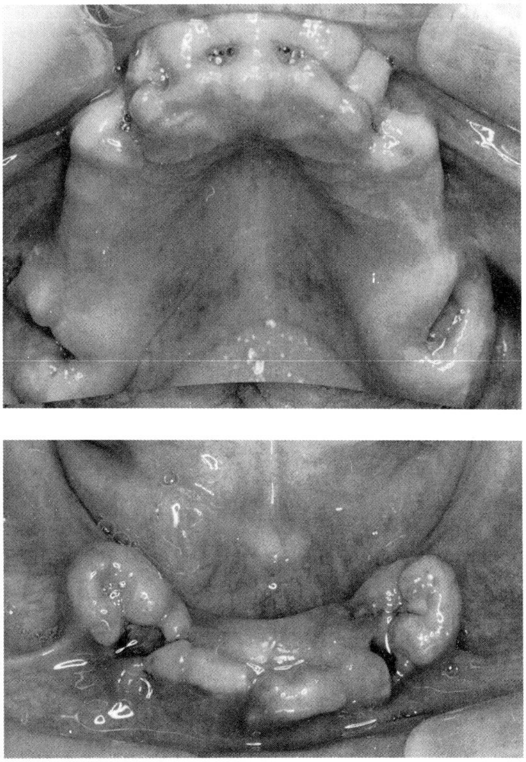

Figure 26.2 Immediate dentures. Examples of careless surgery and prosthetic technique. Preservation of soft tissues and alveolar bone is essential in immediate denture treatment

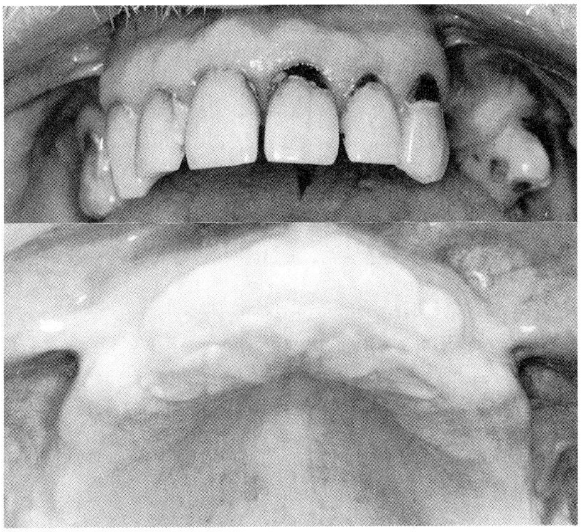

Figure 26.3 Complete upper and lower immediate dentures. View of upper denture-bearing area four weeks after careful forceps extraction without alveolectomy. Dentures made with labial flanges and occlusion carefully balanced

Labial flange with alveolectomy (excision)

Indications

1. Prominent pre-maxilla which (a) would prevent insertion of a flanged denture, and (b) would give a poor appearance if socketed teeth were used.
2. Limited anterior interalveolar space and deep vertical overlap.

Contraindications

1. Fairly severe surgical task.
2. Increase in resorption following labial cortical bone removal.

Labial flange with alveolotomy (incision)

A modification of the above where the operation of trans-septal alveolectomy or intraseptal alveolotomy is carried out. This consists of collapsing the anterior buccal plate by surgical means in order to eliminate the undercut.

Advantages

1. No cortical bone is removed and post-surgical resorption is reduced.
2. Surgery is less traumatic than alveolectomy.
3. Less interference with facial form.

Disadvantages

1. The undercut cannot always be completely eliminated.
2. Bone, even though it is mainly cancellous, is removed and, from the point of view of alveolar ridge preservation, that should always be avoided if possible.

Post-immediate or delayed immediate dentures

These can be used to replace posterior and anterior teeth at the same time and are useful where extensive bridges or implants have to be removed or where there is pathology such as a large cyst present.

In this seldom-used technique trial dentures are prepared on casts where the teeth have been cut off and the ridge smoothed. The teeth are then extracted and, after a day or two, the trial dentures are inserted in the mouth with a zinc oxide–eugenol (ZOE) paste or elastomeric wash and impressions made in the closed mouth position. The dentures are processed and fitted the same day.

This method is useful where many teeth have to be extracted in theatre and hospitalization is recommended.

A large amount of resorption may take place in the first few weeks, although this depends on the pre-extraction state and the type of surgery.

Immediate partial denture

Any of the above methods may be used in this service and the most obvious indication is for aesthetic reasons or space maintenance. Socketed dentures, with proper follow-up treatment, are commonly used prior to construction of a fixed bridge and also following injury and trauma.

Clinical procedure

Stages

1. The advantages and limitations of immediate dentures must be explained to the patient beforehand. The extra expense involved must be agreed and the possibility of rebase in a few months emphasized, together with the necessity for replacement dentures at a later period.
2. The teeth are scaled and cleaned and the oral hygiene brought up to a reasonable standard.
3. The posterior teeth are now extracted, having decided which teeth are to be retained as a guide to correct jaw relationship, i.e. usually the four first premolars, if these are present, but the incisors and canines may suffice if their contact coincides with a stable intercuspal occlusion at an acceptable occlusal face height. The extraction of the posterior teeth can be carried out under local or general anaesthesia. This is best done in a minimum of two visits, extracting only the posterior teeth on one side at each visit. At the time of extraction the interdental and interradicular alveolus is smoothed and toilet of the area completed by adequate suturing. This unilateral extracting and care of the part promotes healing, reduces the time of the partially edentulous period, and leads to better future denture support.
4. The patient is then dismissed.
5. The waiting period before recall varies. If there were edentulous areas already present, and the number of posterior teeth recently extracted is few, then about three weeks may be sufficient as the already existing edentulous areas will give good support to the immediate dentures. If, however, all the posterior teeth have been extracted then about six to eight weeks will be required to give adequate support. Up to six months after extraction fairly active alveolar resorption can be expected which will obviously reduce the usefulness of the immediate denture. The bone condition, with sites of pathology, will also affect the time. Therefore, the waiting period depends upon various factors and differs in different cases.
6. Preliminary impressions are made in alginate and stock trays.

7. Individual trays are prepared (these may not be necessary if the preliminary impression and casts are deemed accurate).
8. Master impressions are made in alginate or elastomer, being especially careful of peripheral trimming. An alternative impression is a compression impression, i.e. composition and impression paste of the edentulous parts and alginate of the remaining teeth, which will ensure a well-trimmed periphery and some functional loading of the denture-bearing area.
9. Record blocks are prepared on the stone casts.
10. The jaw relations are registered in retruded contact position. A facebow record of the maxillary cast may be made. Shade of teeth is noted. If the patient's anterior teeth are to be reproduced exactly a small local alginate impression is taken in a sectional tray and wax poured into this. These teeth are then invested and processed individually. Drawings of the anterior teeth may be made to indicate the presence of fillings, stains, or any peculiar characteristics.
11. The posterior teeth are set on a moving-condyle articulator and balanced occlusion is obtained if possible (the standing teeth, at this stage, may prevent this).
12. The partial wax dentures are tried in the mouth, the occlusion verified and the anterior teeth checked for shade, shape and form.
13. The patient is prepared for the next visit, i.e. type of anaesthesia and general procedure. The occlusion is now balanced on the articulator. The dentures are processed, remounted and then finished in the laboratory.
14. The anterior teeth are removed under local or general anaesthesia. With the latter healing is more rapid and there is little disturbance to the tissue as there is with the injection of local anaesthetic. With local, however, the tissues are anaesthetized which aids initial tolerance of the denture. The dentures are inserted as soon after the extractions as possible. Adjustments to the dentures involving the occlusion or base is contraindicated at this stage because of the patient's limited tolerance and, therefore, the dentures should be scrupulously inspected (and scrubbed with soap and water) before insertion.

    The patient is dismissed with certain instructions: the dentures must be kept in the mouth until the next visit which, as a routine in all immediate denture cases, should be 24 h; if the dentures are left out of the mouth for more than a few minutes they may be very difficult to re-insert; the diet should consist of easily masticated food; pain is controlled by analgesics.
15. At the next visit the denture is removed and cleaned. The patient is given a suitable demulcent mouthwash. The tissues at this time may be exceedingly tender and much care is needed. A sensitive patient may be embarrassed by having to show an unclean denture. The denture must be cleaned after every meal but otherwise never left out of the mouth.
16. The next visit is about three to five days later when the occlusion is checked and perfected by selective grinding.
17. The patient is recalled in two to three months and rebase of the dentures is now considered. A rebase, if required, is often only necessary in the area of the extractions.
18. Replacement dentures are constructed 6–12 months later and, in most cases, the shape and tooth position of the immediate dentures should be imitated.

General points

The previous description relates to the delivery of complete upper and lower immediate dentures in one stage. This can be rather a severe ordeal for a patient, considering the added bulk, the speech upset, the change in eating habits, the number of extractions and pain. Consequently, anything the clinician can do to reduce this ordeal is welcomed by the patient.

For example, in a patient requiring total extractions and who has never worn dentures, one could, having extracted the posterior teeth and allowed for healing, either (a) Fit transitional partial dentures to allow the patient to become accustomed to dentures: after a few weeks anterior teeth are added to the partial dentures and delivered as immediate dentures; or (b) An upper immediate denture only may be made in conjunction with a partial lower denture: when the patient is used to this, the immediate complete lower denture can be made.

Various combinations of treatment can be used but the decision often depends upon economic as well as prosthetic factors (Figures 26.4, 26.5 and 26.6).

Laboratory procedures

Removing the plaster teeth and carving the cast

This is done after the partial wax dentures have been checked in the mouth. The alternate teeth are removed one at a time and the acrylic tooth set in position.

With anterior teeth socketed

1. Remove the plaster tooth to the level of the gingival margin, but preserve the latter.
2. Deepen the socket 1–2 mm leaving the margins intact.

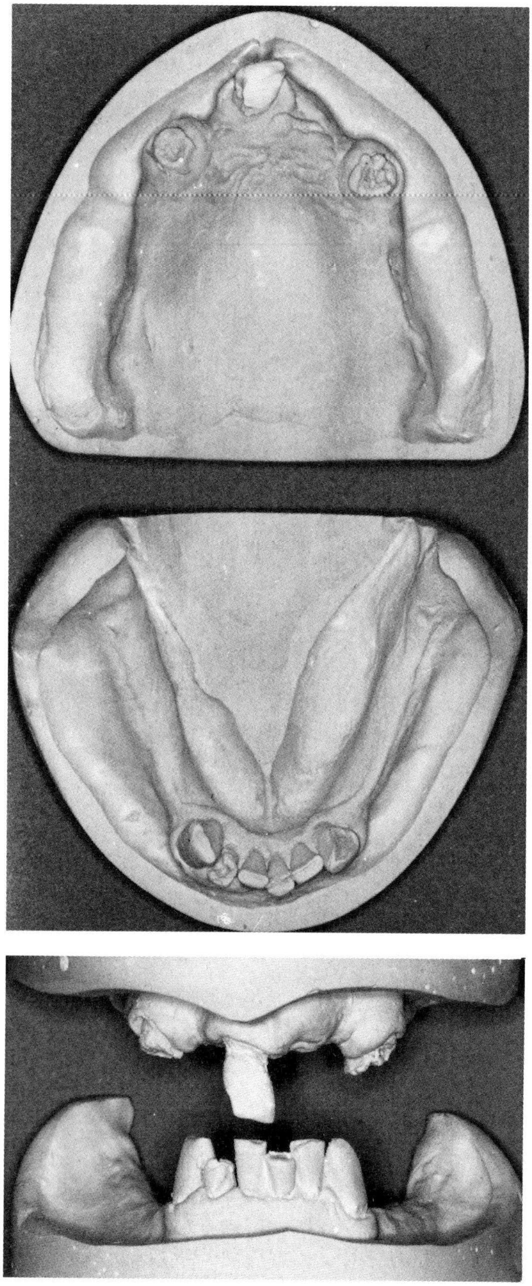

Figure 26.4 Patient at time of presentation wearing loose acrylic partial dentures

3. Deepen the labial part of the socket a further 1–2 mm and lightly scrape the labial margin. The direction of this socketing should follow the long axis of the tooth being replaced. The bulk of the tooth should not occupy all the socket otherwise an irregular ridge will result. Only the labial aspect occupies the socket.

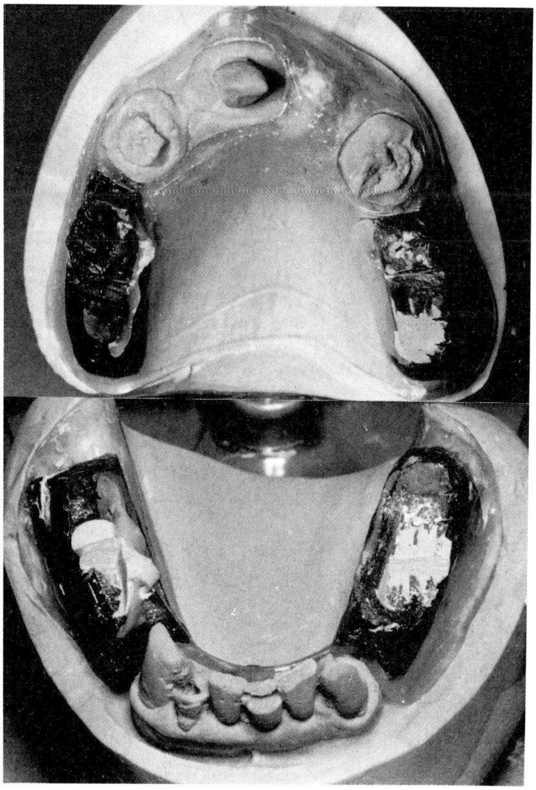

Figure 26.5 Same case as Figure 26.4. Acrylic bases and composition occlusal rims with ZOE paste as RCP recording medium

4. If deep periodontal pocketing is present in the mouth then slightly deeper carving may be permitted than stated above.

Never socket a lower denture which is always better made with a labial flange.

When fitting a socketed denture the interdental septae may require reduction in the mouth otherwise the denture may rock over them.

Labial flange without alveolectomy

Sockets are not carved but left proud by about 2 mm. The labial part of the gingival margin is scraped to allow for collapse of the soft gingival border after extraction. A good ridge shape will result if the cast is properly prepared.

Labial flange with alveolectomy

Sockets are carved a little deeper and the labial plate is reduced by scraping in the area of the attached mucosa. Avoid the fraenum and reflected mucosa. Reduce interdentally and scrape the ridge to form a smooth rounded labial contour. Do not scrape

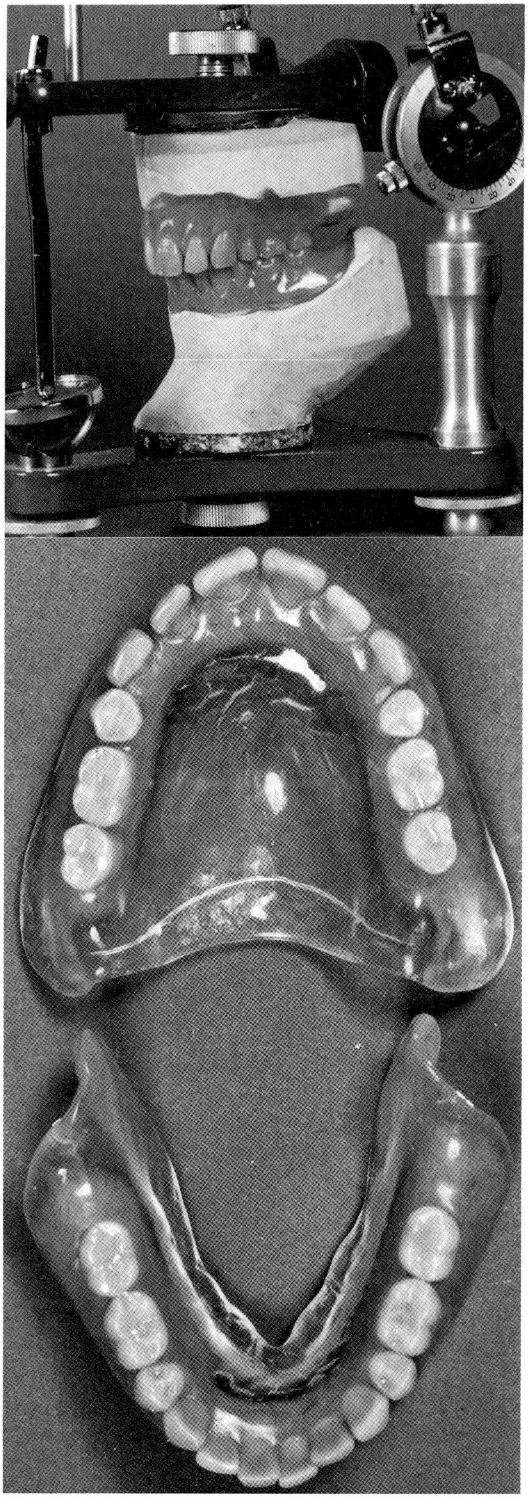

Figure 26.6 Same case as Figures 26.4 and 26.5. Plaster teeth removed after trial stage and complete immediate dentures finished by curing pink acrylic to clear acrylic bases

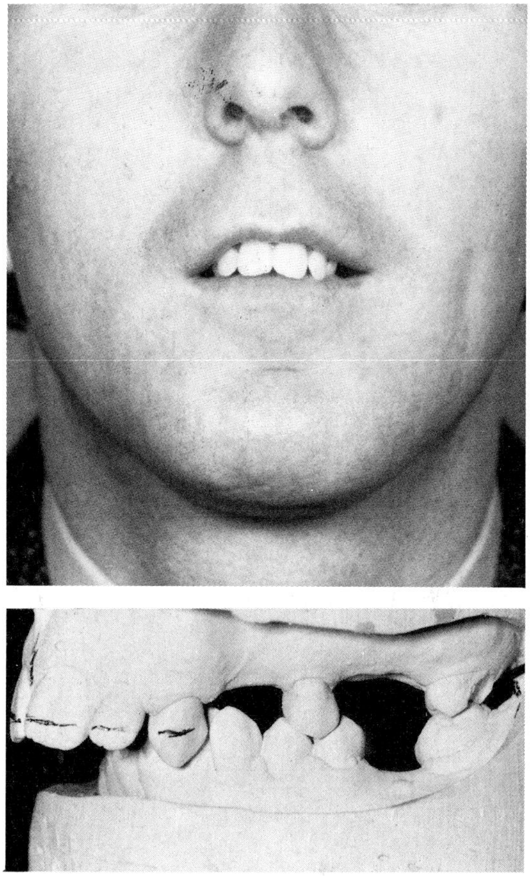

Figure 26.7 Complete upper immediate denture. Pre-extraction Angle class II division 1 malocclusion. Pencil line on cast shows planned level of incisors on denture

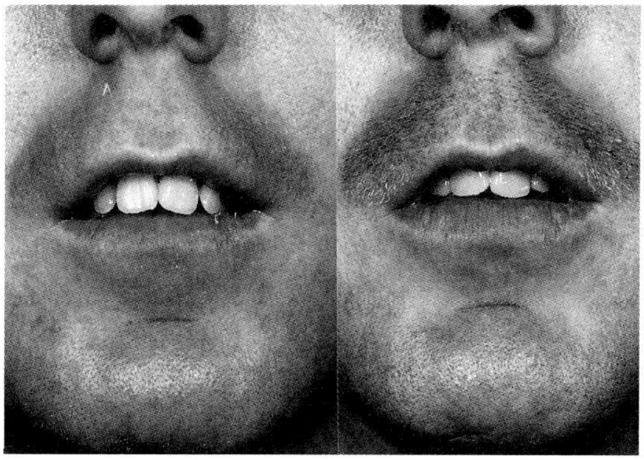

Figure 26.8 Same case as Figure 26.7. Pre- and post-extraction result with maxillary immediate denture *in situ*

lingually or palatally. A duplicate cast is now made of this and a clear acrylic base-plate is processed on the duplicate. This base-plate may be used during the alveolectomy as a guide to the removal of bone. The denture is processed on the master cast.

When the alveolectomy is carried out it is important to remove sufficient bone.

Set the teeth at approximately the same distance from the front of the ridge but at a higher level in those cases where the maxillary anterior teeth are excessively prominent, as in an Angle class II division 1 malocclusion, and where an aesthetic improvement is desired (Figures 26.7 and 26.8).

Post-immediate technique

1. Record master impressions of the dentate jaws in alginate or elastomer. In some cases stock trays are adequate for this as long as a bubble-free periphery is obtained together with a good impression of the tuberosity vestibular space, the hamular notch region and the retromylohyoid space. If this degree of accuracy with stock trays is not possible then acrylic individual trays are made. A lot depends on the clinical ability and laboratory services.
2. Pour the impressions in dental stone.
3. Duplicate the casts in stone for reference during the construction of the dentures and future record purposes.
4. Mount the casts with a facebow on an adjustable articulator in either the intercuspal or retruded contact position. Whichever position is selected it should be reproducible.
5. Take a shade and note any particular characteristics of the teeth and their arrangement. The clinician may elect to change the midline or occlusal level.
6. Make trial dentures in the laboratory without any further reference to the patient. This is the important part as far as the laboratory is concerned as there is no room for error. The bases can be made in either heat-cure or cold-cure acrylic with undercuts blocked out. The periphery is kept slightly short of the cast periphery and the teeth are set with a sticky wax or a cold-cure acrylic foundation so that they will not come off at the next clinical visit.
7. A few days after the teeth have been extracted both dentures are rebased in the mouth in occlusion. Any suitable material, such as ZOE or one of the elastomers, is used. ZOE takes up little space but is is rather messy and tends to get mixed up with the healing sockets; the elastomers tend to slip on the viscous saliva and are rather uncontrollable and slow to set. The choice depends on the operator and the question of asepsis applies in all cases. The healing sockets may be tender and care is needed.
8. As soon as the closed-mouth impressions have been recorded pour casts and finish the dentures without delay. If the wax-up has been done carefully the dentures can be put in the flask directly without having to mount them up. This is an obvious advantage as it prevents any further laboratory errors. The important factor is to return the dentures to the mouth quickly because the postoperative changes are rapid. There is no reason why the dentures should not be finished within hours of the time of the rebasing impressions.
9. The main advantage of a post-immediate technique is that a large number of teeth can be extracted at one time, preferably in theatre, with minimum inconvenience to the patient. The purpose of the rebasing impressions is to allow for any problems that may occur in the surgical technique such as fractured roots, loss of buccal bone, expansion of the buccal plate, and so on. The technique is extremely versatile but it is worth emphasizing that the clinical and laboratory techniques have to be foolproof because there is little room for error or mistakes.

Chapter 27

Overlay and onlay dentures; overdentures and hybrids

An overlay (or onlay) denture is one which is designed to alter the shape and height of the occlusal surfaces of the teeth over which it fits.

Overlay dentures may form part of a conventional partial denture, or be fitted in a mouth in which no teeth are missing. They may be constructed of acrylic, gold alloy, cobalt–chromium alloy or combinations of these.

Conditions requiring an overlay

Overlay dentures are used to correct faults of occlusion and articulation in the natural dentition and six broad classes of such faults may be identified.

1. Correction of a reduced occlusal face height and appearance caused by tooth surface loss due to attrition, abrasion or erosion (Figure 27.1; see Chapter 29).
2. Where an irregular occlusal table due to early extraction and subsequent tooth drift opposes an edentulous jaw (see Single denture later in this chapter).
3. Those occlusions causing damage to the tissues. Figure 27.2 illustrates a case in which the occlusion was such that the upper incisors were biting into the labial gingivae of the lower incisors, and the lower incisors were traumatizing the palatal mucosa. The fitting of an overlay on the occlusal surfaces of the upper teeth protected the palatal gingivae and prevented the damage continuing.
4. Those cases in which the occlusion is such that the lower teeth occlude palatally to the uppers (Figure 27.3). Such a condition makes it difficult or impossible for the individual to chew efficiently. Making an overlay on the upper teeth, shaped to occlude with the lower teeth, enables the patient to masticate.

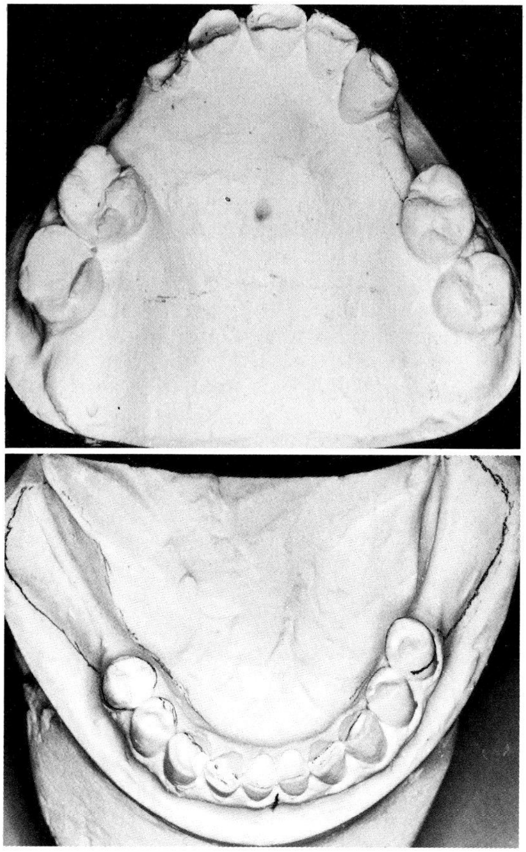

Figure 27.1 Tooth surface loss of natural dentition

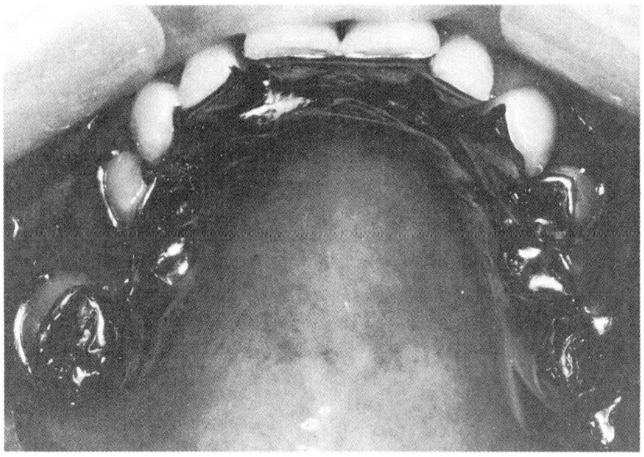

Figure 27.2 An incisal relationship that traumatized palatal and lower labial gingivae. Yellow gold (type II) maxillary overlay covering all teeth with occlusion developed by functionally generated path. Retention by occlusally-approaching clasps

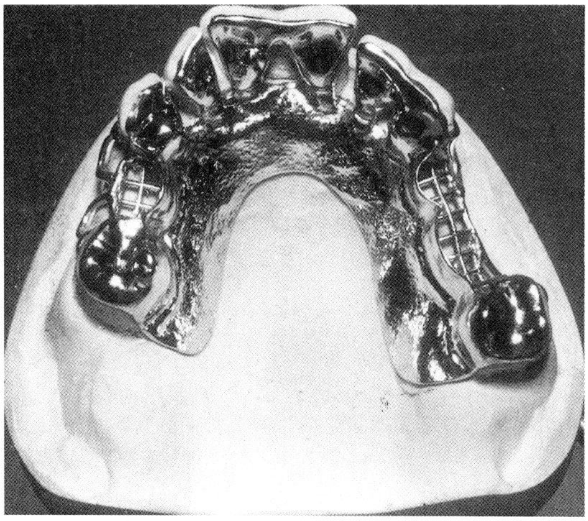

Figure 27.3 Cobalt–chromium overlay made to equilibrate the occlusion. This design protects the maxillary teeth from mandibular incisor trauma and acts as a periodontal splint. Note the alloy cut away in the diastemata and the close fit into the incisal edges

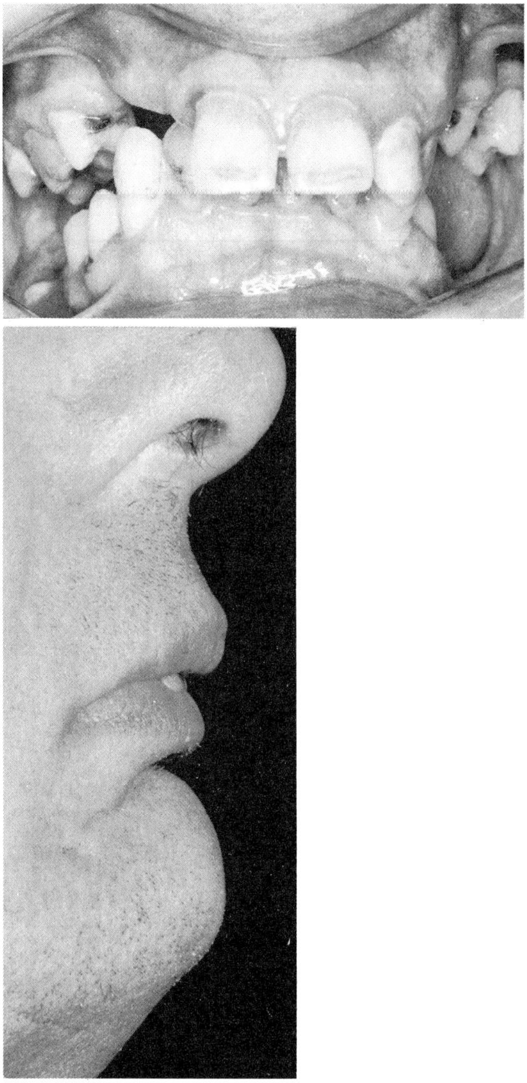

Figure 27.4 Marked malocclusion of natural teeth at the beginning of the opening movement showing traumatic relationship. Profile view of patient

5. Those cases in which the occlusion is locked in the position of retruded occlusion and attempts to make lateral chewing movements cause excessive loads to be imposed on the periodontal membranes of the teeth with consequent damage to these tissues. A traumatic occlusion of this type can frequently be corrected by fitting an overlay to the upper teeth thus providing a change in the cuspal relationships which allows lateral movements to be made (Figure 27.4).
6. Those cases in which pain or derangement of function of the temporomandibular joints is associated with faults in the occlusion. A concept of the articulation of the mandible with the skull is that of a triad of joints, muscles and occlusion and not merely two isolated joints. The mandible, moved by muscles, articulates with the skull through the two temporomandibular joints and through the occlusal and incisal surfaces of all the teeth. For efficient and comfortable function therefore these three components must be in harmony. The muscle activity controlling the mandible should be stable, and harmonize with the movement affected by the joint anatomy and tooth surfaces. If one of the triad fails to fit functionally with the other two then a condition of stress will develop which may produce symptoms of dysfunction and pain. So far as the

treatment of these conditions is related to overlays, we are concerned here only with the dysharmony of the occlusion and articulation of the teeth in relation to the muscles and joints. The position of the mandible when the teeth are in contact is determined by the incisor relationships and the interdigitation of the molar and premolar cusps which act as inclined planes and which, under the influence of the powerful muscles of mastication, seat the mandible in a definite relationship to the skull on each closure. If this position of the mandible is directed by faults in the occlusion at the expense of the temporomandibular joints and muscles, then the joints and muscles will be forced to take up strained or abnormal positions, and dysfunction of either or both may supervene.

A common example of this latter situation occurs when one or both condyles are forced to retrude further into the glenoid fossae than the normal laxity of the joint structures will allow. Such a condition may develop as a result of gradual loss of posterior teeth. In Figure 27.5 the relationship of the occluding surfaces is illustrated before any teeth were lost. The premolars and first molars are extracted over the years, and as a result of the extra stress induced in them and their lack of occlusal support, the second molar teeth tilt. This results in the lower incisors sliding upwards and backwards along the inclined palatal surfaces of the upper incisors each time the teeth are occluded. This means that part of the power of the muscles of mastication is directed to moving the mandible, and consequently the condyles, upwards and backwards, and therefore on closure the mandible assumes a more retruded position. The backward movement is usually made worse by the cusp inclines of the tilted molars (Figure 27.6). In a majority of cases this condition never develops because the positions of the upper and lower incisors alter under the extra load applied to them, allowing the upper incisors to tilt forwards and the lowers lingually. If the pressure of the muscles of the lips and tongue is great or the attachments of these teeth is extremely firm, however, such tilting may not occur, and it is in these cases that symptoms of temporomandibular joint pain and dysfunction may develop. The insertion of a partial denture with an overlay in such cases is aimed at restoring the occlusal relationship of the mandible with the maxilla to the original position, and allowing the condyles to assume their normal relationship to the glenoid fossae.

A similar condition of dysharmony can develop without the prior extraction of teeth. The relationship of the condyles to the glenoid fossae when the mandible is in the relaxed or rest position is illustrated in Figure 27.7. From this position to closure the teeth may not interdigitate (Figure 27.8) and when the muscle power is increased the inclined planes of the teeth act as wedges. The lower cusps slide up the upper cusps, forcing the mandible distally or laterally and the heads of the condyles backwards in the fossae (Figure 27.9).

As described in the previous example, the teeth usually adjust their individual positions by moving, and thus accommodate to the joint and muscle position of the mandible, but in some instances the muscle power is so great, or the attachment of the teeth to the jaw so rigid, that no adjustment is made. It is in these cases that the reshaping of the occlusal surfaces by means of an overlay may be of value.

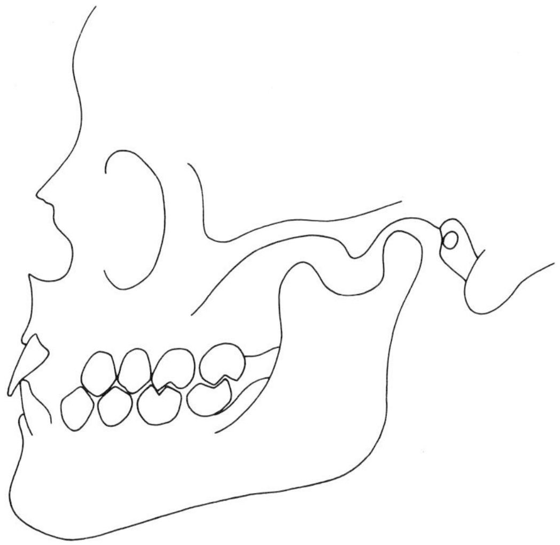

Figure 27.5 Anterior and posterior teeth in occlusion. Note relationship of condyle to glenoid fossa

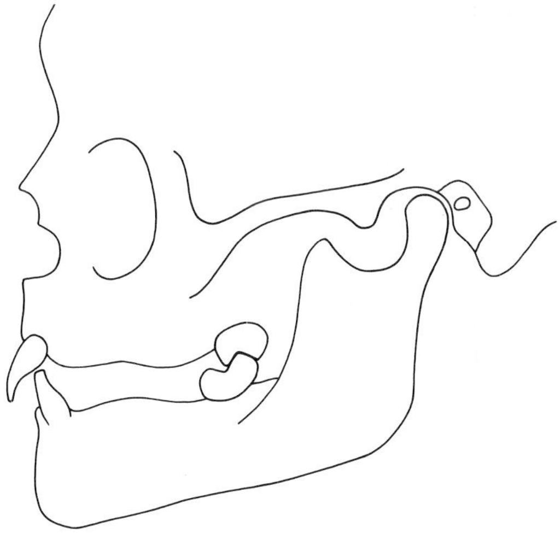

Figure 27.6 Loss of posterior teeth may lead to a backward position of the mandible. Compare condyle/fossa relationship with Figure 27.5

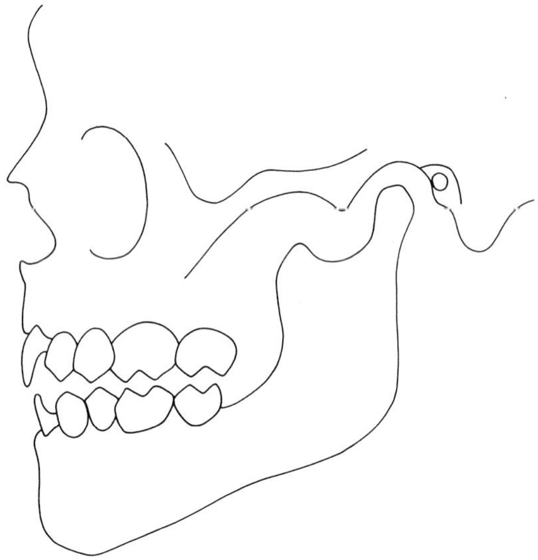

Figure 27.7 Mandible in rest position with teeth apart. Note position of condyle in the glenoid fossa

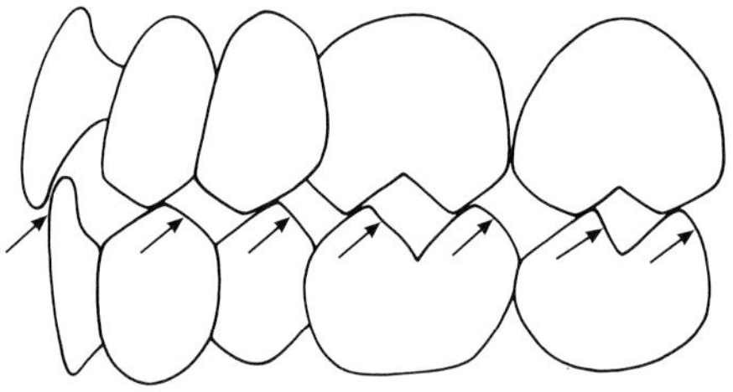

Figure 27.8 Enlarged view of teeth in Figure 27.7. From the rest position the teeth may not interdigitate. When muscle power increases the inclined planes of the cusps guide the mandible distally or laterally

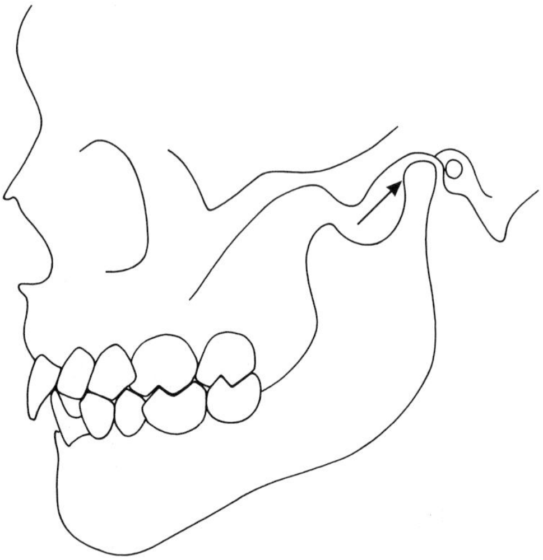

Figure 27.9 Mandibular position resulting from tooth relationship shown in Figure 27.8. Note distal movement of condyle

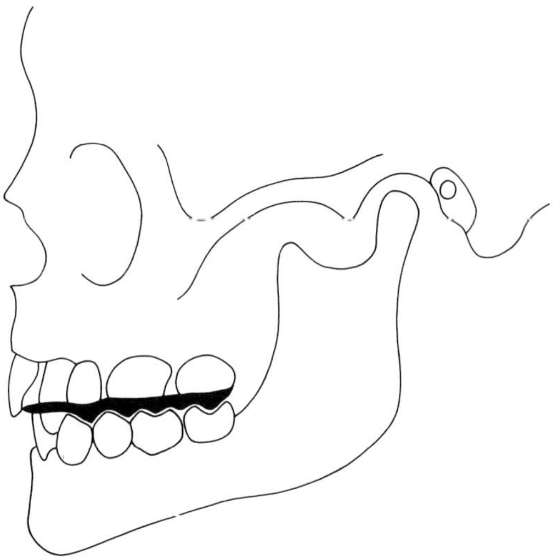

Figure 27.10 Diagram of overlay denture to prevent distal and upward movement of the mandible

Figure 27.10 shows how this is effected. It should be emphasized that a diagnosis of temporomandibular joint dysfunction syndrome cannot be made from a malocclusion only and there are many morphological malocclusions that are perfectly stable and symptom-free. Therefore overlay dentures should never be prescribed for cases of temporomandibular joint dysfunction unless definite evidence of an occlusal aetiology can be demonstrated.

Use of articulator

In all cases where the construction of an overlay denture is being considered an essential requirement is to mount the casts on an articulator to assess the circumstances and plan the design.

A facebow is used to mount the upper cast on the articulator in the correct relationship to the hinge axis. A check record of softened wax is made with the patient lying flat and relaxed and the teeth closed into but not through the record. The rationale behind this is that when the mandible is closed from the position in which it is held by the relaxed muscles into the wax, the mandible is following the path directed by the muscles and the temporomandibular joints. As it is not closed completely through the wax the cusps of the opposing teeth do not come into contact, and therefore no cuspal guidance occurs to divert the mandible from the muscle and joint path of closure. If now, using this wax record, the lower cast is related to the upper cast already mounted by the facebow, and the wax record removed, the casts can be closed through the 1 or 2 mm which separate the occlusal surfaces of the teeth with fair assurance that they are following the same path that the patient's mandible would follow as guided by the joints and muscles. This is because the last few millimetres of closure of the mandible is a hinge movement with the condyles acting as the centres of rotation. When the teeth are occluded on the articulator, it can be observed whether or not they interdigitate correctly, or meet in such a manner that a major shift of the mandible is necessary to effect intercuspation. The effects of occlusal faults are best seen on an adjustable articulator where movements of the articulator condyles, if any, can be measured during occlusal contacts of the casts.

It is then that an overlay can be designed and constructed to reshape the occlusal surfaces in harmony with the joint and muscle path of closure and thus prevent any deflective cuspal guidance affecting mandibular position.

General remarks

Overlay dentures should preferably be constructed to fit the upper teeth. The reason for this is that by carrying an alloy or acrylic platform behind the upper incisors a surface is presented with which the tips of the lower incisors can occlude, and this prevents any possibility of their over-eruption. The contact of the overlay with the palatal surfaces of the upper incisors also helps to prevent their movement. If the overlay is constructed on the lower teeth, it may be necessary to carry it over the incisors to prevent over-eruption and this produces an unsightly appearance which is avoided with a maxillary overlay.

Overlay dentures should not normally obliterate the freeway space, although their presence will obviously reduce it, and they should never be built higher than is absolutely necessary. Some patients have so small a freeway space that even a shallow overlay will completely obliterate it but, in these cases, it is usually found that after a short time a freeway space develops again. This may be due either to the fact that, in the first instance, the patient was not fully relaxing the mandible, and therefore giving an inaccurate recording of the true freeway space, or the presence of the overlay has caused the teeth to be depressed into the alveolus. This latter occurrence severely disrupts the occlusion and should be avoided by more careful mounting of casts.

In a case in which it is considered that an overlay might be a suitable form of treatment, the first appliance may be constructed in acrylic. Such an appliance might be termed a diagnostic overlay. After it has been worn by the patient with comfort and abatement of the signs or symptoms for which it was made, then it can be assumed that it is a suitable form of treatment, and can be replaced in due course by an alloy overlay which is more robust, more accurate and takes up less space. If, on the other hand, no improvment of signs or symptoms occurs after a few weeks wear then the acrylic diagnostic appliance may be discarded and no great loss of time or effort will have occurred.

It is important that overlay dentures and the natural teeth are kept scrupulously clean by the patient. A strict fluoride regimen is advantageous.

In general, patients tend to dislike overlay dentures because they lie beyond the normal anatomical boundaries of natural teeth and therefore always tend to feel bulky. For this reason clasps should be unobstrusive and connectors made as thin as possible without jeopardizing strength.

Single complete denture

Overlay dentures are particularly useful in patients where one jaw is edentulous and the other jaw has a number of natural teeth with an irregular occlusal table caused by early extraction and subsequent tooth drift (Figure 27.11). The difficulty in such cases is to balance the occlusion of the single complete denture, an essential requirement if pain and looseness of the denture are to be avoided.

Three techniques may be used.

Functionally generated path

Where the irregularity of the occlusal table of the natural teeth is only mild it is best treated by a functionally generated path technique without resort to an overlay.

Use acrylic posterior teeth and build the occlusion on the articulator as far as possible. Cut out mesiodistal channels and reduce the upper denture

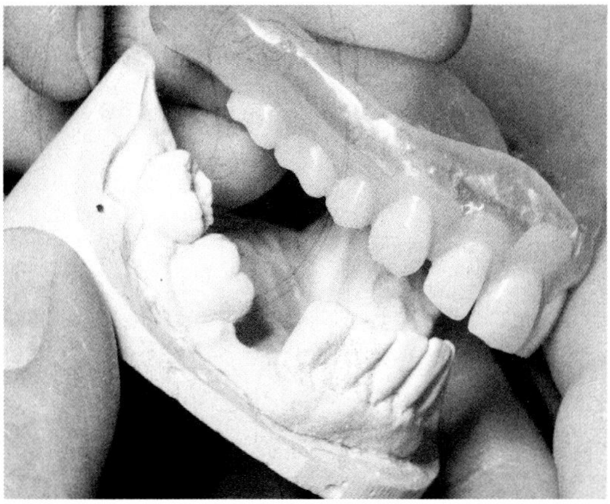

Figure 27.11 The single denture problem. Irregular occlusal table caused by loss of natural teeth poses problems of occlusal balance and looseness of complete denture

teeth out of contact with the teeth on the lower cast. Fill the channels with impression compound and make centric stops. Check in the mouth for all-round contact in the retruded position. Build the remainder of the upper teeth in hard wax on the articulator. Return the denture to the mouth and take the patient through working, non-working and protrusive excursions to shape the wax to these eccentric contacts. The centric stops prevent closure of the vertical dimension. In the laboratory pour occlusal registers, remove the hard wax and compound, replace with casting wax, sprue and cast in yellow gold alloy (Figure 27.12). Polish the castings and attach them to the denture with EBA (ortho-ethoxy benzoic acid) cement. (See also 'gold occlusals' later in this section)

Overlay

Where the occclusal table of the lower teeth is irregular, usually with a number of missing teeth (Figure 27.13), an overlay is useful. Record blocks are made (Figure 27.14), the lower extending over the posterior teeth in the form of a thin sheet. The upper denture teeth are set, checked in the mouth and the retruded contact position verified (Figure 27.15). The lower cast is prepared and duplicated to form the refractory model on which the planned overlay denture is cast. The occlusion is refined on the articulator (Figure 27.16) before delivering the finished dentures to the mouth.

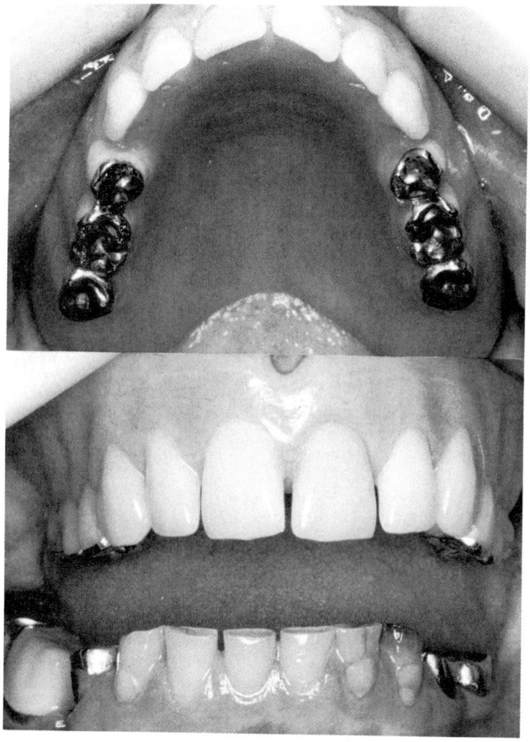

Figure 27.12 Gold occlusal surfaces of posterior maxillary denture teeth developed by a functionally generated path technique against irregular lower natural teeth

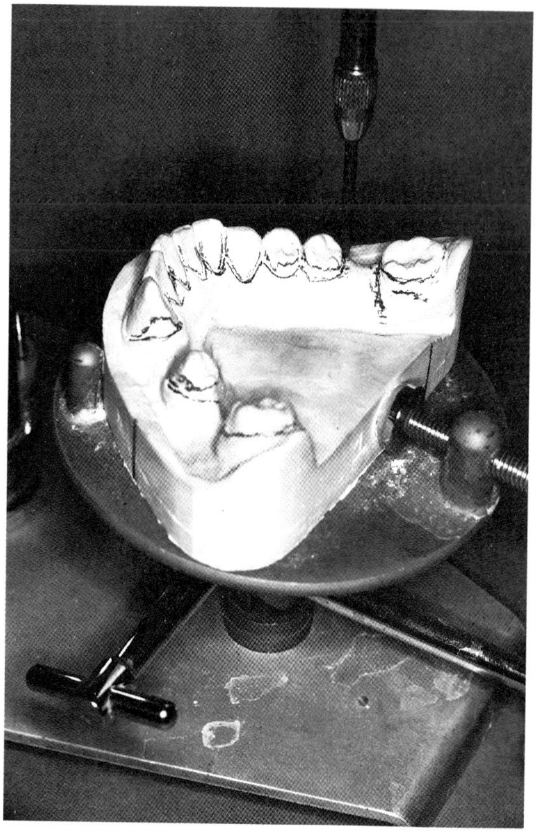

Figure 27.13 Irregularity of lower natural teeth producing problems of occlusion

The occlusal form and design of such an overlay denture depends on the particular circumstances of the case. In most situations the upper posterior teeth are made in porcelain and the overlay in cobalt–chromium alloy. In some cases, where there is enough interocclusal space and the overlay sufficiently thick, the occlusal surface can be made in acrylic with the opposing upper posterior teeth also in acrylic (Figure 27.17). The problem then, of course, is that the acrylic occlusal surfaces wear and it is not long before the occlusion is no longer balanced. There are, however, tooth-coloured polymers, such as heat-cured dimethacrylate, which have a reasonably high abrasion resistance.

Fixed bridges

In single denture cases the most efficient method of correcting occlusal problems is to construct bridges, preferably with an occlusal design fabricated by a

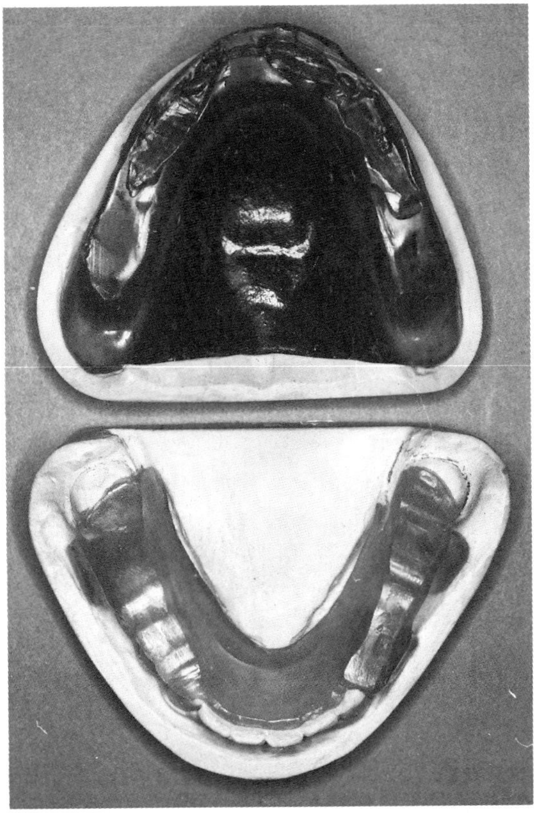

Figure 27.14 Same case as in Figure 27.13. Record blocks are made. Care is taken that the lower surface does not distort

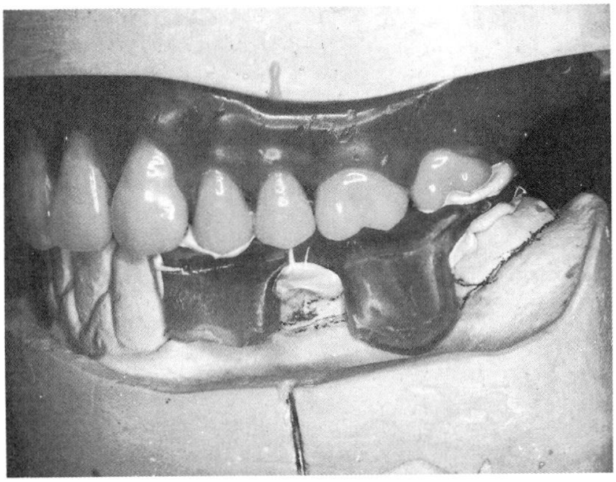

Figure 27.15 Same case as in Figure 27.13. Maxillary teeth are set and the retruded contact position verified at the chairside with quick-setting ZOE paste

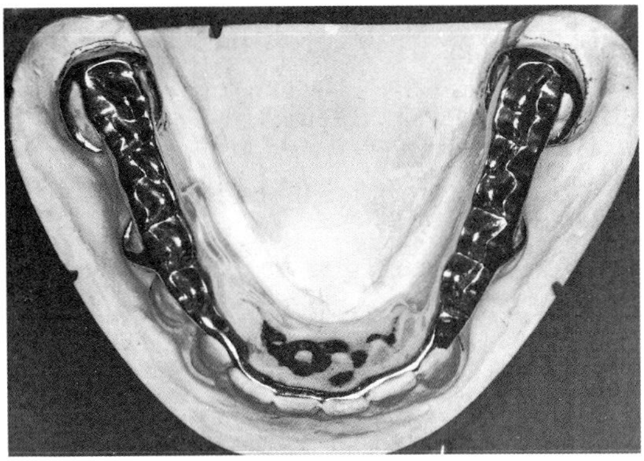

(*a*)

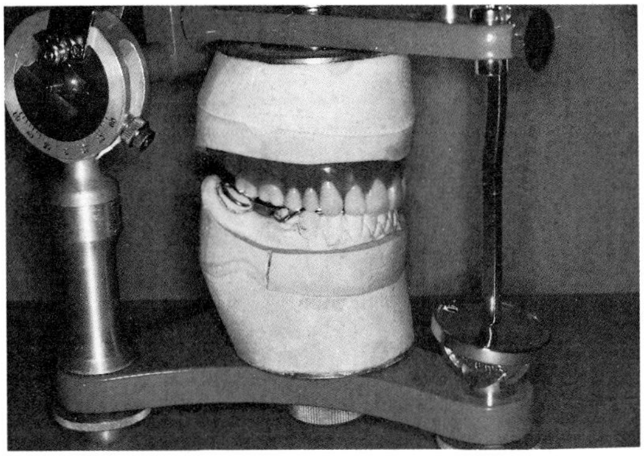

(*b*)

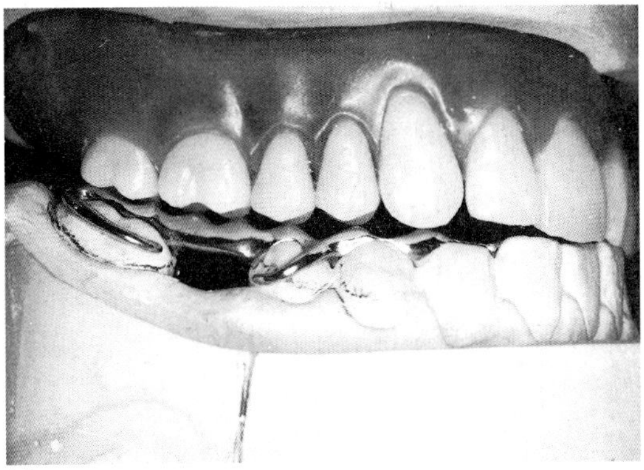

(*c*)

Figure 27.16 Same case as in Figure 27.13. The cast cobalt–chromium overlay is made (*a*) and the occlusion refined on the articulator (*b*). Contact in working, protrusive and non-working (*c*) positions is essential to produce a satisfactory complete upper denture

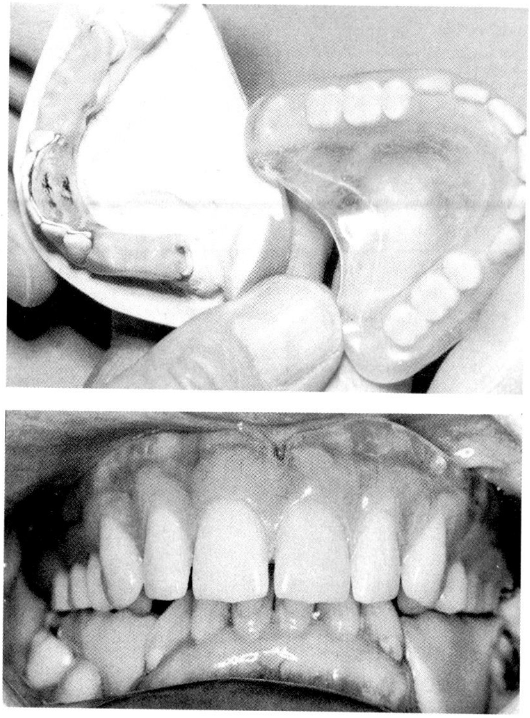

Figure 27.17 Acrylic overlay denture (same case as in Figure 27.11). The apparent difference in shade between the upper and lower anterior teeth is due to the horizontal overjet being about 12 mm in this case

functionally generated path technique. If the occlusal surfaces of the bridges are made of porcelain then porcelain teeth should be used on the denture. If gold alloy forms the occlusal surfaces of the bridges then acrylic teeth may be set on the denture with their occlusal surfaces formed in gold alloy as a thin veneer. Such a technique is sometimes referred to as gold occlusals.

After the denture with acrylic teeth has been worn in the mouth for a few weeks and the occlusion is deemed to be satisfactory, the denture is remounted on the articulator against the opposing cast. An impression of the occlusal surfaces of the denture teeth is made in refractory material which is then removed and filled with casting wax to a depth of no more than 1 mm. Attach retention loops, sprue and cast in gold alloy. Reduce the acrylic teeth and attach the castings with acrylic cement in correct occlusion against the opposing cast. This method copies exactly the acrylic teeth, the occlusal surfaces of which have already been verified in the mouth.

Overdentures and hybrids

Overdentures, also known as hybrids or tooth-supported dentures, have been used in various forms for many years, but recently have become more popular for a number of reasons:

1. The increased age of the population with teeth being retained longer.
2. Improved methods of tooth conservation and endodontics.
3. Better hygiene measures.
4. Changing attitudes to preservation of natural teeth.
5. Improved standards of dental materials and technology.

Definitions

An overdenture is a complete or partial denture supported by mucoperiosteum and prepared teeth or roots.

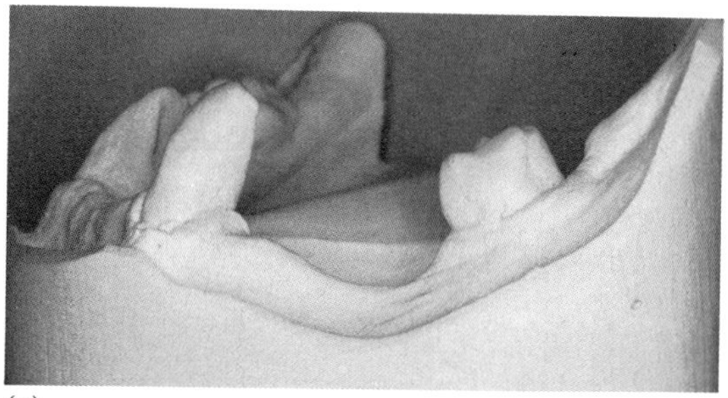

(*a*)

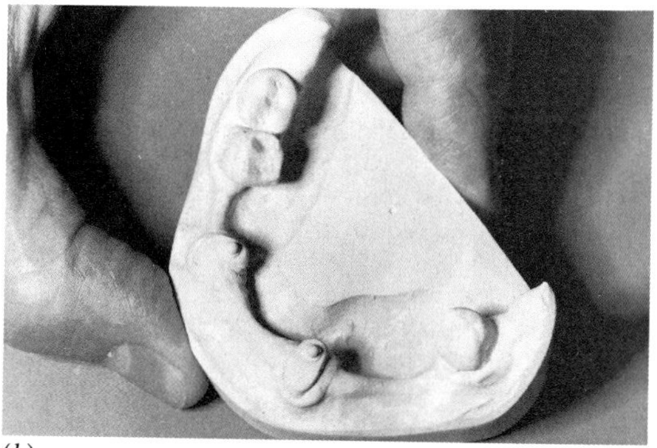

(*b*)

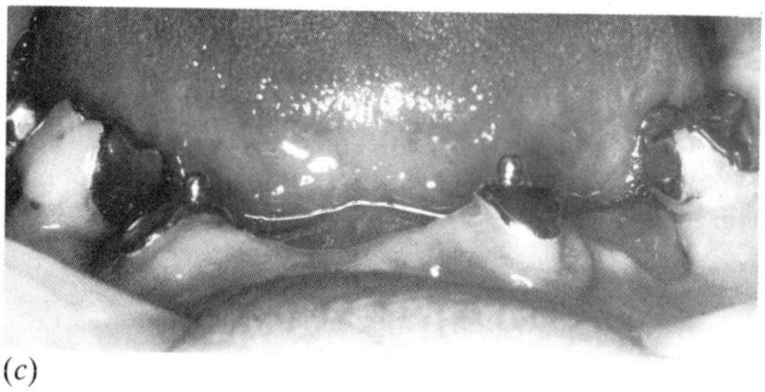

(*c*)

Figure 27.18 Partial overdenture (*a*) Lower cast showing retroinclined canines and mesially-inclined molars. (*b*) Cast of prepared mouth with endodontic treatment of canines and stud attachments; molars restored with inlays and vertical guiding surfaces. (*c*) Abutments in the mouth

A hybrid is a type of overdenture that looks like a complete denture but is retained and supported by natural teeth for which prefabricated or precision attachments have been made.

A partial overdenture is similar to a partial denture except that some part or parts cover natural teeth that have been prepared or modified for that purpose (Figure 27.18).

The difference between an overlay denture and a partial overdenture is not always clear-cut and the words are often used interchangeably.

Benefits

1. Maintenance of tactile discrimination which is otherwise diminished with loss of teeth.
2. Preservation of alveolar bone which resorbs after the loss of teeth.
3. Better support because of the presence of periodontal membrane on the remaining abutments.
4. Improved retention, especially in hybrids by the use of attachments.
5. Masticatory efficiency which is often diminished with total loss of teeth and complete dentures.
6. Psychological, which in some patients is particularly important as the loss of all natural teeth takes on a significance of premature ageing and senility.

Drawbacks

1. Maintenance of good oral hygiene is too difficult for some patients; caries, gingivitis and denture plaque lead to failure.
2. Increased cost and length of treatment.
3. Undercuts around abutments pose problems of insertion of flanges.
4. Lack of denture space leads to difficulty in placing denture teeth and to structural weakness of the overdenture.

Indications for overdenture treatment

1. When few natural teeth remain and it is envisaged that the patient will have difficulty in adapting to complete dentures. Parkinson's disease is an example, but retention of natural teeth has to be balanced against the difficulty of maintenance of oral hygiene in such cases.
2. Maxillo-facial patients, e.g. congenital or acquired cleft palate, have a deficiency of tissue and retention of a few abutments increases the retention and stability of the overdenture and obturator.
3. When the remaining teeth are considered unsuitable as partial denture abutments because of position, angulation or state of the crowns.
4. When the prognosis of the teeth, because of mobility, is poor. Retaining a few teeth for overdenture treatment acts as a transition between partial dentures and complete dentures when eventually all teeth are extracted.
5. In cases of tooth surface loss by attrition, erosion or abrasion, the crown height is already diminished. These teeth are not always suitable for restorative treatment because of the mutilated and shortened crowns. Intentional reduction and preparation of the crowns for an overdenture is a logical form of treatment, although the cause of the original tooth loss may in turn damage the overdenture.

Selection of abutments

Any tooth or root will serve as an abutment for an overdenture but canines and molars are best. In many cases it is not possible to choose the ideal because of previous tooth loss. In both mandible and maxilla two canines and two second molars, decoronated and prepared, provide good tooth support, but many overdentures perform well where only one or two abutments remain. Wherever possible the abutments should be positioned so that a line between them is approximately at right angles to the sagittal plane; diagonally-placed teeth lead to a rocking effect of the overdenture.

Patients with rampant caries are seldom suitable for this treatment because of the history of inadequate hygiene and while it may be possible to salvage one or two teeth, and their roots, the ultimate prognosis is not good. The same is probably true where there is advanced periodontal disease but the prognosis is usually better in such cases in spite of the fact that the supporting bone is diminished in amount. It is, however, this last fact that makes overdenture treatment so useful in periodontal cases because retention of a number of roots ensures preservation of alveolar bone, at least for a number of years.

In selecting abutments the need to remove the crowns must be considered in relation to the probability of endodontic treatment which may complicate the treatment planning because of patient attitudes, time, cost and other sequelae of root canal therapy.

The teeth in the opposing jaw should be considered when selecting abutments. If natural teeth are present in one jaw then an overdenture in the other, with a few well-selected retained roots, will help to preserve against alveolar bone loss, a common sequel in an edentulous jaw opposite natural teeth.

A problem can arise if abutments are opposite one another because when the overdentures are out of the mouth the patient may brux on the prepared teeth and damage them.

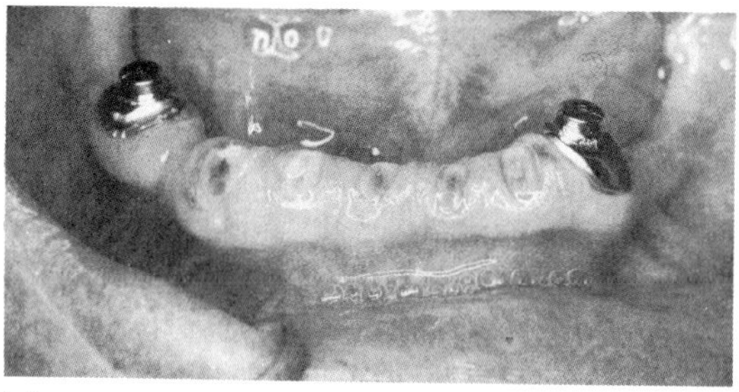

(*a*)

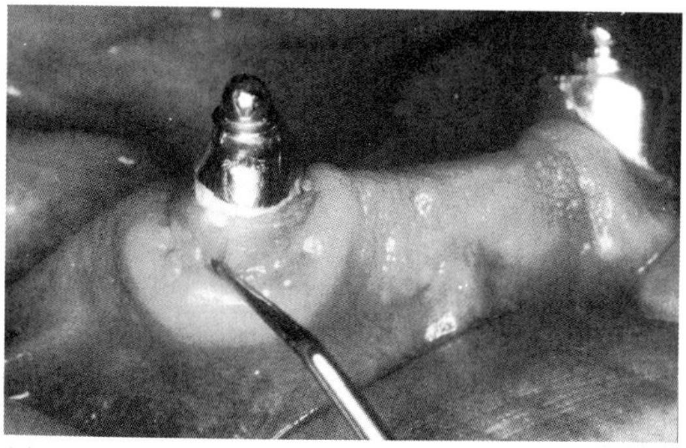

(*b*)

Figure 27.19 Various attachments may be used in overdenture treatment. (*a*) Remaining lower anterior teeth reduced to cervical level as a means of preserving alveolar bone (endodontic treatment not required in this case). (*b*) Leverage on overdentures is often excessive, leading to fracture of abutment root

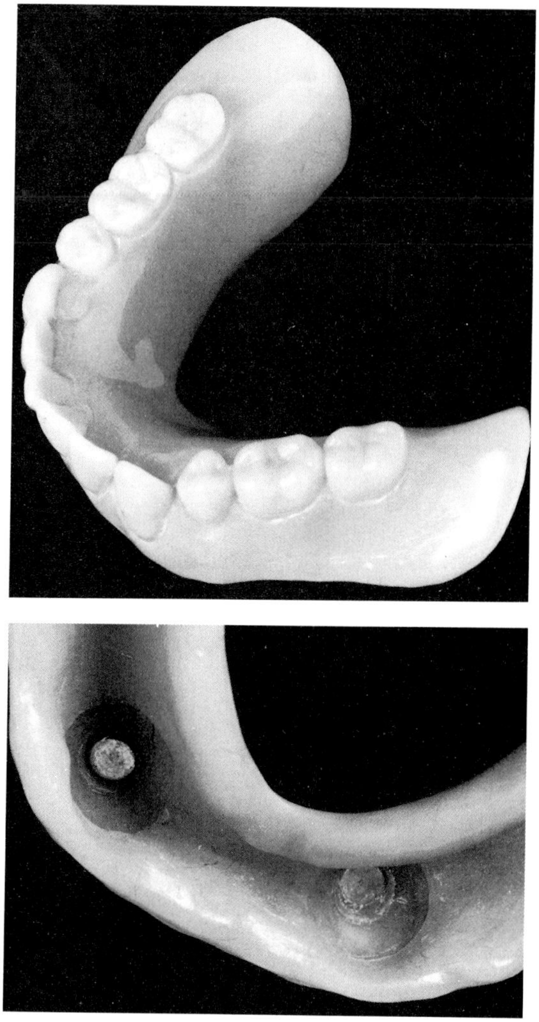

Figure 27.20 Complete mandibular overdenture retained by magnets. Although magnets tend to be bulky this denture has been carefully designed to produce a satisfactory prosthesis

Abutment preparation

Dentine

In most cases the simpler the preparation the better. The aim should be to avoid endodontic treatment and reduce the crown to a rounded supragingival dome. This takes up minimum space and is easily cleaned by the patient. The dentine becomes polished in time as the overdenture rolls over the abutment face. This simple preparation is particularly useful in those cases where hygiene may not be reliable, as little clinical time is lost if the abutments have to be subsequently extracted because the patient is not maintaining oral health. Where endodontic treatment has been done the root face may be obturated with amalgam, glass-ionomer cement or glass-cermet cement.

Alloy

There are various designs of abutment piece that can be used. The crown may be reduced in the form of a jacket preparation and a yellow gold thimble cemented. This provides retention to the overdenture if the walls are nearly parallel and good lateral bracing results from this technique. On the other hand the crown–root ratio may be unfavourable.

A better preparation is a gold alloy dome attached by a cast or wrought post in the root-filled tooth. This is particularly useful where the dentine is deemed to require protection and where further caries is likely. The edge of the alloy should be supragingival.

Various prefabricated attachments may be used if retention is considered important (Figure 27.19). There are many different designs of studs, rings and intraradicular attachments and wherever possible one should be selected that occupies minimum space and that requires minimum maintenance.

Magnets are used in overdentures in the form of rare earth metals such as samarium or neodymium alloyed with cobalt or iron and boron (Figure 27.20). These magnets may offer up to 750 g breakaway strength but are not effective against sudden withdrawing forces and so their use is limited. They also tend to be rather bulky.

Maintenance

One of the biggest problems with overdentures is the maintenance of oral health after delivery. It should be remembered that these patients have already lost the majority of their teeth and poor oral hygiene probably contributed to this. Therefore it is common to find, after a few months, gingivitis, caries, plaque or calculus deposits which all begin to signal failure of the treatment.

It is imperative that good instruction is given to each patient, including a strict fluoride regimen. A regular recall system is essential if any long-term success is expected in the overdenture treatment.

Chapter 28

Cleft palate from the prosthetic aspect

Definition

A cleft palate may be defined as a lack of continuity of the palate. It may be congenital or acquired as a result of injury or disease.

Development

The palate is developed from the maxillary and pre-maxillary growth centres, union of the three segments commencing at the region of the nasal floor represented in full development by the incisive foramen. Union from this point proceeds backwards until both the hard and soft palates and uvula have united, and forwards along the line of the future maxillary pre-maxillary sutures, eventually uniting with the developing lip on either side.

Classification

Failure of union at any stage will result in a congenital cleft palate which may be classified, according to Veau, as:

Class 1 Clefts involving soft palate only.
Class 2 Clefts involving soft and hard palates up to incisive foramen.
Class 3 Cleft of soft and hard palates, forwards through alveolar ridge and continued into lip on one side.
Class 4 Same as Class 3 but associated with bilateral cleft-lip.

Another useful classification has relevance to the surgically repaired congenital cleft lip and palate and also to acquired clefts which, by nature of their origin from injury or elective surgery, are very varied in extent. This is as follows:

1. Enclosed defects (Figure 28.1):
   (a) Soft palate.
   (b) Hard palate.
   (c) Hard and soft palate.
2. Open-end defects (Figure 28.2):
   (a) Anterior unilateral (or, very rarely, bilateral).
   (b) Posterior.
   (c) Anteroposterior.

Problems of congenital cleft palate

The basic problem of a cleft palate from which all the others stem is the inability to close at will the nasopharynx from the oropharynx. In the normal person this closure is effected by raising the soft palate into intimate contact with the posterior and lateral pharyngeal walls (Figure 28.3). This airtight separation of the two cavities is essential to the functions of normal swallowing and speech.

Swallowing

In swallowing, the food bolus or liquid is held in the depressed centre of the tongue, the sides of which are pressed hard against the lateral aspects of the hard palate. Peristaltic-like waves then travel along the tongue from before backwards and propel the food or liquid towards the pharynx. The soft palate which is already raised into contact with the walls of the pharynx prevents the escape of food into the nose and directs it towards the oesophagus; the pharyngeal walls contract to propel it on its way.

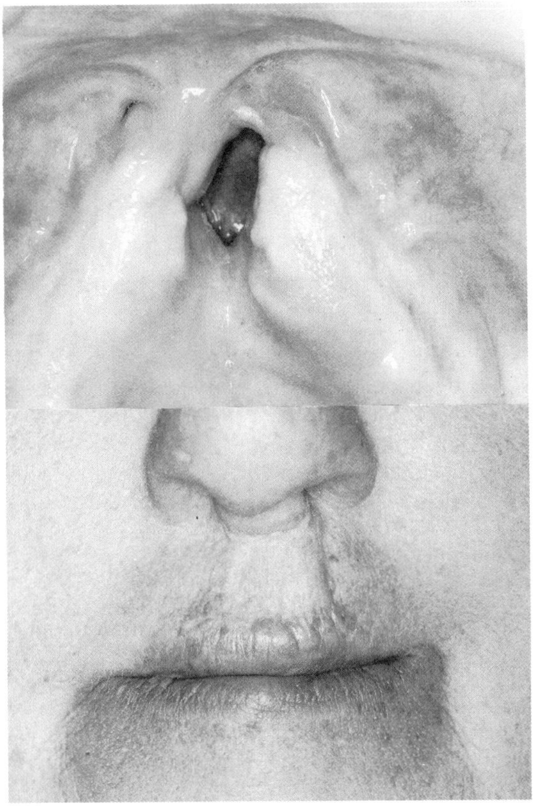

Figure 28.1 Enclosed defect of palate following surgical repair of congenital cleft lip and palate

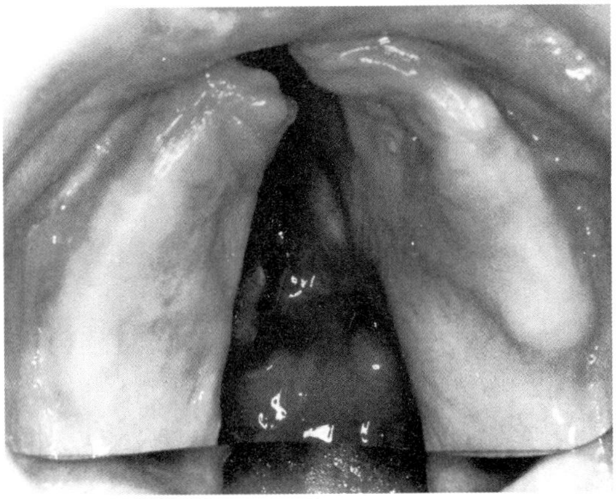

Figure 28.2 Anteroposterior open end defect of palate

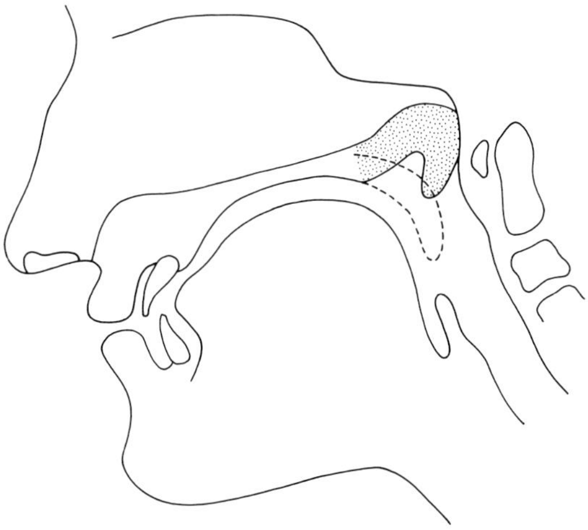

Figure 28.3 Dotted line indicates relaxed position of soft palate. Continuous line indicates position of raised soft palate in contact with pharynx. Note that it is above anterior arch of atlas

Speech

The production of all oral sounds requires the air stream to be under some degree of pressure and this can only be maintained, and the air stream correctly directed through the cavities of the mouth, if the soft palate and pharyngeal walls are producing an airtight seal to nasal escape. In the person with a cleft palate this is not possible and the air stream escapes through the nose. In an attempt to prevent this the back of the tongue is thrust into the cleft and, if the treatment of the cleft either by surgical or prosthetic means is delayed much after the second year (which is the age when rapid speech development occurs), this tongue habit becomes well-established and even after treatment has been given makes correct speech difficult, because the tongue is a potent factor in the shaping of the modulating cavities and its free play, especially forwards, is vital to good speech (Figure 28.4).

Appearance

The effect of a cleft on the appearance of an individual will depend on whether the lip is cleft as well as the palate.

When the lip is cleft

A cleft lip may be unilateral or bilateral and the pre-maxilla may be detached entirely from the maxilla in bilateral clefts. The cleft will involve the alveolar process and in most cases the lateral incisor tooth will either be missing or deformed.

The cleft lip is repaired surgically about six weeks after birth, and results in a functional lip of good appearance, but a repaired lip produces more tension than a normal lip on the anterior maxillary ridges and a degree of malocclusion. If the lateral incisor is missing the gap tends to close and orthodontic treatment will be necessary to restore

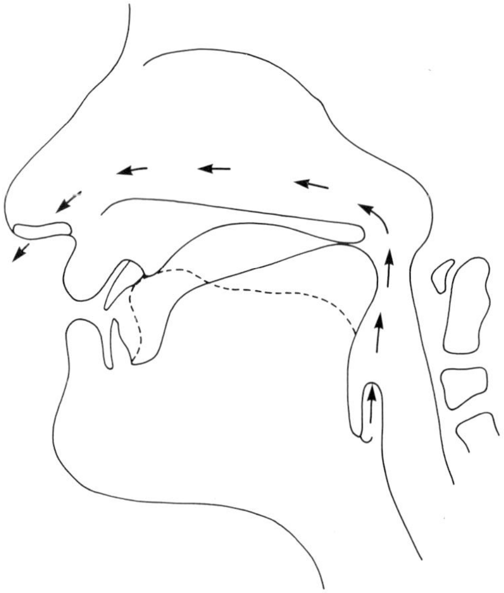

Figure 28.4 Dotted line shows how the tongue and maxillary teeth should make the stop for the T sound, but the palate is cleft and therefore the vibrating air stream escapes through the nose. In an effort to prevent this escape the cleft patient pushes the tongue into the pharynx (continuous line) and develops a major fault of tongue position and thus of speech

the form of the arch and bring the teeth into correct occlusion with the mandibular teeth which will not have suffered any deformity. Thereafter a simple denture will be necessary to maintain the expansion and replace the lateral incisor prior to more permanent restoration of the tooth and adjacent tissue.

When the hard palate is cleft

If the cleft in the hard palate is repaired surgically there is nearly always a reduction in the lateral and forward growth of the maxillae as a result of the tension in the scar tissue of the repair. Orthodontic treatment will reduce this contraction of the arch and in doing so frequently open up parts of the cleft. A denture may be necessary to maintain the expansion and obturate the open cleft.

Modern surgery has reduced the resulting contraction of the arch which formerly occurred, but it is essential that orthodontic treatment is instituted early and is maintained. If for some reason no orthodontic treatment is given, severe deformity of the maxilla may result. Even more severe deformation is occasionally seen in older patients treated by the more traumatic surgical techniques employed in the past. The effect on the appearance of the individual is marked; the middle third of the face is flattened and contracted and the deformation resulting from uranoplasty is made worse if the lip repair was poorly done and has resulted in a tight immobile lip.

Prosthetic treatment of malaligned dental arches

The treatment of patients if they are past the age when orthodontic treatment is likely to be effective is to construct a denture over the misplaced teeth to restore the arch to normal. The lower jaw will usually not have suffered any deformation and if the denture teeth are set to occlude with the lower teeth an improvement in appearance will be effected. In some cases the forward placement of the denture teeth is difficult because of the tightness of the lip (see Figure 29.11).

General remarks

The treatment of cleft palate is a combined effort by the plastic surgeon, orthodontist, prosthodontist and speech therapist. The child should be examined by all four and a combined plan of treatment formulated. The surgeon's main problem will be to repair the lip at about six weeks after birth if the infant's physical condition allows. Early repair of the lip simplifies feeding. Next the repair of the soft palate should be considered: this is of vital importance because on its success or failure will depend the ability of the child to speak clearly. Surgical repair of the soft palate is obviously superior to the fitting of a prosthesis. This is only true however if surgery can produce a functional soft palate and this will depend on the amount of muscular tissue present in the remnants of the soft palate, particularly of the levator muscles.

If the cleft is wide, and the muscular remnants poorly developed, consideration should be given to abandoning surgery and treating the cleft entirely by prosthetic obturation. If surgery can only produce a united soft palate which is non-functional, the patient may be worse off than if no surgery had been performed, because the problem of fitting an obturator in cases with a repaired and non-functional soft palate is greater than in those cases which have received no surgical treatment. If, in addition, a pharyngoplasty has been done, the pharyngeal ring mechanism, on the function of which a successful obturator depends, may have been irreparably damaged. If surgical repair is decided upon this will usually be performed before the end of the second year because it is between the second and third years that the child really commences to talk and if repair is delayed beyond this time faulty habits of speech will have developed which are so difficult to eradicate.

If it is decided that surgery is unlikely to be successful then it is at about two years of age that the first obturator should be made. Finally when the question of the treatment of the lip and soft palate has been decided, consideration should be given to the repair of the hard palate. This is the least important problem of all because the cleft in it can be covered so easily and with extremely successful results by means of a simple acrylic or alloy prosthesis. If the cleft in the hard palate is wide its repair by surgery may result in contraction of the dental arch and maxilla and the cleft may be disturbed by the subsequent orthodontic treatment.

Prosthetic treatment of soft palate clefts

The treatment of clefts in the soft palate is by means of an obturator, sometimes called a speech bulb. Its method of function and its form are described later but, basically, it is a smooth acrylic appliance lying in the plane of maximal pharyngeal contraction so that when the pharynx is relaxed there is a space between it and the appliance allowing free passage of air to and from the nose, and when the pharynx is contracted it grips the acrylic, producing an airtight seal of the nasopharyngeal isthmus.

Types of obturator

Obturators are of three varieties:

1. Fixed pharyngeal.
2. Hinged pharyngeal.
3. Meatal.

The fixed is an extension of a denture projecting into the pharynx at about the level of the anterior arch of the atlas and shaped so that it can be gripped by the pharyngeal walls. The hinged is attached to the posterior border of a denture by a hinge and its lateral borders are shaped so that they may be gripped by the remnants of the soft palate and be raised and lowered with them. The meatal obturator is an extension of the back of the denture, upwards at right angles to it, so that it occludes the opening of the posterior nares. Prosthetists employ the fixed pharyngeal obturator almost always and this is the only one which will be described. The reasons for this are as follows: the hinged obturator is supposedly designed to function as a substitute soft palate and imitate the movements of the normal soft palate but, as will be seen later, this is impossible to achieve; the second criticism of the hinged obturator is that the hinge is a source of weakness and frequently comes out of alignment.

The meatal obturator is only used in cases presenting a very large cleft and is extremely difficult to adjust so that it prevents the nasal escape of air when speaking the oral consonants and yet does not produce hyponasality of the nasal consonants and vowels; also this obturator does not help the patient when swallowing.

Anatomy of the soft palate and pharynx

The soft palate is a curtain of soft tissue attached anteriorly to the lower surface of the posterior border of the hard palate and laterally to the walls of the pharynx. Its posterior border is free and hanging centrally from it is the uvula. The soft palate is composed mainly of extrinsic muscles and covered with mucous membrane, ciliated on its nasal surface and squamous on its oral surface and distal part of the nasal surface.

The muscles inserted into the soft palate are paired, one entering from each side as follows.

Tensor palati descend from their origins on the base of the skull and lateral surface of the cartilaginous part of the pharyngotympanic tube and, curving by means of tendons round the hamular processes of the medial pterygoid plates, fan out into the aponeurosis of the soft palate which they themselves help to form. Their function is to lower and tense the soft palate from side to side. They are the first to contract in any movement of the palate because they tense the aponeurosis and provide a firm base upon which the other muscles can act; they are particularly active in swallowing.

Levator palati originate from the base of the skull and medial surface of the cartilaginous part of the pharyngotympanic tube and, descending slightly forwards and inwards, are inserted into the soft palate over a wide area of the middle third. If the mouth is opened widely when saying ‘ah’, two depressions can be seen on the oral surface of the soft palate which coincide with the nasal insertions of the levators. The levators raise the soft palate and pull it backwards into contact with the posterior pharyngeal wall.

Palatopharyngeus muscles have two insertions into the soft palate, one above and one below the insertion of the levators. They curve laterally and posteriorly into the walls of the pharynx with some fibres descending to their origin from the thyroid cartilage. Covered with mucous membrane, this pair of muscles forms the posterior pillars of the fauces. Their function is to lower the sides of the soft palate and to approximate them. They are particularly active in swallowing.

Palatoglossus muscles originate from the sides and base of the tongue and, curving outwards and upwards, enter the undersurface of the soft palate. Covered with mucous membrane they form the anterior pillars of the fauces. They function to raise the back of the tongue and lower the soft palate and are most active in swallowing.

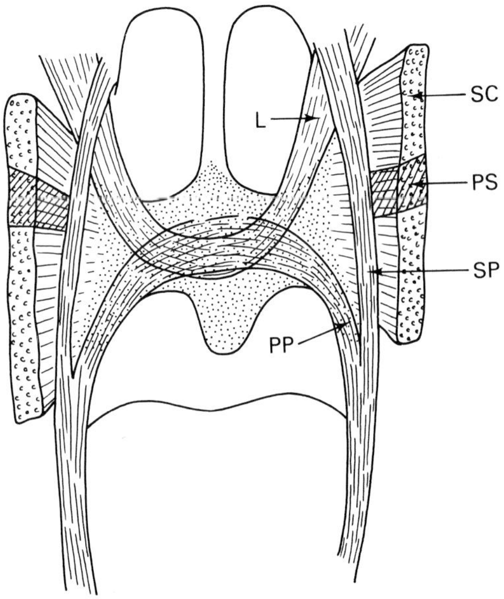

Figure 28.5 Diagrammatic representation of muscles of soft palate and pharynx seen from behind. SC, lateral wall of superior constrictor; PS, palatopharyngeal sphincter; SP, salpingopharyngeus; PP, palatopharyngeus; L, levator palati

Pharynx: the upper part of the pharynx is surrounded by the superior constrictor muscle which is slung by its central raphe and pharyngobasilar fascia from the base of the skull. Its anterior border continues downwards and forwards to be attached to the posterior edge of the medial pterygoid plate. Below this, fibres are inserted into the aponeurosis of the soft palate and the hamular process. These muscle fibres circle the pharynx to form the palatopharyngeal sphincter of Whillis. Below this level the superior constrictor is inserted into the pterygomandibular raphe and finally at its lower border into the mylohyoid ridge with some fibres running inwards to be inserted into the tongue.

The space between the upper border of the superior constrictor and the base of the skull is filled by the pharyngobasilar fascia. Looked at from above in horizontal section the superior constrictor muscle is roughly pear-shaped. Lying in the lateral corners of the pharynx and running downwards from their origin on the inferior part of the pharyngotympanic tube to mingle with the fibres of the palatopharyngeus muscle are the salpingopharyngeus muscles which, covered with mucous membrane, form the salpingopharyngeal folds (Figures 28.5 and 28.6).

Action of the pharynx and soft palate

The action of the pharynx is complex but basically it contracts from side to side and its posterior surface moves forwards. It is capable of local contractions at various levels, mainly used in speech, and also peristaltic type of contractions which travel downwards and which are employed during swallowing. The inward movement of the sides of the pharynx is markedly reinforced by the salpingopharyngeus muscles. The function of the soft palate and pharynx must be considered as one because they act in unison to form a combination between a flap valve and a sphincter. The various muscles of the palatopharyngeal complex act rapidly and accurately together to open and close the nasopharyngeal isthmus.

Speech

The tensor muscles contract to tense the aponeurosis to form a firm base from which the other muscles may act. The lateral walls of the pharynx contract and move inwards reinforced by the salpingopharyngeus muscles. The levator muscles raise the middle third of the soft palate and bunch it up so that it

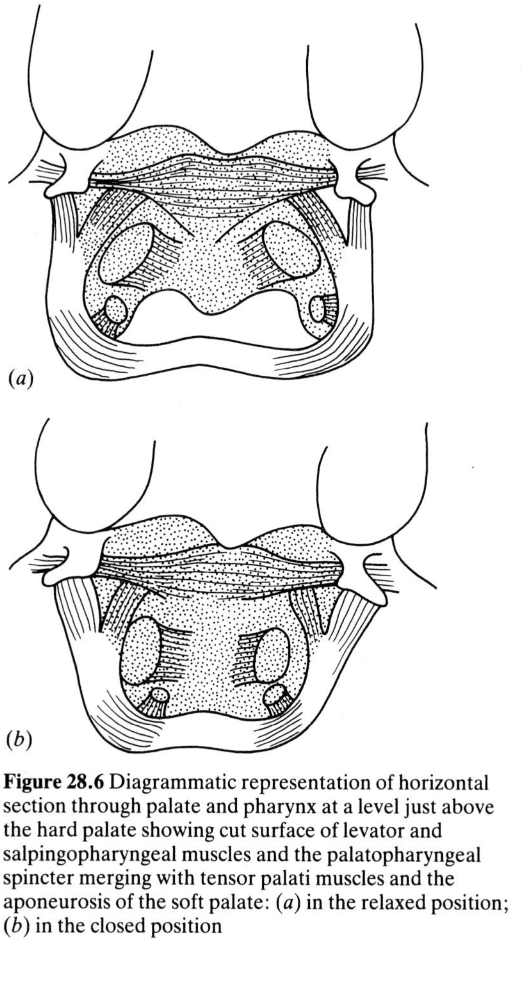

Figure 28.6 Diagrammatic representation of horizontal section through palate and pharynx at a level just above the hard palate showing cut surface of levator and salpingopharyngeal muscles and the palatopharyngeal spincter merging with tensor palati muscles and the aponeurosis of the soft palate: (*a*) in the relaxed position; (*b*) in the closed position

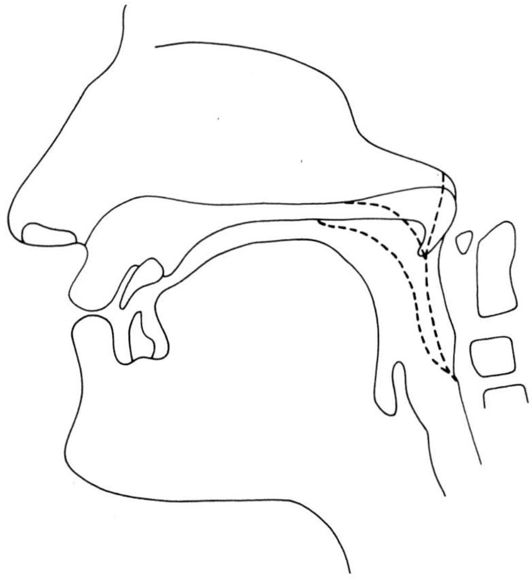

Figure 28.7 Illustrates positions of soft palate and posterior pharyngeal wall during speech. Dotted line indicates both when swallowing. Note marked forward shift of pharyngeal wall in swallowing position

becomes thicker from above downwards than when relaxed. The posterior third of the soft palate hangs downwards and the uvula curves away from the posterior pharyngeal wall. This position of the palate and pharynx is a preparatory position and when speech commences short rapid movements of raising and lowering the palate, brought about by the levator muscles, close and open the nasopharyngeal isthmus a limited amount depending on the sound which is being produced. The more explosive the sound the higher the palate rises. The forward movement of the pharynx during speech is small and the area of contact of the palate and pharynx during speech is well above the anterior arch of the atlas, i.e. well above the area of the palatopharyngeal sphincter of Whillis (Figure 28.7).

Swallowing

The tensor muscles contract lowering the anterior third of the soft palate so that the palate grips the bolus of the food between itself and the tongue. The lateral walls of the pharynx contract and the posterior wall moves forwards. The levator muscles pull the middle third of the palate backwards and the palatopharyngeus muscles pull the palate downwards and inwards into contact with the posterior pharyngeal wall. The posterior third of the tongue is raised upwards and backwards, thus contributing to the protection of the opening into the pharynx. The palatopharyngeal sphincter contracts to produce a circular muscular ring at the level of the anterior arch of the atlas which grips the soft palate (Figures 28.8; 28.9). Waves of contraction then travel down the pharynx from this level. The ring-like contraction of the palatopharyngeal sphincter produces the ridge of Passavant. Contact of the soft palate with the pharynx during speech occurs in the normal person at a higher level than the ridge of Passavant.

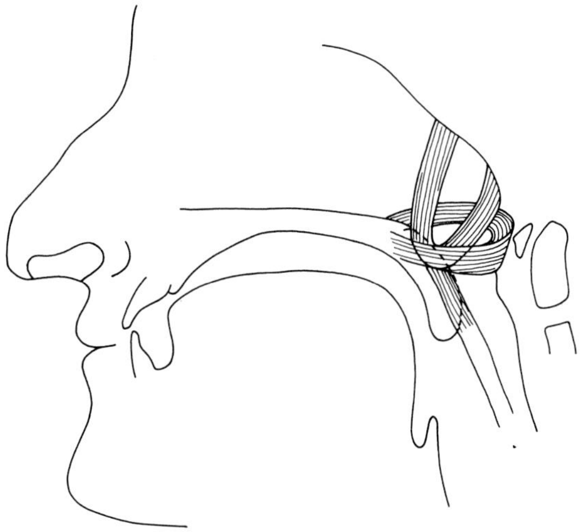

Figure 28.8 Diagrammatic representation of the action of the levator and palatopharyngeal muscles and the sphincter when closing the pharynx for swallowing: in the relaxed position

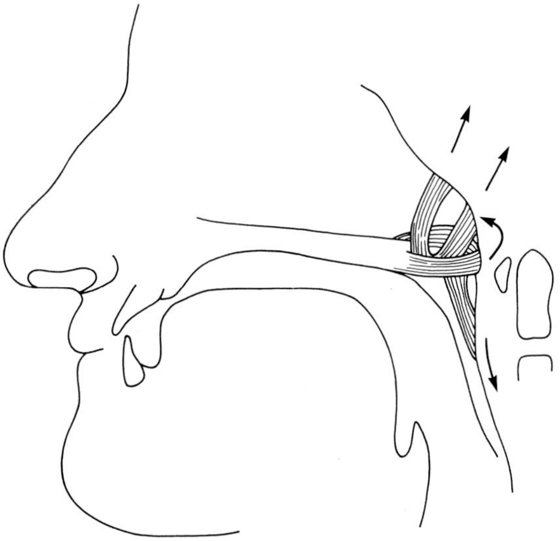

Figure 28.9 See Figure 28.8. The closed position in swallowing. The direction of contraction of the various muscles is indicated by the arrows

Action of the muscles in clefts

The function of the muscles is similar to the normal but the results are different. The contraction of the tensor muscles, palatoglossus and palatopharyngeus, tends to draw the two halves of the soft palate away from one another in the area of their insertions. The contraction of the levators, although tending to pull the remnants of the palate away from one another while drawing them upwards and backwards, tends, by the increase in the bulk of the middle third of the palate which this contraction produces, to close the cleft to some extent. In an attempt to overcome this disability the palatopharyngeal sphincter invariably hypertrophies and endeavours to squeeze the muscles of the soft palate together and close the cleft. In cases of a small cleft this action may be reasonably successful. The other method employed by a patient with a cleft palate to close the gap, is to push the dorsum of the tongue into the space and swallow down the sides of the tongue. It is this action and habit which has such a disastrous effect on speech. Another habit which the patient acquires in an attempt to prevent the nasal escape of air is to contract the nares and, in untreated or uncompensated cases of cleft palate, this action is most noticeable, although its results are quite unsuccessful.

This is the basic muscular pattern therefore into which an obturator has to be fitted and, although marked individual variations exist, the basic task of the dentist is to place the obturator so that the muscles of the remnants of the soft palate and pharynx can grip it and thus enable the patient to close off the nasopharynx from the oropharynx at will.

Obturator position

The position of an obturator should accommodate the cleft in both the functions of speaking and swallowing even though the shape and action of the pharynx differs so much in these two actions. The fact that the method by which a patient uses an obturator is entirely by gripping it with his ring or sphincter mechanism and squeezing the remnants of the soft palate against it means that the plane of location of the obturator must be in the plane of action of the palatopharyngeal sphincter or ridge of Passavant. In practice an obturator is shaped by luting a piece of softened gutta-percha to a wire loop extending from the posterior border of the denture along the midline of the cleft into the pharynx. The gutta-percha is then shaped by the muscles as they function. Details of this technique are given later.

Horizontal plane

When the muscles contract the palatopharyngeal sphincter produces the ridge of Passavant on the posterior wall of the pharynx. It runs laterally outside the salpingopharyngeal muscles which form raised vertical ridges in the corners of the pharynx before going lateral to the remnants of the soft palate containing the levator muscles. Figure 28.10 shows in horizontal section at the level of the hard palate the relationship of the levator and salpingopharyngeal muscles and the sphincter in both the relaxed and contracted positions when an unrepaired cleft is present and illustrates how an obturator positioned in the plane of the palatopharyngeal sphincter will be related to these structures both when relaxed and when contracted. It will be observed that in the first diagram there is a space between the obturator and its related structures which allows air to pass freely to and from the nose, whereas in the second diagram the surrounding musculature grips the periphery of the obturator firmly, producing an efficient seal of the oronasal isthmus.

Shape of obturators

It will be observed that the obturator illustrated in Figure 28.10 is T-shaped and this is because the remnants of the soft palate are well-developed and

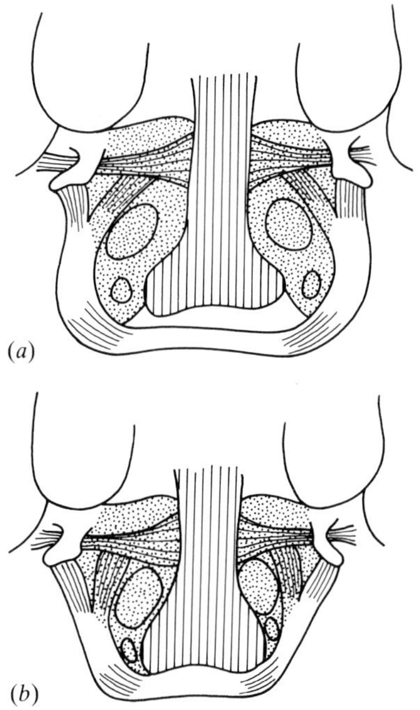

Figure 28.10 Horizontal section through the pharynx and palate at the level of the hard palate. (*a*) The obturator in position with the remnants of the soft palate and pharynx relaxed. Note space for air to pass from nasopharynx to oropharynx. (*b*) Palatal remnants and pharynx constricted tightly round obturator sealing off nasopharynx from oropharynx

their contained levator muscles, being bulky when squeezed inwards by the palatopharyngeal sphincter, produce a neck between the posterior border of the denture and the pharyngeal section of the obturator. The width and anteroposterior dimension of the obturator will vary from patient to patient depending on the size of the pharynx and the degree of hypertrophy of the palatopharyngeal sphincter. In some cases, two small horn-like processes develop on the obturator as it is shaped. These result from the extension of the obturator into the lateral pharyngeal recess which in some patients appears to be inactive. The inactivity is probably due to the weakness of the salpingopharyngeal muscles which normally close this area of the pharynx and it is probable that closure of the pharynx will be quite effective without them. In the first instance the obturator should always be tried without these processes, only replacing them if an air leak is experienced. This outline of the horizontal form of an obturator may be considered as the basic type and is designated *group A*. There are, however, three other modifications of this basic shape depending on the form and activity of the enveloping tissues.

Group B: those which develop when the soft palatal remnants are small and inactive. This group also includes those cases where surgical intervention has been unsuccessful and resulted in deformed remnants which are partially or completely bound to the lateral pharyngeal walls by scar tissue and are partially or completely immobile.

Group C: those cases in which a good union of the soft palatal remnants has been achieved, but where the resultant palate is too short or insufficiently functional to close the oronasal isthmus completely.

Group D: those cases in which the united soft palate is functional posteriorly at the expense of a palatal cleft between the posterior border of the hard palate and the anterior border of the united soft palate.

The modification in the horizontal form of the obturator group B is entirely the result of the inactivity or smallness of the levator muscles which therefore do not produce the neck and have a horizontal form which is pear-shaped or circular.

Group C differ from the preceding types mainly by the fact that the neck section joining the obturator to the denture does not function as part of the obturator by occluding the palatal section of the cleft but merely acts as a bridge to unite the pharyngeal section to the denture. The pharyngeal bulb of the obturators in this class is moulded by the pharynx and palatopharyngeal sphincter on their posterior and lateral surfaces in the same way as the other classes, but the anterior surface of the bulb is moulded by the posterior border of the united soft palate and the degree of moulding will depend on the degree of activity of the muscles of the palate. The general form of such obturators is that of a flattened ellipse which varies in size depending on the degree of failure of the soft palate to close with the pharyngeal walls.

Group D obturators are mainly static and not moulded by any muscle action at all except perhaps to a limited amount on their posterior border by the slight rise and fall of the anterior border of the repaired soft palate as its posterior section functions to close the oronasal isthmus.

The sagittal shape of the upper and lower surfaces of obturators is discussed more fully later.

To make an obturator or not?

To make such a decision it is convenient to divide patients into three classes:

(a) Those not suitable for surgical closure of the soft palate.
(b) Those who have grown up without any surgical treatment.
(c) Those who have had unsuccessful surgical treatment.

Class (a) patients should be fitted with an obturator as soon as they are old enough to allow it to remain in place. In most cases this will be between the second and third year. The fitting of an obturator should not be delayed later than this otherwise bad habits of speech will be developed.

Class (b) patients require very careful consideration because there are three possibilities and it is important that the correct one be selected.

The first possibility is that no treatment at all be given. Some individuals who have reached maturity with no treatment for their cleft have adapted to the disability remarkably well. They can swallow liquids and solids competently with no nasal escape and their speech, although exhibiting marked hypernasality, is sufficiently intelligible for them to be understood. Others however suffer from such degradation of speech that they are quite unintelligible. The possible lines of treatment for these patients are a denture carrying an obturator, or surgical repair of the cleft, both aimed primarily at improving speech. The success of either treatment will depend on the intelligence and acuity of hearing of the patient and his desire to improve his speech because, in adult life, improvement of speech demands the eradication of faulty habits.

Class (c) is perhaps the most difficult class of case in which to make a decision as to whether an obturator will benefit as surgery has produced a united soft palate but without any marked improvement of speech. In these cases a diagnosis must be made as to the cause of failure. It may be due to faults of speech which the patient has been unable to eradicate either because of lack of perseverance or of desire to improve or because of dullness of hearing or lack of intelligence. It may, on the other hand, be due to failure of function of the palate which, although it appears from examination through the mouth to be long enough and sufficiently functional to occlude the nasopharyngeal isthmus, is in fact neither of these.

Examination of palatopharyngeal contact by observation through the mouth is misleading because the main area of contact of the palate with the pharynx is in the middle third of the palate which is bunched up by the action of the levators and this cannot be seen by observations through the mouth. A palate which appears long enough may in fact entirely lack this bunching up action. Another test of palatopharyngeal closure (which in many cases is valueless) is blowing up a balloon or manometer, although frequently an individual with palatal insufficiency, or even a patent cleft, can produce a quite impressive rise of mercury by pushing the short palate up with the back of the tongue. Two tests which are valuable, however, are the snoring test and a lateral cephalograph.

Snoring results from drawing air in through the nose and by its passage to the lungs forcefully separating the raised soft palate from the pharyngeal wall. The air passes in a series of short puffs causing the soft palate to vibrate producing the snoring sound. If the soft palate is incapable of making firm contact with the pharynx snoring is impossible.

A lateral cephalograph is taken after several drops of barium solution have been introduced into each nostril while the individual is lying down and the head gently moved from side to side to spread the barium over the palate and pharynx. The exposure should be made while the patient is making the action of sounding a prolonged 'P' but without actually parting the lips. This will cause the soft palate to rise to its high level if it is capable of so doing. Several cephalographs may be needed to produce convincing evidence of palatal position and function and frequently reveal what appears from oral examination to be an adequate palate to be merely a thin sheet of soft tissue completely out of contact with the posterior pharyngeal wall. At other times, it reveals a fully functional and competent palate. In the former case an obturator shaped and placed to occlude the space which exists between the repaired soft palate and the pharynx is justified and frequently produces excellent results.

Clinical techniques

There are some differences in the technique for making an obturator for those cases where the cleft is patent along the length of the soft palate or hard and soft palates, and those where surgery has produced a united but incompetent soft palate. The differences in technique only apply up to the point of commencing to trim the speech bulb but thereafter they are similar. Up to this point therefore they will be described separately.

Unrepaired cleft of hard and soft palates

A compound impression is taken in a stock tray. There is no need to extend this impression much beyond the posterior border of the hard palate as nothing is to be gained at this stage by trying to obtain a comprehensive impression of the remnants of the soft palate and the pharynx. In cases with unrepaired clefts involving both the hard and soft palates the compound will of its own accord flow upwards into the cleft in the hard palate.

An acrylic individual tray is made to straddle the cleft in the hard palate but not contoured into it. In this tray an alginate or elastomer impression is made. Normally no impression material is placed in the cleft because, if an adequate amount is put on the tray, sufficient flows into the cleft to give a satisfactory impression and if too much material is present it may flow excessively on to the nasal side of the cleft of the hard palate and when the tray is removed the material will tear, leaving the nasal section of the impression *in situ*. If this does happen, in most cases it can be retrieved by inserting a probe deeply into the remnant of the impression and sliding it back towards the soft palatal cleft where it can be brought downwards into the mouth. Sometimes, however, the nasal section becomes locked into place and then has to be removed piecemeal which can be a trying procedure for both the patient and the dentist and, as nothing is gained by obtaining an excessive impression of the nasal cavities, it is wiser to limit the impression material in this region. In wide clefts problems are not usually encountered with excess material, but in narrow ones, or those where surgery has left a hole or series of holes in the palate, it is wise to pack these with petroleum jelly gauze prior to the impression, for if alginate does flow into the nose through a small defect, serious difficulty may be experienced in its removal (Figure 28.11).

The working cast from this master impression is produced in stone. The cleft in the hard palate is filled in with plaster to reproduce the contour of a normal palate and a record block constructed.

At the trial stage a nickel silver wire loop is bent to shape and attached to the base of the denture. This loop should lie along the centre of the cleft of the soft palate, completely out of contact with its remnants or with the posterior pharyngeal wall when a prolonged 'Ah' is sounded, and its plane should be slightly above that to which the soft palate remnants rise when the 'Ah' sound is made. It should be adjusted by bending and altering its position on the base until it satisfies these require-

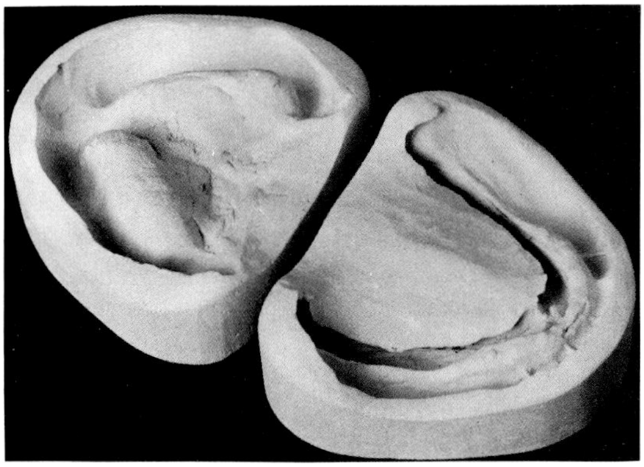

Figure 28.11 Preliminary casts of small enclosed defect of hard palate showing how cleft was occluded with gauze prior to recording alginate impression

ments. If the loop is made of nickel silver wire it is more easily adjusted than if made of stainless steel. When the trial denture is satisfactory it is returned to the cast and plaster flowed around the wire loop to hold it in position and the case processed and finished. The denture is now ready for the trimming of the speech bulb.

In those cases where difficulty with regard to wearing the denture is anticipated it is sometimes desirable to leave the wire loop off the denture altogether and allow the patient to wear the denture for a week or two until it is quite comfortable. The wire loop may then be added to the denture with cold-cure acrylic.

Repaired but incompetent soft palates

After the denture has been completed and fitted, a tailpiece must be made and positioned so that when attached to the posterior edge of the denture it crosses the united soft palate at a level just below that which the latter assumes when fully relaxed. If the tailpiece is at a higher level when the soft palate relaxes it will rest on the tailpiece which, being narrow, will cause discomfort and areas of pressure. If, on the other hand, the plane of the tailpiece is much below that assumed by the relaxed soft palate, then it will cause discomfort by obstructing the movements of the tongue.

The technique of locating the plane of the tailpiece is as follows: to the posterior edge of the denture a piece of pink base-plate wax is luted with sticky wax, this wax being about 9 mm wide and long enough to cross the soft palate into the pharynx. The denture carrying the wax is then inserted into the mouth and the patient asked to relax and breathe through the nose. If left in place for a few minutes the wax will be moulded by the relaxed soft palate above and the tongue below to conform to the plane and contour of the relaxed palate. The denture is carefully removed and the wax chilled thoroughly. The denture is then replaced in the mouth and a check made of the plane of the wax in relation to the relaxed soft palate when observed with the mouth open. To do this the patient is asked to open the mouth, to relax fully and breathe through the nose; if there is any appearance of the wax supporting the soft palate the shaping technique as previously described should be repeated. When the plane and contour of the wax is satisfactory, a plaster cast is poured under the palatal side of the wax and extending sufficiently far under the denture to enable it to be located.

When the plaster is set, and this will only take a few minutes if an accelerator is used, the wax is removed, the plaster painted with sodium alginate separator and a thin mix of cold-cure acrylic is run on to the plaster in place of the wax and carried on to the back of the denture which has been roughened sufficiently to ensure a firm union. When the cold-cure acrylic has hardened it is trimmed, rough polished and tried in the mouth to ensure it is in the same relation to the soft palate as was the wax. The pharyngeal end of the cold cure tailpiece is then grooved, holes bored in it and a piece of gutta-percha, softened in boiling water, firmly secured to the tailpiece and roughly shaped into a flattened ellipse, with its long axis lying laterally.

The denture carrying this tailpiece and gutta-percha is then inserted into the mouth and the gutta-percha gently pressed upwards, behind the soft palate, into the region of the nasopharynx and the patient requested to swallow, say 'Ah' and move the head from side to side. A drink of warm water, or preferably hot tea, will facilitate swallowing. This action will bring the muscular pressure of the posterior and the lateral walls of the pharynx and the posterior border of the soft palate to bear on the softened gutta-percha and shape it to conform to the space which exists in the nasopharyngeal isthmus due to the incompetence of the soft palate.

The denture is then removed and the gutta-percha inspected; it will probably have increased in dimension from above to below and become flattened anteroposteriorly and show evidence of moulding. Its periphery, where the gutta-percha has been squeezed into the nasopharynx, should be trimmed slightly with a very hot wax knife which will cut the gutta-percha easily without dragging. The gutta-percha should then be dipped into very hot water and tested for temperature on the back of the hand because gutta-percha, being a very poor thermal conductor, holds its heat. The denture is inserted into the mouth and the trimming routine repeated. In order to check that the gutta-percha has been moulded by the delicate tissues of the palate instead of distorting them, some pressure-indicating paste is applied to the dried palatal surface of the acrylic tailpiece and the anterior surface of the gutta-percha, the whole reinserted and the trimming routine repeated. On removal, a completely unbroken film of white paste with clear-cut evidence of tissue moulding should be evident. If the black gutta-percha or acrylic has penetrated the white film this is evidence of distortion of the tissues by the hard material and some of it should be removed in the area indicated, the denture reinserted and retrimmed.

When this impression is satisfactory, a plaster cast is poured, including the fitting surface of the denture, the palatal surface of the tailpiece and the anterior surface of the gutta-percha pharyngeal section as one piece. When the plaster has set a second plaster core is poured to the posterior surface of the pharyngeal section after the first cast has been painted with separator to prevent union of the core. This technique ensures that the gutta-percha can be removed from the pharyngeal part of the cast easily by separating the two halves of the cast. When the plaster is set the whole is placed in hot water to soften the gutta-percha, then the cast is divided, and the gutta-percha and the denture removed. This plaster cast is an accurate reproduction of the position of the central area of the relaxed soft palate and the deficient area of the pharynx when contracted and to it an accurately shaped and fitting tailpiece in cast metal can be made.

Construction of the permanent tailpiece

The temporary acrylic tailpiece is cut from the denture and the back and lingual surfaces of the denture grooved to receive the retaining tag of the permanent tailpiece which is outlined on the cast as a flat, fairly narrow bar and as thin as is commensurate with adequate strength. Casting wax is laid down to this outline and carried into the tag grooves of the denture and extended into the pharyngeal section of the impression to within 3 mm of the posterior pharyngeal wall. To the undersurface of the wax in this region a wax post 6 mm long and 3 mm diameter is attached, extending centrally upwards into the nasopharynx. To this the final speech bulb will be attached. The completed wax pattern is cast in cobalt–chromium, trimmed and polished and attached to the denture with cold cure acrylic. The assembly is now ready for the final trimming of the speech bulb.

Shaping the speech bulb

In both the case of the patent cleft and the repaired but incompetent palate, the speech bulb is formed in gutta-percha and fully adjusted to fit the movements of the pharynx and palatal remnants before being processed in acrylic.

A ball of gutta-percha is roughly adapted with the fingers to either the wire loop or tailpiece and conformed to the shape of the deficiency as it appears on the master cast, i.e. T-shaped, pear-shaped or a flattened ellipse.

The denture is inserted into the mouth and gutta-percha pressed with the fingers upwards and backwards into the pharynx. The patient should be given a cup of hot tea to drink; the heat of the tea will tend to maintain the ability of the gutta-percha to flow. The swallowing action this initiated will cause the palatopharyngeal sphincter to contract and the muscles of the soft palate to function and they will mould the gutta-percha so that it fills the space and adapts to the form of the functioning muscles. After several sips of tea the denture is removed and the gutta-percha inspected. A limited change will have taken place in its shape and it should show evidence of having been moulded; the posterior border should show a tendency to be flattened, the lateral corners a tendency to roundness and, in the case of a T-shaped cleft, the lateral surfaces a tendency to narrowing. The pear-shaped clefts will produce less or no narrowing at all, but show evidence of a side-to-side flattening while the repaired soft palate type will show evidence on its anterior surface of moulding by the posterior border of the unrepaired palate.

If the amount of gutta-percha is excessive, the excess will have been forced mostly up into the nasopharynx but a little may have escaped downwards, between the back of the tongue and the posterior pharyngeal wall. If insufficient gutta-percha was present to fill the cleft, none will have been forced into the nasopharynx and some of its surfaces will show no evidence of moulding. The moulded surfaces will develop a matt appearance and those not moulded will still retain some of the shiny appearance of the gutta-percha as originally inserted. Where evidence of excess gutta-percha is present it should be removed with a hot wax knife. Where a deficiency appears more soft gutta-percha should be added by drying and flaming both the surfaces to be united. After these adjustments the gutta-percha bulb should be dipped in hot water for about a minute and, after testing for temperature, reinserted in the mouth and more tea drunk. This routine should be carried out several times and on each removal further evidence of moulding or lack of it will be evident with its need for removal or addition of gutta-percha.

When swallowing has impressed a definite form on the gutta-percha, movements of the head should be instituted because these have an effect on the shape of the pharynx, and if the gutta-percha is not moulded to accommodate them the finished speech bulb will cause pressure and probably ulceration when such movements are made. The patient is therefore requested to bend the head forward and then move it from side to side. These actions should be performed several times. Next the action of speaking should be induced to mould the gutta-percha and the patient should be asked to say some of the explosive consonants, which produce the greatest action of the pharynx and palate, as forcefully as possible. By this time the gutta-percha bulb will have developed a definite form around its periphery, but its superior and inferior surfaces and its thickness will be variable. These should now be adjusted and to do this the ridge of Passavant should be evoked by asking the patient to say 'Ah' with the mouth open and the ridge painted with disclosing paste. The denture is replaced and the patient asked to say 'Ah' and swallow. When the denture is removed the area of action of the ridge of Passavant will be visible as a white smudge on the back of the gutta-percha and the bung should then be trimmed superiorly and inferiorly so that it is 3 mm above the highest plane and 1.5 mm below the lowest plane of travel of the ridge.

The form of the inferior surface should be gently concave looking downwards because this shape will allow the greatest amount of room for the dorsum of the tongue and also deflect the airstream from the larynx into the mouth. The upper surface should curve as steeply as possible towards the pharynx so that nasal secretions can flow backwards towards the throat.

By now the gutta-percha bulb should be of comfortable proportions with the patient tolerating it easily. It is softened in hot water once more and then the patient dismissed to wear it for 24 h.

When the patient returns it will be found in most cases that the bulb has undergone further moulding, especially in the areas within the grasp of the palatopharyngeal sphincter and, in the case of T-shaped bulbs, in the region of the levator muscles. Excess gutta-percha which has been squeezed upwards and downwards by this action should be trimmed away and the patient questioned regarding the feel of the speech bulb. If a complaint of soreness is made the whole bulb should be coated with paste and the patient given more tea to drink. Pressure spots should be trimmed with a hot wax knife and more paste applied. This should be continued until the black gutta-percha remains covered by the white paste. If swallowing becomes more difficult with the bulb in place it may be due to the fact that the inferior surface of the bulb is too concave and part of the food bolus lodges in it. A flattening of the concavity should be effected. In most cases where nasal breathing is impeded it will be found by the white paste test that the whole bulb is over size so that the tissues are unable to relax away from it and produce a breathing space. In these cases the whole bulb should be re-softened and the whole cycle of trimming movements vigorously and persistently repeated. If any doubt exists that the bulb is not fully or correctly adapted it should be wiped clear of white paste, fully re-softened and the patient dismissed for another 24 h.

When the bulb appears to have reached a final shape, and no hard areas of gutta-percha are visible through the paste, the whole is invested in plaster, the gutta-percha and paste removed and the resulting cavity filled with wax and processed in acrylic. If the denture is well-retained and the speech bulb is not too large the latter can be made of solid acrylic. If the denture is poorly retained or the speech bulb is large, then to reduce the weight of the appliance the speech bulb can be made hollow.

After-care of patients

It will take time for a patient to adapt to wearing an obturator for a soft palate defect and he must be encouraged to learn to grip the bulb when speaking as in the act of swallowing.

The only improvement in the voice to be anticipated when the obturator is fitted is in the tone: the deeply ingrained faults of articulation will only be rectified by speech training given by an experienced therapist, to whom the patient should be referred when the obturator has been fitted. Close cooperation with the speech therapist will ensure any adjustment in the shape of the speech bulb which may be necessary as progress in voice production is made.

Silicone retentive obturator

In congenital clefts of the hard palate, enclosed or open-ended, and in many acquired clefts, a useful form of obturator is made of silicone (or latex rubber) which is attached to the denture by studs. The fact that the obturator is removable and replaceable is good from the point of view of hygiene and also means that adjustments and alterations can be made to the obturator independently of the denture itself. The design is particularly useful in the edentulous cleft patient but is also very helpful in large acquired defects of the palate where retention is a major problem.

The stages are as follows (Figures 28.12–28.18):

1. Cut a postdam 5 mm from the edge of the cleft on the master cast (Figure 28.12).
2. Fill the cleft with wax and carve to the contour of a normal palate.
3. Add a sheet of wax.
4. Embed two studs (Figure 28.13).
5. Take an impression of the cast in elastomer (Figure 28.14).
6. Add two studs to the impression (Figure 28.15) and pour it to produce a working cast (Figure 28.16).

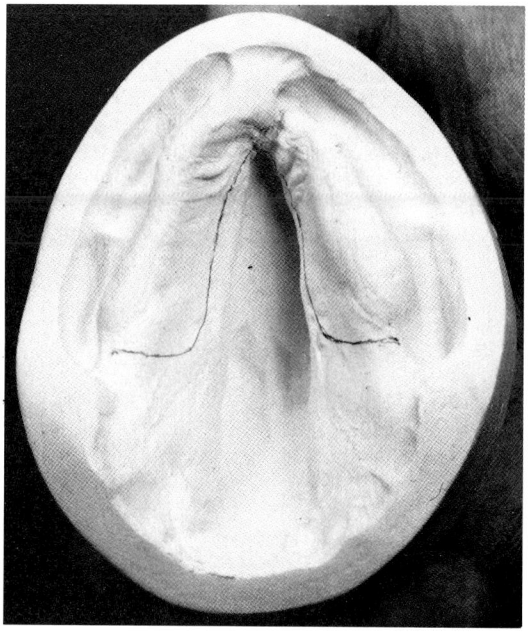

Figure 28.12 Open-end defect in a congenital cleft. Marking the outline of the postdam

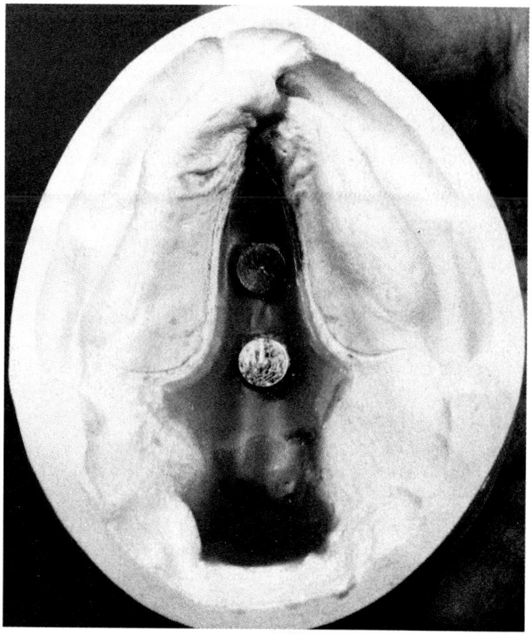

Figure 28.13 The cleft is filled with wax and two studs are located

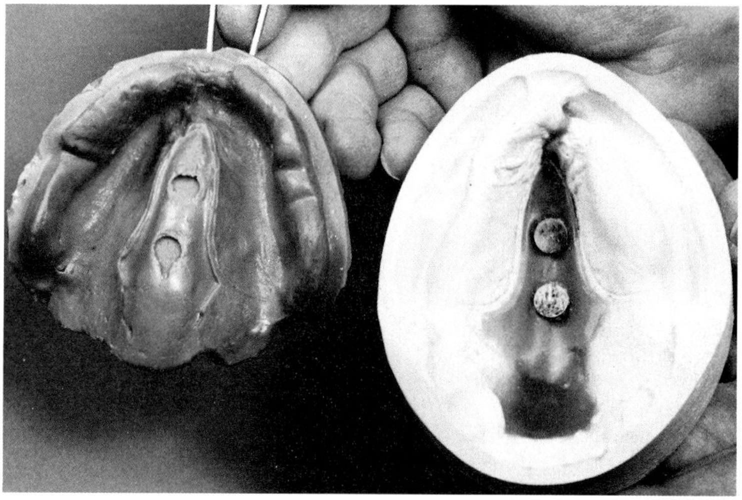

Figure 28.14 An elastomeric impression is made

7. Use the working cast to make a complete denture (Figure 28.17).
8. Pour a plaster register to the master cast to hold the studs in relation to the cleft.
9. Fill the cleft with silicone rubber to produce the obturator which is retained on the studs on the denture (Figure 28.18).
10. The master cast serves as a permanent mould for replacement obturators.
11. If soft palate obturation is required then gutta-percha can be added to the silicone obturator and, after moulding in the mouth, returned to the master mould and studs prior to making a new, accurate mould.

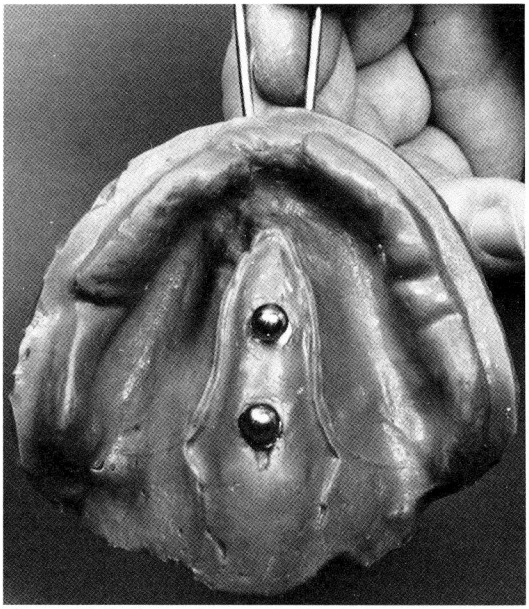

Figure 28.15 Two studs are tacked to the impression. Note postdam and butt edge round cleft

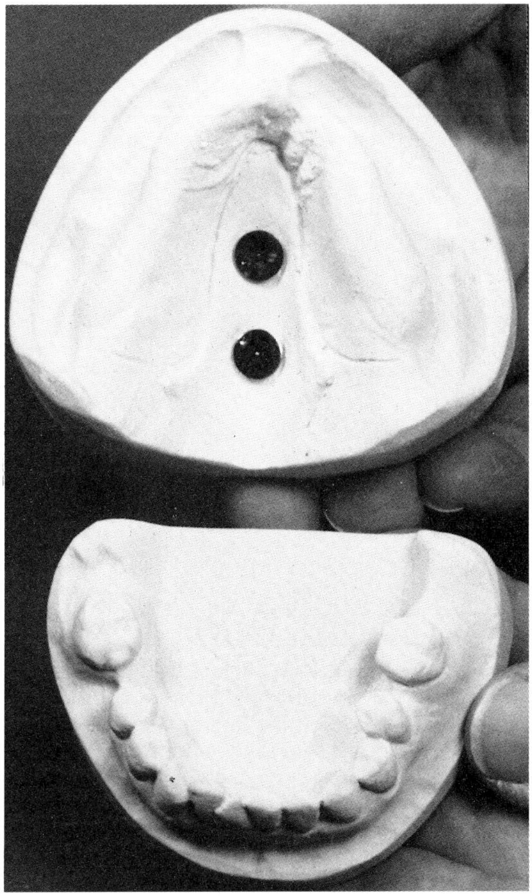

Figure 28.16 The working cast

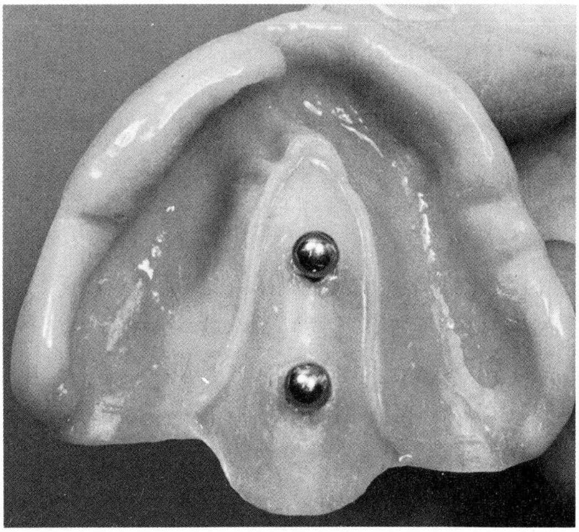

Figure 28.17 The finished acrylic denture. The wide labial flange will assist in restoring the repaired cleft lip

Acquired clefts

The replacement of tissue lost from the mouth as the result of trauma, such as road accidents, gunshot wounds or surgery for the removal of malignancy, all comes within the province of prosthetic dentistry and the following section gives information on some appliances needed for the treatment of these conditions.

A common cause of tissue loss results from the removal of neoplastic tissue. Elective surgery frequently involves the alveolar process and part of the palate, resulting in a defect which may be either enclosed or open-ended.

In the enclosed type the facial contour is not affected and the retention of an obturator is not usually a problem although support of an appliance may be very difficult if the defect is large.

In the open-ended type there may be difficulties with speech, appearance and the design of the appliance because of poor retention and stability. Problems are usually greater if the defect is large and if the obturator is not retentive then speech is almost certainly impaired.

The prosthetic treatment for these conditions demands a preoperative and postoperative appliance.

The preoperative appliance consists of an acrylic base-plate made to an impression of the upper jaw taken preoperatively. Immediately after surgical removal of tissue the plate is inserted, the purpose

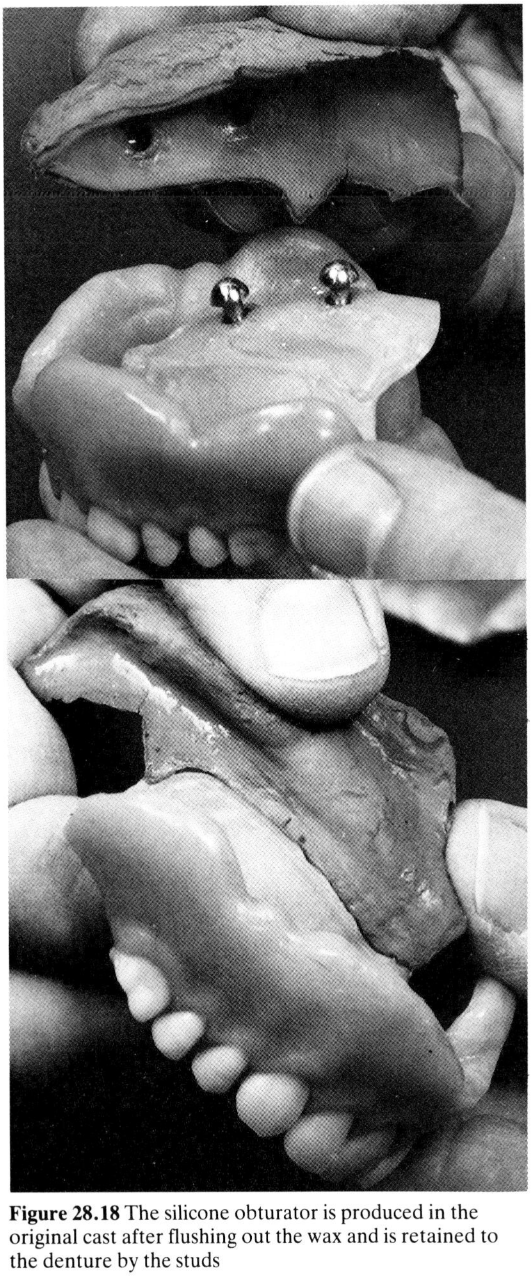

Figure 28.18 The silicone obturator is produced in the original cast after flushing out the wax and is retained to the denture by the studs

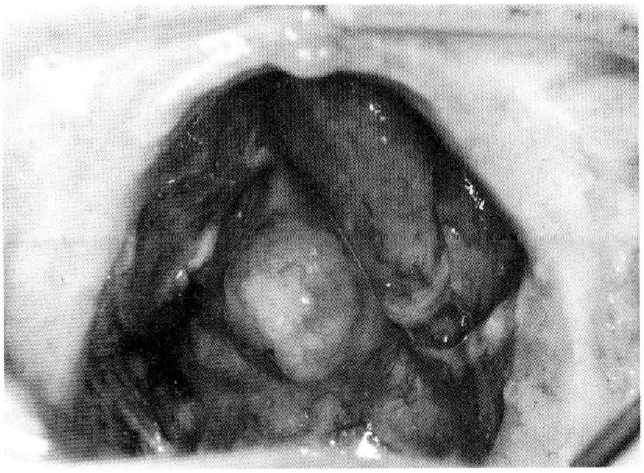

(*a*)

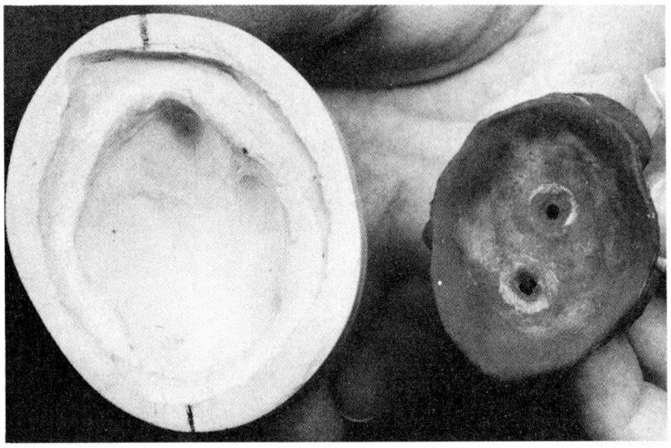

(*b*)

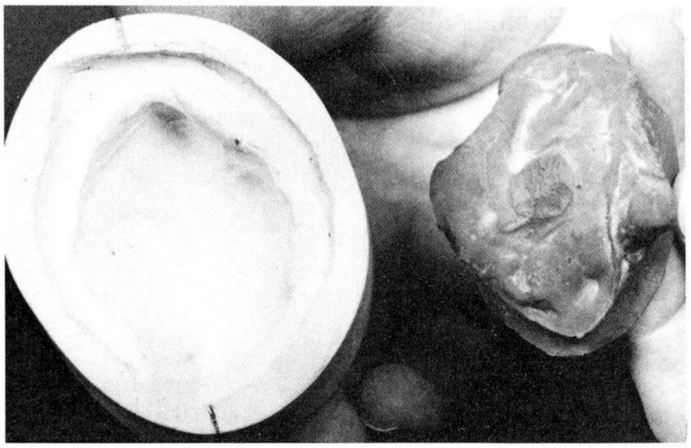

(*c*)

Figure 28.19 (*a*) Enclosed palatal defect resulting from surgical treatment of neoplasm. (*b*), (*c*) The cleft is obturated with hollow silicone retained to the denture by studs

of which is to maintain space and facial form and to enable the patient to speak, eat and drink normally. As soon as the wound has healed sufficiently and is no longer painful an impression is made in an individual tray, care being taken that excess alginate or elastomer does not flow into the nasal cavities and become locked in so that part remains in place on removal of the main impression. Judgment of the amount of impression material used is the simplest way to ensure this, but petroleum jelly gauze can be packed into parts of the nasal cavity if necessary.

On the cast poured from this impression an acrylic base-plate is constructed to the normal outline of an upper denture, penetrating into the cavity for as short a distance as is necessary to produce a seal. On this base-plate the jaw relation records and trial are carried out and then the denture is finished by processing teeth.

The retention of the denture will depend to some extent on the size of the cleft. If this is small the denture can be retained normally by selective adhesion and peripheral seal, although the latter is unreliable. Tooth position and design of the polished surface are important for muscular control.

In cases of extreme loss of tissue, such as when the whole of the palate is removed, the appliance may require to be made hollow to reduce its weight (Figure 28.19).

Enclosed defects

If more than one-third of the denture bearing area is missing the defect may be considered large; if less, then it is considered small, although no less important.

In large defects the nasal structures should be assessed for support and wherever possible the antral walls and roof should be used rather than the midline structures. If the obturator is to be load-bearing the impression should be taken in one piece if possible, although the entrance to the mouth, and the exit, may make this difficult. A one-piece impression, however, is always more reliable than a sectional as the part of the impression in the depth of the cleft may shift, albeit slightly, when the main impression is located to it in the mouth. If a sectional impression is taken the two parts are pinned together with stainless steel wire before pouring. The same is true of the appliance; a one-piece is better than a sectional mainly because it is easier for the patient to manage. The nasal part is made in silicone rubber and preferably hollowed to reduce its weight. This nasal part is made first on a sectional cast and tried in the mouth. It is then returned to the cast and an impression of this is made to produce a working cast on which the denture is constructed. This method prevents movement of the nasal portion in the mouth.

If the obturator is load-bearing and made in two separate pieces, then it is best to use an acrylic shell construction, rather than a bulb, and a split pin attachment.

In a large enclosed defect it is often not possible to make the obturator load-bearing. In such a case the impression material should extend about 1 cm into the nasal floor but obstruction of the nasal airway should be avoided. A useful appliance is a silicone retentive obturator with three or four studs. It is often better to use latex rather than silicone because it is lighter in weight and, in cases where radiation necrosis or healing is a problem, a hollow latex obturator is a good design.

In small enclosed defects, which may be acquired or congenital, impressions can be made with spoon-shaped metal trays made especially for this procedure in dentate patients. In edentulous patients, of course, impression of the cleft would usually be taken as part of the overall impression. Care must be taken not to lose impression material on the nasal side of the cleft. On the finished denture the obturator may either be retained as a heat-cured silicone or by studs, and before the denture is processed in acrylic, a postdam should be cut around the perimeter of the cleft to aid the development of peripheral seal (Figure 28.20).

Open-end defects

In anterior open-end defects the lip will have been repaired but the alveolar ridge is either absent or

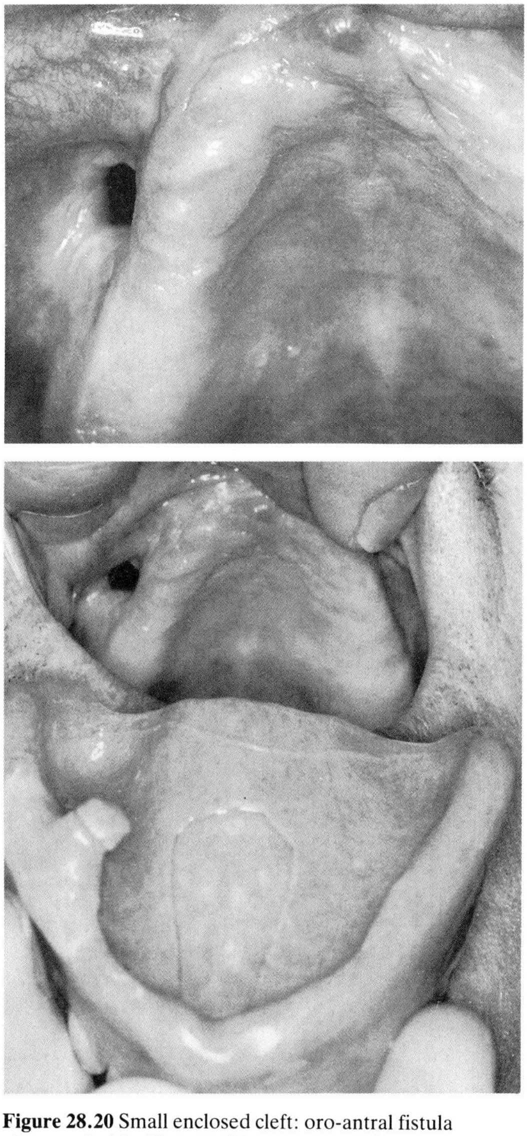

Figure 28.20 Small enclosed cleft: oro-antral fistula obturated with silicone rubber processed directly to complete denture

deficient. This, together with lack of nasal support, poses the main problem as load on the anterior part of the appliance is not resisted. An important feature of such cases is the escape of fluid through the nostrils from the anterior end of the vestibule and maximum obturation should be obtained to reduce this problem. If there is little undercut present to aid retention the denture and obturator are made in acrylic, but otherwise a silicone retentive obturator should be used.

In posterior open-end defects the main problem in edentulous cases is the lack of resistance to backward movement of the appliance especially where there is marked resorption of the anterior alveolar ridge. This is one of the main reasons for retaining as many natural teeth as possible in cleft patients, especially where the defect is an open-end posterior one. The most useful appliance is a silicone retentive obturator with or without soft palate obturation depending on whether speech can be improved or not.

Chapter 29

Complex prostheses and attachments

Strictly speaking a complex partial denture is one with some fixed parts (crowns or bridges) and some removable parts but the definition can be extended to include the wide range of appliances and prostheses that not only present problems in design but also are technically difficult to make in the laboratory.

In prosthetic dentistry it is often tempting to design complicated appliances to meet the difficult problems presented in clinical practice and many dentures over the years are admirable examples of engineering and technical skills. Unfortunately their complexity either makes them clinically unmanageable or some component fails to function in the hostile oral environment. For successful treatment, therefore, it is always best, while obeying the principles of denture design, to make the design as simple and streamlined as possible. To do this properly the importance of accurate and careful technology must be emphasized.

Swinglock partial dentures

This design is commonly used in mandibular bilateral free-end saddle cases where support and retention are often difficult (Figure 29.1). It is also useful in other cases, such as overlays (Figure 29.2).

The design consists of a labial hinged bar which locks into the major component of the denture (Figure 29.3). In the case of mandibular dentures a lingual plate is used in conjunction with the labial bar.

The labial bar usually has vertical struts which contact each abutment tooth apical to its greatest curvature. This provides splinting of the teeth and excellent retention of the denture. The design also avoids the use of clasps and provides resistance to lateral and posterior displacement, tipping action and rotary movements.

The design is particularly useful where the remaining anterior teeth are periodontally weak or are deemed to be unsuitable for restorative procedures (Figure 29.4). In maxillo-facial prosthodontics, where cases often present severe retention problems, a swinglock is recommended.

The labial bar with its struts is sometimes aesthetically displeasing and in such cases the struts are replaced by an acrylic veneer, a method particularly useful where there is loss of interdental papillae or severe gingival recession. The only drawback with the labial veneer is gingival damage and the need for even better oral hygiene.

A swinglock design is liable to damage the remaining natural tissues if it is made without adequate tooth support. Merely designing a lingual plate connector to lie against the lingual surfaces of the lower incisors will not provide tooth support and such a denture will tend to slip gingivally, as will the labial bar. Rest seats must be prepared in the remaining teeth, therefore, to prevent damage.

Sectional partial dentures

In some partially edentulous patients, particularly those with multiple bounded saddle areas, problems arise in selecting a suitable path of insertion of the denture. When the casts are surveyed undercuts are found opposing each other and so a single path of insertion is only possible if some of the undercuts are blocked out. If this is done then unsatisfactory spaces are produced when the denture is in the mouth. These are unsightly and cause food to dislodge.

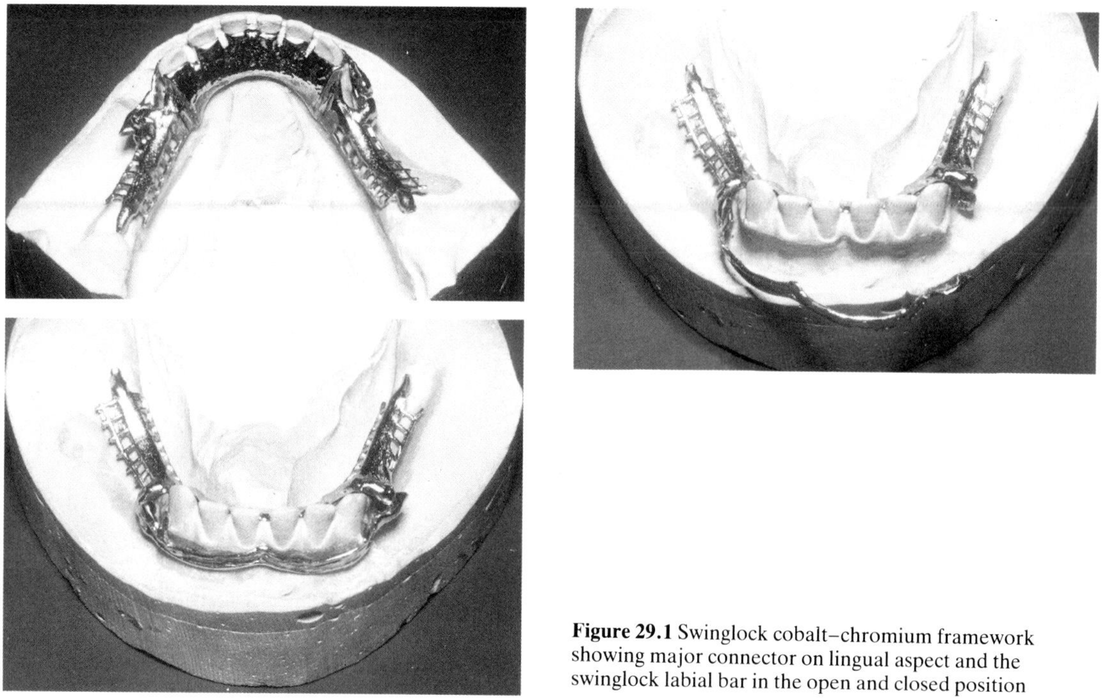

Figure 29.1 Swinglock cobalt–chromium framework showing major connector on lingual aspect and the swinglock labial bar in the open and closed position

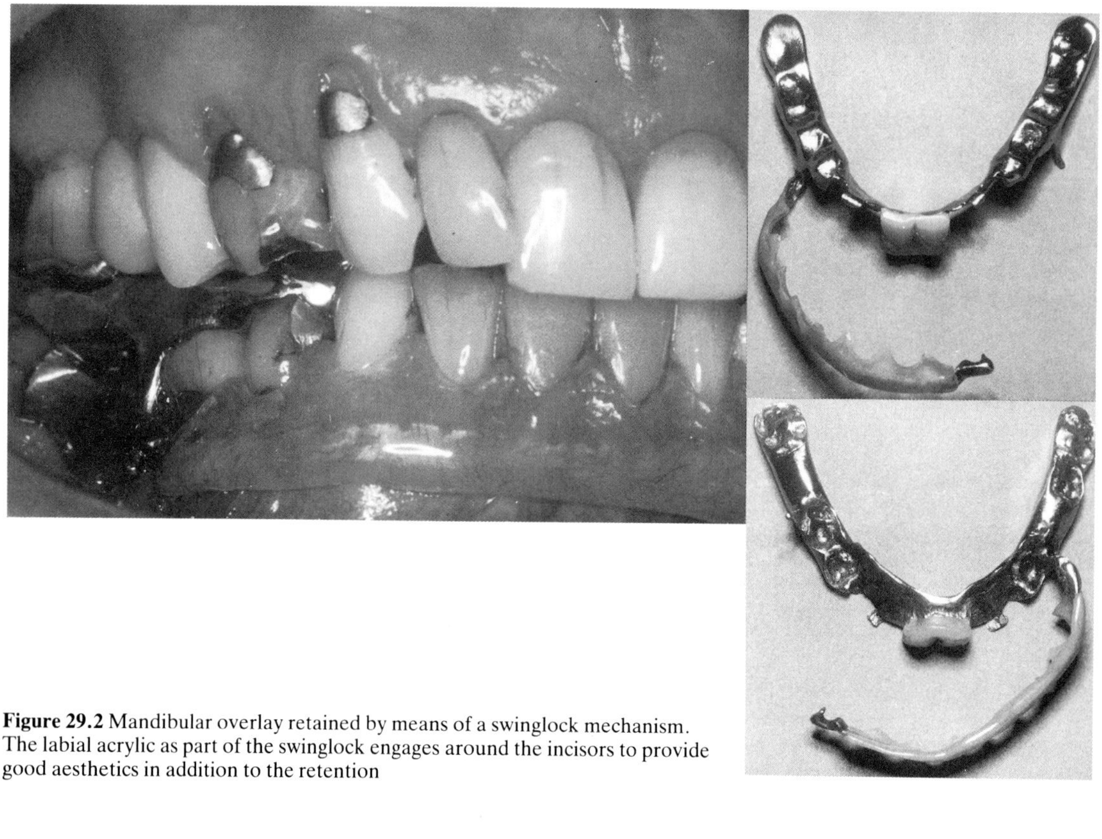

Figure 29.2 Mandibular overlay retained by means of a swinglock mechanism. The labial acrylic as part of the swinglock engages around the incisors to provide good aesthetics in addition to the retention

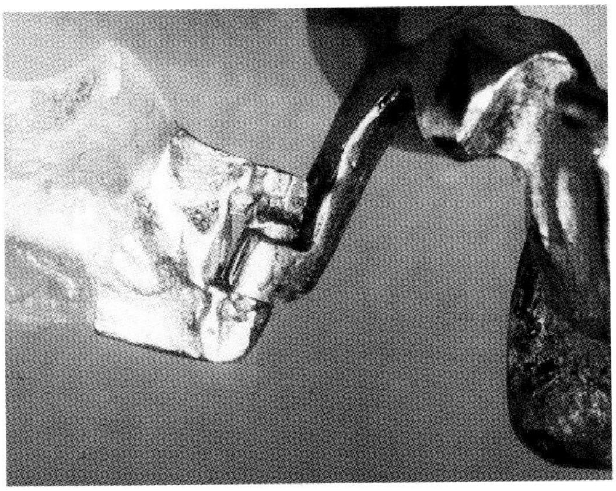

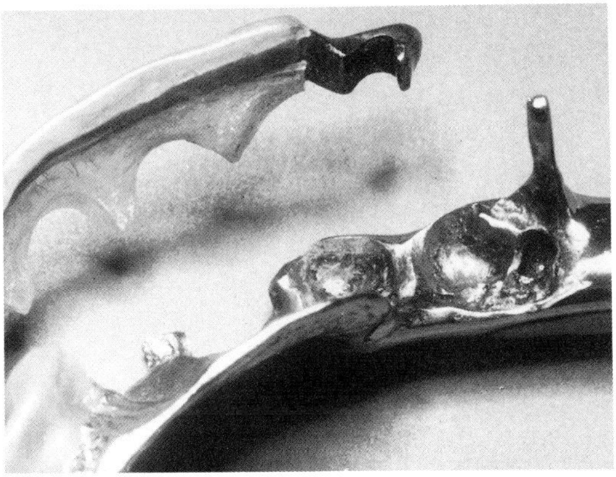

Figure 29.3 Close-up of the hinge and locking mechanism of a swinglock denture

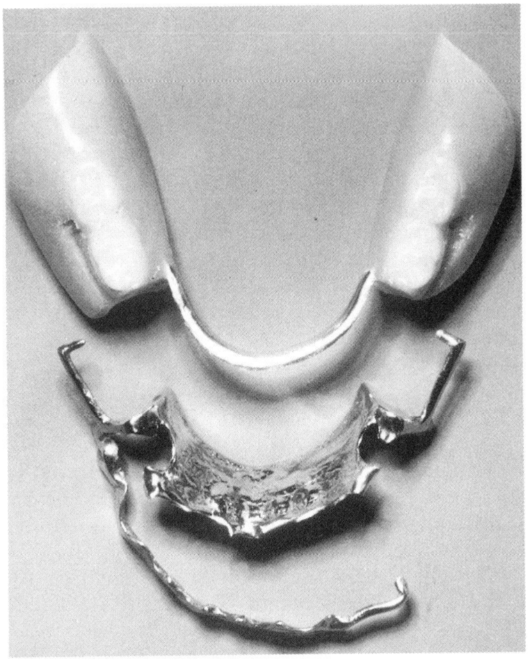

Figure 29.4 A swinglock is particularly useful in a disjunct denture as it provides excellent retention while obviating the need for clasps. This retention gives the necessary indirect support to the stress-breaking design

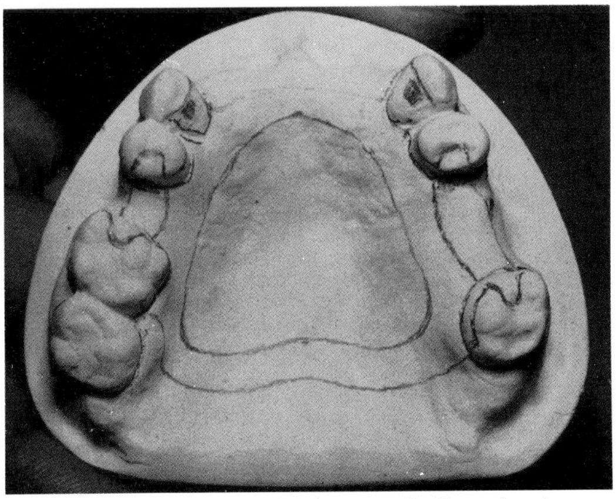

Figure 29.5 Sectional partial denture. Outline of major component

If the conflicting undercuts are very mild the proximal enamel of the abutment teeth may be ground to form favourable guiding surfaces and thus produce a single path of insertion. In most cases, however, the undercuts are too deep or too divergent to allow for this procedure.

A convenient solution is to use a sectional denture which inserts in two different paths. It has the advantage of filling all the spaces and providing a very positive retention because all the undercuts are utilized. The appearance is also better, particularly as many of these designs use a reduced number of clasps.

Most sectional dentures are in two parts although occasionally three parts are used. There is a danger in complicating the design because then patients find them difficult to manage. In some designs the two parts are separate, assembled by the patient in or out of the mouth and locked together by split pins, locking bolts, tubes and clips and similar devices. In other designs, the denture is assembled permanently but the two parts move on a hinge and, after seating in the mouth, the two parts are locked together. This latter type is usually easier for the patient to manage.

Figure 29.5 shows a maxillary cast with three bounded saddles. If the anterior saddle and flange is inserted upwards and backwards the undercuts on distal first premolars would have to be blocked out and thus leave unsightly spaces; the major component of the planned tooth-borne denture is outlined.

The casting is made with a labial spur which houses the locking bolt, the anterior teeth are assembled and the labial flange waxed around the bolt (Figure 29.6). When the denture is finished in acrylic (Figure 29.7) the lock is opened and the labial flange disengaged by pulling straight forward. The patient inserts the major component vertically, the labial flange horizontally and then locks the two parts by engaging the bolt.

Detailed instructions are given to patients on the management and hygiene of sectional dentures which because of their greater complexity must be treated with care if damage is to be avoided.

Prefabricated attachments

A prefabricated attachment, sometimes referred to as a precision attachment or retainer, is a device manufactured commercially and fixed to a denture to provide retention and/or support.

These have been used in prosthetic dentistry for many years and there are between 100 and 200

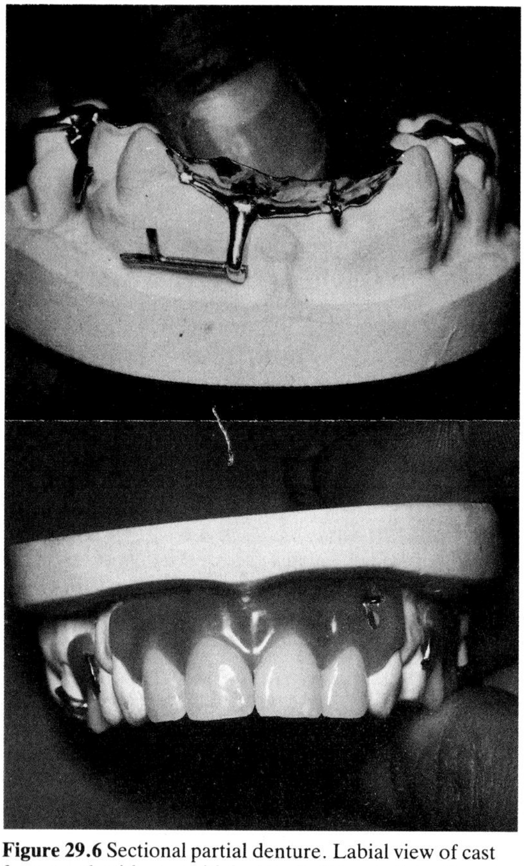

Figure 29.6 Sectional partial denture. Labial view of cast framework with spur with locking bolt located; teeth and wax added prior to flasking

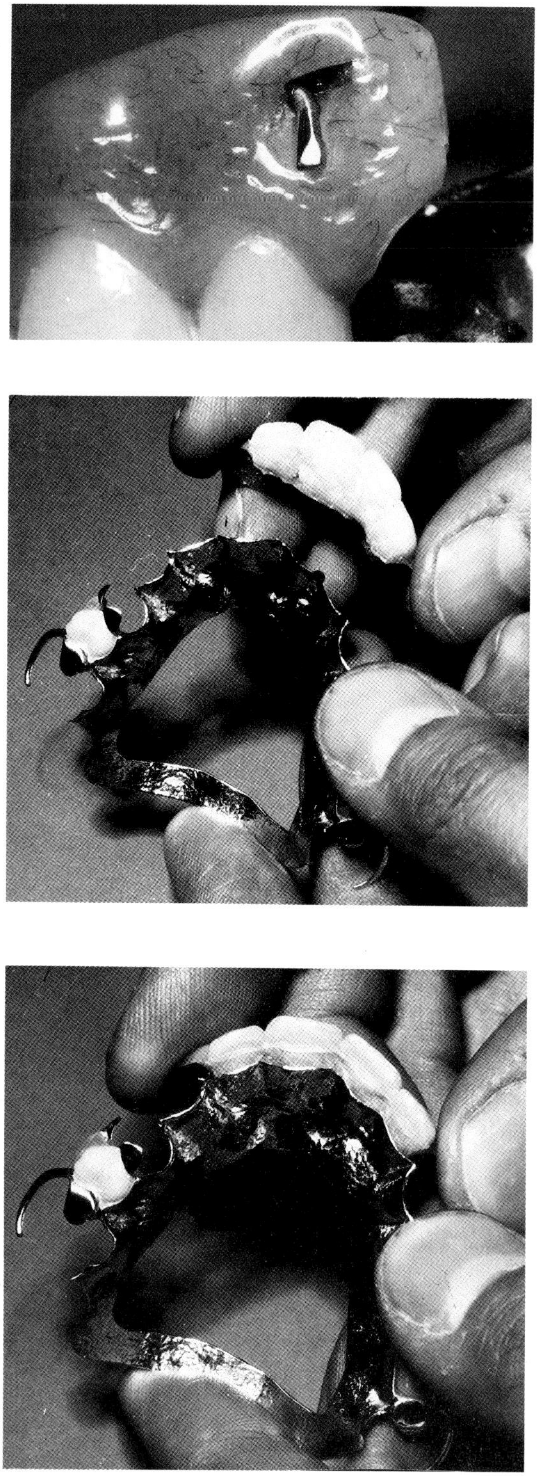

Figure 29.7 Sectional partial denture. Locking bolt in closed position. The patient opens the bolt, disengages the labial part, inserts the major component, engages the labial part, and closes the bolt

different typcs, many of which arc known by the name of the designer. Most attachments are made of alloys of noble metals, but many have additional parts made of a polymer, such as nylon.

In those attachments involving movement between the components a classification sometimes used is as follows:

1. Disjunctors consist of two parts, one being incorporated in the main component of the denture, the other in the free-end saddle, particularly of lower dentures. The purpose of disjunctors is to allow vertical or ball and socket movement between the differently-supported parts of a denture.
2. Hinges also consist of two parts usually joined by a pin or threaded screw inserted from the buccal side so that the assembled attachment operates like a door hinge.
3. Conjunctors in which one part is soldered on to, or cast into, an inlay or crown cemented to an abutment tooth, while the other part is attached or housed within the saddle of a removable denture. Conjunctors may take the form of studs, bars or channels.

A better classification, because it covers the whole range of attachments, is given below.

1. Intra-coronal attachments lie within the anatomical crown of the abutment tooth (Figure 29.8). The matrix is incorporated in an inlay or crown, the patrix in the denture. The frictional fit between the matrix and patrix provides the retention while the support is obtained by the contact of the patrix on the base of the matrix channel. Lateral bracing is a feature of these H-shaped attachments because of the accurate fit between the components, although in long-bounded saddles additional bracing arms should be used on the buccal and lingual aspects of the abutments. One of the problems of intra-coronal attachments is that of limited space within the abutment to accommodate the matrix in the inlay or crown. Teeth with sufficient crown height are necessary and care must be taken not to damage the pulp. One of the great assets of attachments is the streamlined result in that all the restorations are contained within the anatomy of the natural teeth. Some designs work within the root of the abutment after endodontic treatment: the maxtrix forms a blind end in the root while the patrix is contained in the denture. Such attachments are known as intra-radicular.
2. Extra-coronal attachments are specifically designed to be soldered on to the surface of a crown on an abutment tooth or, in some cases, joined to it during casting. The part of the mechanism lying outside the crown incorporates the hinge or spring mechanism which allows the attachment to function when linked to a free-end saddle. There is some danger to the gingival margin under the attachment and good hygiene is essential. Because the bulk of the attachment is outside the crown there is less danger of pulp involvement than with intra-coronal attachments.
3. Studs are used on abutment teeth which have been root-filled. A post and diaphragm are then made to carry a patrix which is lined up in the selected path of insertion of the partial denture or overdenture. The matrix of the attachment is contained within the denture (Figure 29.9) and the assembled attachment provides both retention and support. This method of treatment is useful when the prognosis of an abutment tooth

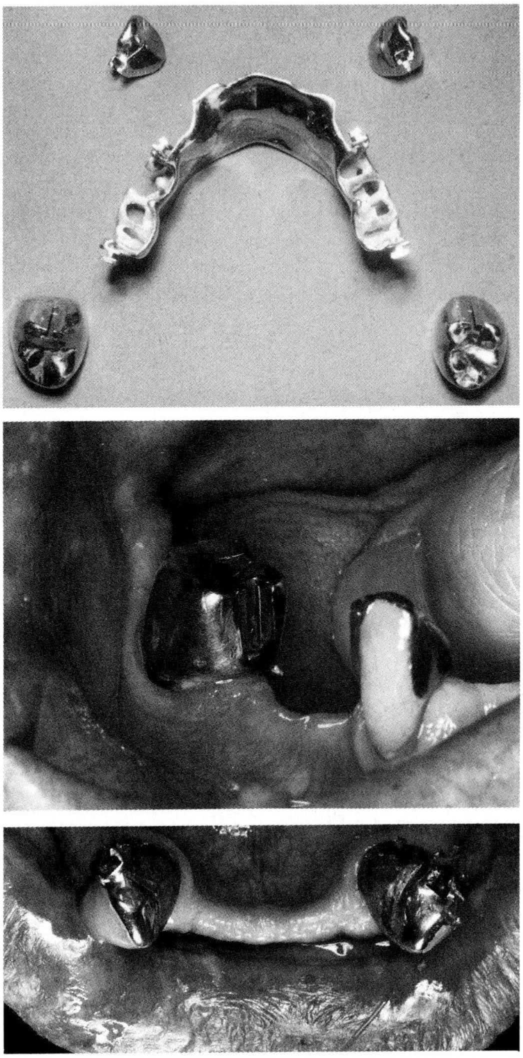

Figure 29.8 Intracoronal channel attachments

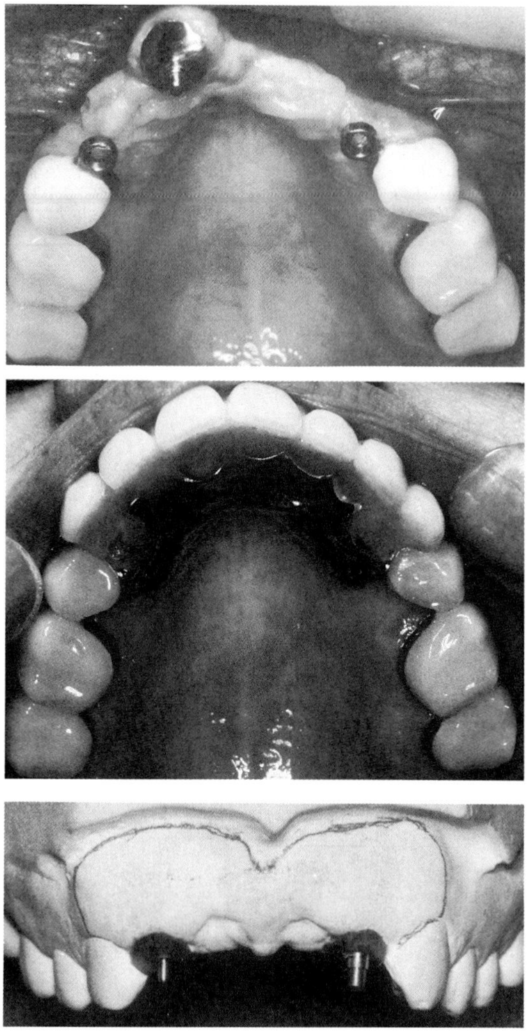

Figure 29.9 Stud attachments

is unfavourable because of its crown–root ratio; by removing the crown and applying load on the stud which is almost at gingival level, damaging forces are reduced.

4. Bars of various types and designs are used in bounded saddles (Figures 29.10 and 29.11). These are usually known by the name of the originator, e.g. Dolder, Andrews, Gilmore, Ceka, Ackermann. The bars are either soldered directly to the cast crowns or attached to the abutment piece by screws. Whatever method is used the result is a fixed bridge to which the denture is attached by spring clips or cone-shaped patrices that fit matrices set into the bar.
5. There are many miscellaneous attachments some of which act as auxiliaries to the principal attachments:

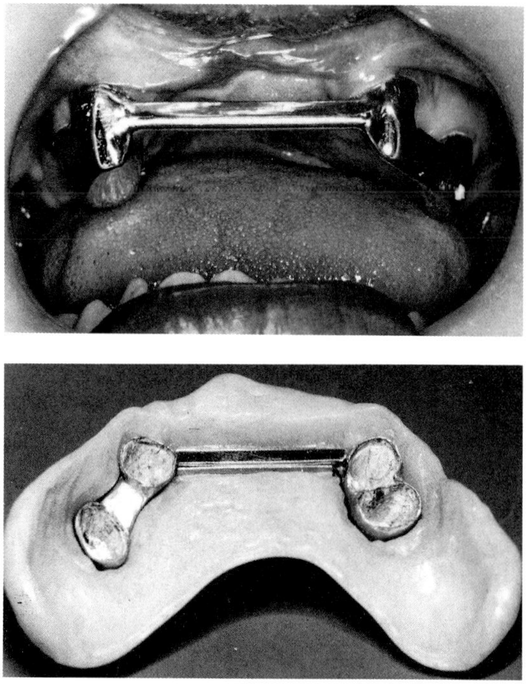

Figure 29.10 Prefabricated bars. Congenital cleft lip and palate. Full veneer crowns prepared on 43/35 with soldered Dolder bar. Overdenture with crowns and bar prior to cementation (see Figure 29.11)

(a) Spring-loaded patrices engage small prepared dimples on the proximal surfaces of abutment teeth to act as retainers (Figure 29.12).
(b) Screw retainers are used to retain parts of fixed partial dentures. These cannot be removed by the patient but they are intended to be removable by the dentist.
(c) Milled attachments are not purchased commercially but are prepared in the dental laboratory. They involve the preparation of full veneer crowns to receive a matching component contained within the denture. The two components fit accurately together and act as retainers by frictional force and the location of pins in drilled holes. These preparations are, in effect, a more refined stage of telescopic crowns which have been used in prosthetic dentistry for years.

Benefits of prefabricated attachments

1. The absence of clasps means that the aesthetics are better.
2. The dentures are much more streamlined because of the absence of extra-coronal clasps and rests, particularly as most attachments are contained within the crowns of the natural teeth.

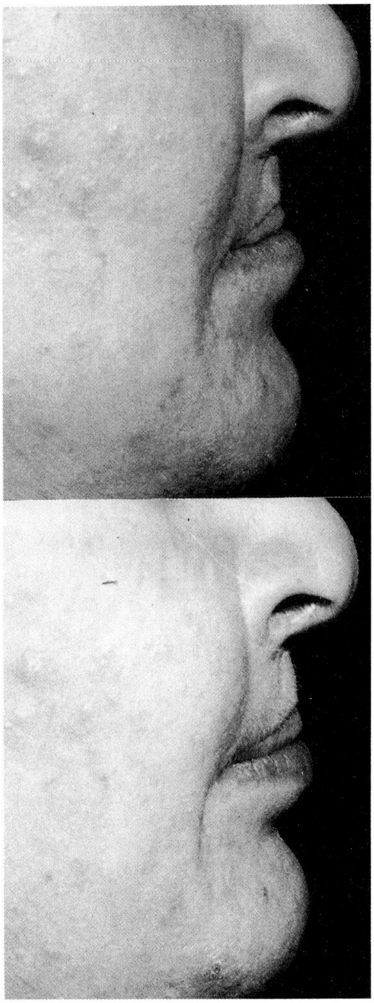

Figure 29.11 Same case as Figure 29.10. The repaired cleft lip was severely scarred but the resistance offered by the bar enabled the denture to restore the lip to a reasonable profile

3. Loads applied to the denture, and therefore to the attachments, are more favourably applied to the abutment teeth as the loads are directed along the long axes of the teeth.
4. Horizontal loads are more favourably applied to the teeth although this usually means that bracing elements should be added as many attachments, particularly channel attachments, do not have sufficient bracing against lateral loading.
5. Retention is normally better, compared with ordinary clasps, because the frictional fit of a manufactured attachment is extremely good except that this close contact tends to wear and reduce in time.

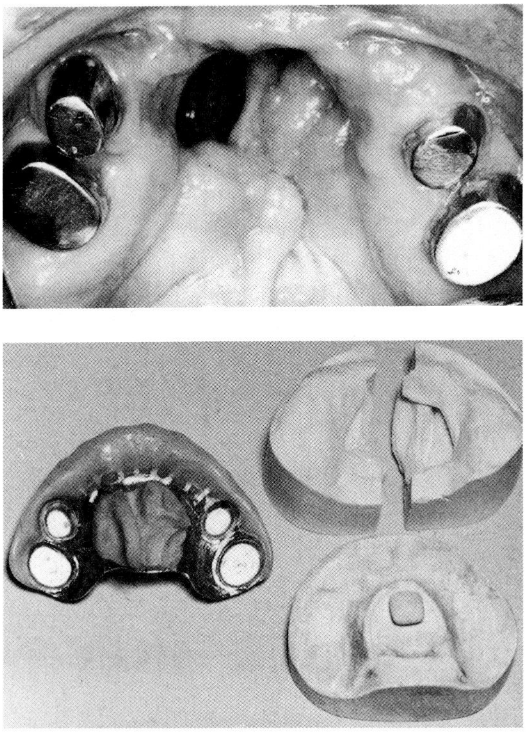

Figure 29.12 In this repaired congenital cleft spring-loaded patrices in the denture engage dimples on the surfaces of the full veneer crowns (the cleft is obturated with silicone attached by a stud to the denture)

6. They are particularly effective in preventing rotational and backward movements of the denture base, a problem common to unilateral and bilateral free-end saddle cases.

Drawbacks of prefabricated attachments

1. Tooth preparation is required, often for a large number of abutment teeth.
2. Teeth with vital and large pulps are somewhat at risk because of the large amount of tooth structure that has to be removed to contain the matrix of the attachment.
3. Crowns with a short height are usually unfavourable, particularly with channel attachments, because the sliding fit of a matrix and patrix of only a few millimetres is inadequate.
4. They present problems in free-end saddle cases because of the complexity of movement and their so-called stress-breaking action which is often theoretically unsound.
5. Cost and time are high and the technical expertise required is considerable, both clinically and in the laboratory.

Palatal training appliances

Patients with restricted or uncoordinated movements of the soft palate may present problems to the speech therapist. These may occur after cleft palate surgery but may also occur in palates with normal structure. In either case the problem lies in the failure of the soft palate to elevate fully, and thus to nasal escape of air. This leads to hypernasality in speech sounds and interference with the playing of certain wind instruments, such as the clarinet, where full soft palate lift is essential.

Intra-oral training appliances, also called palatal lift or Selley appliances, have been used for a number of years, the object being, as the name implies, to assist in the elevation of the soft palate. These appliances generally consist of a U-shaped piece of stainless steel wire attached to an acrylic base-plate, the wire extending to touch the resting soft palate in the region of normal maximum lift.

It is usually found that very little gagging or retching occurs with these appliances and patients soon adapt to wearing them. The presence of the wire contacting the palate assists in the voluntary lift of the palate in the patient's attempt to block off the oronasal pharynx.

The main problem with an acrylic base-plate is retention because, of course, the weight and activity of the soft palate against the extended wire loop creates a very unfavourable downward force tending to dislodge the appliance. Retention is usually obtained by multiple crib clasps on the molars and premolars and, in young people where the crown height is usually short, the best type of crib is the Adams design. An alternative design is shown in Figure 29.13 where a cast cobalt–chromium base was made with multiple occlusally-approaching clasps engaged in every possible undercut, including the canines. Aesthetics is not normally a problem with these appliances as they are worn only during training periods or while playing the musical instrument.

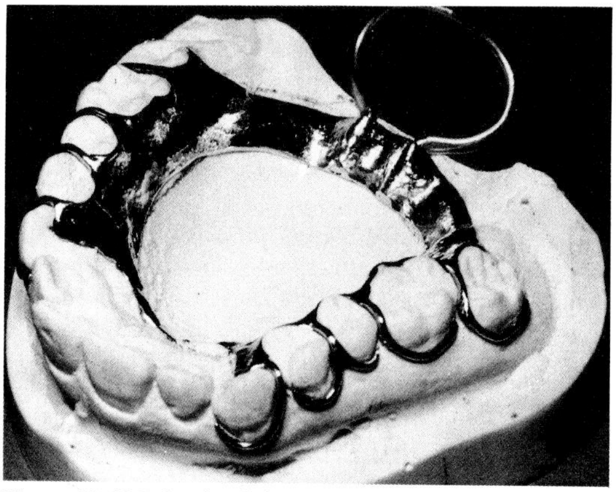

Figure 29.13 Palatal training appliance. Cast cobalt–chromium with multiple retention by occlusally-approaching clasps. The wire loop, engaging tubes in the posterior palatal bar, can be removed and adjusted to effect greater palatal lift as required. The wire is covered with polythene tube to lessen trauma against the soft palate mucosa

Tooth surface loss

Attrition, abrasion and erosion of natural teeth is becoming more common nowadays and there is no doubt the longer teeth are retained the more likely will the problem become. The improvement in dental health and the upsurge of preventive dentistry brings in its wake the loss of the hard dental tissues in some patients.

Tooth wear is not always uniform. The surface loss may affect only a few teeth while the rest remain relatively normal (Figure 29.14). In other patients,

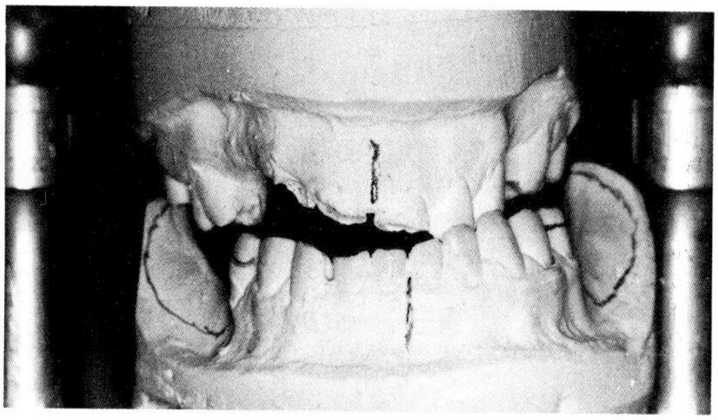

Figure 29.14 Tooth surface loss may affect only a few natural teeth

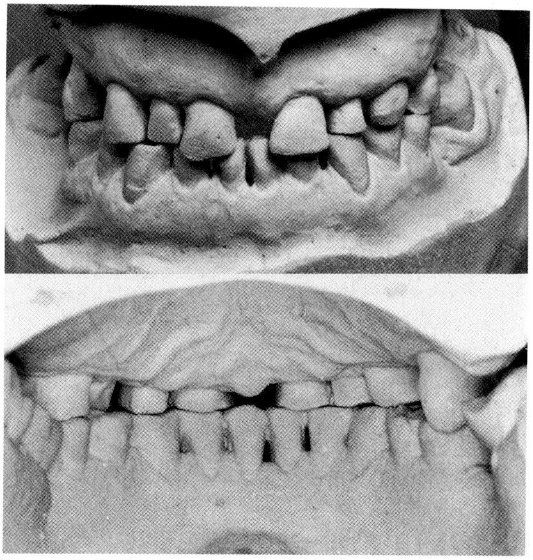

Figure 29.15 Tooth surface loss. Labial and lingual view of case where a large number of teeth is involved in destruction

the majority of the teeth are worn although not necessarily to the same degree (Figure 29.15).

The most common reason for a dental consultation in these cases is appearance, either on the part of the patient himself or pressure from a relative or friend. There are occasionally difficulties with eating, and less commonly with speech, but there is usually secondary dentine laid down and so the pulps are protected, bony alveolar growth to maintain the occlusal face height and adaptation of masticatory muscles. All these changes usually mean that oral function remains remarkably efficient and normal. For these reasons the most common need for prosthodontic treatment is in connection with aesthetics.

Wear of teeth may be due to loss of other teeth particularly in the posterior segments of the arches. The patient then chews and contacts on the anterior

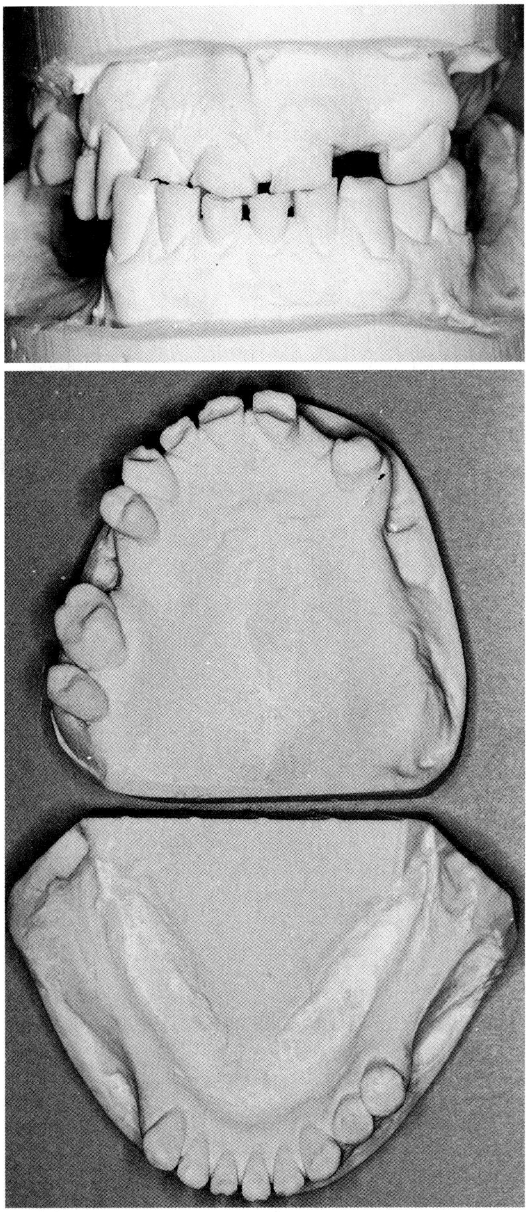

Figure 29.16 A 54-year male patient with missing teeth, tooth surface loss and disrupted occlusion (see Figure 29.17)

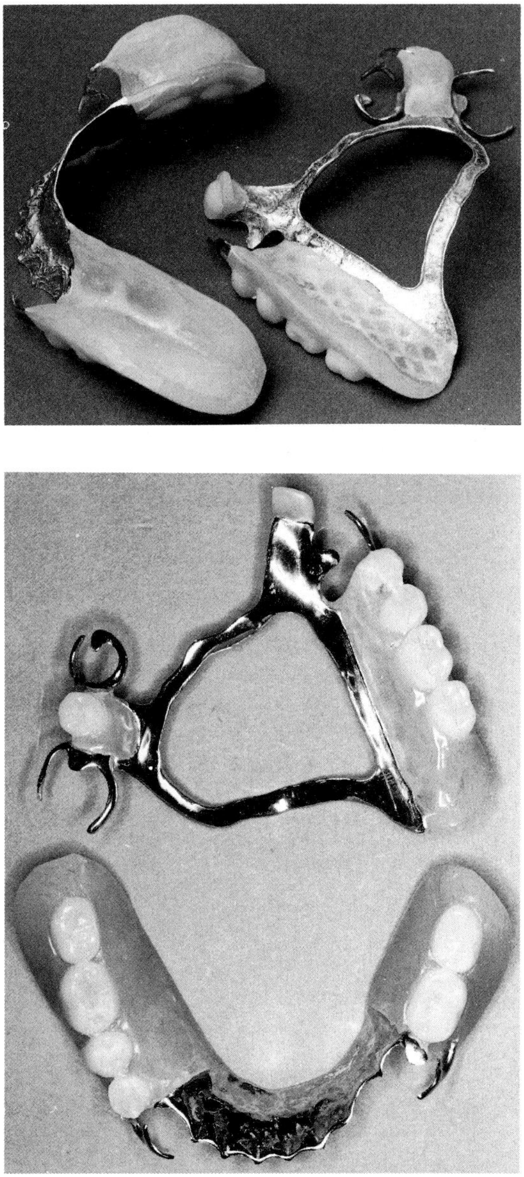

Figure 29.17 Unsatisfactory partial dentures made for patient shown in Figure 29.16. These designs attempted to replace the missing teeth but effected no improvement in the tooth surface loss, the occlusion or the appearance

teeth only, the tooth wear becoming greater as the mandible postures forwards. In such cases there is little point in making partial dentures merely as space fillers without regard to mandibular function, the already worn anterior teeth or the future prognosis of the case. Patients in this category are unlikely to understand the purpose of this partial denture treatment which does little to improve the appearance and because of the continuing occlusal instability damage is likely to continue (Figures 29.16 and 29.17).

Bruxism and parafunctional habits account for tooth surface wear, although it is often difficult to be certain of either the cause or the actual habit movement. Study casts, mounted on an adjustable articulator, are usually essential to analyse the particular movement causing the tooth wear.

There is little doubt that previous fillings, or any fixed or removable restoration, can give rise to a bruxist habit because of occlusal faults which the patient attempts to eliminate, often subconsciously, by contact with opposing teeth.

In all cases of tooth surface loss, full mouth radiographs and study casts should be made as soon

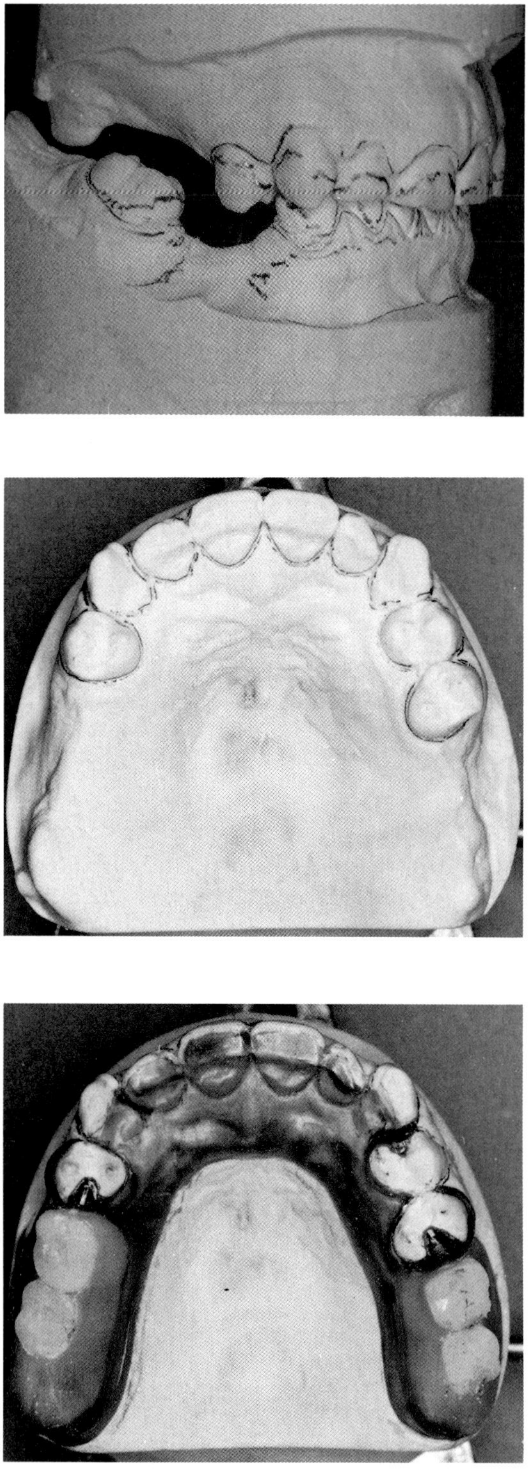

Figure 29.18 Study casts mounted on the articulator and diagnostic wax-up is a useful method of approaching treatment planning in cases with tooth surface loss

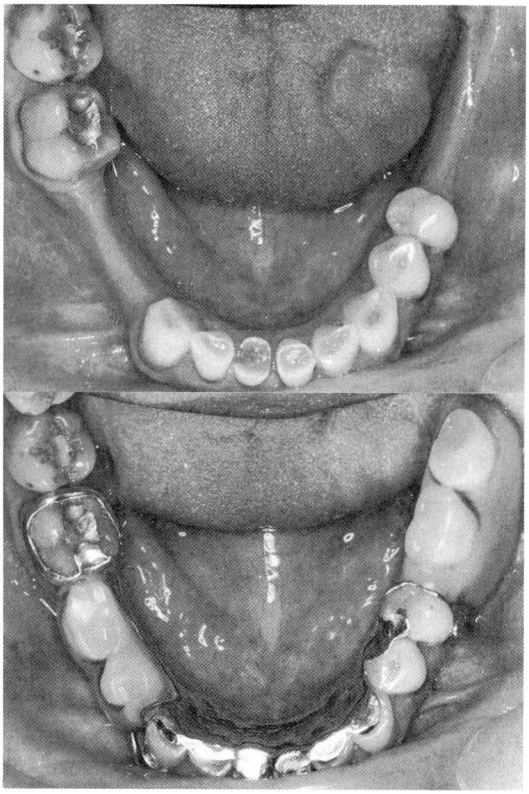

Figure 29.19 Mandibular teeth with attrition of incisors protected by a removable partial denture. This is a simple but effective treatment

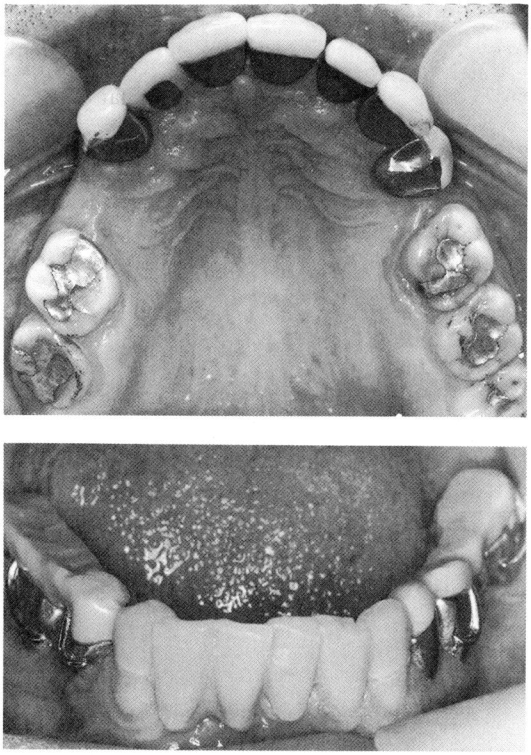

Figure 29.20 Marked tooth surface loss. Maxillary anterior teeth restored by porcelain bonded crowns. Mandibular teeth restored by shallow full veneer crowns and removable overlay

as a medical and dental history is recorded. It is generally true that the teeth are firm and the periodontal state good, although there is often evidence of oral neglect. The radiographic bone picture is usually very favourable so that the quality of supporting tissue for any planned prosthesis is excellent.

At the second visit the casts should be mounted on an adjustable articulator. A D-shaped wax record is made for the maxillary cast which is mounted with a facebow. The lower cast is mounted in the retruded position in a midline position just short of tooth contact. While this is being done an assessment is made of the occlusal face height by watching the mandibular movement during speech with particular reference to the closest speaking space. It is unlikely that any planned prosthesis can be made which will invade this space.

It is sometimes suggested that a provisional or diagnostic appliance is made in acrylic in order to assess the level of tolerance of the patient, particularly with regard to any increase in occlusal face height. Such appliances, however, by nature of the material and the way they are made, are bulky and relatively crude so that in themselves are of little help to the patient or the clinician in reaching a definite clinical decision. It is best to make a definitive appliance in cast alloy from the start if such a restoration is deemed necessary. It is for this reason that study casts, accurately mounted are essential in reaching a treatment plan. In the laboratory a diagnostic wax-up, including any modification of existing teeth, can be carried out on the study casts which should be duplicated for record purposes (Figure 29.18). From this laboratory plan, and having discussed it with the patient as it may involve preparation and restoration of a number of teeth, an alloy base can be finally made to effect an improvement both in occlusion and appearance (Figure 29.19).

In all cases of tooth surface loss it is always best to plan for fixed restorations wherever possible, but it is important to remember that many of these patients are careless about dental health and oral

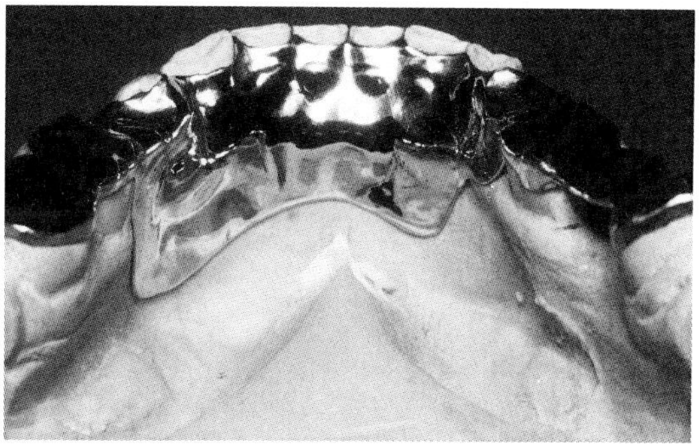

Figure 29.21 Mild tooth surface loss restored by removable yellow gold alloy overlay denture

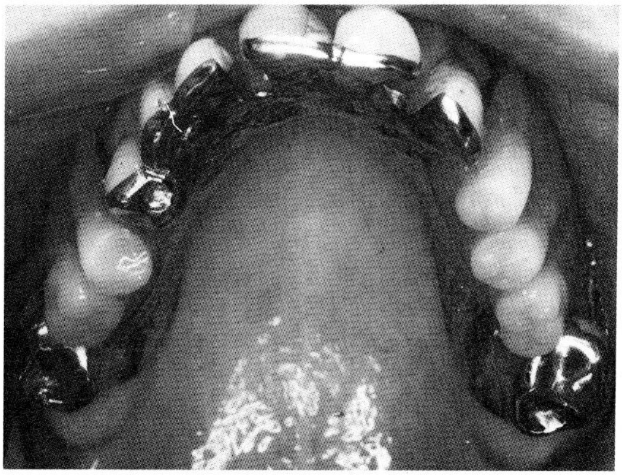

Figure 29.22 Mild tooth surface loss restored by removable cobalt–chromium overlay. A close fit of alloy against the incisal edges is difficult but very important for patient comfort

hygiene otherwise they would not have allowed so much deterioration to occur before seeking treatment. For this reason fixed partial denture treatment must not be embarked on lightly and it should be planned in such a way that the patient can be allowed to discontinue if he tires of the length of treatment. Very often, however, a combination of fixed and removable partial dentures produces a very good result, particularly where the amount of tissue loss is great and where the interocclusal clearance is large (Figure 29.20).

In patients where the tooth surface loss is relatively mild and involving a large number of teeth, and particularly where there is a known history of bruxism, an alloy overlay partial denture is a suitable protective restoration. It is best made on the jaw which presents with the greatest amount of tooth wear. Yellow gold alloy (Figure 29.21) is the most pleasant of the alloys for patients to use but cobalt–chromium (Figure 29.22) offers the most abrasion resistance. In either case great care is needed to develop the occlusal surface to be compatible with the patient's particular mandibular movements and opposing occlusal anatomy. A functionally generated path is the technique of choice. If the occlusal scheme of the overlay is wrong there is a possibility that the bruxism will become worse rather than better.

Chapter 30

Implant dentures

Prosthodontists have long sought a means of increasing the retention, stability, efficiency and comfort of complete dentures for those patients presenting with grossly resorbed edentulous ridges. The life of such patients is often made miserable by the continual instability of their dentures or by the pain caused by pressure on thin, friable mucosa overlying an irregular bone surface or on a mandibular or mental nerve which has come to lie near the surface as a result of the excessive resorption.

It has long been obvious that were it possible in such cases to anchor a denture to the bone by means of a metal insert then a great deal could be achieved. Such a metal insert attached to the bone with abutment posts penetrating the mucosa is termed an implant and during the last century attempts have been made with a variety of metals, alloys, polymers and ceramics, employing a large number of techniques, to perfect such implants. Most failed because the implant was rapidly exfoliated or sepsis intervened.

One of the main reasons for this failure was the electrolytic incompatibility of such metals and alloys with oral tissues. This major disadvantage partially disappeared with the advent of the cobalt–chromium alloys. The use of these alloys in general surgery in the form of plates and screws for positioning the ends of fractured bones is well-known.

About 40 years ago a method was developed for inserting cobalt–chromium into the jaws in the form of subperiosteal implants to provide a firm stable base to support dentures in cases presenting major problems of stability or discomfort. To the present day there have been successes and failures and many variations of the technique have been tried, modified or abandoned, but the general principles of the method are still relevant in spite of the advent of other forms of dental implant.

Technique of subperiosteal implants

Preliminary

The normal prosthetic procedure for constructing complete upper and lower dentures is carried out until the dentures have reached the trial stage. At this point the occlusion and appearance of the dentures are carefully checked and the upper denture is finished in the normal way, the lower denture being retained in the wax stage. In the laboratory the first molars and the canines are removed from the wax lower denture and an instrument pushed through the wax in the areas occupied by these teeth until it penetrates the surface of the ridge of the cast. These marks on the cast locate the positions of the abutments of the implant. A piece of base-plate wax is adapted to the cast, contoured to the shape of a denture base and then withdrawn and processed in clear acrylic. This template is replaced on the cast and holes are drilled through it in the areas marked for the future abutments.

Two impression trays are made on the cast and they will be used to take the impression of the bone surface when the mucoperiosteum has been reflected.

An acrylic record block is also constructed to occlude with the finished upper denture. Rims are only built in the premolar and molar regions, and wire staples are inserted into the acrylic in the premolar regions to facilitate its manipulation. This record block will be used lined with gutta-percha to record the jaw relationship when the mucosa has been reflected to enable the cast of the bone impression to be correctly related to the upper denture.

For an implant to be successful it must fit the surface of the bone accurately and so it is constructed to an impression of the bone. There are two surgical stages. The first consists of the reflection of the mucoperiosteum, two impressions of the surface of the bone, and the recording of the occlusion taken with the record block fitting the bone. The second stage, which is usually about three to six weeks after the first, consists of the reflection of the mucoperiosteum and the insertion of the implant substructure.

First surgical stage

Under anaesthesia the template is positioned on the lower ridge and a probe locates the position of the future abutment posts. Shallow pits are drilled into the surface of the bony ridge to locate the positions of the posts on the cast poured from the bone impression. The mucoperiosteum is now reflected to expose the mylohyoid ridges, the external oblique ridges, the genial tubercles and the mental nerves which are carefully identified. As wide a reflection of the flap as possible is desirable.

The bone impressions are now made, an over-extended impression being far better than an underextended one. The tray is loaded with composition in an even thickness of about 4 mm and inserted under the mucoperiosteal flaps. When fully in place the composition is chilled, removed and inspected. It should show impressions of the mylohyoid ridges, the external oblique ridges, the mental nerves and the genial tubercles, and should be well-extended over the labial surface of the ridge. The surface of the composition is dried, covered with rubber-base or silicone impression material and again inserted and held in place until the impression material has fully set. The composition stage can be omitted and the rubber used alone if desired. A second bone impression is then made. It is essential that two impressions are taken because it is difficult to assess their absolute accuracy and therefore it is a safe precaution to have two implants made, one to each impression.

The fitting surface of the acrylic record block is lined with softened gutta-percha and a little soft wax placed on the occlusal surfaces of the blocks. The gutta-percha is located on the bone surface and the mandible closed on the softened wax against the teeth of the finished upper denture previously inserted. The stabilizing of the record block is facilitated by inserting the fingers on the wire staples in the premolar regions of the block. The final stage of the first operation is the careful approximation of the mucoperiosteal flaps with sutures.

Laboratory procedure

1. The cast from the bone impression is mounted with the upper denture by means of the record block.
2. The cast is duplicated in refractory investment.
3. The substructure of the implant is outlined on the refractory model. The abutment posts are positioned as indicated by the small location pits in the model and the bars of the framework are kept as narrow as possible commensurate with strength. The periphery of the framework is located on or over the external oblique ridges, and well short of the mylohyoid ridges, because if it protrudes lingually beyond these structures it will ulcerate through the thin lingual mucosa. It is kept well clear of the mental nerves and is carried as deeply as possible down the labial surface of the ridge. The struts joining the abutment posts to the periphery of the framework are kept narrow and the spaces between them wide. Any additional struts required for strengthening the substructure should be as few as possible and little or no metal should be placed in or across the incision line.
4. The wax implant is prepared to the proposed outline. The abutment posts should be shaped with a neck of 2.5–3 mm diameter and with a depth slightly greater than the thickness of the mucosa. The height of the abutment posts above the mucosa should be such that they will be well short of the occlusal surfaces of the upper teeth. The diameter of the base of the abutment posts should be about 4 mm in the canine regions and 6 mm in the molar regions and each post should have a 5° taper. The patterns of the posts can be made in either wax or acrylic resin. Casting of the

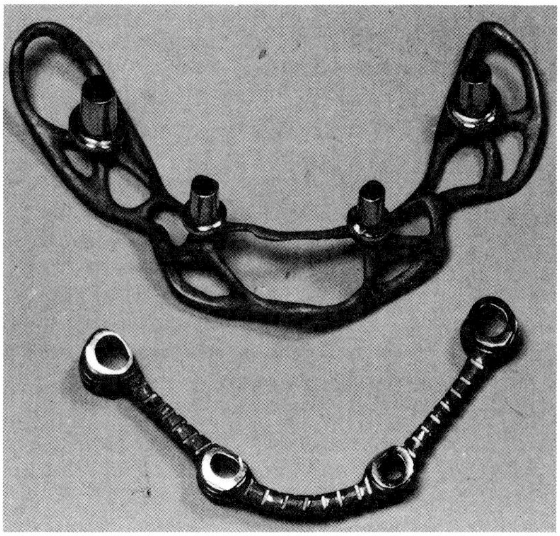

Figure 30.1 Subperiosteal implant. The cobalt–chromium framework and superstructure

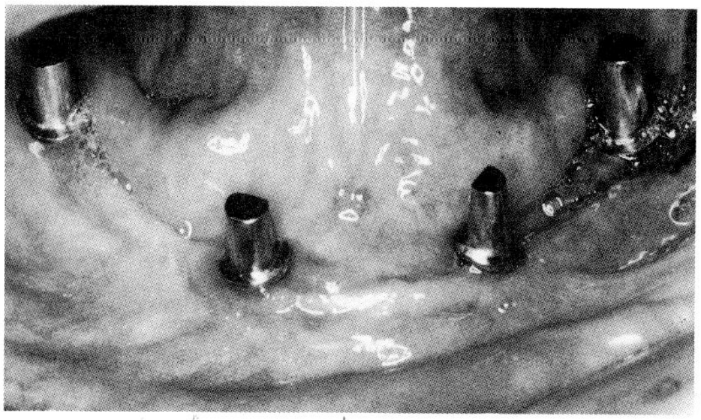

(*a*)

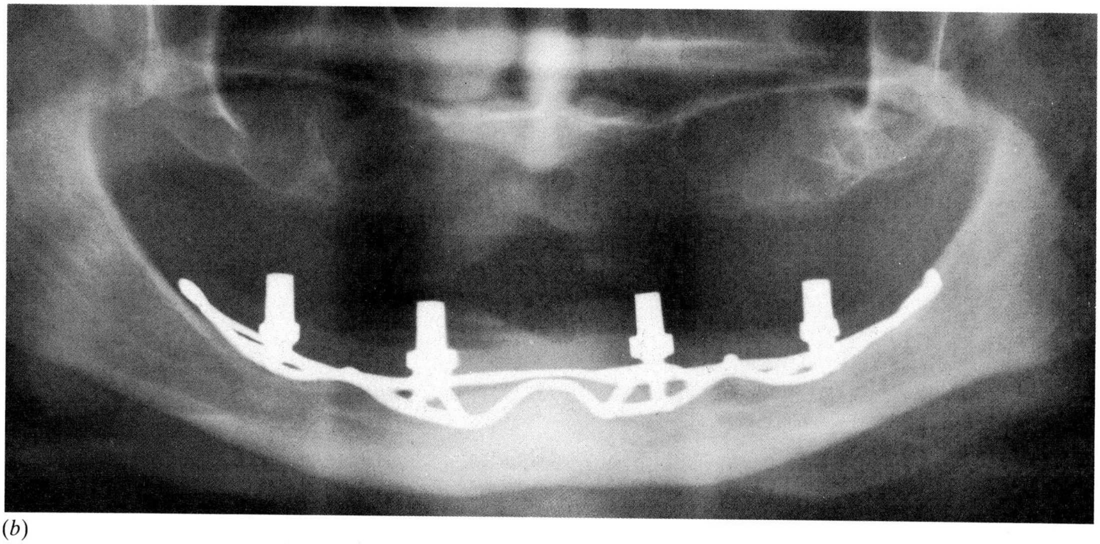

(*b*)

Figure 30.2 (*a*) Subperiosteal implant *in situ* after initial healing of surgical wound. (*b*) Radiograph shows framework location to the mandible

pattern is made with a nickel-free cobalt–chromium alloy. The casting is trimmed and finished with a sand blasted surface, but the abutment posts and necks are highly polished. A radiograph of the casting is made for evidence of any internal porosity.

5. The implant is positioned on the cast, thimbles waxed to the abutment posts and joined by wax bars. The whole is cast in cobalt–chromium to form the superstructure (Figure 30.1).
6. The cast superstructure is seated on the abutment posts and the lower denture waxed around it. This denture carries six anterior teeth, but the posterior teeth are represented by blocks built to occlude with the molars and premolars of the upper denture. The reason for this is that such a procedure simplifies any occlusal adjustment which may be necessary after the fitting of the implant and the flat surfaces of the lower blocks cause little or no lateral force to be applied to the implant. Some clinicians make no lower denture until the tissues have healed around the implant but fitting the denture to the substructure as soon as it is placed has two advantages; first it covers the wound, protecting it from the tongue, and second, and perhaps more important, each time the patient occludes it tends to seat the implant firmly on to the bone surface. The waxed denture is processed in acrylic.

Second surgical stage

This takes place three to six weeks after the first operation. The mucoperiosteum is reflected but not so widely as previously. The implant should fit the bone surface accurately all round the area of the framework and lie completely inert when pressure is applied to each abutment post successively. The more suitable of the two implants is selected for insertion.

When the implant has been positioned, the mucoperiosteum is carefully united with sutures. The lower denture is then placed in position, and its occlusion with the upper denture carefully adjusted to be quite even in the retruded contact position.

Provided all the stages have been accurately carried out the healing of the tissues over the substructure and around the abutments should be uneventful. It is important that while the denture is a firm frictional fit on the abutment posts it is not so tight that undue force is needed to remove it (Figure 30.2).

General remarks

Numerous subperiosteal implants have been inserted throughout the world during the last 40 years. Many of these have been in place and highly successful for five years or more. If an implant is successful the benefit to the patient is considerable. Many implants have been failures for one or more of the following reasons:

1. Inaccurate fit on the surface of the bone.
2. Incorrect outline and inadequate extension of the substructure framework.
3. Shape of the denture leading to uneven pressure being applied to it by the surrounding muscles or occlusal faults.
4. Careless surgical technique.
5. General health of the patient and careless oral hygiene.

In some areas, although the general healing of the tissues over the substructure has been good, the tissues have failed to cover the alloy. In some a status quo has developed and the implant has remained in place, but in others it has had to be removed. An implant is held by the periosteal fibres around the framework binding it firmly in place. In a well-fitting properly extended implant the firmness is very great.

A gingival margin similar in many respects to that surrounding a natural tooth develops but it is important that the patient keeps the posts free of plaque by scrupulous use of a toothbrush and dental tape. Care of the denture is also equally important.

Endosseous implants

Endosseous implants, consisting of metal pins, screws or blades inserted directly into the residual alveolar bone of the maxilla or mandible, have been used for a number of years (Figure 30.3). They are made in many different shapes and sizes but they all have a trans-mucosal post or cylinder on which the denture or crown fits. The mucosa is intended to form a gingival seal or cuff around the post.

Some endosseous implants are, to all intents and purposes, metallic screws although some are developed in the form of spirals. Others are blade-shaped with spaces or mesh built into the design to form vents, hence the general term, blade-vent. Some incorporate a combination of screw and vent. Others take the form of a ship's anchor, the belief being that its mechanical shape will more likely resist removal from the bone. The purpose of the vents is that after surgical insertion osteoblastic activity will form callus in and around the implant thus securing its position. The pin design usually comprises three, or occasionally four, separate pins which are driven in at different angles to meet at an apex on which the abutment post is fitted. The pins are divergent to provide a firmer foundation and also to avoid important structures such as the maxillary antrum and mandibular canal. Other pin implants are used when natural teeth are still present and are termed endodontic pin implants as they are inserted into the root canal and through the apex to enter the apical alveolar bone for a prescribed distance thereby anchoring an otherwise mobile tooth which can then be used as an abutment.

Materials

Metals may have a high tensile and compressive strength but often have poor fatigue characteristics which are important in the often severe cyclic stresses used in mastication. For corrosion resistance the metals or alloys most commonly used are stainless steel, cobalt–chromium, titanium and tantallum. The natural tendency of metal is to revert from the stable metallic state to the oxide or other compounds and this tendency to corrosion is enhanced by the action of stress. Saliva, a highly corrosive and aggressive medium, varies consider-

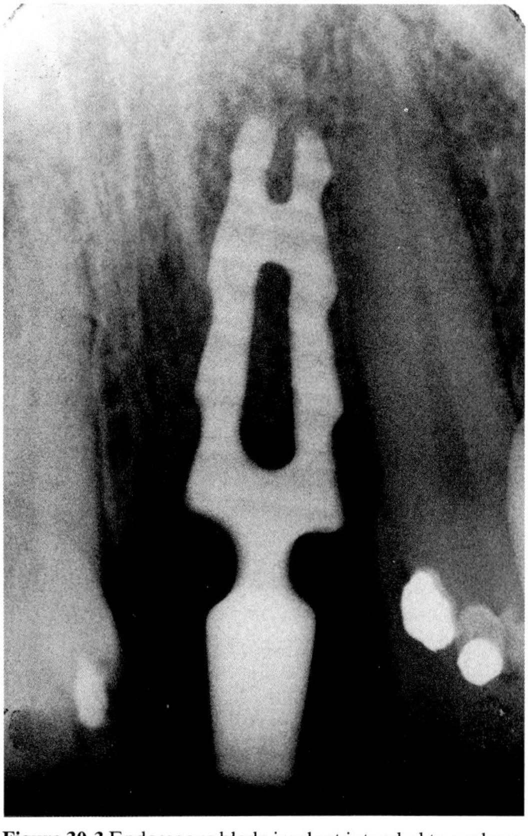

Figure 30.3 Endosseous blade implant intended to replace missing maxillary incisor

ably in composition and pH in different people and at different times during the day. Metal such as stainless steel, titanium and others rely for their corrosion resistance on the presence of a film of oxide. This film may be disrupted through mechanical or chemical damage and localized corrosion or pitting occurs where passivity has broken down. If tensile stresses are present then severe cracking and failure of metals can also occur, known as stress corrosion cracking. Corrosion of metals has two effects on the body. First, wastage and thinning of the metal occurs, decreasing the strength of the implant. Second, metallic ions and metallic particles are released and may lead to adverse tissue response. The release of metal ions by passive metals is determined by the polarization behaviour of the metal. Stainless steel exhibits a greater passive current density than titanium or tantallum and therefore a greater release of metallic ions will occur. This may be the cause of the more ready rejection of implants made of stainless steel than those made of titanium and tantallum.

Cobalt–chromium alloys have been used for blade implants in the mouth for several years and recent experimental studies have shown bony ingrowth within the metal openings but the adaptation is only a fibrous capsule and not an attachment. With endosseous implants such as blades, pins and screws there is a general localized reaction in the adjacent soft tissues and the bone rapidly resorbs away from the alloy. The major problem is probably the lack of a seal around the exposed portion of the implant.

To encourage osteogenesis and to eliminate fibrous connective tissue between bone and implant, metallic endosseous implants have been coated with a layer of pure aluminium oxide ceramic. Aluminium oxide ceramics do not appear to initiate pathological host reactions. If the alumina ceramic has pores greater than 100 μm in diameter, ingrowth of osseous tissue occurs and the implant becomes 'locked or ankylosed' by the host tissues. When subjected to functional loads, however, such implants again tend to be encapsulated by connective tissue leading ultimately to instability.

General comment

It is generally accepted that endosseous implants of the types described above are clinically unsatisfactory and should not be used. It is not only the materials which are in doubt but also the surgical methods and biomechanics. For example, a blade-vent implant is inserted into a prepared gutter in the residual alveolar bone and finally tapped into place; after initial healing it is subject to many unfavourable forces, often due to occlusal problems; it is difficult for the patient in many cases to cleanse the mucosa-post interface. For these reasons the prognosis of endosseous implants is never good but even before they are lost there may well be considerable sepsis and pathology of which the patient may be unaware.

Osseointegrated implants

The most recent and rewarding concept in implantology is that of osseointegration whereby the implant is directly connected to remodelling bone without any intermediate soft tissue component and so provides a direct transfer of loads to the anchoring bone. The metal used is titanium and the oxide layer formed on the surface of the implant appears to be responsible for its tissue integration. The oxide layer is clinically inert and the highly polarizable surface gives the implant a great affinity for various biomolecules. The implant surface appears to blend into a thin organic ground substance that serves to cement viable cells to the implant, although the actual method of attachment is still not clearly understood.

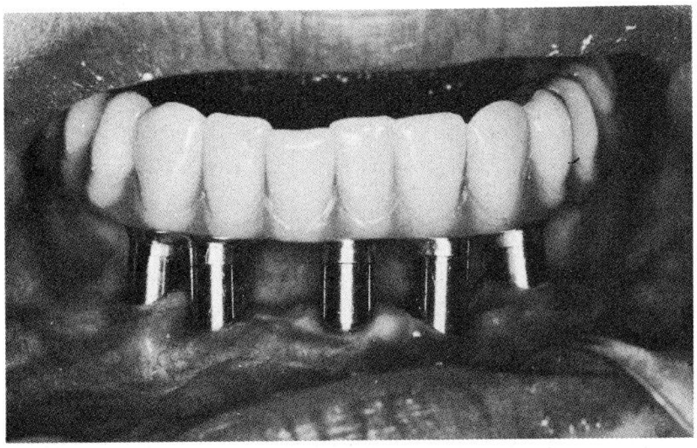

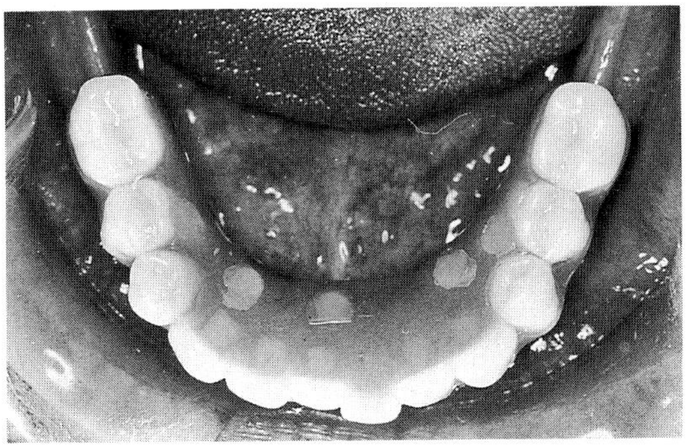

Figure 30.4 Osseointegrated implant. Labial and occlusal view of denture supported on five fixtures. This denture or bridge cannot be removed by the patient. Note the self-cleansing nature of the design, the health of the gingival margins and the fact that the pontic extends no further distally than the first molar

Fundamental to the technique are careful surgical placement of the titanium implants, the subsequent osseointegration between the bone and titanium oxide film and meticulous care in the prosthetic and occlusal aspects of the treatment.

Technique

A two-stage procedure is used whereby the endosseous implant is surrounded by bone in the first stage and connected to the oral cavity via a transmucosal post in the second stage.

In the first stage, threaded titanium implants or fixtures are inserted into alveolar bone by careful surgical methods designed to preserve the health of existing bone. Once the implants are located, they are covered by the mucoperiosteum and left *in situ* for a number of months during which time bone forms in direct contact with the oxide surface of the implant, hence the term osseointegration. At the end of this period the implants are uncovered and the transmucosal posts fitted to act as supports for the denture superstructure. In some cases the denture (or bridge) is fixed to the abutments and can only be removed by the dentist, while in others the denture is removable by the patient (Figure 30.4).

As in all implant patients, strict oral hygiene is essential to maintain mucosal health immediately adjacent to the fixtures.

Bibliography

Complete dentures

ANDERSON, J. N. and STORER, R. (1981) *Immediate and Replacement Dentures,* 3rd edn, Blackwell, Oxford.

BASKER, R. M., DAVENPORT, J. C. and TOMLIN, H. R. (1983) *Prosthetic Treatment of the Edentulous Patient,* 2nd edn, Macmillan, London.

HEARTWELL, C. M. and RAHN, A. O. (1986) *Syllabus of Complete Dentures,* 4th edn, Lea & Febiger, Philadelphia.

HICKEY, J. C., ZARB, G. A. and BOLENDER, C. L. (1985) *Boucher's Prosthodontic Treatment for Edentulous Patients,* 9th edn, Mosby, St Louis.

HOBKIRK, J. A. (1985) *A Colour Atlas of Complete Dentures,* Wolfe Medical, London.

HOBKIRK, J. A. (1986) *Complete Dentures,* Wright, Bristol.

MORROW, R. M., RUDD, K. D. and RHOADS, J. E. (1986) *Dental Laboratory Procedures, Vol. 1: Complete Dentures,* 2nd edn, Mosby, St Louis.

NEILL, D. J. and NAIRN, R. I. (1983) *Complete Denture Prosthetics,* 2nd edn, Wright, Bristol.

WATT, D. M. and MacGREGOR, A. R. (1986) *Designing Complete Dentures,* 2nd edn, Wright, Bristol.

WINKLER, S. (1987) *Essentials of Complete Denture Prosthodontics,* 2nd edn, PSG Publishing, Massachusetts.

Partial dentures

BAKER, J. L. and GOODKIND, R. J. (1981) *Theory and Practice of Precision Attachment Removable Partial Dentures,* Mosby, St Louis.

BATES, J. F. (1978) *Removable Partial Denture Construction,* 2nd edn, Wright, Bristol.

BATES, J. F., NEILL, D. J. and PREISKEL, H. W. (1984) *Restoration of the Partially Dentate Mouth.* Quintessence, Chicago.

BOUCHER, L. J. and RENNER, R. P. (1982) *Treatment of Partially Edentulous Patients,* Mosby, St Louis.

DAVENPORT, J. C., BASKER, R. M., HEATH, J. R. and RALPH, J. P. (1987) *A Colour Atlas of Removable Partial Dentures,* Wolfe, London.

DYKEMA, R. W., GOODACRE, C. J. and PHILLIPS, R. W. (eds) (1986) *Johnston's Modern Practice in Removable Partial Prosthodontics,* 4th edn, Saunders, Philadelphia.

HENDERSON, D., McGIVNEY, G. P. and CASTLEBERRY, D. J. (1985) *McCracken's Removable Partial Prosthodontics,* 7th edn, Mosby, St Louis.

LAMMIE, G. A. and LAIRD, W. R. E. (1986) *Osborne and Lammie's Partial Dentures,* 5th edn, Blackwell, Oxford.

NEILL, D. J. and WALTER, J. D. (1983) *Partial Dentures,* 2nd edn, Blackwell, Oxford.

PREISKEL, H. W. (1984) *Precision Attachments in Prosthodontics: The Application of Intracoronal and Extracoronal Attachments.* Vol. 1. Quintessence, Chicago.

PREISKEL, H. W. (1985) *Precision Attachments in Prosthodontics: Overdentures and Telescopic Prostheses.* Vol. 2. Quintessence, Chicago.

PULLEN-WARNER, E. and L'ESTRANGE, P. R. (1978) *Sectional Dentures,* Wright, Bristol.

RUDD, K. D., MORROW, R. M. and RHOADS, J. E. (1986) *Dental Laboratory Procedures: Vol. 3: Removable Partial Dentures,* 2nd edn, Mosby, St. Louis.

STEWART, K. L., RUDD, K. D. and KUEBKER, W. A. (1983) *Clinical Removable Partial Prosthodontics,* Mosby, St Louis.

WATT, D. M. and MacGREGOR, A. R. (1984) *Designing Partial Dentures,* Wright, Bristol.

ZARB, G. A., BERGMAN, B., CLAYTON, J. A. and MACKAY, H. F. (1978) *Prosthodontic Treatment for Partially Edentulous Patients,* Mosby, St Louis.

General

BATES, J. F., ADAMS, D. and STAFFORD, G. D. (1984) *Dental Treatment of the Elderly,* Wright, Bristol.

BRANEMARK, P.-I., ZARB, G. A. and ALBREKTSSON, T. (1985) *Tissue-integrated Prostheses,* Quintessence, Chicago.

COHEN, B. and THOMSON, H. (1986) *Dental Care for the Elderly,* Heinemann, London.

GRANT, A. A. and JOHNSON, W. (1983) *An Introduction to Removable Denture Prosthetics,* Churchill Livingstone, Edinburgh.

HUNTER, B. (1987) *Dental Care for Handicapped Patients,* Wright, Bristol.

LAMB, D. J. (1987) *Appearance and Aesthetics in Denture Practice,* Wright, Bristol.

LANEY, W. R. and GIBILISCO, J. A. (1983) *Diagnosis and Treatment in Prosthodontics,* Lea & Febiger, Philadelphia.

WILSON, H. J., MANSFIELD, M. A., HEATH, J. R. and SPENCE, D. (1987) *Dental Technology and Materials for Students,* 8th edn, Blackwell, Oxford.

Index